Scientific Evidence for Musculoskeletal, Bariatric, and Sports Nutrition

Scientific Evidence for Musculoskeletal, Bariatric, and Sports Nutrition

Edited by
Ingrid Kohlstadt, M.D., M.P.H., F.A.C.N.

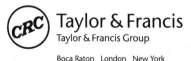

Taylor & Francis
Taylor & Francis Group

Boca Raton   London   New York

A CRC title, part of the Taylor & Francis imprint, a member of the
Taylor & Francis Group, the academic division of T&F Informa plc.

Published in 2006 by
CRC Press
Taylor & Francis Group
6000 Broken Sound Parkway NW, Suite 300
Boca Raton, FL 33487-2742

International Standard Book Number-10: 0-8493-3724-0 (Hardcover)
International Standard Book Number-13: 978-0-8493-3724-6 (Hardcover)
Library of Congress Card Number 2005052908

Library of Congress Cataloging-in-Publication Data

Scientific evidence for musculoskeletal, bariatric, and sports nutrition / edited by Ingrid Kohlstadt.
    p. ; cm.
  Includes bibliographical references and index.
  ISBN 0-8493-3724-0 (alk. paper)
  1. Nutrition. 2. Musculoskeletal system--Diseases--Nutritional aspects. 3. Obesity--Nutritional aspects. 4. Sports--Nutritional aspects. I. Kohlstadt, Ingrid.
  [DNLM: 1. Musculoskeletal Diseases--etiology. 2. Nutrition Disorders--complications. 3. Evidence-Based Medicine. 4. Musculoskeletal Diseases--diet therapy. 5. Obesity--diet therapy. 6. Sports--physiology. WE 140 S4163 2006]

QP141.S3485 2006
612.3--dc22   2005052908

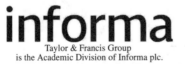

Taylor & Francis Group
is the Academic Division of Informa plc.

Visit the Taylor & Francis Web site at
http://www.taylorandfrancis.com

and the CRC Press Web site at
http://www.crcpress.com

Preface

Scientists and clinicians who want to broaden their understanding of the musculoskeletal system should read this book, whether their patients are top-placed marathon runners or persons for whom taking ten steps out of bed is a marathon.

As a society, we are very accustomed to the visible functions of muscle, fat, bone, and connective tissue. We frequently refer to the musculoskeletal system when describing a person — frail, strong, brittle-boned, big, lean, short, agile, muscular, skinny, fit, and so on. Minutes after a child's birth we proudly announce those two key musculoskeletal parameters of height and weight.

Contrast what meets the eye to the unseen critical functions of the musculoskeletal system. The human body is a veteran of famine, deprivation, and procreation. In its millennia of experience, maintaining blood pH and temperature, fueling the brain and vital organs, and defending against foreign invaders have been afforded top priority and receive minute-by-minute attention. One may think of it like this: the musculoskeletal system is analogous to a bank account on which the body draws to satisfy its top priorities. Millions of "transactions" occur each second and are known collectively as our metabolism. Only if funds are available does the body maintain muscle for strength, bone for structure, fat for shape, and connective tissue for motion.

Insufficiency of nutrients for muscle and bone health usually has a gradual onset. In some circumstances, the process begins in the womb. Then one day, seemingly out of the blue, the gradual process reveals itself: the favorite jeans are too tight, the rotator cuff tear does not heal, the small slip results in a hip fracture, the dentist diagnoses periodontal disease, or the muscle strain does not heal in time for the last game of the season. Discovering a musculoskeletal weakness can be as upsetting as finding out that the bank account is not FTC (Federal Trade Commission) insured. Neither is the musculoskeletal system FTC (fitness and total conditioning) insured, except with strategic nutrition.

The treatment of musculoskeletal conditions is widely shared among specialties:

- Preventive medicine corrects short-term dips in the musculoskeletal reserves, while integrative medicine corrects longer-term dips in the musculoskeletal reserves associated with pathology. Furthermore, preventive, integrative, functional, holistic, antiaging, complementary, naturopathic, and alternative medicine practitioners are championing the transition from an acute health care system to a system of chronic disease management more inclusive of nutrition.
- Sports, military, aerospace, and occupational medicine anticipate the extreme environment of their patients, and optimize muscle and bone-sparing nutrition accordingly.

- Pediatricians diligently monitor patients' growth; abdominal girth, weight and height are important health indicators at all ages. Early environments of the womb, infancy, and childhood shape future musculoskeletal health.

- Endocrinologists have identified the pathways that build muscle and bone and metabolize fat. Adipose tissue is now credentialed as an endocrine organ. Bariatricians and bariatric surgeons similarly pioneer ways to metabolize fat.

- Surgeons pioneer understanding of how nutrition enhances outcomes and have said, "Repairing a shoulder without muscle is like nailing a chiffon pie to the wall." Dentists are surgeons for a uniquely visible component of the musculoskeletal system. They can identify nutritional deficiencies by keenly observing oral markers on the initial visit, and dentists are credited for first warning how sugar harms bone (tooth) health.

- Pain management specialists, osteopathic physicians, physical therapists, massage therapists, chiropractors, and acupuncturists have partnered with nutrition specialists to relieve pain, especially for fibromyalgia.

- Life expectancy is increasing, and at the same time degenerative conditions of the muscles, joints, and tissues are beginning earlier. Consequently, the fields of antiaging medicine and geriatrics both focus on treating sarcopenia, obesity, osteoporosis, and arthritis.

- Nutritionists work tirelessly to help patients navigate through a dizzying array of boxes and cans and when needed, voice the verdict "That's not food!" Behavioral medicine buttresses the efforts of nutrition specialists; many people who set out to make healthy choices are thwarted by food cravings, habits, social norms, and marketing schemes.

- Public health has long advocated good nutrition and identified community risk factors for practicing clinicians. Food processing techniques and contamination with xenobiotics pose new broad-sweeping challenges to the musculoskeletal system. Recently, anthropologists have stepped into public health nutrition with an insightful variation on the turn of phrase "You are what you eat." The health of bones from our evolutionary ancestors coincides with dietary history.

Nutrition has long been the missing link in the daily treatment of the various musculoskeletal conditions by the health professionals listed above. The often-stated reason for giving nutrition short shrift is the lack of evidence. Here it is!

This textbook is a reference for the evidence-based integration of nutrition into medical treatment. It includes the biologic rationale, animal studies, epidemiology, clinical trials, ongoing research initiatives, and food industry statistics. Several contributors have privileged and intimate knowledge of the food industry. Most of us in medicine are not taught how our food is prepared, neither is the information readily available in our peer-reviewed journals. Dramatic shifts in food quality in recent decades have led to pervasive and quantifiable shifts in the very nutrients needed for musculoskeletal health, and provide extremely compelling evidence not customarily found in medical textbooks.

The most important advances in the science of medicine may be those that enhance the art of medicine. Knowledge of the molecular processes that underlie chronic disease equips a clinician to help patients walk their unique path back to health.

Putting nutrition into practice can be straightforward. This textbook explains how new technology can be integrated. It elaborates on foods and nutraceuticals with effects similar to medications. Information is organized into 100 tables and figures designed for easy reference. The text also includes pearls from clinicians who have achieved world renown for nutritional innovations in fibromyalgia, sports medicine, extreme environments, osteoporosis, and obesity.

This intellectual work generously contributed by 40 scientists and clinicians seems analogous to a mosaic or impressionist painting; as one steps away from it, a masterful image of musculoskeletal health emerges.

Ingrid Kohlstadt, M.D., M.P.H., F.A.C.N.
Physician Nutrition Specialist

About the Editor

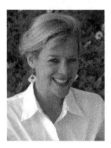

Ingrid Kohlstadt, M.D., M.P.H., F.A.C.N. is the founder and director of INGRIDients, Inc., which provides nutrition information to colleagues and consumers. Dr. Kohlstadt earned her bachelor's degree in biochemistry at the University of Maryland and Universität Tubingen in 1989, and her medical degree at Johns Hopkins University in 1993. Board-certified in general preventive medicine, she became convinced that nutrition is a powerful and underutilized tool to prevent disease. She therefore continued her training in nutrition with fellowships at The Centers for Disease Control and Prevention and at Johns Hopkins.

Dr. Kohlstadt's clinical work and nutrition consultancies have spanned all seven continents and include the U.S. Antarctic Program, Amazon Basin tribes, Alaskan Inuit, African refugees, displaced persons in the Caucasus, Native American nations, and Central Asian governments. For her contribution to medical anthropology, she has been elected to The Explorers Club.

Citing obesity as the primary national nutrition challenge, in 1999 Dr. Kohlstadt focused her career on the medical, public health, anthropologic, and biochemical aspects of fat metabolism. She has worked as a bariatric physician at the Johns Hopkins Weight Management Center and the Florida Orthopaedic Institute. She currently instructs and conducts research at Johns Hopkins University. Dr. Kohlstadt has been elected a Fellow of the American College of Nutrition.

Contributors

Stephen Alway, Ph.D.
Professor and Chair
Division of Exercise Physiology
West Virginia University School of Medicine
Morgantown, West Virginia

Richard A. Anderson, Ph.D.
Nutrient Requirements and Functions Laboratory
Beltsville Human Nutrition Research Center
Beltsville, Maryland

David J. Baer, Ph.D.
Diet and Human Performance Laboratory
Beltsville Human Nutrition Research Center
Beltsville, Maryland

John D. Bagnulo, Ph.D., M.P.H.
Assistant Professor of Nutrition and Exercise Physiology
University of Maine
Farmington, Maine

Fereydoon Batmanghelidj, M.D.
Global Health Solutions
Vienna, Virginia

Jeffrey S. Bland, Ph.D., F.A.C.N.
Metagenics Inc.
Gig Harbor, Washington

Susan E. Brown, Ph.D., C.N.S.
Director
Osteoporosis Education Project
East Syracuse, New York

Luke R. Bucci, Ph.D., C.C.N., C.N.S.
Weider Nutrition
Salt Lake City, Utah
InnerPath Nutrition
Reno, Nevada

Aileen P. Burford-Mason, Ph.D.
Research Consultant
DRS Consulting
Toronto, Ontario, Canada

See Wai Chan, M.D., M.P.H.
Assistant Professor of Pediatrics,
OB/GYN and Reproductive Sciences
University of Pittsburgh, School of Medicine
Pittsburgh, Pennsylvania

Carlo Contoreggi, M.D.
Intramural Research Program
National Institute on Drug Abuse
National Institutes of Health
Baltimore, Maryland

Altoon S. Dweck, M.D., M.P.H.
Johns Hopkins University, Bloomberg School of Public Health
Baltimore, Maryland

Mary G. Enig, Ph.D.
Enig Associates
Silver Spring, Maryland

Kevin Gebke, M.D.
Indiana University Center for Sports Medicine
Indiana University Medical Center
Indianapolis, Indiana

Paula J. Geiselman, Ph.D.
Department of Psychology
Louisiana State University and
Pennington Biomedical Research Center
Baton Rouge, Louisiana

Lawrence B. Godwin, M.Ac., L.Ac.
Virginia Acupuncture
Alexandria, Virginia

Gabriel Keith Harris, Ph.D.
Diet and Human Performance Laboratory
Beltsville Human Nutrition Research Center
United States Department of Agriculture
Beltsville, Maryland

Tony Helman, M.B. B.S., Dip.Obst. R.C.O.G.,
Mast. Med., D. Hum. Nutr., M.R.A.C.G.P.
School of Health Sciences
Deakin University
Melbourne, Victoria, Australia
School of Public Health,
Curtin University
Perth, Western Australia

Michael F. Holick, Ph.D., M.D.
Section of Endocrinology
Department of Medicine
Boston University School of Medicine
Boston, Massachusetts

Russell Jaffe, M.D., Ph.D., C.C.N., N.A.C.B.
Senior Fellow
Health Studies Collegium
Sterling, Virginia

Ian Janssen, Ph.D.
School of Physical and Health Education, and
Department of Community Health and Epidemiology
Queen's University
Kingston, Ontario, Canada

Vilma A. Joseph, M.D., M.P.H.
Montefiore Medical Center/Albert
Einstein College of Medicine
Weiler Hospital
Bronx, New York

Ingrid Kohlstadt, M.D., M.P.H., F.A.C.N.
INGRIDients, Inc.
Tampa, Florida
and Johns Hopkins University
Baltimore, Meryland

Joseph J. Lamb, M.D.
The Integrative Medicine Works
Alexandria, Virginia

Helyn Luechauer, D.D.S.
Private Practice
Vallejo, California

Wayne C. Miller, Ph.D.
Department of Exercise Science
The George Washington University Medical Center
Washington, D.C.

David I. Minkoff, M.D.
BodyHealth, Inc.
Clearwater, Florida

Laurie Mischley, N.D.
University Health Clinic Specialty Care and Research Center
Seattle, Washington

David Musnick, M.D.
Bastyr University and University of Washington
Seattle, Washington

Karen Mutter, D.O.
Integrative Medicine Healing Center LLC
Clearwater, Florida

Craig Nadelson, D.O.
Indiana University Center for Sports Medicine
Indiana University Medical Center
Indianapolis, Indiana

Gilberto Pereira, M.D.
Department of Pediatrics
The Children's Hospital of Philadelphia
University of Pennsylvania School of Medicine
Philadelphia, Pennsylvania

Matthew A. Pikosky, Ph.D., R.D.
Military Nutrition Division
U.S. Army Research Institute of Environmental Medicine
Natick, Massachusetts

Kathryn Poleson, D.M.D., F.A.C.D.
Editor, WAGD Today
Clark College, School of Dental Hygiene
Vancouver, Washington

Arline D. Salbe, Ph.D., R.D.
Research Nutritionist
Obesity and Diabetes Clinical Research Section
National Institute of Diabetes and Digestive and Kidney Diseases
National Institutes of Health
Phoenix, Arizona

Marlene B. Schwartz, Ph.D.
Department of Psychology
Yale University
New Haven, Connecticut

Eric Schweitzer, D.P.T., M.T.C.
Florida Orthopaedics
Tampa, Florida

Kevin R. Short, Ph.D.
Assistant Professor
Endocrine Research Unit
Mayo Clinical College of Medicine
Rochester, Minnesota

Steven R. Smith, M.D.
Pennington Biomedical Research Center
Louisiana State University
Baton Rouge, Louisiana

Jacob Teitelbaum, M.D.
Annapolis Research Center for Effective
CFS/Fibromyalgia Therapies
Annapolis, Maryland

Andrew J. Young, Ph.D.
Military Nutrition Division
U.S. Army Research Institute of Environmental Medicine
Natick, Massachusetts

Contents

Section IV: Muscle Tissue

Section V: Soft Tissue

Section VI: Bone

Section I

Frontiers and Technologic Advances

1 Body Composition: Quantifying the Musculoskeletal System

Ian Janssen, Ph.D.

CONTENTS

INTRODUCTION

A central aspect of the field of nutrition and musculoskeletal health is establishing the body composition characteristics of humans. This chapter provides an overview of concepts and methodology related to quantifying human body composition, particularly as they pertain to measuring the quantity and distribution of fat, fat-free mass (FFM), and the skeleton. This chapter will also briefly discuss the influence of growth and development, aging, race, and gender on the musculoskeletal system, and in so doing will set the stage for many of the subsequent chapters.

BODY COMPOSITION RULES

FIVE-LEVEL BODY COMPOSITION MODEL

The human body can be organized into five distinct levels of increasing complexity: atomic, molecular, cellular, tissue, and whole body.[1] Figure 1.1 illustrates the primary components of the five levels. There are two key concepts of the five-level body composition model. The first is that components at higher levels are composed of lower-level components. Consider, for example, adipose tissue, a tissue level component that includes (but is not limited to) adipocytes at the cellular level, lipids at the molecular level, and carbon at the atomic level.

The second key concept of the five-level body composition model is the existence of relations among components that are relatively constant within a given individual over time (e.g., before and after weight loss) and among different individuals (e.g., similar in overweight and lean individuals). For instance, there is a relatively stable relation between total body water at the atomic level and FFM at the molecular level (FFM = total body water $\times$ 1.37).[2] The existence of these stable relations is fundamental to the body composition field as they allow investigators to estimate an unknown component based on a measured component. Thus, in the

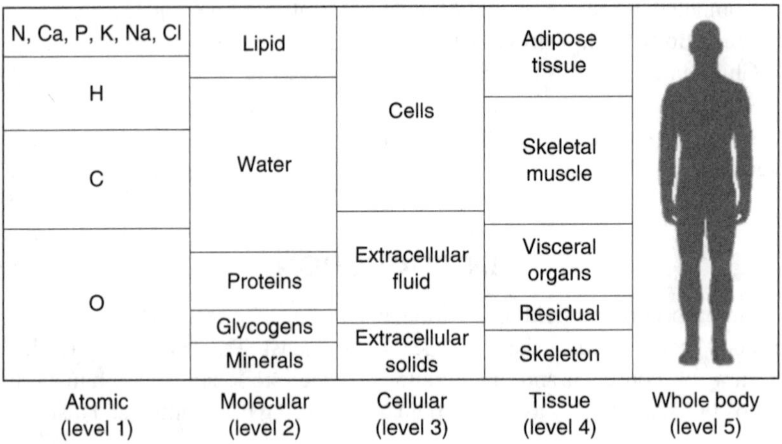

N, Ca, P, K, Na, Cl	Lipid	Cells	Adipose tissue	
H			Skeletal muscle	
C	Water		Skeletal muscle	
O	Proteins	Extracellular fluid	Visceral organs	
O	Glycogens	Extracellular fluid	Residual	
O	Minerals	Extracellular solids	Skeleton	
Atomic (level 1)	Molecular (level 2)	Cellular (level 3)	Tissue (level 4)	Whole body (level 5)

FIGURE 1.1 Five-level body composition model. (Adapted from Wang, Z.M., Pierson, R.N., Jr., and Heymsfield, S.B., *Am. J. Clin. Nutr.*, 56, 19–28, 1992.)

aforementioned example, FFM could be estimated based on total body water measures.

The next five sections will provide a brief description of each body composition level. Interested readers are referred to a more detailed description of the five-level body composition model and of the specific levels.[1]

ATOMIC LEVEL

Elements are the building blocks of all biological organisms. There are about 50 elements contained in the human body, most of which are required for growth and maintenance.[1] Four elements (O, C, H, and N) account for over 95% of the body mass, and an additional seven (Na, K, P, Cl, Ca, Mg, and S) over 99.5% of the body mass.[1] Although the elements themselves are rarely an outcome of interest in body composition or nutrition research, they are at times measured to gain an insight into the quantity of one or more of the components at the molecular, cellular, or tissue level. That is, elements maintain relatively stable relationships with body composition components at higher levels, and these known relationships allow components at body composition levels 2 through 4 to be estimated based on the measurement of elements at level 1. For instance, the potassium (atomic level) to skeletal muscle (tissue level) ratio in the human body is approximately 120 mmol/kg. Thus, skeletal muscle mass can be estimated with a high degree of accuracy based on measured quantities of total body potassium.[3]

MOLECULAR LEVEL

The molecular level components can be subdivided into five main groups: lipids, water, proteins, carbohydrates, and minerals. Triglycerides, which are also referred to as nonessential lipids in the body composition field, are the most abundant lipid species in humans. Triglycerides serve as energy storage compounds in large amounts in adipose tissue and in smaller amounts in many other tissues such as skeletal muscle and liver. The remaining lipid species (phospholipids, sphingolipids, steroids) are often referred to as essential lipids, and these lipids are involved in a number of biochemical and physiological processes.

The nonlipid molecular level components consist of water (which can be subdivided into intracellular and extracellular compartments), proteins (e.g., actin and myosin proteins in skeletal muscle), glycogen (<1 kg stored in skeletal muscle and liver), and minerals (bone and soft-tissue minerals). These nonlipid molecular components are often combined or lumped together in body composition methods. For instance, the classic "two-compartment" model is based on the concept that the body can be divided into FFM (water + protein + glycogen + minerals) and fat mass (essential lipids + nonessential lipids). The two-compartment model has been a widely applied body composition model for over 50 years.[4] More recently, multicompartment models have been developed that are based on fractioning the body into more than two components at the molecular level.[5] These multicompartment models are useful in situations where the composition of FFM is altered (e.g., sarcopenia or osteoporosis). In these situations, one of the fundamental assumptions of the two-compartment model (e.g., similar ratio between the various FFM molecules across individuals) is violated.

CELLULAR LEVEL

The cellular level consists of cell mass, extracellular fluids, and extracellular solids. The extracellular solids consist primarily of bone minerals and collagen, reticular, and elastic fibers. The extracellular fluid includes water and dissolved electrolytes and proteins. The cell mass is of a greater nutritional interest, and includes organelles, mitochondria, and triglycerides. Because cells are the basic functioning biological units, evaluating the three major components of the cell level allows insight into a number of biological processes.

TISSUE LEVEL

The primary tissue level compounds are adipose tissue, skeletal muscle, bone, visceral organs, brain, and a residual component (e.g., tendons, skin). Adipose tissue is further subdivided into subcutaneous (adipose tissue directly underneath the skin), visceral (adipose tissue surrounding the organs of the gastrointestinal tract), and interstitial (marbled adipose tissue between muscle fibers and bundles) depots. Over the past 15 years there has been a great interest in discerning the separate effects of the various adipose tissue depots on obesity-related health risk.[6,7]

Editor's Note

Obesity is an epidemic of allometry, the disproportionate growth of one part of an organism. A disproportionate decrease in lean to nonlean tissue is a relatively early sign of the metabolic imbalances which lead to obesity, sarcopenia, and arthritis. Clinicians can use the technologic advances in body composition assessment to quantify the musculoskeletal health of their patients.

BODY COMPOSITION METHODS

This section describes various methods for estimating human body composition. Only commonly employed body composition methods that are used to measure the three tissues of interest in this book — fat (or adipose tissue), lean soft tissues (primarily skeletal muscle), and the skeleton — will be covered. More detailed descriptions of these and other body composition methods have been presented in earlier publications.[8,9] A brief overview of basic measurement method principles is provided before specific body composition techniques are discussed.

MEASUREMENT METHOD PRINCIPLES

The ideal approach for measuring a specific body composition component is to measure it directly. Unfortunately, with the exception of simple anthropometric measures (e.g., height, body mass), direct measurement of human body composition can only be achieved by cadaver analysis. Even medical imaging methods such as magnetic resonance imaging (MRI) and computed tomography (CT) are indirect methods. With MRI and CT, cross-sectional images (pictures) are obtained at specific levels in the body. Because the tissue size is measured in the cross-sectional images and not *in vivo*, these imaging methods are considered indirect body composition measures.

Most body composition methods are far more indirect than MRI and CT as they rely on a mathematical transformation, whereby the measured property is transformed into the body composition component of interest. Two basic types of mathematical transformations exist.[10] The first is based on stable relationships between measured properties and body composition components, many of which can be understood from their underlying biological basis. As an example, FFM = total body water × 1.37.[2] The second is based on a statistically derived relationship between the measured property and the body composition component, whereby the measured property is mathematically transformed into the body composition component. That is, a statistically derived regression equation for predicting the body composition component, as measured by a reference method, is derived in a group of individuals in whom both the body composition component and the measured property were obtained. The constant and coefficients from this regression model can then be applied to the measured properties of other individuals, who did not have their body composition measured by the reference method, to estimate the body composition component of interest. For instance, bioelectrical impedance analysis (BIA) measures of current resistance can be entered into a regression model along with other measured properties (e.g., height, weight, age, sex) to predict FFM as determined by underwater weighting.[11] These simple, quick, and inexpensive BIA measures could then be used to predict FFM in cases where it is not suitable to obtain the more cumbersome, time-consuming, and expensive underwater weight measures.

The precision of a body composition prediction equation refers to its performance within the sample from which it was derived, while the accuracy refers to the performance of the equation when it is applied to a new subject group or individual. A number of factors influence the precision and accuracy of body composition prediction equations including the magnitude of the error involved in obtaining the measured (independent) and body composition component (dependent) variables (as error increases the precision and accuracy decrease), the strength of the biological and statistical relations between the independent and

TABLE 1.1
Classification of adiposity status in adults according to BMI and waist circumference

Classification	BMI (kg/m^2)	Morbidity and mortality risk	
		Low waist (men ≤ 102 cm, women ≤ 88 cm)	High waist (men > 102 cm, women > 88 cm)
Underweight	<18.5	Increased	NA
Normal range	18.5–24.9	Low	Increased
Overweight	≥25		
Preobese	25–29.9	Increased	High
Obese class I	30–34.9	High	Very high
Obese class II	35–39.9	NA	Very high
Obese class III	≥40	NA	Extremely high

Note: NA = not applicable. All underweight individuals have a low waist circumference and virtually all class II and class III obese individuals have a high waist circumference.

Source: Adapted from National Institutes of Health National Heart Lung and Blood Institute, *Obes. Res.*, 6, S51–S210, 1998.

dependent variables (as the strength of the relationships increases, the precision and accuracy increase), the size of the sample in which the equation was developed (as the sample size increases, the precision and accuracy will tend to increase), and the degree to which the characteristics of the sample in whom the equation was developed are comparable to the characteristics of the sample or individual in whom the equation is being applied (the greater the difference between samples, the poorer the accuracy).[11]

ANTHROPOMETRY

Anthropometric instruments are portable and inexpensive. Further, procedures are non-invasive and minimal training is required. This makes anthropometry practical for application in the clinical setting and in large epidemiological studies. In its simplest form, anthropometry includes direct measures of height and body mass. The body mass index (BMI), a simple index of weight-for-height (kg/m^2), is commonly employed in both research and clinical settings as a measure of adiposity status. The globally accepted BMI classification system for adults is shown in Table 1.1.[12] This classification system is based on the relation between BMI, chronic disease, and mortality. The BMI cut-points are the same for both sexes and are age independent. These BMI values can be used for all racial groups, with the exception of Asian populations in whom a BMI of 23 kg/m^2 denotes overweight and a BMI of 27 kg/m^2 denotes obesity.[14]

In children, BMI changes substantially with age, rising steeply during infancy, falling during the preschool years, and then rising again continuously into adulthood. For this reason, overweight and obesity in children and adolescents is determined using age-specific BMI cut-points. Numerous countries have produced BMI-for-age growth curves, which allows an individual's BMI to be expressed as an age- and sex-specific percentile. Historically, the 85th and 95th percentiles have been used to determine overweight and obesity status, respectively, in children and adolescents.[12] International BMI standards for defining overweight and obesity in youth have also been developed by regressing the adult BMI cut-points of 25 and 30 kg/m^2 at age 18 back through the growth curve.[15] This approach also provides age- and sex-specific BMI cut-points that, from a global perspective, may be the most appropriate means for defining overweight and obesity in children and adolescents.

Although BMI is a decent correlate of fat mass, the relation between BMI and fat mass is influenced by a number of factors including race, age, genetic factors, and fitness level. In fact, somewhere in the order of 25 to 50% of the interindividual variation in fat mass within each sex is not accounted for by BMI.[16] Not surprisingly, more direct anthropometric measures of body fat obtained via skinfold thickness explain an additional 15% of the variance in fat mass than BMI.[16]

Skinfold thickness measures are obtained by grasping the skin and adjacent subcutaneous adipose tissue between the thumb and forefinger, pulling it away from the underlying muscle, and using a skinfold caliper to measure the thickness of the subcutaneous adipose tissue at that site. A precision of about 5% for skinfold thickness measures can be attained by properly trained and experienced individuals.[17] Typically, skinfold thickness measures are obtained at five to seven sites that cover the torso, arms, and legs. These skinfold thickness measures can then be summed (e.g., sum of five skinfolds)[16] or inserted into a number of different body fat prediction equations[17] to be used as an index of adiposity status. Table 1.2 lists cut-points for underweight, normal weight, overweight, and obesity based on the sum of five skinfolds and percent body fat (% body fat = fat mass/body mass × 100) values that correspond to the commonly used cut-points based on BMI.[16,18]

Although it may be more appealing to use indirect estimates of fat mass derived from skinfold prediction equations than directly measured sum of skinfold measures, skinfold thickness prediction equations need to be applied with great caution. These equations make the assumption that there is no interindividual variation in the proportion of subcutaneous adipose tissue to total fat mass, which is incorrect. For instance, the ratio of subcutaneous to visceral adipose tissue varies by race, sex, age, and physical activity level. Thus, skinfold prediction equations should be restricted to individuals with similar characteristics to the subject pool in which the equations were derived. This is a daunting task as numerous skinfold equations exist,[17] although most of these are specific to healthy young and middle-aged Caucasian populations.

Body circumference measurements have also been used to measure body fat and its distribution. In addition to total fat mass, the distribution of fat within

TABLE 1.2
Classification of adiposity status in adults according to BMI, sum of five skinfolds, and percent body fat

Classification	BMI (kg/m²)	Sum of five skinfolds (mm)[a]		% Body fat	
		Men	Women	Men	Women
Underweight	<18.5	<25	<46	<13	<23
Normal range	18.5–24.9	25–54	46–83	13–21	31–37
Overweight (preobese)	25–29.9	55–77	84–113	21–25	31–37
Obese	30–34.9	>77	>113	≥26	≥38

[a]Sum of five skinfolds = subscapular + biceps + triceps + iliac crest + calf skinfolds.

Source: Adapted from Janssen, I., Heymsfield, S.B., and Ross, R., *Can. J. Appl. Physiol.*, 27, 396–414, 2002, and Food and Nutrition Board (Institute of Medicine), *Dietary Reference Intakes for Energy, Carbohydrate, Fiber, Fat, Fatty Acids, Cholesterol, Protein, and Amino Acids (Macronutrients)*, National Academies Press, Washington, DC, 2003.

the body is an important determinant of obesity-related health risk. In particular, the two abdominal fat depots — abdominal subcutaneous and visceral adipose tissue — are involved in the pathogenesis of numerous cardiovascular disease and diabetes risk factors.[12,13] The accumulation of excess visceral adipose tissue is believed to be of particular relevance. In this regard, waist circumference is a simple anthropometric measurement that is an approximate index of abdominal subcutaneous and visceral adipose tissue content.[16] Furthermore, changes in waist circumference reflect changes in abdominal fat.[19] Thus, waist circumference is a useful clinical tool that can be used to identify individuals at increased health risk due to abdominal obesity.

Ideally, waist circumference should be used in combination with BMI as an anthropometric indicator of health risk, as waist circumference explains an additional component of morbidity and mortality than is explained by BMI alone. The U.S. National Institutes of Health[13] have proposed that waist circumference values of ≥ 102 cm (40 in.) in men and ≥ 88 cm (35 in.) in women can be used within the BMI categories listed in Table 1.1 to differentiate between those with and without abdominal obesity. For example, a class I obese man with a waist circumference of < 102 cm would be considered to have a "normal" abdominal fat content and a "high" health risk, whereas a class I obese man with a waist circumference of ≥ 102 cm would be considered to have a "high" abdominal fat content and a "very high" health risk. The added effect of waist circumference is illustrated in a representative sample of American men in Figure 1.2, which demonstrates the prevalence of the metabolic syndrome — a constellation of cardiovascular disease risk factors — according to waist circumference classification

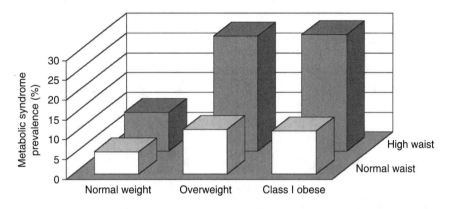

FIGURE 1.2 Prevalence of the metabolic syndrome according to BMI status (normal weight, overweight, or class I obese) and waist circumference status (normal or high) in American men. (Adapted from Janssen, I., Katzmarzyk, P.T., and Ross, R., *Arch. Intern. Med.*, 162, 2074–2079, 2002.)

within normal weight, overweight, and class I obese BMI categories.[20] In this example the prevalence of the metabolic syndrome is more than doubled in men with a high waist circumference compared to men with a normal waist circumference within each of the three BMI categories.

In addition to fat mass and distribution, skinfold and circumference measures have also been employed to predict the quantity of skeletal muscle. Historically, this has been done from a malnutrition perspective using estimates of skeletal muscle size in the upper arm. Because skeletal muscle is the body's primary protein reserve, muscle wasting is a reflection of malnutrition.[21] Although the circumference of the upper arm alone does not yield a precise diagnosis of malnutrition, the circumference of the upper arm (C_a) corrected for the thickness of the triceps skinfold (S) can be used to estimate the upper-arm muscle circumference (C_m) as $C_m = C_a - \pi S$.

Anthropometric measures have also been used in prediction equations to estimate whole-body skeletal muscle mass in adults using upper-arm, forearm, thigh, and calf limb circumferences corrected for subcutaneous skinfold thickness.[22] Corrected muscle circumferences in these four regions are squared and multiplied by height to obtain a three-dimensional (volume or mass) skeletal muscle measure using a prediction equation derived from a reference-method dependent procedure. Assessment of skeletal muscle size in adults has important applications in a number of disciplines. Most notably, geriatricians are interested in examining the influence of aging on muscle wasting, a universal age-related phenomenon that has been named "sarcopenia," as will be discussed in greater detail in Chapter 17. Although sarcopenia is a universal process, with 100% of the population losing muscle with increasing age, cut-points have been developed to denote significant muscle loss. Although there is no universal agreement on what cut-points should

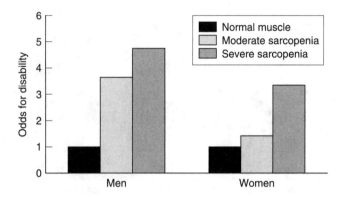

FIGURE 1.3 Odds ratio for physical disability according to skeletal muscle mass (normal, moderate sarcopenia, or severe sarcopenia) in older American men and women. (Adapted from Janssen, I., Baumgartner, R.N., Ross, R., Rosenberg, I.R., and Roubenoff, R., *Am. J. Epidemiol.*, 159, 413–421, 2004.)

be employed, recently height-adjusted skeletal muscle mass cut-points of 5.76 to 6.75 kg/m^2 in women and 8.51 to 10.75 kg/m^2 in men have been proposed to denote a moderate level of sarcopenia, and cut-points of ≤5.75 kg/m^2 in women and ≤8.50 kg/m^2 in men have been proposed to denote a severe level of sarcopenia.[23] Sarcopenia, as defined using this cut-points approach, is strongly related to the functional impairment and physical disability that are common among elderly persons, as illustrated in Figure 1.3 for a representative sample of American men and women aged 60 and above.[23]

DENSITOMETRY

The measurement of body density is often considered the "gold standard" in the measurement of human body composition. This is a reflection of the early development and widespread use of this method, as a number of more accurate and valid methods for measuring human body composition are presently available, such as MRI, CT, dual-energy x-ray absorptiometry (DXA), and multicompartment models.[8,9] The most commonly used approach for determining body density is underwater weighing, which has been employed in body composition research for over 60 years.[24] This method requires the subject to be completely immersed in water, and the volume of displaced water and the subject's weight underwater (corrected for residual lung volume), in combination with their body mass, are used to calculate the density of the body according to Archimedes principle as density = body mass/body volume. The body density in turn can be used to estimate body composition according to the two-compartment model as % body fat = (495/density) − 4.50.[25]

FFM has a greater density than fat mass (1.1 vs. 0.9 kg/l). Thus, the greater the body density, the lower the percent body fat. The measurement of body density is based on the assumption that the densities of fat mass (0.9 kg/l) and FFM (1.1 kg/l) are relatively constant. This is a reasonable assumption for fat mass, but not for FFM as there are variations in FFM density with sex and race, as well as individual changes that occur in response to aging, physical activity, and disease.[9] Normal variations in hydration, protein content, and mineral content can also influence FFM density.[9] The individual error for densitometry derived measures of fat mass is in the order of 3 to 4% of body mass.[25]

In recent years, air-displacement plethysmography has started to replace underwater weighing as a means of measuring body density.[26] In this technique the subject is placed in an egg-shaped, closed air-filled chamber called the "Bod Pod." The volume of the chamber is altered slightly, and the pressure vs. volume relationship is used to calculate the volume and density of the subject. With this technique the subject does not have to be submerged in water, which is a clear advantage over underwater weighing. However, all the limitations that are inherent to the body density and composition prediction equations that were originally developed for underwater weighing remain true for air-displacement plethysmography.

BIOELECTRICAL IMPEDANCE ANALYSIS

BIA is one of the most frequently used body composition methods due to the inexpensive cost of the instrumentation, its ease of operation, and portability. BIA reflects the ability of tissues and the whole body to conduct an electrical current. Typically, BIA measurements are performed using four gel electrodes (e.g., ECG electrodes) — two are attached at the right wrist and two at the right ankle. A weak (~50 kHz) alternating current is passed from the BIA apparatus through the outer wrist and outer ankle electrodes. The currents travel across the body, and the drop in current voltage, from which the BIA resistance value is derived, is measured by the BIA apparatus using the inner pair of electrodes. In addition to the classic arm-to-leg BIA apparatus, a variety of leg-to-leg BIA machines have been developed. These scale-like machines use contact electrodes (steel plate on top of the scale) instead of gel electrodes, and the electrical current flows across the legs. Thus, BIA resistance obtained on a leg-to-leg apparatus reflects the voltage drop as the current travels from one foot to the other, and does not reflect the voltage drop across the whole body as is obtained from the classic arm-to-leg BIA apparatus.

When the BIA current flows through the body it is partitioned among different tissues according to their individual volume resistances to current flow. Because skeletal muscle has both a large volume (largest tissue in most people) and low resistance (owing to its high electrolyte content), most of the current in a whole-body BIA measure flows through skeletal muscle, and most of the BIA resistance is explained by muscle mass.[27] Conversely, adipose tissue and bone have poor conductance properties (owing to their low electrolyte content) and thus have a minimal impact on BIA resistance.[27] Further, because the trunk is of little concern in whole-body BIA measures (e.g., the large diameter of the trunk will create little resistance), visceral organ mass also has a minimal impact on BIA resistance.[27]

All currently used BIA approaches are reference-method dependent. That is, BIA resistance measures must be mathematically transformed into the body composition component of interest using a prediction equation. Numerous equations exist for predicting FFM based on BIA measures. Fat mass can subsequently be determined by subtracting FFM from body mass. The vast majority of the studies in which the BIA-FFM equations were developed used underwater weighting or DXA as the reference method.[11] Many BIA equations also exist for predicting total body water, as at the molecular body composition level (level 2, Figure 1.1) BIA resistance is determined by water content. For development of the total body water prediction equations the isotopic dilution of tritium, deuterium, or oxygen-18 was used as the reference method.[9] Finally, BIA measures can also be used to estimate skeletal muscle mass as measured by MRI.[28] In most cases BIA prediction equations are population specific, and great care should be taken to select an appropriate equation for the individual or group of interest. Also, because BIA measures are dependent on hydration status, it is important to control for the consumption of food and fluids and recent exercise, as variations in these factors may temporarily influence hydration status and consequently have a strong impact on estimates of body composition.[29]

As stated in the preceding paragraph, BIA is a commonly employed method for measuring total body water, as well as its distribution into the intracellular and extracellular compartments.[11] The body can gain or lose significant amounts of water in certain clinical situations (e.g., dialysis), with certain drugs, and in response to physiological strains (e.g., dehydration). Thus, the measurement of body water has important clinical implications.

DUAL-ENERGY X-RAY ABSORPTIOMETRY

The measurement of bone mineral density *in vivo* was introduced in 1963.[30] This technique, which later became known as single-photon absorptiometry, permitted bone mineral content to be measured in the wrist. With the emergence of osteoporosis as an important clinical entity (refer to Chapters 26 to 28), numerous technological advances in the measurement of bone mineral density have since been achieved. At present, DXA is the primary clinical method used for the diagnosis of osteoporosis. Although DXA measures were initially limited to the specific regions that are the most important in osteoporosis (e.g., lumbar spine, femoral neck, and forearm), DXA has been extended to allow for the study of the total skeleton in addition to its regional parts.[31] Further, advancements in DXA technology have also permitted for the measurements of soft-tissue composition in addition to bone mineral content and density.[31] Thus, three components can be measured with a whole-body DXA scan: bone mineral mass, fat mass, and bone-free FFM (FFM – bone mineral mass).

Whole-body DXA measurements that are used in the body composition field are relatively quick (15 min or less), noninvasive, precise, and reproducible. Further, the body composition results are operator independent and are available immediately after the DXA scan is complete. The DXA instrument is composed of a generator emitting x-rays of two energies, a scanning table, a detector, and a computer system. The DXA procedure induces a small dose of radiation, equivalent to that received on a transcontinental flight. The basic physical principle behind DXA is the measurement of the transmission of a low-photon (~40 keV) and a high-photon (~80 keV) x-ray through the body. The x-rays are generated beneath the body; when the x-rays pass through the body the intensity of the photons is attenuated, and the intensity of the attenuated x-rays is measured by the detector. The attenuation of the x-rays through bone, bone-free lean tissue, and fat is different, reflecting their differences in density and chemical composition.[32] As the difference in the attenuation properties for these tissues is greater with a low-photon x-ray than a high-photon x-ray, use of both a low- and a high-photon x-ray allows the mass of bone, fat, and bone-free FFM to be estimated by the DXA computer based on a number of complex assumptions and mathematical equations.[32] These body composition estimates, while comparable, differ slightly depending on the DXA manufacturer, model, and software employed.[9,32]

The primary application of DXA has been to obtain site-specific measures of bone mineral density (ratio of bone mineral content to bone area, both of which are measured by DXA) at the lumbar spine, femoral neck, and forearm. DXA is the predominant method used for the clinical diagnosis of osteoporosis and osteopenia (the predecessor of osteoporosis). According to the World Health Organization, individuals whose bone mineral density values are below −2.5 standard deviations relative to the DXA manufacturers' normative data for a young population (aged 20 to 29 years) are considered to have osteoporosis,[33] while those who fall from −1.0 to −2.5 standard deviations are considered to have osteopenia.[33] With this approach, individuals will be categorized differently according to the site of measurement, the DXA equipment, and the manufacturers' reference population.[33] For instance, someone who is diagnosed with osteoporosis based on a lumbar spine measure from a Hologic DXA scanner would not necessarily be diagnosed with osteoporosis based on a femoral head measure from a Lunar DXA scanner. Thus, there are some inconsistencies in the clinical diagnosis of osteoporosis and osteopenia.

One of the primary advantages of employing DXA for soft-tissue assessment is the capacity to obtain both whole-body and regional analyses. The standard regions that are analyzed include the head, arms, legs, pelvic region, and trunk. For fat mass, assessment of the trunk fat mass is of particular interest given the effect of abdominal fat on the risk of diabetes and cardiovascular disease. For bone-free FFM, the assessment of lean mass in the arms and legs is of particular importance. The vast majority of bone-free FFM in the arms and legs is composed of skeletal muscle, and with the emergence of sarcopenia as an important public health issue, DXA is increasingly being used to estimate muscle mass.[34]

Computed Tomography and Magnetic Resonance Imaging

CT and MRI imaging methods are the most accurate means available for *in vivo* quantification of body composition at the tissue level. Although access and cost remain obstacles to routine use, these imaging approaches are now used extensively in body composition research. CT and MRI are the methods of choice for calibration of field methods designed to measure adipose tissue and skeletal muscle, and are the only methods available for measurement of internal organs.

The basic CT system consists of an x-ray tube and receiver that rotate in a perpendicular plane to the subject. The x-ray tube emits x-rays that are attenuated as they pass through tissues.[35] A receiver detects the attenuated x-rays, and a cross-sectional image is reconstructed with mathematical techniques. Tissue density is the main determinant of attenuation, and it is the tissue difference in attenuation values that provides tissue contrast in CT images. An example of an abdominal CT image is shown in Figure 1.4.

Cross-sectional CT images are composed of picture elements or pixels, usually 1 by 1 mm squares. For each of the pixels that compose a cross-sectional CT image, the x-ray attenuation value is expressed as a Hounsfield unit (HU). The lower the density of the tissue the lower the HU values for the pixels that make up that tissue. For example, adipose tissue is a low-density tissue with pixel intensity values that range from about − 190 to − 30 HU. Conversely, skeletal muscle, a higher-density tissue, has pixel intensity values that range from about 0 to 100 HU.[36]

The acquisition of MRI images is different from that of CT. Unlike CT, MRI does not use ionizing radiation. Instead, it is based on the interaction between

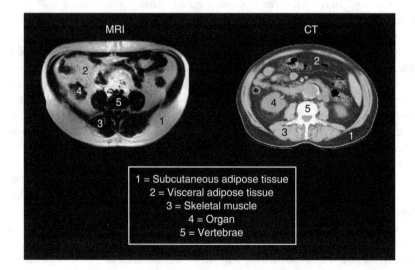

FIGURE 1.4 MRI and CT abdominal images. In the MRI image the lean tissues are dark and the adipose tissue is light. In the CT image the lean tissues are light and the adipose tissue is dark.

hydrogen nuclei (protons), which are abundant in all biological tissues, and the magnetic fields generated and controlled by the MRI system. Hydrogen protons, which are abundant in all tissues, behave like tiny magnets. When a person is placed inside an MRI unit, where the magnetic field strength is typically 15,000 times stronger than the earth's, the magnetic moments of the protons in their body align themselves with the magnetic field. With the protons aligned in a known direction, a radiofrequency pulse is applied by the MRI system, which causes a number of hydrogen protons to absorb energy. When the radiofrequency pulse is turned off, the protons gradually return (relax) to their original positions, in the process releasing energy that is absorbed by the MRI unit in the form of a radiofrequency signal. The MRI unit uses this signal to generate the cross-sectional images. Because different tissues have different relaxation properties, they release different amounts of energy. Manipulating the radiofrequency parameters allows one to exploit the differences in relaxation properties between various tissues, and in so doing, provides the necessary tissue contrast for high-quality cross-sectional images. An example of an abdominal MRI image is shown in Figure 1.4.

After acquisition, CT and MRI images must be analyzed using special computer software. This can be a very time-consuming and laborious process, depending on the analysis technique employed and the number of images acquired. Three techniques are routinely employed to measure tissue size on CT and MRI images, and these techniques vary considerably in terms of computer automation, manual editing, and the anatomical expertise required by the individual analyzing the images. Details of these procedures are provided elsewhere.[37] Briefly, these procedures all begin by identifying pixels that belong to different tissues. After the pixels for a given tissue have been identified, the area (cm^2) of the tissue is calculated by multiplying the number of pixels for a given tissue by the surface area of the individual pixels. If multiple CT or MRI images are obtained, tissue volumes can be calculated by integrating the cross-sectional area data from consecutive images, which can be obtained contiguously (typically 10-mm-thick images) or with interslice gaps between images (e.g., space between the top of one image and the bottom of the next image), which usually range from 20 to 40 mm. Tissue volumes are then calculated based on the tissue areas in the cross-sectional images and the distance between adjacent images.[37] Because there are little interindividual tissue densities for adipose tissue, skeletal muscle, and organs, CT and MRI volume measures can be converted to mass units by multiplying the volume by the assumed density values for that tissue. For example, the constant densities for adipose tissue and skeletal muscle are 0.92 and 1.04 kg/l, respectively.[38]

REFERENCE BODY COMPOSITION DATA

CHILDREN

The amount of body composition data available for preschool children is limited. This reflects the difficulty in obtaining physical measures (e.g., cooperation from

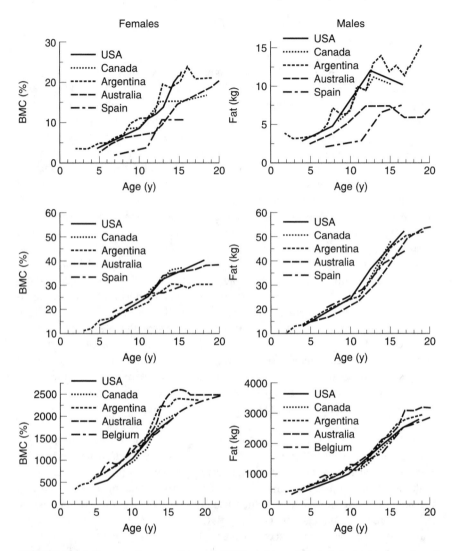

FIGURE 1.5 Influence of age on fat mass, FFM, and bone mineral content in samples of 5- to 18-year-old children and adolescents from different countries. (From Ellis, K.J., *Physiol. Rev.*, 80, 649–680, 2000.)

the child) and the concerns about the accuracy of techniques for such small body sizes.[9] There is, however, a considerable amount of body composition data available for school-aged children and adolescents. A summary of body composition data for pediatric studies conducted around the world is presented in Figure 1.5.[9] As shown in this figure, there is a marked increase in FFM, fat mass, and bone mineral content during the growing years independent of sex and nationality.

Countries throughout the world experienced a marked increase in the prevalence of overweight and obese children, and adolescents from the 1980s into the 21st century. A recent study compared the prevalence of overweight and obesity (as defined according to the International Obesity Task Force child cut-points) in school-aged youth from 34 industrialized countries.[39] These findings, which are presented in Figure 1.6, speak of the magnitude of the childhood obesity epidemic. (*Note*: In this study BMI was based on self-reported height and weight, and the prevalences of overweight and obesity were likely underestimated.) A more detailed discussion on childhood obesity is contained in Chapter 15.

ADULTS

Until recently there was an absence of representative body composition data for adults. However, national reference body composition data for the United States were recently published based on the BIA data from the Third National Health and Nutrition Examination Survey.[40] The mean FFM, fat mass, and % body fat values are plotted in Figure 1.7 according to sex, race or ethnicity, and age. These findings indicate that men have, on average, more FFM than women regardless of age and racial or ethnic status. Conversely, women have a higher fat mass and % body fat than men for a given age. Further, independent of sex and race or ethnicity, fat mass increases with advancing age until approximately 60 years. Conversely, FFM decreases with advancing age after approximately 50 years.

As with children, overweight and obesity are at epidemic proportions in adults. In developed countries the prevalence of adult obesity is often 10 to 20%.[41] In the United States, the prevalence of obesity in 20- to 74-year-olds has more than doubled in the past 30 years from 15% in 1976 to 1980 to 31% in 1999 to 2000.[42] Approximately 65% of U.S. adults were either overweight or obese at the turn of the century.[42] The age-related prevalence of obesity as determined by BMI tends to follow age-related patterns in fat mass, with an increase from the third to seventh decades and a decrease after age 70.[42] In the United States, the prevalence of obesity is slightly higher in women than in men (33 vs. 28%) and is higher in ethnic minorities for both men and women.[42]

As with BMI, a number of factors influence fat distribution. For a given level of total fat, men have more abdominal and visceral fat than women,[43] older adults have more abdominal and visceral fat than younger adults,[43,44] Caucasians have more abdominal and visceral fat than African–Americans,[43] and physically inactive and unfit individuals have more abdominal and visceral fat than physically active and fit individuals.[45]

Using the cut-points approach for defining sarcopenia, as explained previously in this chapter, it was recently reported that 53.1% of American men aged 60 or greater have a moderate level of sarcopenia and that 11.2% have a severe level of sarcopenia.[23] For American women aged 60 or greater, 21.9% have moderate sarcopenia and 9.4% have severe sarcopenia.[23] Within the elderly population, there is also an increasing prevalence of sarcopenia with advancing age, with the

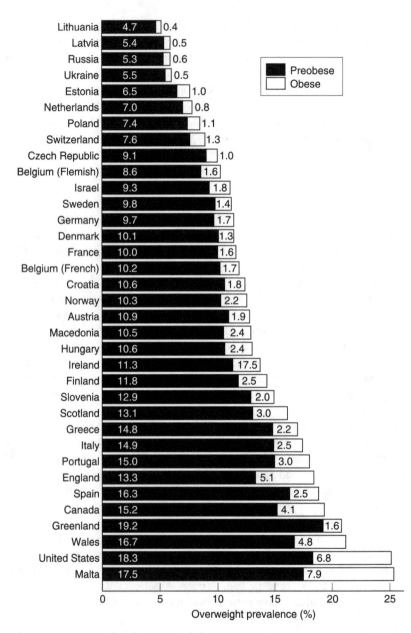

FIGURE 1.6 Prevalence of overweight and obesity in 10- to 16-year-old children from 34 industrialized countries. (From Janssen, I., Katzmarzyk, P.T., and Boyce, W.F. et al., *Obes. Rev.*, 6, 123–132, 2005.)

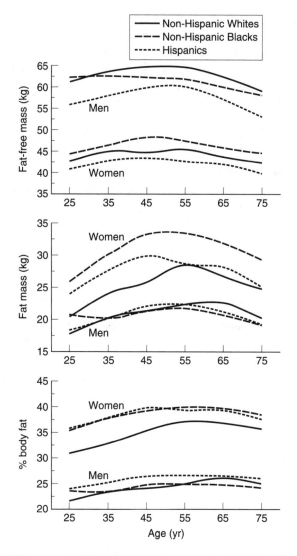

FIGURE 1.7 Differences in FFM, fat mass, and percent body fat from 25 to 75 years of age in American men and women. (Adapted from Chumlea, W.C., Guo, S.S., Kuczmarski, R.J. et al., *Int. J. Obes. Relat. Metab. Disord.*, 26, 1596–1609, 2002.)

prevalence rates being highest in the oldest old.[46] Sarcopenia prevalence rates tend to be higher in ethnic minorities such as Mexican–Americans.[46]

The prevalence of osteoporosis is quite high in the elderly population. Based on femoral bone mineral density values and the World Health Organization approach for defining osteoporosis and osteopenia, it has been estimated that

13 to 18% of American women aged 50 years of age or older have osteoporosis and that 37 to 50% have osteopenia.[47] Based on male-specific cut-points, it has been estimated that 3 to 6% of American men aged 50 years or above have osteoporosis and that 28 to 47% have osteopenia.[47] Within the population aged 50 years and above, the prevalence of osteoporosis increases with advancing age such that the highest prevalence rates are in the oldest old.

SUMMARY AND CONCLUSION

At present a number of methods can be used to quantify human body composition. The method selected for the specific research project or clinical application will depend on many factors, which include but are not limited to the body composition components being measured, the reproducibility and accuracy of the body

TABLE 1.3
Summary of advantages and disadvantages of body composition methods

Body composition method	Components measured	Cost	Technical expertise	Accuracy/ reproducibility	Portable equipment
Anthropometry	Height, weight, BMI Skinfolds, circumferences FFM, fat mass, muscle	Low	Low	Low to moderate	Yes
Densitometry (underwater weight, air displacement)	FFM, fat mass	Moderate	Moderate	Moderate	No
BIA	FFM, fat mass, muscle, total body water	Low	Low	Low to moderate	Yes
DXA	Total and regional FFM, fat mass, bone mineral content, and density	High	High	High	No
Imaging (CT, MRI)	Specific fat (subcutaneous, visceral) and lean tissue (muscle, organ) depots	Very high	Very high	Very High	No

composition measures required for the specific application, the cost of purchasing and maintaining the body composition equipment, the technical expertise required to operate the equipment and obtain the body composition measures, the degree of inconvenience and invasiveness that the subject or patient is willing to endure, the time required to obtain and analyze the body composition measures, and the portability of the equipment. A summary of how the various body composition methods covered in this chapter compare for these variables is provided in Table 1.3.

In addition to outlining a number of specific body composition techniques, this chapter has reviewed basic body composition rules and the methodological principles that form the basis of the various body composition techniques. Because it is necessary to establish body composition characteristics in most fields of nutrition and musculoskeletal health, the concepts and ideas discussed in this chapter will provide a background for many of the subsequent chapters in this book.

REFERENCES

1. Wang, Z.M., Pierson, R.N., Jr., and Heymsfield, S.B., The five-level model: a new approach to organizing body-composition research, *Am. J. Clin. Nutr.*, 56, 19–28, 1992.
2. Pace, N. and Rathbun, E.N., Studies on body composition. III. The body water and chemically combined nitrogen content in relation to fat content, *J. Biol. Chem.*, 158, 685–691, 1945.
3. Wang, Z., Zhu, S., Wang, J., Pierson, R.N., Jr., and Heymsfield, S.B., Whole-body skeletal muscle mass: development and validation of total-body potassium prediction models, *Am. J. Clin. Nutr.* 77, 76–82, 2003.
4. Keys, A. and Brozek, J., Body fat in adult men, *Physiol. Rev.*, 33, 245–325, 1953.
5. Pietrobelli, A., Heymsfield, S.B., Wang, Z.M., and Gallagher, D., Multi-component body composition models: recent advances and future directions, *Eur. J. Clin. Nutr.*, 55, 69–75, 2001.
6. Wong, S., Janssen, I., and Ross, R., Abdominal adipose tissue distribution and metabolic risk, *Sports Med.*, 33, 709–726, 2003.
7. Goodpaster, B.H., Measuring body fat distribution and content in humans, *Curr. Opin. Clin. Nutr. Metab. Care*, 5, 481–487, 2002.
8. Heymsfield, S.B., Wang, Z., Baumgartner, R.N., and Ross, R., Human body composition: advances in models and methods, *Annu. Rev. Nutr.*, 17, 527–558, 1997.
9. Ellis, K.J., Human body composition: *in vivo* methods, *Physiol. Rev.*, 80, 649–680, 2000.
10. Wang, Z.M., Heshka, S., Pierson, R.N., Jr., and Heymsfield, S.B., Systematic organization of body-composition methodology: an overview with emphasis on component-based methods, *Am. J. Clin. Nutr.*, 61, 457–465, 1995.
11. Guo, S.S., Chumlea, W.C., and Cockram, D.B., Use of statistical methods to estimate body composition, *Am. J. Clin. Nutr.*, 64, 428S–435S, 1996.
12. World Health Organization, *Obesity: Preventing and Managing the Global Epidemic*, Report of a WHO Consultation on Obesity, Geneva, 1998.

13. National Institutes of Health National Heart Lung and Blood Institute, Clinical guidelines on the identification, evaluation, and treatment of overweight and obesity in adults: the evidence report, *Obes. Res.*, 6, S51–S210, 1998.

14. WHO Expert Consultation, Appropriate body-mass index for Asian populations and its implications for policy intervention, *Lancet*, 363, 157–163, 2004.

15. Cole, T.J., Bellizzi, M.C., Flegal, K.M., and Dietz, W.H., Establishing a standard definition for child overweight and obesity worldwide: international survey, *Br. Med. J.*, 320, 1240–1243, 2000.

16. Janssen, I., Heymsfield, S.B., and Ross, R., Application of simple anthropometry in the assessment of health risk: implications for the Canadian Physical Activity, Fitness and Lifestyle Appraisal, *Can. J. Appl. Physiol.*, 27, 396–414, 2002.

17. Lukaski, H.C., Methods for the assessment of human body composition: traditional and new, *Am. J. Clin. Nutr.*, 46, 537–556, 1987.

18. Food and Nutrition Board (Institute of Medicine), *Dietary Reference Intakes for Energy, Carbohydrate, Fiber, Fat, Fatty Acids, Cholesterol, Protein, and Amino Acids (Macronutrients)*, National Academies Press, Washington, DC, 2003.

19. Ross, R., Dagnone, D., Jones, P.J. et al., Reduction in obesity and related comorbid conditions after diet-induced weight loss or exercise-induced weight loss in men. A randomized, controlled trial, *Ann. Intern. Med.*, 133, 92–103, 2000.

20. Janssen, I., Katzmarzyk, P.T., and Ross, R., Body mass index, waist circumference, and health risk: evidence in support of current national institutes of health guidelines, *Arch. Intern. Med.*, 162, 2074–2079, 2002.

21. Jelliffe, E.F. and Jelliffe, D.B., The arm circumference as a public health index of protein-calorie malnutrition of early childhood, *J. Trop. Pediatr.*, 15, 179–192, 1969.

22. Lee, R.C., Wang, Z., Heo, M., Ross, R., Janssen, I., and Heymsfield, S.B., Total-body skeletal muscle mass: development and cross-validation of anthropometric prediction models, *Am. J. Clin. Nutr.*, 72, 796–803, 2000.

23. Janssen, I., Baumgartner, R.N., Ross, R., Rosenberg, I.R., and Roubenoff, R., Skeletal muscle cutpoints associated with elevated physical disability risk in older men and women, *Am. J. Epidemiol.*, 159, 413–421, 2004.

24. Behnke, A.R., Freen, B.G., and Welham, W.C., Specific gravity of healthy men, *J. Am. Med. Assoc.*, 118, 495–498, 1942.

25. Siri, W.E., Body composition from fluid spaces and density: analysis of methods, in *Techniques for Measuring Body Composition*, Brozek, J. and Henschel, A., Eds., National Academy of Sciences National Research Council, Washington, DC, 1961, pp. 223–244.

26. Dempster, P. and Aitkens, S., A new air displacement method for the determination of human body composition, *Med. Sci. Sports Exerc.*, 27, 1692–1697, 1995.

27. Foster, K.R. and Lukaski, H.C., Whole-body impedance — what does it measure? *Am. J. Clin. Nutr.*, 64, 388S–396S, 1996.

28. Janssen, I., Heymsfield, S.B., Baumgartner, R.N., and Ross, R., Estimation of skeletal muscle mass by bioelectrical impedance analysis, *J. Appl. Physiol.*, 89, 465–471, 2000.

29. Kushner, R.F., Gudivaka, R., and Schoeller, D.A., Clinical characteristics influencing bioelectrical impedance analysis measurements, *Am. J. Clin. Nutr.*, 64, 423S–427S, 1996.

30. Cameron, J.R. and Sorenson, J., Measurement of bone mineral *in vivo*: an improved method, *Science*, 142, 230–232, 1963.

31. Mazess, R.B., Barden, H.S., Bisek, J.P., and Hanson, J., Dual-energy x-ray absorptiometry for total-body and regional bone-mineral and soft-tissue composition, *Am. J. Clin. Nutr.*, 51, 1106–1112, 1990.

32. Pietrobelli, A., Formica, C., Wang, Z., and Heymsfield, S.B., Dual-energy x-ray absorptiometry body composition model: review of physical concepts, *Am. J. Physiol.*, 271, E941–E951, 1996.

33. WHO Expert Committee, World Health Organization (WHO) 1994 Assessment of Fracture Risk and its Application to Screening for Postmenopausal Osteoporosis: Reports of a WHO Study Group, WHO, Geneva, 1994.

34. Kim, J., Wang, Z., Heymsfield, S.B., Baumgartner, R.N., and Gallagher, D., Total-body skeletal muscle mass: estimation by a new dual-energy x-ray absorptiometry method, *Am. J. Clin. Nutr.*, 76, 378–383, 2002.

35. Sprawls, P., *The Physical Principles of Diagnostic Radiology*, University Park Press, Baltimore, 1977.

36. Chowdhury, B., Sjostrom, L., Alpsten, M., Kostanty, J., Kvist, H., and Lofgren, R., A multicompartment body composition technique based on computerized tomography, *Int. J. Obes. Relat. Metab. Disord.*, 18, 219–234, 1994.

37. Ross, R., Computed tomography and magnetic resonance imaging, in *Human Body Composition*, 2nd ed., Heymsfield, S.B., Wang, Z., and Going, S., Eds., Human Kinetics, Champaign, IL 2005, pp. 89–108.

38. Snyder, W.S., Cooke, M.J., Manssett, E.S., Larhansen, L.T., Howells, G.P., and Tipton, I.H., Report of the Task Group on Reference Man, Pergamon Press, Oxford, 1975.

39. Janssen, I., Katzmarzyk, P.T., Boyce, W.F. et al., Comparison of overweight and obesity prevalences in school-aged youth from 34 countries and their relationships with physical activity and dietary patterns, *Obes. Rev.*, 6, 123–132, 2005.

40. Chumlea, W.C., Guo, S.S., Kuczmarski, R.J. et al., Body composition estimates from NHANES III bioelectrical impedance data, *Int. J. Obes. Relat. Metab. Disord.*, 26, 1596–1609, 2002.

41. Seidell, J.C., Obesity, insulin resistance and diabetes — a worldwide epidemic, *Br. J. Nutr.*, 83 (Suppl. 1), S5–S8, 2000.

42. Flegal, K.M., Carroll, M.D., Ogden, C.L., and Johnson, C.L., Prevalence and trends in obesity among US adults, 1999–2000, *J. Am. Med. Assoc.*, 288, 1723–1727, 2002.

43. Hill, J.O., Sidney, S., Lewis, C.E., Tolan, K., Scherzinger, A.L., and Stamm, E.R., Racial differences in amounts of visceral adipose tissue in young adults: the CARDIA (Coronary Artery Risk Development in Young Adults) study, *Am. J. Clin. Nutr.*, 69, 381–387, 1999.

44. DeNino, W.F., Tchernof, A., Dionne, I.J. et al., Contribution of abdominal adiposity to age-related differences in insulin sensitivity and plasma lipids in healthy nonobese women, *Diabetes Care*, 24, 925–932, 2001.

45. Janssen, I., Katzmarzyk, P.T., Ross, R. et al., Fitness alters the associations of BMI and waist circumference with total and abdominal fat, *Obes. Res.*, 12, 525–537, 2004.

46. Baumgartner, R.N., Koehler, K.M., Gallagher, D. et al., Epidemiology of sarcopenia among the elderly in New Mexico, *Am. J. Epidemiol.* 147, 755–763, 1998.

47. Looker, A.C., Orwoll, E.S., Johnston, C.C., Jr. et al., Prevalence of low femoral bone density in older U.S. adults from NHANES III, *J. Bone Miner. Res.*, 12, 1761–1768, 1997.

2 Nutrigenomics: Strategic Prevention of Musculoskeletal Disorders of Aging

Jeffrey S. Bland, Ph.D.

CONTENTS

DEFINING NUTRIGENOMICS

Nutrigenomics, which has recently been entered into Webster's dictionary, is a term that has far-reaching implications. It suggests that a specific diet consumed by an individual influences his or her function in a unique way because of the information in the food. Food is information molecules that contain a dietary signature. Food is much more than calories and the prevention of nutrient-deficiency diseases; it influences gene expression, proteomic function, and ultimately, metabolism.

The foundation for nutrigenomics was laid in the 1950s by investigators such as Pauling, Williams, Watson, and Crick. These investigators pioneered what is now being called the age of molecular medicine. Discoveries from these investigators have led to the recognition that the "book of life" is encoded in our genes. Each of us has a slightly different book based on the uniqueness of genetic inheritance.

There are many story lines, and how the story unfolds and the ultimate message delivered from it depends on the environment in which the book is read. Within each of our genes is the potential for a healthier or less healthy lifespan, depending on the selections we may make and how we set the environment for the expression of our genes.

Genetic expression is the term applied to how the messages encoded in our genes are read by our cells to shape our phenotype. What is now being recognized is that phenotype — the functional look, feel, and capabilities of an individual — is not determined solely by the genotype. Phenotype is determined by how the genes are expressed in the context of metabolism. This results in what has been termed the "triology of omics," where genomics give rise to proteomics that give rise to metabolomics, which, in turn, give rise to our phenotype, or phenomics.

THE NUTRITIONAL ENVIRONMENT

Over the past decade, the environment, and specifically the nutritional environment, has been recognized as a major modulator of genetic expression, proteomics, and ultimately, the control of metabolism. Food is information. The field of nutrigenomics is exploding in this area, and both basic and clinical research have started to develop a better understanding of the relationship between the information molecules in food and how they influence the triology of omics in the individual.

The environment plays a larger role in phenotypic expression than was previously acknowledged. For example, as Dr. Chan discusses in Chapter 3, adult body composition is influenced by the *in utero* environment. This is powerful and encouraging information for clinicians, because while we cannot change our genes, we can change the environment in which the genes are expressed. Carrying a gene that encodes for high cholesterol is not a sentence for premature death by heart disease. Rather, it indicates that this genetic uniqueness will respond differently in specific environments, in either a more harmful or a less harmful way. Emerging data suggest that many age-related musculoskeletal conditions such as osteoarthritis, sarcopenia, and osteoporosis may manifest as a consequence of the expression of the genes in a specific environment.

Editor's Note

Nutrition changes the environment, which changes gene expression. Nutrigenomics is not an evaluation of good genes and bad genes; it teaches us how strategic nutrition can create an environment that builds muscle, metabolizes fat, strengthens bone, and repairs cartilage.

As pointed out in a landmark article by James Fries of Stanford University School of Medicine in 1980, "[Aging is] not a function. Aging can be defined as an endogenous, progressive deterioration in age-specific components of fitness. It is instead a secondary effect of the decline in the force of natural selection with age."[1] Lifestyle and nutrition play significant roles in how the aging process is manifested in the individual. In the 1980 article, Dr. Fries proposed that we could compress illness into the last short period of a person's life, and maximize their survival and healthy function, thereby increasing their "health span" through intervention with lifestyle, nutrition, and exercise programs.

In 1998, Vita et al. presented evidence collected from a study of 1741 University of Pennsylvania alumni over a period of 32 years that a healthy lifestyle delivers not only increased years of life, but more importantly, improved function[2] and compressed morbidity. In an accompanying editorial, the results of this study were summarized:

> In the group with the lowest level of risk, the onset of functional disability was postponed by about 5 years. In the group with the highest level of risk — those who had a body mass index of 26 or higher, smoked 30 or more cigarettes per day, and got no regular vigorous exercise — there was both an earlier onset of disability and a greater level of cumulative disability, as well as more disability in the final year of life for the 10% of the cohort that had died.[3]

Historically, most individuals have believed that we age by a genetically pre-determined process that is beyond our control, and that age-associated diseases are a manifestation of our genetic inheritance. Therefore, taking this as a presumption, for the past few decades medical professionals and the lay public have believed that we could do little to prevent these associative illnesses of aging. However, in the past 15 years, as researchers have deciphered the genome locked into our 23 pairs of chromosomes, this deterministic model of sickness has been replaced by a more plastic view of the genes or environment connection. Genes are not found to be a code for specific diseases of aging; instead, they are a code for various strengths and weaknesses in an individual's constitution that give rise to resistance or susceptibility factors for specific age-related diseases. Some people get the luck of the draw and have more resistance genes to factors associated with 21st century living. Other individuals, like the Pima Indians, may have genes that were effective for the environment in which they evolved over several million years, but are maladapted to today's diets, which are high in sugar, fat, alcohol, indoor activity, and inactivity. We often say that the Pima Indians have "diabetic genes," when in reality, they have "warrior genes." That is, their genes were adapted to provide fitness for the natural environment in which they lived throughout most of their cultural history. Only recently, within the past 100 years, have these genes been exposed to an environment that has given rise to the expression patterns of obesity, diabetes, and heart disease.

In a 2002 article in *Science* magazine, Walter Willett from the Harvard School of Medicine, Department of Nutrition, asserted: "Genetic and environmental factors, including diet and lifestyle, both contribute to cardiovascular disease, cancers, and other major causes of mortality, but various lines of evidence indicate that environmental factors are most important."[4]

Following this theme, Nada Abumrad pointed out that "Nutritional support can be tailored to the individual genotype to favor beneficial phenotypic expression or to suppress processes that lead to later pathology."[5]

The important theme the environment plays in determining genetic expression resulting in disease was driven home in an article published in 2000 in *The New England Journal of Medicine* describing research by the investigators at the Karolinska Institute in Sweden, who reported on 44,788 pairs of identical twins. This study showed that identical twins do not experience cancer at the same rate. In fact, the study reported that "inherited genetic factors make a minor contribution to susceptibility to most types of neoplasms. This finding indicates that the environment has the principal role in causing sporadic cancer."[6]

In 1950, Roger Williams published an article in *The Lancet* titled, "The Concepts of Genetotrophic Disease," in which he advanced the bold concept that a number of diseases whose origins were unknown at that time could be understood as conditions associated not with malnutrition, but with undernutrition based on the individual's unique genetic needs. He postulated that diabetes, mental disease, arthritis, and even alcoholism could be considered to have a "genetotrophic origin."[7]

In 2002, Bruce Ames, Professor Emeritus of Biochemistry from the University of California at Berkeley, provided the 21st century substantiation of Williams' concepts. Ames showed, in his detailed review paper, that "as many as one-third of mutations in a gene result in the corresponding enzyme having an increased Michaelis constant, or K_m, (decreased binding affinity) for a coenzyme, resulting in a lower rate of reaction." Some people carry polymorphisms that are more critical in determining the outcome of their health histories. Ames goes on to argue that studies have shown that administration of higher than dietary reference intake levels of cofactors (specific vitamins and minerals) to people with these polymorphic genes restores activity to near-normal or even normal levels. He concludes that nutritional interventions to improve health are likely to be a major benefit of the genomics era.[8] If a disease-related gene expression involves specific genetic variations, one preventive option might be to use nutritional agents targeted to these genetic variations.[9]

As pointed out by Muller and Kersten,

> In the past decade, nutrition research has undergone an important shift in focus from epidemiology and physiology to molecular biology and genetics. This is mainly a result of three factors that have led to a growing realization that the effects of nutrition on health and disease cannot be understood without a profound understanding of how

nutrients act at the molecular level ... there has been a growing recognition that micronutrients and macronutrients can be potent dietary signals that influence the metabolic programming of cells and have an important role in the control of homeostasis.[10]

NUTRIGENOMICS AND THE HEALTH CARE SYSTEM

Nutrigenomics is a concept forwarding the present-day nutrition and lifestyle movement in medicine.[4] Nutrigenomics can improve clinical outcomes for chronic, age-related, degenerative diseases, while also reducing unnecessary health care expenditures. "All of us should have in mind doing everything we can for our health, not relying on medicines as the only answer. We could do more with diet and exercise," advises Dr. Frank Williams, Scientific Director for the American Federation for Aging Research and a specialist in geriatrics.[11]

In his recent book *Is It in Your Genes?* Philip R. Reilly explains how genetic medicine can change health care:

> Most people think of genetic diseases as rare conditions caused by muta-tions in a single gene that generally afflict children. This impression is 20 years out of date. It's simply no longer accurate. Extraordinary advances in our understanding of human genetics are changing how physicians think about the causes of disease. Today, we know that vir-tually all the diseases and disorders that afflict humans are influenced by the genes with which they are born.
>
> We have entered the era of genetic medicine. It is a new field, still in its infancy; but over the next couple of decades, thanks to the success of the Human Genome Project and countless other research efforts, it will substantially change the nature of health care ... As we cross that boundary, we will enter a new world which some scientists and physi-cians are already calling Personalized Medicine.[12]

Dr. Reilly concludes the book on genetic susceptibility to disease with a very insightful and prescient view of the future:

> Nutritional genetics will be a central feature of wellness programs. Motivated individuals will adhere to diets and consume particular nutraceuticals based on compatibility with their genetic profile. The rapidly growing nutrition business will be based on far more credible scientific evidence than it is today. Nutritional counseling will be replete with genetic analysis. Much of the focus will be on using a combination of genetic information, dietary choice, and fitness regimes to pursue a robust wellness into the ninth decade ... Knowledge of one's genetic profile will be crucial to a long and vigorous life. The

concept of medicine will be broadened, and the line between drugs and nutritional substances will be almost completely erased. In the economically powerful nations, most of medicine will be aimed at maximizing the chances of living vigorously until 100. Individuals who have the resources and good sense to incorporate genetic risk information into their lives, much as do people today who are committed to healthy diets and logical exercise regimens, will be far more likely to reach that goal.[13]

Jones et al. pointed out that physicians face a complex set of challenges when interweaving the emerging knowledge about aging and disease, environment, genomics, and proteomics with the existing health care model.[14] Physicians are now starting to learn that the risk of disease and age-related decline in function are unique to each patient, and the phenotype appears to be more vulnerable to environmental pressures than to genetic influence.

The medicine that helps patients achieve genetic potential through nutrition has been called personalized medicine. The clinician matches the patient's history and genetics with interventions tailored specifically for that individual, thus modulating the health of a patient and improving the realization of his or her maximum genetic potential for healthy longevity. Most clinical practices have not yet caught up with this knowledge. For example, less than 1 in 5 of the 6712 patients received appropriate counseling and health education in a report published in *The New England Journal of Medicine* in 2003.[15]

In considering how nutrigenomics might influence health care delivery, it may be important to recognize that the change is not new. In 400 B.C. Hippocrates described the interaction of one's constitution (the genetics and genomics of today) and the environment. Hippocrates explained the resulting health care system as follows:[16]

Wherefore I say that such constitutions as suffer quickly and strongly from errors in diet are weaker than others that do not and that a weak person is in a state very nearly approaching to one of disease.

And this I know, moreover, that to the human body it makes a great difference whether the bread be fine or coarse, of wheat with or without the hull, whether mixed with much or little water, strongly wrought or scarcely at all, baked or raw ...

Whoever pays no attention to these things, or paying attention does not comprehend them, how can we understand the diseases that befall man?

For by every one of these things, a man is affected and changed in this way and that, and the whole of his life is subjected to them, whether in health, convalescence or disease.

Nothing else, then, can be more important or more necessary to know than these things.

In conclusion, applying nutrigenomics to clinical practice compels the clinician to diagnose and treat underlying mechanisms. It is not enough to intervene with a single agent that focuses on a specific risk factor. It is more important to intervene with a diet and lifestyle that "tickles" many genes that control the phenotype associated with lowering the risk of CVD, diabetes, stroke, and musculoskeletal disorders. Following are the concepts that nutrigenomics addresses.

SHARED MECHANISMS

Health care focuses on care of the sick and classifies patients into various disease-specific categories. Nutrigenomics helps identify common molecular pathways, such as inflammation or nutrient deficiency. Conditions as divergent as low back strain, obesity and periodontal disease may be ameliorated by a single therapy and treated by the same clinician.

Nutrigenomics moves clinical medicine from disease-specific niches to common underlying disease mechanisms. One set of genetically influenced biochemical pathways associated with muscle loss is inflammation. The loss of muscle and the gain in fat has recently been associated with specific nutrigenomic changes. These include the impact of specific nutrients on the genetic expression of genes specific to the immune inflammatory response.

The immune system is in part divided into the thymus dependent lymphocytes type 1 (Th1) and type 2 (Th2). Like many biochemical systems, not only the absolute concentration but also the ratio of the two concentrations is important. The balance between Th1 and Th2 is influenced by several genes, which individualizes response to the environment. Imbalance of the equilibrium between Th1 and Th2 results in alterations in inflammatory mediators. Increasing evidence now suggests that any condition that increases the levels of Th1 inflammatory cytokines can have adverse impact on protein synthesis and muscle function.[17] Recent studies have shown that cytokines can directly influence skeletal muscle contractility independent of changes in muscle protein content.

In situations in which there is an increase in inflammatory signals, production of interleukin 1 (IL-1), IL-6, and tumor necrosis factor alpha (TNF-α) in white cells is enhanced, as is that of nuclear factor kappa B (NFκB). NFκB has been implicated in autoimmune disorders, inflammatory disorders, and infections. Its production is increased as a consequence of an inflammatory event that shifts toward the proinflammatory TH1 cytokines.[18] In situations of increased expression of NFκB and downstream elaboration of proinflammatory cytokines, there is an alteration in muscle protein metabolism and function.

Under conditions of physiological stress, there is increasing production of proinflammatory mediators and loss of muscle, which has been called sarcopenia (*sarc* — flesh, *penia* — loss of).[19] The relationship between inflammatory mediators and conditions such as obesity, sarcopenia, arthritis, and muscle loss is shown in Figure 2.1.

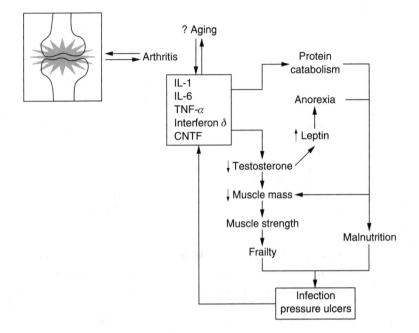

FIGURE 2.1 The vicious cycle of cytokine-induced frailty. CNTF, ciliary neurotrophic factor.

The fat cell, the adipocyte, produces the same inflammatory cytokines. Obesity, therefore, may be viewed as a low-grade systemic inflammatory disease.[20] Obese children and adults have elevated serum markers of inflammation including high-sensitivity C-reactive protein, IL-6, TNF, and leptin. Extreme obesity is associated with heart failure through similar immune mechanisms.[21,22]

Many diseases of muscle loss are thought to have not only pathophysiology, but also shared interventions. Humoral mediators, including the TH1 cytokines, appear to influence protein nutritional status by directly impairing the regulation of skeletal muscle protein turnover. Extensive research is currently ongoing in an effort to identify specific nutritive factors that can influence cytokine production and promote regular catabolic activity on the muscle cell.

MEASURING NUTRIGENOMIC FACTORS

Loss of muscle and replacement by body fat occurs well before an individual exhibits a significant alteration in body mass index. Measurement, therefore, has clinical applications. While nutritional testing may involve extensive biochemical assays and genetic testing may involve DNA probes on a patient's extended family, nutrigenomic testing can be inexpensive and noninvasive and is performed in the clinic with the patient present.

Inexpensive and noninvasive measures would be useful to assess the patient's body composition and ability to build muscle. Bioimpedance assays (BIA) may offer precisely that, as described by Dr. Janssen in the chapter on body composition. Briefly, BIA send a current through the body and measures how quickly it returns. Since hydrophilic muscle is a conductor and hydrophobic fat - an insulator, the more muscle, the more quickly the current returns. In this way BIA characterize body composition. Additionally, BIA assess membrane potential at the tissue level measured by the phase angle. Phase angle is defined as the relationship between the two vector components of impedance: resistance and reactance. The wider the phase angle the more beneficial the cellular reduction potential. As the phase angle decreases, there is loss of electrochemical gradient and lowered bioenergetics at the cellular level. Both percent body fat and phase angle can be useful tools in determining the overall cell signaling process and physiological status in the whole organism.

A number of studies looking at BIA of individuals from young to older ages have shown a general trend toward lower fat-free mass after the age of 50 years.[23] A recent study used BIA to assess body composition of 995 acutely or chronically ill patients at hospital admission and found that the fat-free mass was significantly lower, and fat mass significantly higher in the patients, as compared to 995 healthy age and height matched controls.[24] A study comparing 131 patients on chronic hemodialysis with 272 age and sex matched healthy controls found that a change in phase angle was the strongest predictor of poor prognosis in the hemodialysis patients. It seemed to be a reliable detector of clinically overt depletion of lean body mass and changes in intracellular electrolyte and fluid balances.[25] Another study demonstrated that patients with both overt and subclinical thyroid disease had altered phase angle and bioimpedance values. This study suggests that it may be a useful tool in the management of patients with complex endocrine metabolic dysfunctions.[26] Heber et al. at the Division of Clinical Nutrition of UCLA School of Medicine used BIA to identify a high prevalence of sarcopenic obesity among premenopausal women at increased risk of breast cancer. These women had normal body height-to-weight ratios, but upon analysis of body composition by BIA, presented increased levels of body fat and decreased muscle.[27]

Another example of a nutrigenomic test is phosphorus 31 nuclear magnetic resonance (NMR) spectroscopy. This helpful research technology does not require muscle biopsy and can be done in real time with a person exercising the muscle within a spectrometer to examine the effects of exercise on bioenergetics. In a study of individuals who were suffering from disorders associated with malnutrition and increased levels of proinflammatory cytokines, Khursheed Jeejeebhoy and colleagues found that phosphorus 31 NMR spectroscopy was capable of detecting bioenergetic changes in muscle.[28] Phosphorus 31 NMR spectroscopy is used to evaluate the ATP dynamics in muscle because it can evaluate the presence of ATP, ADP, AMP, and inorganic phosphorus, as well as phosphocreatine in muscle.

Hormone testing also is within the realm of nutrigenomics. Hormones orchestrate the genetic expression to conduct the dietary symphony to build either muscle or fat. Physical changes in aging have been considered related to sarcomere physiology but there is evidence that some of these changes are related to decline in hormonal activity.[29] Lamberts points out in his article "The Endocrinology of Aging," that "Three hormonal systems show decreasing circulating hormone concentrations during normal aging: (i) estrogen (in menopause) and testosterone (in andropause), (ii) dehydroepiandrosterone and its sulfate (in adrenopause), and (iii) the growth hormone/insulin-like growth factor I axis (in somatopause). In certain circumstances hormones can be assayed noninvasively, by sampling saliva and urine."

ACHIEVING HEALTHSPAN

The emerging genetic priority in understanding the aging process is to define the endogenous and exogenous factors that influence the gene transcription and proteomic expression regulating catabolic and anabolic factors. Agents that up-regulate proinflammatory processes alter the anabolic–catabolic balance and shift physiology into a catabolic state, with increased apoptosis occurring in postmitotic tissue such as brain, heart, and muscle.[30]

For example, there is a long-held belief that older men lose muscle principally as a consequence of lowered protein biosynthetic capability. For that reason, most people have felt that there is little an individual can do about that loss. Muscle loss and fat replacement of muscle are not the result of a poor-quality diet and lack of exercise alone. Nor are they entirely functions of aging. The shift in physiognomy is the result of a complex interaction between cellular physiology and cellular messengers that may induce loss of muscle function and integrity, resulting in a reduced fat-free mass. A study by Volpi et al., described in further detail in Dr. Short's chapter on sarcopenia, demonstrates this concept.[31] The researchers found that net muscle protein balance was similar in young and old men. Differences in mean muscle protein synthesis and breakdown were smaller than expected between healthy older and younger men. The most important result is that differences in basal muscle protein turnover between younger and older men do not explain the muscle loss that occurs with chronologic age. Instead, other secondary factors influence the physiology of the muscle cell, which may contribute to loss of muscle protein with age. In a companion editorial titled "Sarcopenia — Understanding the Dynamics of Aging Muscle," Roubenoff and Castaneda describe this process.[32] Commenting on the Volpi paper, the authors wrote:

> These observations strongly suggest that sarcopenia is not due to inadequate basal (fasting) protein synthesis. More likely, aging muscle fails to respond to stimuli that are anabolic to young muscle — e.g., diet and exercise — perhaps because of hormonal or immunological changes that occur with age and no longer favor anabolism ... Taken together, these two studies [this and a previous study Volpi's group]

implicate insulin resistance or immune factors, such as catabolic cytokines or other hormonal or immunological factors, acting primarily in the postprandial state as an important cause of sarcopenia.[33]

The mechanism by which cellular mediators such as insulin, inflammatory cytokines, NFκB, and excess production of nitric oxide induce loss of muscle protein appears to be a consequence of uncoupling of mitochondrial oxidative phosphorylation in the myocyte.[33] Mitochondrial uncoupling proteins have been discovered over the past several years with uncoupling protein 3 (UCP3) now appearing to have a putative role in uncoupling of mitochondrial respiration, thereby increasing the production of reactive oxygen species and altering the regulation of glucose metabolism in skeletal muscle.[34] The inflammatory cytokines appear to activate the expression of UCP3 and therefore increase the production of mitochondrial oxygen species, which increases oxidative stress and altered bioenergetics.

Altered mitochondrial oxidative phosphorylation results in declining muscle protein synthesis, lowered energy, and lowered cognitive function. The reason is that muscle and neurological tissue both depend on mitochondrial oxidative phosphorylation for the production of ATP, which is involved in the contractility of muscle and generation of neurotransmitters.[35] There is a strong correlation between mitochondrial uncoupling and the recognition that many degenerative diseases associated with aging are the result of lowered mitochondrial activity.[36,37] Declining mitochondrial bioenergetics is a unifying concept underlying many chronic age-related disorders associated with sarcopenic obesity and inflammation. Stimuli that trigger the release of the inflammatory mediators create a cellular environment in postmitotic tissue, such as in the myocyte, cardiocyte, and neuron, in which oxidative injury occurs, leading to degeneration and apoptosis.

PERSONALIZED MEDICINE

Nutrigenomics offers a personalized medicine, using nutrient, dietary, and lifestyle interventions to mitigate adverse biochemical pathways. Here is an example of a nutrigenomic intervention that allows the practitioner to restore a muscle-building environment: Some statin medications used to treat heritably elevated cholesterol may deplete mitochondrial enzyme function and coenzyme Q10, which results in mitochondrial energy uncoupling, oxidative stress and subsequent cell death.[38,39] The use of coenzyme Q10 supplements has been suggested to improve mitochondrial function in muscle and reduce myopathic pain in patients who have adverse response to statins.[40–43] This intervention utilizes coenzyme Q10 as a conditionally essential nutrient to replete a critical biomolecule necessary for proper mitochondrial function. This is an example of personalizing the nutrient intake for the specific gene–environment relationship of the patient.

Another application to direct patient care is the use of strategic nutrition to enhance insulin sensitivity. The stress response prompts the adrenal glands to release glucocorticoids. Chronic stress results in chronic elevations in cortisol and eventually abdominal fat and insulin resistance.[38,44] The resulting visceral obesity increases the production of inflammatory mediators such as TNF-α and IL-6. Patients caught in this cycle of inflammation and adiposity may need a clinician's help to reverse the unfavorable environment. Nutritional interventions such as improved-quality carbohydrates, vitamin D, magnesium, and chromium, each discussed in later chapters, can improve insulin sensitivity and, eventually, phenotypic expression.

Hormones that deliver anabolic messages may be repleted as part of premature aging. As Dr. Teitelbaum suggests, in the chapter on fibromyalgia, laboratory tests should be evaluated within the personalized context of the individual patient and can be used to optimal levels within age-specific parameters.

Strategic nutrition and an exercise prescription, such as those elaborated in later chapters, can measurably improve the early markers of disease and, eventually, phenotypic expression. Hackman and colleagues evaluated modestly overweight women who were placed on a medical food intervention program, along with a regular walking regimen. After following this program for several weeks, phosphorus 31 NMR spectroscopy revealed that the women had significantly improved body composition, lowered body fat and increased fat-free mass (muscle mass gain), as well as increased mitochondrial bioenergetics.[45] The program resulted in preservation of muscle energy function, loss of fat mass, and preservation of lean muscle mass. A companion study used the same nutritional supplement that is high in soy protein with phytonutrients, vitamins, and minerals in another group of modestly overweight women. This program resulted in a reduction in blood cholesterol, increased muscle mass, and lowered body fat. This study compared the nutritional supplement to an over-the-counter weight-loss product. Although the two programs resulted in the same weight loss over 12 weeks, most of the weight lost using the commercially available, over-the-counter product came as muscle loss and not as fat loss. The nutrient-dense, phytonutrient-rich product, in contrast, resulted not only in the loss of weight as fat, but also in a reduction in blood cholesterol.[46]

Evans and his colleagues have developed an approach for managing sarcopenic obesity through regular strength and aerobic conditioning exercise. A controlled trial found that strength training improved functional capacity and muscle physiology, and reduced sarcopenia in 90-year-old men.[47] Physiology research has demonstrated that properly prescribed and implemented resistance training increases the production of anabolic hormone messengers and reduces inflammatory mediators.

Sarcopenia is partly a consequence of mitochondrial uncoupling that results from oxidative stress after exposure to proinflammatory mediators, such as TNF-α, IL-6, and NFκB. Nutritional intervention using a diet augmented with nutrients that help lower the inflammatory potential and support redox function at the mitochondrial level may be important in managing these conditions. Redox-active nutrients include vitamin E, selenium, lipoic acid, coenzyme Q10,

N-acetylcysteine, and *N*-acetylcarnitine. Dr. Richard Weindruch, from the University of Wisconsin, proposed that interventions based on the possibility that oxidative stress contributes to sarcopenia may prove useful in managing patients with inflammation-induced muscle loss.[48]

Sarcopenia is related to the altered functional capacity of the individual. The symptoms in those with sarcopenic obesity are weakness, fatigue, depression, immune hypersensitivity, and inflammation. Altered aerobic capacity, altered immunological function, and altered hormone levels are commonly associated with increased inflammatory signaling associated with changes in diet, activity patterns, and lifestyle.[49] Reversing dietary, activity, and lifestyle factors varies from individual to individual. Addressing them needs to be a personalized form of medicine.

CONCLUSION

The new genomic model of personalized medicine will enable individuals to nourish themselves to optimize their quality of life for years. The tools of medicine will include food-derived substances, as well as exercise prescriptions that modulate genetic expression and promote proper function. As new inexpensive laboratory tests to assess genetic predispositions and physiological function become available, a personalized form of medicine will become a reality. The doctors of the 21st century will need to understand how to assess patients' genotypes and personalize treatment for their individual needs. They will also need to know how to help patients improve their lifestyles and environments to minimize the risks of age-related chronic diseases and achieve their genetic potential through nutrition.

REFERENCES

1. Fries. J.F., Aging, natural death, and the compression of morbidity, *N. Engl. J. Med.*, 303, 130–135, 1980.
2. Vita, A.J., Terry, R.B., Hubert, H.B., and Fries, J.F., Aging, health risks, and cumulative disability, *N. Engl. J. Med.*, 338, 1035–1041, 1998.
3. Campion, E.W., Aging-better, *N. Engl. J. Med.*, 338, 1064–1066, 1998.
4. Willett, W.C., Balancing life-style and genomics research for disease prevention, *Science*, 296, 695–698, 2002.
5. Abumrad, N.A., The gene-nutrient-gene loop, *Curr. Opin. Nutr. Metab. Care*, 4, 407–410, 2001.
6. Lichtenstein, P., Holm, N.V., Verkasalo, P.K. et al., Environmental and heritable factors in the causation of cancer — analyses of cohorts of twins from Sweden, Denmark, and Finland, *N. Engl. J. Med.*, 343, 78–85, 2000.
7. Williams, R.J., Beerstecher, E., Jr., and Berry, L.J., The concept of genetotrophic disease, *Lancet*, 1, 287–289, 1950.
8. Ames, B.N., Elson-Schwab, I., and Silver, E.A., High-dose vitamin therapy stimulates variant enzymes with decreased coenzyme binding affinity (increased K_m): relevance to genetic disease and polymorphisms, *Am. J. Clin. Nutr.*, 75, 616–658, 2002.

9. Kornman, K.S., Martha, P.M., and Duff, G.W., Genetic variations and inflammation: a practical nutrigenomics opportunity, *Nutrition*, 20, 44–49, 2004.

10. Muller, M. and Kersten, S., Nutrigenomics: goals and strategies, *Nat. Rev./Genet.*, 4, 315–322, 2003.

11. Hawthorne, F., *The Merck Druggernaut: The Inside Story of a Pharmaceutical Giant*, John Wiley & Sons, Inc., Hoboken, NJ, 2003, p. 107.

12. Reilly, P.R., *Is It in Your Genes?* Cold Spring Harbor Laboratory Press, Cold Spring Harbor, NY, 2004, p. xi.

13. Reilly, P.R. *Is It in Your Genes?* Cold Spring Harbor Laboratory Press, Cold Spring Harbor, NY, 2004, p. 243–244.

14. Jones, D.S., Bland, J.S., and Quinn, S., Healthy aging and the origins of illness: improving the expression of genetic potential, *Integr. Med.*, 2, 16–25, 2004.

15. McGlynn, E.A., Asch, S.M., Adams, J. et al., The quality of health care delivered to adults in the United States, *N. Engl. J. Med.*, 348, 2635–2645, 2003.

16. Labadarios, D. and Meguid, M.M., Nutrigenomics: unraveling man's constitution in relation to food, *Nutrition*, 20, 2–3, 2004.

17. Zoico, E. and Roubenoff, R., The role of cytokines in regulating protein metabolism and muscle function, *Nutr. Rev.*, 60, 39–51, 2002.

18. Holmes, M.M., Nuclear factor kappa B signaling in catabolic disorders, *Curr. Opin. Clin. Nutr. Metab. Care*, 5, 255–263, 2002.

19. Morley, J.E., Anorexia, sarcopenia, and aging, *Nutrition*, 17, 660–663, 2001.

20. Das, U.N., Is obesity an inflammatory condition? *Nutrition*, 17, 953–966, 2001.

21. Kenchaiah, S., Evans, J.C., Levy, D. et al., Obesity and the risk of heart failure, *N. Engl. J. Med.*, 347, 305–313, 2002.

22. Massie, B.M., Obesity and heart failure — risk factor or mechanism? *N. Engl. J. Med.*, 347, 358–359, 2002.

23. Kyle, U.G., Genton, L., Slosman, D.O., and Pichard, C., Fat-free and fat mass percentiles in 5225 healthy subjects aged 15 to 98 years, *Nutrition*, 17, 534–541, 2001.

24. Kyle, U.G., Unger, P., Dupertuis, Y.M., Karsegard, V.L., Genton, L., and Pichard, C., Body composition in 995 acutely ill or chronically ill patients at hospital admission: a controlled population study, *J. Am. Diet Assoc.*, 102, 944–948, 2002.

25. Maggiore, Q., Nigrelli, S., Ciccarelli, C., Grimaldi, C., Rossi, G.A., and Michelassi, C., Nutritional and prognostic correlates of bioimpedance indexes in hemodialysis patients, *Kid. Int.*, 50, 2103–2108, 1996.

26. Seppel, T., Kosel, A., and Schlaghecke, R., Bioelectrical impedance of body composition in thyroid disease, *Eur. J. Endocrinol.*, 136, 493–498, 1997.

27. Heber, D., Ingles, S., Ashley, J.M., Maxwell, M.H., Lyons, R.F., and Elashoff, R.M., Clinical detection of sarcopenic obesity by bioelectrical impedance analysis, *Am. J. Clin. Nutr.*, 64, 472S–477S, 1996.

28. Thompson, A., Damyanovich, A., Madapallimattam, A., Mikalus, D., Allard, J., and Jeejeebhoy, K.N., 31P-nuclear magnetic resonance studies of bioenergetic changes in skeletal muscle in malnourished human adults, *Am. J. Clin. Nutr.*, 67, 39–43, 1998.

29. Lamberts, S.W., van den Beld, A.W., and van der Lely, A.J., The endocrinology of aging, *Science*, 278, 419–424, 1997.

30. Hasty, P. and Vijg, J., Genomic priorities in aging, *Science*, 296, 1250–1251, 2002.

31. Volpi, E., Sheffield-Moore, M., Rasmussen, B.B., and Wolfe, R.R., Basal muscle amino acid kinetics and protein synthesis in health young and older men, *J. Am. Med. Assoc.*, 286, 1206–1212, 2001.

32. Roubenoff, R. and Castaneda, C., Sarcopenia — understanding the dynamics of aging muscle, *J. Am. Med. Assoc.*, 286, 1230–1231, 2001.
33. Adams, V., Gielen, S., Hambrecht, R., and Schuler, G., Apoptosis in skeletal muscle, *Front. Biosci.*, 6, d1–d11, 2001.
34. Schrauwen, P., Skeletal muscle uncoupling protein 3 (UCP3): mitochondrial uncoupling protein in search of a function, *Curr. Opin. Clin. Nutr. Metab. Care*, 5, 265–270, 2002.
35. Korzeniewski, B. and Mazat, J.P., Theoretical studies on the control of oxidative phosphorylation in muscle mitochondria: application to mitochondrial deficiencies, *Biochem. J.*, 319, 143–148, 1996.
36. Fosslien, E., Review: mitochondrial medicine — molecular pathology of defective oxidative phosphorylation, *Am. Clin. Lab. Sci.*, 31, 25–67, 2001.
37. Wallace, D.C., *A Mitochondrial Paradigm for Degenerative Diseases and Ageing. Ageing Vulnerability: Causes and Interventions*, Vol. 235, Novartis Foundation Symposium, Wiley, Chichester, 2001, pp. 247–266.
38. Baker, S.K., Molecular clues into the pathogenesis of statin-mediated muscle toxicity, *Muscle Nerve*, Feb. 14, 2005.
39. DeAngelis, G., The influence of statin characteristics on their safety and tolerability, *Int. J. Clin. Pract.*, (10), 945–955, 2004.
40. Mabuchi, H., Haba, T., Tatami, R., Miyamoto, S., Sakai, Y., Wakasugi, T., Watanabe, A., Koizumi, J., and Takeda, R., Effects of an inhibitor of 3-hydroxy-3methylglutaryl coenzyme a reductase on serum lipoproteins and ubiquinone-10 levels in patients with familial hypercholesterolemia, *Atheroscler. Suppl.*, (3), 51–55, 2004.
41. Silver, M.A., Langsjoen, P.H., Szabo, S., Patil, H., and Zelinger, A., Statin cardimyopathy? A potential role for co-enzyme Q10 therapy for statin-induced changes in diastolic LV performance: description of a clinical protocol, *Biofactors*, 18, 125–127, 2003.
42. Wolters, M. and Hahn, A., Plasma ubiquinone status and response to six-month supplementation combined with multivitamins in healthy elderly women — results of a randomized, double-blind, placebo-controlled study, *Int. J. Vitam. Nutr. Res.*, 73, 207–214, 2003.
43. Ellis, C.J. and Scott, R., Statins and coenzyme Q10, *Lancet*, 361, 1134–1135, 2003.
44. Wolf, G., Glucocorticoids in adipocytes stimulate visceral obesity, *Nutr. Rev.*, 60, 148–151, 2002.
45. Hackman, R.M., Ellis, B.K., and Brown, R.L., Phosphorus magnetic resonance spectra and changes in body composition during weight loss, *J. Am. Coll. Nutr.*, 13, 243–250, 1994.
46. Bland, J.S., Diaabiase, F., and Ronzio, R., Physiological effects of a doctor-supervised versus an unsupervised over-the-counter weight loss program, *J. Nutr. Med.*, 3, 285–293, 1992.
47. Hurley, B. and Roth, S.M., Strength training in the elderly, *Sports Med.*, 30, 249–268, 2000.
48. Weindruch, R., Interventions based on the possibility that oxidative stress contributes to sarcopenia, *J. Gerontol.*, 50A, 157–161, 1995.
49. Evans, W.J. and Campbell, W.W., Sarcopenia and age-related changes in body composition and functional capacity, *J. Nutr.*, 123, 465–468, 1993.

3 Early Environments: Fetal and Infant Nutrition

See Wai Chan, M.D., M.P.H. and
Gilberto Pereira, M.D.

CONTENTS

INTRODUCTION

The *in utero* environment is crucial for normal fetal development. Derangements in intrauterine nutrient provision due to maternal, placental, and fetal factors may alter fetal growth and development. Furthermore, the intrauterine environment may alter programming for gene expression predisposing growth discrepant individuals to adult onset chronic diseases. This chapter reviews normal fetal growth, alterations in body composition, and fetal growth discrepancies and its consequences. In addition, this chapter provides information on nutritional requirements for neonates and infants and on the methods of delivering nutrients during the immediate postnatal period for both term and preterm infants. Last, this chapter reviews the various types of infant feedings that are available for neonates.

Editor's Note

The nutritional environment interprets an individual's genetic code, beginning in the womb. Premature birth, *in utero* toxin exposure, maternal insulin resistance, *in utero* exposure to famine, and bottle feeding vs. breast feeding have been shown to influence musculoskeletal health into adulthood. In this age of the genome, it is easy to mistake "nurture" for "nature." The crucial role of nutrition begins before conception.

FETAL GROWTH AND ALTERATIONS IN BODY COMPOSITION

After conception, the embryo undergoes rapid growth during embryonic and fetal life. Embryonic and early fetal periods are critical for tissue growth and organogenesis. It is thought that during these periods, the fetus grows via increasing its cell number rather than its cell size. Later in fetal life, the fetus achieves growth via increasing both cell number and cell size. This phase of growth continues, in an organ system specific manner, throughout infancy and adolescence with increases in both cell number and cell size. It is not until adulthood that the final stage of growth is reached, with a sole increase in cell size.

The absolute growth rate of the fetus, both in weight and in length, further accelerates during the last trimester of pregnancy. It has been reported that the average fetal weight increases from 45 g at 12 weeks of gestation to 820 g at 24 weeks of gestation, and up to 2900 g at 36 weeks of gestation. The growth in fetal length as measured by fetal crown–rump length is equally dramatic. The fetal crown–rump length increases from 87 mm at 12 weeks of gestation to 230 mm at 24 weeks of gestation, and finally to 340 mm at 36 weeks of gestation.[1]

The rapid fetal growth phase brings along changes in fetal body composition. In 1976 Ziegler reported that the human fetus, at early third trimester, has up to 89% of its body weight as water, mostly extracellular water. However, with fetal growth, the body water content, especially the extracellular water content, decreases, and the total body protein and fat increase. The accumulation of body fat is slow until the third trimester, when rapid accumulation occurs. The fetal body mineral contents also change with the decrease in fetal body water, especially extracellular water, and increase in intracellular water content. The fetal sodium and chloride contents decline with the decline in extracellular water. Coincident with the increase in intracellular water, the fetal potassium content increases. Accumulation of minerals important to skeletal development, such as calcium, phosphorus, and magnesium, increases dramatically with growth of the fetal skeletal mass during the third trimester.[2,3] In fact, fetal serum concentrations of these minerals exceed the maternal serum levels, and it is believed that the fetal accretion occurs via active placental transport systems against concentration gradients.[4,5] The fetus acquires two thirds of its final calcium stores during the third trimester by increasing its daily calcium accretion rate, from approximately 50 mg at midgestation to 330 mg at 35 weeks gestation. The average daily accretion rate of calcium during this period is 200 mg.[6]

REFERENCE FETAL GROWTH CURVES

Since the 1960s, fetal growth curves had been derived from regional, ethnic, and racial specific data. Some of these fetal growth curves are still widely used by obstetricians and pediatricians for the assessment of fetal growth.[7–10] However, they had been criticized for their geographically, ethnically, and racially derived data, which may not be reflective of the population norms for all live-born infants across the United States. In 1996, a national reference for fetal growth was reported utilizing 1991 live-birth records from the National Center for Health Statistics for all single live births to resident mothers of the United States. Figure 3.1 contains the average birth-weight curves for each completed week of gestation, derived from 1991 birth records of over 3.5 million single live births across ethnic and racial backgrounds, and geographic locations in the United States.[11] The American Academy of Pediatrics recommends that growth standards for premature infants should reflect growth and composition of weight gain of a fetus of the same gestational age.[12]

DEFINITION OF FETAL GROWTH DISCREPANCIES

The assessment of inappropriate fetal growth varies with definitions and references. Some may define fetal growth restriction or fetal overgrowth by a set cutoff reference weight irrespective of population norms and gestational age of the fetus. For example, birth weight of less than 2500 g had been defined as low birth weight. However, a newborn with a birth weight of less than 2500 g may be appropriate for his/her gestational age. Newborns from different ethic or racial background, from various geographic locations may have different population references, due to genetic growth potentials. Thus, fetal growth discrepancies are more appropriately defined by birth weights above or below two standard deviations of the population references at specific gestational ages. Figure 3.1 contains

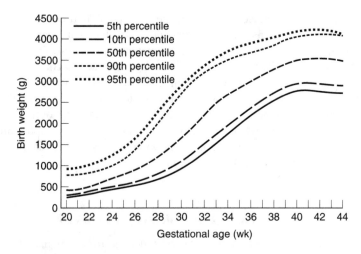

FIGURE 3.1 Smoothed percentiles of birth weight for gestational age. (From Alexander, G.R., Himes, J.H., Kaufman, R.B., Mor, J., and Kogan, M., *Obstet. Gynecol.*, 87, 163–168, 1996.)

the reference birth weights of the 1991 United States national data from 20 to 44 weeks of gestation.[11]

ABERRANT FETAL GROWTH AND THEIR CONSEQUENCES

Maternal, placental, and fetal factors are well known to affect fetal growth. These include disturbances in maternal metabolism, prepregnancy and pregnancy malnutrition, poor maternal adaptation to pregnancy, and medical conditions that affect nutrient delivery to the fetus via the placenta. Maternal medical conditions that reduce placental blood flow and oxygen supply, such as maternal hypertension, cyanotic heart disease, renal insufficiency, or vasculopathies, impact fetal growth by decreasing placental nutrient delivery. Placental factors also affect fetal nutrient delivery and fetal growth. Placentas that are small, malimplanted, and those with reduced placental uterine interface surface area or with structural abnormalities may not be able to support fetal nutrient demand. This is particularly apparent during late gestation when fetal growth and nutrient demands are at their highest. Fetal factors, such as chromosomal abnormalities, intrauterine infections, and exposures to toxins, also may manifest as impaired fetal growth. Environmental factors, such as high altitude, may impact fetal growth. Last, social factors, such as low socioeconomic status, poor education, and maternal age, may have adverse effects on fetal size.[13]

Intrauterine nutritional deprivation results in growth-retarded infants by their birth anthropometric measures for their gestation. Such infants are classified as "small" for gestational age or considered to have intrauterine growth retardation (IUGR). Short-term consequences of IUGR include perinatal hypoglycemia, increased risk of infections due to impaired immunity, higher rate of mortality, impaired postnatal growth, and delayed intellectual development. The long-term impact of IUGR is currently an active area of medical epidemiologic research.

Retrospective cohort studies from individuals conceived and born before, during, and after the Dutch Hunger Winter of 1944 to 1945 provided insights on effects of severe maternal malnutrition and demonstrated the lasting impact of *in utero* undernutrition. An extreme food shortage occurred for 5 months. Food was rationed to less than 1000 cal per capita per day for the general population over 21 years of age in the western Netherlands. The famine-exposed pregnant women experienced weight loss or poor weight gain over the course of their pregnancy. Poor maternal nutrition adversely affected the offspring, as reflected by their birth anthropometric parameters. The impact of severe undernutrition was noted to be trimester specific for both maternal weight gain and offspring birth size. Famine-exposed women during the third trimester experienced weight loss or poor pregnancy weight gain and their offspring were significantly lighter. In contrast, women with famine exposure limited to the first trimester had greater final weight gain and their offspring were as heavy as offspring of mothers without famine exposure.[14–17]

Trimester-specific long-term health consequences were identified in the prenatal famine-exposed Dutch population. Individuals who were small at birth were noted to have higher blood pressures.[18] Their glucose tolerance was reduced as adults, especially for those with late-gestation famine exposure, indicating that there may be permanent alterations in their insulin–glucose metabolism.[19] Their lipid profiles were more atherogenic with significantly higher LDL–HDL cholesterol ratios for those with early-gestation famine exposure.[20] Men with early-gestation famine exposure had a higher rate of obesity as young adults, while middle-aged women with early-gestation famine exposure had a higher body mass index and waist circumference.[21,22] The prevalence of coronary heart disease was notably higher in those individuals with first-trimester famine exposure, especially those with lower birth weights.[23] Last, although a direct relationship between adult mortality rate and famine exposure was not demonstrated, an increase in adult mortality rate is implied because of the link between prenatal famine exposure and increase prevalence of cardiovascular disease risk factors.[24]

In the late 1980s, Barker et al. reported a link between low birth weight and increased risk of cardiovascular disease in the British population and proposed the "fetal and infant origins of disease."[25,26] More recently, epidemiological studies from across the world also reported associations between low birth weight and onset of cardiovascular disease and its risk factors, including obesity, hypertension, adult onset (Type II) diabetes, and hypercholesterolemia.[25–35] Additional studies revealed that individuals at the greatest risk for development of cardiovascular disease are those who were IUGR at birth and demonstrated catch-up growth during infancy and childhood.[26,34,36] Therefore, Barker et al. postulated that *in utero* undernutrition during critical periods of fetal and infant development permanently changed the body structure and metabolism, leading to altered programming of gene expression and resulting in the appearance of diseases in adulthood.[37]

Infants who are large for gestation, as a result of *in utero* oversupply of nutrients, as in the case of maternal diabetes, carry both short- and long-term consequences as well. Fetal overgrowth is the product of exposure to relatively high maternal levels of glucose, amino acids, and fatty acids. Fetal hyperinsulinism, as a result of fetal hyperglycemia, also leads to an increased accumulation of fetal fat and glycogen stores.

The known fetal complications of maternal diabetes, such as macrosomia, polycythemia, hyperbilirubinemia, and hypertrophic cardiomyopathy, are related to fetal hyperinsulinism in response to hyperglycemia. Insulin, being a potent fetal growth factor, causes overgrowth of somatic and visceral organs. The hypoglycemia and electrolyte disturbances observed in the early postnatal period reflect poor adaptation to the extrauterine environment. Furthermore, maternal pregestational diabetes and poor glycemic control at conception have teratogenic effects on the fetus during embryogenesis. Major congenital malformations in infants of diabetic mothers are two to four times more frequent than in the general population, and account for 50% of perinatal deaths.[38-40] Reductions in perinatal complications, including the frequency of congenital anomalies, have been reported with tight maternal pregestational and gestational glycemic control.[41-43]

Long-term complications of infants of diabetic mothers include the propensity for childhood and adolescent obesity and Type II diabetes.[44-49]

NUTRITIONAL REQUIREMENTS FOR NEONATES AND INFANTS

Methods to estimate the nutritional requirements of neonates include: the composition and intake of human milk,[50,52] the growth rates and nutrient accretion rates of the fetus,[2,53] and the net uptake of nutrients by the umbilical circulation.[54] Other methods are nutrient balance studies,[2,55,56] infusion of stable isotopes,[51,57] and the determination of optimal intake that prevents nutritional deficiency and allows for favorable growth and developmental outcome.[58] Nutritional requirements in neonates are known to vary according to the birth weight and gestational age of the infant, the method of feeding (enteral vs. parenteral), and the metabolic alterations caused by some illnesses and their therapies. Compared to full-term infants, premature infants have greater nutritional requirements primarily because of their faster growth rates and their physiological immaturity. Parenteral nutritional requirements differ from enteral nutritional requirements because of differences in absorption, bioavailability, and obligatory losses. Nutritional requirements may also vary according to the type and severity of illness due to changes in metabolic demand. Table 3.1 provides the daily nutritional requirements for neonates, emphasizing differences based on gestational age (term and preterm infants), the route of administration (parenteral vs. enteral), and the specific disease process.

TABLE 3.1
Nutritional requirements for infants

	Premature		Full term	
	Enteral	Parenteral	Enteral	Parenteral
Water (ml/kg/d)[a]	150–200	120–150	120–150	100–120
Energy (kcal/kg/d)[b]	110–130	90–100	100–120	80–90
Protein (g/kg/d)[c]	3–3.8	2.5–3.5	2–2.5	2–2.5
Carbohydrates (g/kg/d)	8–12	10–15	8–12	10–15
Fat (g/kg/d)	3–4	2–3.5	3–4	2–4
Sodium (mEq/kg/d)	2–4	2–3.5	2–3	2–3
Chloride (mEq/kg/d)	2–4	2–3.5	2–3	2–3
Potassium (mEq/kg/d)	2–3	2–3	2–3	2–3
Calcium (mg/kg/d)[d]	210–250	60–90	130	60–80
Phosphorus (mg/kg/d)[d]	112–125	40–70	45	40–45
Magnesium (mg/kg/d)	8–15	4–7	7	5–7
Iron (mg/kg/d)[e]	1–2	0.1–0.2	1–2	0.1–0.2
Vitamin A (IU/d)[f]	700–1500	700–1500	1250	2300
Vitamin D (IU/d)	400	120–260	300	400
Vitamin E (IU/d)[g]	6–12	2–4	5–10	7
Vitamin K (mg/d)	0.05	0.06–0.1	0.05	0.2
Vitamin C (mg/d)	20–60	35–50	30–50	80
Vitamin B_1 (mg/d)	0.2–0.7	0.3–0.8	0.3	1.2
Vitamin B_2 (mg/d)	0.3–0.8	0.4–0.9	0.4	1.4
Vitamin B_6 (mg/d)	0.3–0.7	0.3–0.7	0.3	1
Vitamin B_{12} (μg/d)	0.3–0.7	0.3–0.7	0.3	1
Niacin (mg/d)	5–12	5–12	5	17
Folate (μg/d)[h]	50	40–90	25–50	140
Biotin (μg/d)	6–20	6–13	10	20
Zinc (μg/kg/d)[i]	800–1000	400	830	250
Copper (μg/kg/d)[i,j]	100–150	20	75	20
Manganese (μg/kg/d)[j]	10–20	1	0.75–7.5	1
Selenium (μg/kg/d)[k]	1.3–3	1.5–2	1.6	2
Chromium (μg/kg/d)	2–4	0.2	2	0.2
Molybdenum (μg/kg/d)	2–3	0.25	2	0.25
Iodine (μg/kg/d)	4	1	7	1

[a]Higher fluid requirement may be needed in the immediate postnatal period, especially for the extremely low birth weight infants.

[b]Adjust according to weight gain and stress factors.

[c]Requirements increase with increasing degree of prematurity.

[d]Inadequate amount in total parenteral nutrition solutions due to risk of precipitation.

[e]Initiate between 2 weeks and 2 months of age. Delay initiation in premature infants with progressive retinopathy.

[f]Supplementation might reduce incidence of bronchopulmonary dysplasia.

[g]Supplementation might reduce severity of retinopathy of prematurity.

[h]Not present in oral multivitamin supplement.

[i]Increased requirements in patients with excessive ileostomy drainage or chronic diarrhea.

[j]Removed from TPN solutions in patients with cholestatic liver disease.

[k]Not present in standard trace element solution for neonates.

After birth, the fastest body growth rate is achieved during early infancy. Consequently, the serial monitoring of postnatal growth parameters is commonly the fastest used to assess the adequacy of nutritional intake in neonates. Contemporary postnatal growth curves have been recently published for term infants,[59] preterm infants, and those preterm infants with major medical morbidities.[60]

NUTRITION DURING THE IMMEDIATE POSTNATAL PERIOD

Nutritional care of neonates starts soon after birth. The goals for nutrition support during the immediate postnatal period are maintenance of fluid status, glucose homeostasis, nitrogen balance, and normalization of serum electrolyte and mineral concentrations.

The neonate, especially the very low birth weight neonate, lacks appreciable nutrient stores and has limited capacity to tolerate prolonged starvation. The time that a neonate can tolerate starvation may be inversely related to the degree of prematurity.[61] The severity of medical illness and the extent of malnutrition may further limit the neonate's ability to tolerate starvation. Given the extent of metabolic stress in the face of limited nutrient reserves in these sick neonates, it is crucial to initiate intravenous fluids containing dextrose immediately after birth and parenteral or enteral nutrition support within 24 to 36 h after birth.[62–64] While a significant number of sick infants rely solely on parenteral nutrition during the first weeks of postnatal life, enteral feeding remains the preferred method of nutrition support and therefore, should be initiated as soon as possible.

ENTERAL NUTRITION

While parenteral nutrition is routinely used for initial nutrition support of ill term and preterm neonates, attempts should be made to begin enteral feedings as soon as the gastrointestinal tract is functional. Advantages of enteral feeding over parenteral nutrition include physiologic stimulation and preserved integrity of the gastrointestinal mucosa, reduced rate of complications related to parenteral nutrition, and lower cost. Prior to the initiation of enteral feedings, the critically ill infant should be evaluated for signs that suggest readiness for enteral feedings.[65] These include the absence of abdominal distention, previous passage of meconium stools, and presence of active bowel sounds.

MINIMAL VOLUME TROPHIC ENTERAL FEEDINGS

While the ill term and preterm, especially those extremely preterm, infants are essentially dependent on parenteral nutrition for the first few days to weeks of life, the administration of minimal enteral feeding has gained wide acceptance for the nutritional management of these infants. These trophic feedings are intended to "prime" the gastrointestinal tract prior to the initiation of more substantial enteral nutrition. Intraluminal nutrients appear to stimulate the development of gastrointestinal mucosa, induce maturation of intestinal motor activity,[66–69] and increase secretion of regulatory peptides and hormones.[70–73] Several controlled studies of infants with birth weights less than 1500 g have uniformly documented that the administration of minimal enteral feedings of 2.5 to 20 ml per kg per day result in shorter time to attain full enteral nutrition and a lower incidence of feeding intolerance.[66,72,74–76] Other reported benefits of trophic feedings include lower incidence of cholestasis, lower levels of serum bilirubin and alkaline phosphatase,[74] shorter length of hospitalization,[66] increased calcium and phosphorus retention,[77] shorter intestinal transit time,[77] and improved weight gain.[76]

COMPOSITION OF ENTERAL FEEDINGS

Table 3.2 outlines the feedings commonly given to full-term and preterm neonates. The table describes the composition of various types of infant feedings, the clinical indications for their use, and the guidelines for the use of nutritional supplements.

Human milk is the preferred feeding for term and preterm infants despite reports of slower rate of weight gain during early infancy in breast-fed infants.[50,78,79] Breast-feeding has numerous benefits to both the infant and the mother because of its unique species-specific nutrient composition, increased bioavailability of nutrients, immunological properties, the promotion of maternal–infant attachment, and the presence of hormones, enzymes, and growth factors.[80,81] Breast milk may have a protective role against diabetes mellitus, especially in genetically susceptible individuals.[49,82–87] Breast milk may also reduce the risk of adult cardiovascular disease.[88–93] Despite the aforementioned benefits, there exist a few contraindications to breast-feeding. Breast-feeding is not recommended for infants with galactosemia, mothers infected with viruses, such as human immunodeficiency virus and human T-cell lymphotropic virus, and mothers receiving certain chemotherapeutic agents.[81]

Human milk is a highly variable product and its composition is altered by factors that include maternal diet, maternal age, maternal nutritional status, stage of lactation, gestational age of the infant, the infant's demand for milk, and time of the day. Table 3.3 outlines the general variations in human milk composition for selected nutrients. It remains controversial whether nutritional supplements, notably vitamin D, fluoride, and iron, should be routinely provided to healthy, breast-fed babies younger than 6 months of age.[80,81]

The mother's own preterm human milk is the preferred feed for premature infants. Studies have reported that preterm human milk has a higher concentration of calories, protein, sodium, chloride, and a lower concentration of lactose, when compared to mature human milk.[94,95] These compositional differences, which persist for the first 2 to 4 weeks of lactation, are regarded as nutritionally

TABLE 3.2
Types of infant feedings

Feedings	Indications	Special composition	Comments	Supplements
Mature human milk	Full-term infants with intact GI function	High nutrient bioavailability; immune factors; hormones; growth factors; and low osmolality	Preferred feeding; model for composition of formulas; psychological benefits; and low cost	Vitamin D 200 IU/d; iron 1 mg/kg/d (preferably from iron-fortified foods, starting at 4–6 months of age)
Standard infant formulas Similac, Similac Advance$_1$, Enfamil, Enfamil Lipil$_1$, Gerber, Carnation$_2$, PM 60:40$_2$, and Lactofree$_3$	Full-term infants with intact GI function	Cow's milk protein: casein or whey predominant; lactose-only carbohydrate except$_3$; fat blend with predominance of LCT; long-chain polyun-saturated fatty acid added$_{(1)}$; and low renal solute load$_{(2)}$	Alternative to human milk, promotes adequate growth; commonly used for neonates with cardiac or renal disease$_2$ or lactose intolerance$_3$	Fe 2 mg/kg/d if formula is not Fe fortified
Preterm human milk	Premature infants ($<$37 weeks gestation)	Higher protein, calories, NaCl compared to mature human milk; immune factors; growth factors; hormones; low osmolality	Preferred feeding; special compositional differences persist during first month of lactation; psychological benefits	Liquid fortifier 1:1 ml; powder fortifier, 1 packet/25 ml; Poly-Vi-Sol 0.5 ml/d; Fe 2 mg/kg/d by 1 months of age
Premature infant formulas Similac Special Care$_4$, Similac Special Care Advance$_5$, Enfamil Premature$_6$, and Enfamil Premature Lipil$_7$	Premature infants ($<$37 weeks gestation)	Whey predominant protein; 50% lactose load; 40–50% fat as MCT; high concentration of minerals and vitamins; available at 20 or 24 kcal/oz.; available with and without	Alternative to preterm human milk; enhanced digestion and nutrient absorption by premature infants; preterm discharge formulas recommended prior to hospital discharge	2 mg/kg/d of Fe by age 2 weeks if formula is not Fe fortified; Poly-Vi-Sol 0.5–1 ml/d when intake $<$170 ml/d$_{(4,5)}$, $<$151 ml/d$_{(6,7)}$

TABLE 3.2
Continued

Feedings	Indications	Special composition	Comments	Supplements
		Fe fortification; long-chain polyunsaturated fatty acids added (*5, *7)		
Preterm discharge formulas Neosure, Nosure Advance *8, Enfacare, and Enfacare Lipil *8	Premature infants weighing <1500g after discharge from hospital or >40 weeks of postconceptual age	22 cal/oz.; available with Fe fortification; higher Ca and P contents; long-chain polyunsaturated fatty acids added (*8)	Provide nutrient and mineral contents between premature and standard formulas; recommended use up to 1 year of age; greater linear growth, weight gain, and bone mineralization compared to standard formulas	Fluoride 0.25 mg/d depending on water supply, after 6 months of age
Soy based formulas Isomil, Isomil Advance *9, Prosobee, Prosobee Lipil *9, and Nursoy	Full-term infants with milk protein or lactose intolerance	Soy protein with methionine; lactose free; high phytate; Fe fortified; long-chain polyunsaturated fatty acids added (*9)	Amino acid content not appropriate for preterm infants; phytate binds to Ca and P	
Protein-hydrolysate formulas Pregestimil, Alimentum, Nutramigen, and Portagen *10	Full-term infants cow's milk allergy; lactose intolerance; and malabsorptive syndromes	Protein hydrolysates; variable carbohydrates, and fat sources; easily absorbed; Fe fortified; high osmolality; very high MCT content and low osmolality (*10)	Dilute for initial use; does not meet protein, Ca, P, and vitamin requirements of premature infants; essential fatty acid deficiency may occur in infants with chronic diarrhea (*10)	Poly-Vi-Sol 0.5 ml/d and Ca and P supplements for premature infants

Note: GI, gastrointestinal; LCT, long-chain triglyceride; Fe, iron; NaCl, sodium chloride; MCT, medium-chain triglyceride; Ca, calcium; P, phosphorus.

TABLE 3.3
Variations in human milk composition

Composition of selected nutrients	Gestation		During a feeding		Diurnal		Stage of lactation		Maternal nutritional status	
	Preterm	Mature	Foremilk	Hindmilk	Early (A.M.)	Late (P.M.)	Colostrum (1–5 d)	Mature (>30 d)	Malnourished	Well nourished
Lactose	→	↑	↑	→	→	↑	→	↑	↕	↕
Protein	↑	→	→	↑	→	↑	↑	→	↑	↑
Fat	↑	→	→	↑	→	↑	→	↑	↑	↑
Energy	↑	→	→	↑	→	↑	→	↑	↑	↑
Volume	↕	↕	—	—	→	↑	→	↑	→	→
Water-soluble vitamins	≈	≈	—	—	—	—	↑	↑	→	←
Fat-soluble vitamins	≈	≈	—	—	—	—	↑	↑	→	←
Calcium/phosphorus	↕	↕	—	—	—	—	↑	↕	→	←
Iron	↑	→	—	—	—	—	↑	→	↑	↑
Sodium	↑	→	—	—	—	—	↑	→	↑	↑
Potassium	↕	↕	—	—	—	—	↑	→	↑	↑

Note: ↑, Higher; ↓, lower; →, same; and ≈, variable.

Source: Modified from Groh-Wargo, S. et al., *Nutritional Care for High-Risk Newborns*, 3rd ed.

TABLE 3.4
Comparison of commercially available human milk fortifiers

	Similac human milk fortifier (SHMF)[a]	Enfamil human milk fortifier (EHMF)[b]	Similac natural care[a]
Macronutrient composition	Corn syrup solids, nonfat milk, whey protein concentrate, and MCT	Corn syrup solids, whey protein hydrolysate, milk protein isolate, MCT, and soybean oil	Corn syrup solids, lactose, nonfat milk, whey protein concentrate, MCT, soy, and coconut oil
Energy	3.5 kcal/pkt	3.5 kcal/pkt	24 kcal/oz.
Calcium/phosphorus	Calcium phosphate tribasic, calcium carbonate (contains higher amounts of calcium, but no hypercalcemia has been reported)	Calcium phosphate, calcium gluconate, and calcium glycerophosphate (hypercalcemia has been reported in infants <1000 g)	Calcium phosphate and calcium carbonate
Fat-soluble vitamins	Adequate levels	Adequate levels (monitor vitamin A and D levels if more than 16–20 packets/d are used)	Adequate levels
Mixing	1 pkt/25 ml to human milk for 24 kcal/oz., 1pkt/50 ml to human milk for 22 kcal/oz.	1 pkt/25 ml to human milk for 24 kcal/oz., 1 pkt/50 ml to human for 22 kcal/oz.	23 kcal/oz. added to human milk at 3:1 ratio, 22 kcal/oz. at 1:1 ratio
Maximum caloric density	24 kcal/oz.	24 kcal/oz.	24 kcal/oz. when substituted for human milk
Estimated osmolality (mOsm/kg H$_2$O)[c]	385 for 24 kcal/oz., 343 for 22 kcal/oz.	330 for 24 kcal/oz., 310 for 22 kcal/oz.	288 for 23 kcal/oz., 285 for 22 kcal/oz.
Packaging	Unit dose packets	Unit dose packets	4 oz. bottles

[a]Ross Pediatric Nutritional Products Guide, Ross Products Division, Columbus, OH, March 2003.
[b]Mead Johnson Pediatric Products Handbook, Mead Johnson Nutritionals, Evansville, IN, 2004.
[c]Estimated osmolality using mature preterm human milk.
Source: Modified from Groh-Wargo, S. et al., *Nutritional Care for High-Risk Newborns*, 3rd ed.

beneficial for premature infants. Despite these differences, some studies suggest that preterm human milk does not consistently meet the premature infant's needs for protein, calcium, phosphorus, sodium, iron, copper, zinc, and some vitamins.[96–99] Therefore, supplementation of human milk with a powder or liquid fortifier is recommended after feedings have been well established and the human milk has matured. Fortification of human milk has been shown to improve growth, protein status, and bone mineralization in preterm infants.[96–104] Table 3.4

presents the composition of the three commercially available human milk fortifiers.

When human milk is not available, standard infant formulas are appropriate for enteral feedings in infants with intact gastrointestinal function. Human breast milk has been the "gold standard" and a guide for the establishment of minimum and maximum levels for selected nutrients in infant formulas.[105] In 1976, the American Academy of Pediatrics established standards for the composition of infant formulas to ensure optimal growth during early infancy.[106] Most recently, the addition of very-long-chain polyunsaturated fatty acids to infant formulas was shown to improve growth, development, and visual acuity in infants, especially in premature infants.

The products described in this chapter as standard infant formulas are prepared from modified cow's milk. Within this group there are three infant formulas with special compositions. Two have lower mineral and electrolyte content, which may be suitable for full-term infants with cardiac or renal disease, and one is prepared without lactose for infants with lactose intolerance. Multivitamin supplementation is unnecessary with the use of standard formulas, unless the infant has increased requirements or receives an inadequate volume of formula. Iron supplementation is also unnecessary if iron-fortified preparations are used. Fluoride supplementation is currently recommended for infants older than 6 months who are receiving infant formulas prepared with water fluoridated at suboptimal levels.[107]

Soy-based formulas are lactose free and contain soy-protein isolates instead of cow's milk protein. Soy-based formulas should be used only in infants who are intolerant of lactose and those with IgE-mediated allergy to cow's milk. Soy-based preparations have lower concentrations of essential amino acids and contain phytates, which decrease intestinal absorption of calcium and phosphorus.[108,109]

Protein hydrolysate formulas are indicated for infants who are unable to fully absorb the macronutrients contained in standard formulas. This type of infant formula is preferred for infants with significant malabsorption due to intestinal or hepatobiliary disease or for those with intolerance to cow's milk and soy proteins. These preparations contain protein in the form of casein or whey hydrolysates, fats with a predominance of medium-chain triglycerides, and multiple sources of carbohydrate, including glucose polymers, dextrose, and modified starches. These formulas may not meet the premature infant's requirements for protein, calcium, phosphorus, sodium, and some fat-soluble vitamins. Disadvantages of the protein hydrolysate formulas include poor taste, greater cost, and high osmolality.

In the absence of human milk, premature infant formula is the most appropriate substitute for preterm infants. In comparison to formulas intended for full-term infants, premature infant formulas provide a higher concentration of whey-predominant protein, a reduced lactose load, a blend of medium-chain triglycerides, and a higher concentration of minerals, vitamins, and trace elements. Premature infant formulas are also available in higher caloric densities with larger amount of protein to promote positive nitrogen retention and more rapid weight gain.[110-114] Multivitamin and folic acid supplementation may be necessary, depending on the daily volume of formula ingested by the infant and the individual nutritional status (see Table 3.3).

Preterm discharge formulas are recommended for preterm infants with birth weight less than 1500 g from the time of nursery discharge to the age of 1 year. These products are also indicated for premature infants who remain hospitalized beyond 40 weeks of postconceptual age. The composition of these formulas includes a calorie density of 22 cal per 30 ml and a nutrient and mineral concentration that is between the preterm and the term formulas. Recent studies have shown that the use of these formulas, as compared to full-term formulas, provide greater linear growth, weight gain, and bone mineralization.[115-118]

REFERENCES

1. Moore, K.L., The ninth to thirty-eighth weeks of human development, in *Before We Are Born*, M, K.L., Ed., W.B. Saunders, Philadelphia, 1989, pp. 73–86.
2. Ziegler, E.E., O'Donnell, A.M., Nelson, S.E. et al., Body composition of the reference fetus, *Growth*, 40, 329–341, 1976.
3. Apte, S. and Iyengar, L., Composition of the human foetus, *Br. J. Nutr.*, 27, 305–312, 1972.
4. Husain, S.M. and Mughal, M.Z., Mineral transport across the placenta, *Arch. Dis. Child.*, 67, 874–878, 1992.
5. Greer, F.R., Calcium, phosphorus, magnesium, and the placenta, *Acta. Paediatr. Suppl.*, 405, 20–24, 1994.
6. Forbes, G., Calcium accumulation by the human fetus, *Pediatrics*, 57, 976–977, 1976.
7. Lubchenco, L.O., Hansman, C., Dressler, M., and Boyd, E., Intrauterine growth as estimated from liveborn birth-weight data at 24 to 42 weeks of gestation, *Pediatrics*, 32, 793–800, 1963.
8. Brenner, W.E., Edelman, D., and Hendricks, C.H., A standard of fetal growth for the United States of America, *Am. J. Obstet. Gynecol.*, 126, 555–564, 1976.
9. Williams, R., Intra- and international comparisons with different ethnic groups in California, *Prev. Med.*, 4, 163–172, 1975.
10. Ott, W., Intrauterine growth retardation and preterm delivery, *Am. J. Obstet. Gynecol.*, 168, 1710–1717, 1993.
11. Alexander, G.R., Himes, J.H., Kaufman, R.B., Mor, J., and Kogan, M., A United States national reference for fetal growth, *Obstet. Gynecol.*, 87, 163–168, 1996.
12. American Academy of Pediatrics, Nutritional needs of the preterm infants, in *Pediatric Nutrition Handbook*, K, R.E., Ed., American Academy of Pediatrics, Elk Grove, IL, 2004, pp. 23–54.
13. Charlton, V., Fetal growth: nutritional issues (perinatal and long-term consequences), in *Avery's Diseases of the Newborn*, Taeusch, H.W., Ballard, R.A., Eds., W.B. Saunders, Philadelphia, 1998, pp. 45–55.
14. Smith, C., Effects of wartime starvation in Holland on pregnancy and its products, *Am. J. Obstet. Gynecol.*, 53, 599–608, 1947.

15. Stein, A.D., Ravelli, A.C.J., and Lumey, L.H., Famine, third-trimester pregnancy weight gain, and intrauterine growth: the Dutch famine birth cohort study, *Hum. Biol.*, 67, 135–150, 1995.
16. Stein, A.D., Zybert, P.A., van de Bor, M., and Lumey, L.H., Intrauterine famine exposure and body proportion at birth: the Dutch Hunger Winter, *Int. J. Epidemiol.*, 33, 831–836, 2004.
17. Lumey, L.H., Ravelli, A.C.J., Wiessing, L.G., Koppe, J.G., Treffers, P.E., and Stein, Z.A., The Dutch famine birth cohort study: design, validation of exposure, and selected characteristics of subjects after 43 years follow-up, *Paediatr. Perinat. Epidemiol.*, 7, 354–367, 1993.
18. Roseboom, T.J., van der Meulen, J.H.P., Ravelli, A.C.J., van Montfrans, G.A., Osmond, C., Barker, D.J.P., and Bleker, O.P., Blood pressure in adults after prenatal exposure to famine, *J. Hypertens.*, 17, 325–330, 1999.
19. Ravelli, A.C.J., van der Meulen, J.H.P., Michels, R.P.J., Osmond, C., Barker, D.J.P., Hales, C.N., and Bleker, O.P., Glucose tolerance in adults after prenatal exposure to famine, *Lancet*, 351, 173–177, 1998.
20. Roseboom, T.J., van der Meulen, J.H.P., Osmond, C., Barker, D.J.P., Ravelli, A.C.J., and Bleker, O.P., Plasma lipid profiles in adults after prenatal exposure to the Dutch famine, *Am. J. Clin. Nutr.*, 72, 1101–1106, 2000.
21. Ravelli, G.P., Stein, Z.A., and Susser, M.W., Obesity in young men after famine exposure *in utero* and early infancy, *N. Engl. J. Med.*, 7, 349–354, 1976.
22. Ravelli, A.C.J., van der Meulen, J.H.P., Osmond, C., Barker, D.J.P., and Bleker, O.P., Obesity at age 50 y in men and women exposed to famine prenatally, *Am. J. Clin. Nutr.*, 70, 811–816, 1999.
23. Roseboom, T.J., van der Meulen, J.H.P., Osmond, C., Barker, D.J.P., Ravelli, A.C.J., Schroeder-Tanka, J.M., van Montfrans, G.A., Michels, R.P.J., and Bleker, O.P., Coronary heart disease after prenatal exposure to the Dutch famine, 1944–45, *Heart*, 84, 595–598, 2000.
24. Roseboom, T.J., van der Meulen, J.H.P., Osmond, C., Barker, D.J.P., Ravelli, A.C.J., and Bleker, O.P., Adult survival after prenatal exposure to the Dutch famine 1944–45, *Paediatr. Perinat. Epidemiol.*, 15, 220–225, 2001.
25. Barker, D.J. and Osmond, C., Infant mortality, childhood nutrition, and ischaemic heart disease in England and Wales, *Lancet*, 1, 1077–1081, 1986.
26. Barker, D.J., Osmond, C., Golding, J., Kuh, D., and Wadsworth, M.E.J., Growth *in utero*, blood pressure in childhood and adult life, and mortality from cardiovascular disease, *Br. Med. J.*, 298, 564–567, 1989.
27. Curhan, G.C., Chertow, G.M., Willett, W.C., Spiegelman, D., Colditz, G.A. et al., Congestive heart failure/ventricular hypertrophy/heart transplantation: birth weight and adult hypertension and obesity in women, *Circulation*, 94, 1310–1315, 1996.
28. Curhan, G.C., Willett, W., Rimm, E.B., Spiegelman, D., Ascherio, A.L. et al., Birth weight and adult hypertension, diabetes mellitus, and obesity in US men, *Circulation*, 94, 3246–3250, 1996.
29. Zhao, M., Shu, X.O., Jin, F., Yang, G. et al., Birthweight, childhood growth, and hypertension in adulthood, *Int. J. Epidemiol.*, 31, 1043–1051, 2002.
30. Jarvelin, M., Sovio, U., King, V., Lauren, L., Xu, B. et al., Early life factors and blood pressure at age 31 years in the 1966 Northern Finland birth cohort, *Hypertension*, 44, 838–846, 2004.

31. Rich-Edwards, J.W., Stampfer, M.J., Manson, J.E., Rosner, B. et al., Birth weight and risk of cardiovascular disease in a cohort of women followed up since 1976, *Br. Med. J.*, 315, 396–400, 1997.

32. Eriksson, J.G., Forsen, T., Tuomilehto, J., Osmond, C., and Barker, D.J., Early growth and coronary heart disease in later life: longitudinal study, *Br. Med. J.*, 322, 949–953, 2001.

33. Barker, D.J., Bull, A.R., Osmond, C., and Simmonds, S.J., Fetal and placental size and risk of hypertension in adult life, *Br. Med. J.*, 301, 259–262, 1990.

34. Hales, C.N., Barker, D.J., Clark, P.M., Cox, L.J., Fall, C., Osmond, C., and Winter, P.D., Fetal and infant growth and impaired glucose tolerance at age 64, *Br. Med. J.*, 303, 1019–1022, 1991.

35. Fall, C.H.D., Osmond, C., Barker, D.J., Clark, P.M.S. et al., Fetal and infant growth and cardiovascular risk factors in women, *Br. Med. J.*, 310, 428–432, 1995.

36. Eriksson, J.G., Forsen, T., Tuomilehto, J., Winter, P.D., Osmond, C., and Barker, D.J., Catch-up growth in childhood and death from coronary heart disease: longitudinal study, *Br. Med. J.*, 318, 427–431, 1999.

37. Barker, D., The fetal and infant origins of disease, *Eur. J. Clin. Invest.*, 25, 457–463, 1995.

38. Weintrob, N., Karp, M., and Hod, M., Short- and long-range complications in offsprings of diabetic mothers, *J. Diab. Comp.*, 10, 294–301, 1996.

39. Kucera, J., Rate and type of congenital anomalies among offspring of diabetic women, *J. Reprod. Med.*, 7, 61–70, 1971.

40. Mills, J., Malformations in infants of diabetic mothers, Teratology, 25, 385–394, 1982.

41. Kitzmiller, J.L., Gavin, L.A., Gin, D.G., Jovanovic-Perterson, L. et al., Preconception care of diabetes: glycemic control prevents congenital anomalies, *J. Am. Med. Assoc.*, 265, 731–736, 1991.

42. Jovanovic-Peterson, L., Peterson, C.M., Reed, G.F., Metzger, B.E. et al., Maternal postprandial glucose levels and infant birth weight: the diabetes in early pregnancy study, *Am. J. Obstet. Gynecol.*, 164, 103–111, 1991.

43. Landon, M.B., Gabbe, S.G., Pianna, R., Mennuti, M.T., and Main, E.K., Neonatal morbidity in pregnancy complicated by diabetes mellitus: predictive value of maternal glycemic profiles, *Am. J. Obstet. Gynecol.*, 156, 1089–1095, 1987.

44. Silverman, B.L., Rizzo, T., Green, O.C., Cho, N.H. et al., Long-term prospective evaluation of offspring of diabetic mothers, *Diabetes*, 40, 121–125, 1991.

45. Pettitt, D.J., Knowler, W., Bennett, P.H., Aleck, K.A., and Baird, H.R., Obesity in off-spring of diabetic Pima Indian women despite normal birth weight, *Diab. Care*, 10, 76–80, 1987.

46. Gillman, M.W., Rifas-Shiman, S., Berkey, C.S., Field, A.E., and Colditz, G.A., Maternal gestational diabetes, birth weight, and adolescent obesity, *Pediatrics*, 111, 221–226, 2003.

47. Pettitt, D.J., Aleck, K.A., Baird, R.H., Carraher, M.J., Bennett, P.H., and Knowler, W.C., Congenital susceptibility to NIDDM: role of intrauterine environment, *Diabetes*, 37, 622–628, 1988.

48. Silverman, B.L., Rizzo, T.A., Cho, N.H., and Metzger, B.E., Long-term effects of the intrauterine environment: the Northwestern University Diabetes in Pregnancy Center, *Diab. Care*, 21, 142–149, 1998.

49. Pettitt, D.J. and Knowler, W., Long-term effects of the intrauterine environment, birth weight, and breast-feeding in Pima Indians, *Diab. Care*, 21, B138–B141, 1998.

50. Butte, N.F., Garza, C., and O'Brien-Smith, E., Human milk intake and growth in exclusively breast fed infants, *J. Pediatr.*, 104, 187–195, 1984.

51. DeBenoist, B., Abdulrazzak, Y., Halliday, B.D. et al., The management of whole body protein turnover in the preterm infant with intragastric infusion of 13C leucine sampling of the urinary leucine pool, *Clin. Sci.*, 66, 154–164, 1984.

52. Garza, C. and Butte, N., Energy intake of human-milk fed infants during the first year, *J. Pediatr.*, 117, S124–S131, 1990.

53. Sparks, J., Human intrauterurine growth and nutrition accretion, *Semin. Perinat.*, 8, 74–93, 1984.

54. Pohlandt, F., Studies on the requirement of amino acids in newborn infants receiving parenteral nutrition, in *Nutrition and Metabolism of the Fetus and Infant*, Visser, H.K.A., Ed., Martinus Niijhoff Publishers, The Hague, 1979, pp. 341–364.

55. Zoltkin, S.H., Bryan, M.H., and Anderson, G.H., Intravenous nitrogen and energy intakes required to duplicate *in utero* nitrogen accretion in prematurely born human infants, *J. Pediatr.*, 99, 115–120, 1981.

56. Roy, R.N., Pollnitz, R.P., Hamilton, J.R. et al., Impaired assimilation of naso-jejunal feedings in healthy low birth weight newborn infants, *J. Pediatr.*, 90, 431–434, 1977.

57. Nissin, I., Yudkoff, M., Pereira, G.R. et al., Effect of conceptual age and dietary protein on protein metabolism in preterm infants, *J. Pediatr. Gastroenterol. Nutr.*, 2, 507–516, 1983.

58. Lucas, A., Morely, R., Cole, T.J. et al., Early diet in preterm babies and developmental status in infancy, *Arch. Dis. Child.*, 64, 1570–1578, 1989.

59. Kuczmarski, R.J., O.C., Grummer-Strawn, L.M. et al., Growth Charts, United States Advance Data from Vital and Health Statistics No. 314, National Center for Health and Statistics, Hyatville, MD, 2000.

60. Ehrenkranz, R.A., Younes, N., Lemons, J.A. et al., Longitudinal growth of hospitalized very low birth weight infants, *Pediatrics*, 104, 280–289, 1999.

61. Heird, W.C. and Winters, R.W., Total parenteral nutrition. The state of the art, *J. Pediatr.*, 86, 2–16, 1975.

62. Kashyap, S., Nutritional management of the extremely-low-birth-weigh infant, in *The Micropremie: The Next Frontier*, Report of the 99th Ross Conference on Pediatric Research, Cowen, R.M., Hay, W.W., Eds., Ross Laboratories, Columbus, OH, 1990, pp. 115–119.

63. Toce, S.S., Keenan, W.J., and Homan, S.M., Enteral feeding in very-low-birth-weight infants, *Am. J. Dis. Child.*, 141, 439–444, 1987.

64. Heird, W.C., Craig, L.J., and Gomez, M.R., Practical aspects of achieving positive energy balance in low birth weight infants, *J. Pediatr.*, 120, S120–S128, 1992.

65. LaGamma, E.F. and Browne, L.E., Feeding practices for infants weighting less than 1500 g at birth and the pathogenesis of necrotizing enterocolitis, *Clin. Perinatol.*, 21, 271–306, 1994.

66. Berseth, C., Effect of early feeding on maturation of preterm infant's small intestine, *J. Pediatr.*, 120, 947–953, 1992.

67. Berseth, C., Neonatal small intestinal motility: motor responses to feeding in term and preterm infants, *J. Pediatr.*, 117, 777–782, 1990.

68. Bissett, W.M., Watts, J., Rivers, R.P.A., and Milla, P.J., Postprandial motor response of the small intestine to enteral feeds in preterm infants, *Arch. Dis. Child.*, 64, 1356–1361, 1989.

69. Koenig, W.J., Amarnath, R.P., Hench, V., and Berseth, C.L., Manometrics for preterm and term infants: a new tool for old questions, *Pediatrics*, 95, 203–206, 1995.

70. Gounaris, A., Anatolitou, F., Costalos, C., and Konstantellou, E., Minimal enteral feeding, nasojejunal feeding, and gastrin levels in premature infants, *Acta. Paediatr. Scand.*, 79, 226–227, 1990.

71. Lucas, A., Bloom, S.R., and Ansley-Green, A., Gut hormone and minimal enteral feeding, *Acta. Paediatr. Scand.*, 75, 719–723, 1986.

72. Meetz, W., Valentine, C., McGuigan, J.E. et al., Gastrointestinal priming prior to full enteral nutrition in very low birth weight infants, *J. Pediatr. Gastroenterol. Nutr.*, 15, 163–173, 1992.

73. Shulman, D. and Kanarek, K., Gastrin, motilin, and insulin-like growth factor-1 concentrations in very low birth weight infants receiving enteral and parenteral nutrition, *J. Parent Enterol. Nutr.*, 17, 130–133, 1993.

74. Dunn, L., H.S., Weiner, J., and Kleigman, R., Beneficial effects of early enteral feeding on neonatal gastrointestinal function: preliminary report of a randomized trial, *J. Pediatr.*, 112, 622–629, 1988.

75. Slagle, T.A. and Gross, S.J., Effect of early low-volume enteral substrate on subsequent feeding tolerance in very low birthweight infants, *J. Pediatr.*, 113, 526–531, 1988.

76. Troche, B., Harvey-Wilkes, K., Engle, W.D. et al., Early minimal feedings promote growth in critically ill premature infants, *Biol. Neonat.*, 67, 172–181, 1995.

77. Schanler, R.J., Shulman, R.J., Lau, C. et al., Randomized trial of gastrointestinal priming and tube feeding method, *Pediatrics*, 103, 434–438, 1999.

78. Dewey, K.G., Heinig, M.J., Nommsen, L.A., Peerson, J.M., and Lonnerdal, B., Growth of breast-fed and formula-fed infants from 0 to 18 months: the DARLING study, *Pediatrics*, 89, 1035–1041, 1992.

79. Stuff, J.E. and Nichols, B.L., Nutrient intake and growth performance of older infants fed human milk, *J. Pediatr.*, 115, 959–968, 1989.

80. American Academy of Pediatrics, Work Group on Breastfeeding, Breastfeeding and the use of human milk, *Pediatrics*, 100, 1035–1039, 1997.

81. American Academy of Pediatrics, Breastfeeding, in *Pediatric Nutrition Handbook*, American Academy of Pediatrics, Elk Grove, IL, 2004, pp. 55–85.

82. Borch-Johnsen, K., Mandrup-Poulsen, T., Zachau-Christiansen, B., Joner, G., Christy, M., and Kastrup, K., Relation between breast-feeding and incidence rates of insulin-dependent diabetes mellitus, *Lancet*, ii, 1083–1086, 1984.

83. Virtanen, S.M., Rasanen, L., Aro, A. et al., Infant feeding in Finnish children less than seven years of age with newly diagnosed IDDM, *Diab. Care*, 14, 415–417, 1991.

84. Pettitt, D.J., Forman, M.R., Hanson, R.L., Knowler, W.C., and Bennett, P.H., Breastfeeding and the incidence of non-insulin dependent diabetes mellitus in Pima Indians, *Lancet*, 350, 166–168, 1997.

85. Mayer, E.J., Hamman, R.F., Gay, E.C., Lezotte, D.C., Savitz, D.A., and Klingensmith, G.J., Reduced risk of IDDM among breastfed children, *Diabetes*, 37, 1625–1632, 1988.

86. Kostraba, J.N., Cruickshanks, K.J., Lawler-Heavner, J., Jobim, L.F., Rewers, M.J., Gay, E.C., Chase, H.P., Klingensmith, G., and Hamman, R.F., Early exposure to cow's milk

and solid foods in infancy: genetic predisposition and risk of IDDM, *Diabetes*, 42, 288–295, 1993.

87. American Academy of Pediatrics, Work Group on Cow's Milk Protein and Diabetes Mellitus, Infant feeding practices and their possible relationship to the etiology of diabetes mellitus, *Pediatrics*, 94, 752–754, 1994.

88. Singhal, A., Cole, T.J., Fewtrell, M., and Lucas, A., Breastmilk feeding and lipoprotein profile in adolescents born preterm: follow-up of a prospective randomised study, *Lancet*, 363, 1571–1578, 2004.

89. Singhal, A., Cole, T.J., and Lucas, A., Early nutrition in preterm infants and later blood pressure: two cohorts after randomised trials, *Lancet*, 357, 413–419, 2001.

90. Marmot, M.G., Page, C., Atkins, E., and Douglas, J.W.B., Effect of breast-feeding on plasma cholesterol and weight in young adults, *J. Epidemiol. Commun. Health*, 34, 164–167, 1980.

91. Ravelli, A.C.J., van der Meulen, J.H.P., Osmond, C., and Barker, D.J.P., Infant feeding and adult glucose tolerance, lipid profile, blood pressure, and obesity, *Arch. Dis. Child.*, 82, 248–252, 2000.

92. Plancoulaine, S., Charles, M.A., Lafay, L. et al., Infant-feeding patterns are related to blood cholesterol concentration in prepubertal children aged 5–11y: the Fleurbaix-Laventie Ville Sante study, *Eur. J. Clin. Nutr.*, 54, 114–119, 2000.

93. Owen, C.G., Whincup, P.H., Odoki, K., Gilg, J.A., and Cook, D.G., Infant feeding and blood cholesterol: a study in adolescents and a systematic review, *Pediatrics*, 110, 597–608, 2002.

94. Anderson, D.M., Williams, F.H,, Merkatz, R.B. et al., Length of gestation and nutritional composition of human milk, *Am. J. Clin. Nutr.*, 37, 810–814, 1983.

95. Lemons, J.A., Moye, L., Hall, D., and Simmons, M., Differences in the composition of preterm and term human milk during early lactation, *Pediatr. Res.*, 16, 113–117, 1982.

96. Cooper, P.A., Rothberg, A.D., Davies, V.A., and Argent, A.C., Comparative growth and biochemical response of very low birthweight infants fed own mother's milk, a premature formula, or one of the two standard formulas, *J. Pediatr. Gastroenterol. Nutr.*, 4, 786–794, 1985.

97. Kashyap, S., Schultz, K.F., Forsyth, M. et al., Growth, nutrient retention, and metabolic response of low birth weight infants fed supplemented and unsupplemented human milk, *Am. J. Clin. Nutr.*, 52, 254–262, 1990.

98. Polberger, S.K.T., Axelsson, J.E., and Raiha, N.C.R., Amino acid concentrations in plasma and urine in very low birth weight infants fed protein-unenriched human milk or protein-enriched human milk, *Pediatrics*, 86, 909–915, 1990.

99. Rowe, J., Rowe, D., Horak, E. et al., Hypophosphatemia and hypercalciuria in small premature infants fed human milk: evidence for inadequate dietary phosphorus, *J. Pediatr.*, 104, 112–117, 1984.

100. Bhatia, J. and Rassin, D.K., Human milk supplementation, *Am. J. Dis. Child.*, 142, 445–447, 1988.

101. Greer, F.R. Improved bone mineralization and growth in premature infants fed fortified own mother's milk, *J. Pediatr.*, 112, 961–969, 1988.

102. Moro, G.E., Minoli, J., Fulconis, F. et al., Growth and metabolic response in low birth weight infants fed human milk fortified with human milk protein or with a bovine milk protein preparation, *J. Pediatr. Gastroenterol. Nutr.*, 13, 150–154, 1991.

103. Schanler, R.J. and Garza, C., Improved mineral balance in very low birth weight infants fed fortified human milk, *J. Pediatr. Gastroenterol. Nutr.*, 8, 58–67, 1988.

104. Modanlou, H.D., Lin, M.O., Hansen, J.W., and Sickles, V., Growth, biochemical status, and mineral metabolism in very-low-birth-weight infants receiving fortified preterm human milk, *J. Pediatr. Gastroenterol. Nutr.*, 5, 762–767, 1986.

105. Raiten, D.J., Talbot, J.M., and Waters, J.H., Executive Summary for the Report: Assessment of Nutrient Requirements for Infant Formulas, Life Sciences Research Office, American Society for Nutritional Sciences, Bethesda, MD, 1998, pp. 1–33.

106. American Academy of Pediatrics, Committee on Nutrition, Commentary on breast feeding and infant formulas, *Pediatrics*, 57, 278–285, 1976.

107. American Academy of Pediatrics, Nutrition and oral health, in *Pediatric Nutrition Handbook*, American Academy of Pediatrics, Elk Grove, IL, 2004, pp. 789–800.

108. Lucas, A., Enteral nutrition, in *Nutritional Needs of the Preterm Infant: Scientific Basis and Practical Guidelines*, Lucas, A., Tsang, R.C., Uauy, R., and Zlotkin, S., Eds., Caduceus Medical Publishers, Inc., Pawling, NY, 1993, pp. 209–223.

109. Shenai, J.P., Jhaveri, B., Reynolds, J.W. et al., Nutritional balance studies in very low birth weight infants: role of soy formula, *Pediatrics*, 67, 631–637, 1981.

110. American Academy of Pediatrics, Committee on Nutrition, Nutritional needs of the low-birth-weight infants, *Pediatrics*, 75, 976, 1985.

111. Towers, H.M., Schulze, K.F., Ramakrishnan, R. et al., Energy expended by low birth weight infants in the deposition of protein and fat, *Pediatr. Res.*, 41, 584–589, 1997.

112. Schulze, K.F., Stefanski, M., Masterson, J. et al., Energy expenditure, energy balance, and composition of weight gain in low birthweight infants fed diets of different protein and energy content, *J. Pediatr.*, 110, 753–759, 1987.

113. Fairey, A.K., Butte, N., Mehta, N. et al., Nutrient accretion in preterm infants fed formula with different protein:energy ratios, *J. Pediatr. Gastroenterol. Nutr.*, 25, 37–45, 1997.

114. Chan, G.M., Mileur, L., and Hansen, J.W., Effects of increased calcium and phosphorous formulas and human milk on bone mineralization in preterm infants, *J. Pediatr. Gastroenterol. Nutr.*, 5, 444–449, 1986.

115. Bishop, N.J., King, F.J., and Lucas, A., Increased bone mineral content of preterm infants fed a nutrient enriched formula after discharge from hospital, *Arch. Dis. Child.*, 68, 573–578, 1993.

116. Carver, J.D., Wu, P.Y.K., Hall, R.T. et al., Growth of preterm infants fed nutrient-enriched or term formula after hospital discharge, *Pediatrics*, 107, 683–689, 2001.

117. Cooke, R.J., McCormick, K., Griffin, I.J. et al., Feeding preterm infants after hospital; discharge: effect of diet on body composition, *Pediatr. Res.*, 46, 461–464, 1999.

118. Lucas, A., Bishop, N.J., King, F.J. et al., Randomized trial of nutrition for preterm infants after discharge, *Arch. Dis. Child.*, 67, 324–327, 1992.

Section II

Key Nutrients

4 Fat

Mary G. Enig, Ph.D. and Ingrid Kohlstadt, M.D., M.P.H.

CONTENTS

Low-fat diets have been promoted since the late 1950s. The premise was that fat, especially saturated fat and cholesterol, is harmful. Today, science has demonstrated that fat contains fat-soluble vitamins and certain fats are themselves vitamins adequate dietary intake of which is essential to health.

The total amount of fat in the American diet, and most other Western diets, remains more or less unchanged. Americans consume more calories today than they did in the 1950s; the ratio of fat to other macronutrients has decreased slightly. The health effects of dietary fat in the past half-century do not lie in the quantity of fat consumed, but in the historically unprecedented shift in the type of fat. This chapter will review the classification of fat, important considerations in food preparation and fat selection for optimizing musculoskeletal health.[1,2]

This text refers to dietary fat in the singular when referring to fat as a macronutrient and the plural is used when referring to unique functions of various fats. The term "lipid" is mentioned in discussions of biochemistry and "adipose" refers to human fat tissue.

OVERVIEW OF LIPID BIOCHEMISTRY

Dietary fat is converted into triglycerides, which are used primarily for energy; phospholipids, which have primarily structural roles; and steroids such as

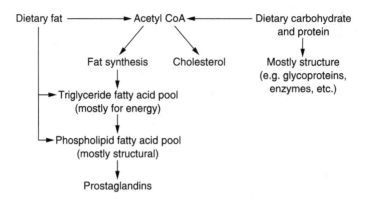

FIGURE 4.1 Overview of dietary fat and its metabolic pathways.

prostaglandins and cholesterol. An overview of fat metabolism is shown in Figure 4.1. Figure 4.1 additionally demonstrates that dietary carbohydrate and protein can also be used to synthesize lipids. Therefore, limiting dietary fat intake does not necessarily limit triglyceride synthesis. In fact, increasing dietary fat and lowering carbohydrate is a recommended dietary intervention to reduce triglycerides.[3]

Triglycerides are composed of three fatty acids attached to a glycerol backbone. Phospholipids contain two fatty acids. Fats are generally classified according to free fatty acids in several ways: (1) classes with subclasses, (2) families, (3) geometric conformation, and (4) dependence on dietary sources. Each definition highlights certain lipid characteristics, which have direct clinical applications.

1. Fatty acid classes are saturated, monounsaturated, and polyunsaturated fats. The term "saturated" refers to the carbons being saturated with hydrogen. In other words, there are no double bonds. Saturated fatty acids are subclassified by carbon chain length as short, medium, and long. "Unsaturated" means that at least one carbon–carbon double bond is present.
2. Unsaturated fats are classified into families, based on the location of the first double bond along the carbon backbone. Further biochemical processing of the fatty acid occurs at the double bond(s), so fats of the same family are processed in a similar manner. The descriptor "omega" is used to identify the first double bond when counting from the methyl (tail) end of the fatty acid, the portion that does not attach to glycerol. When the first double bond is after the third carbon, the fatty acid is placed into the omega-3 family, also symbolized as n-3

and ω-3. The metabolic pathways for two polyunsaturated fats, omega-3 and omega-6, are presented in Figure 4.2 and Figure 4.3, respectively. The omega-3 pathway begins with α-linolenic acid, a polyunsaturated fat with 18 carbons and 3 double bonds. The omega-6 pathway begins with linoleic acid, a polyunsaturated fat with 18 carbons and 2 double bonds. The placement and number of double bonds determines the molecule and its metabolism.

3. Another important aspect of the double bond involves its geometry. The naturally occurring monounsaturated and polyunsaturated bonds are *cis* double bonds with the hydrogens that belong to the double bond on the same side of the molecule. The *cis* geometry creates a U-shaped bend in the molecule. The U-shaped bend can be observed in the fatty acids depicted in Figure 4.2 and Figure 4.3. In the *trans* geometry the hydrogen molecules of the double bond are on opposite sides. The *trans* geometry does not create the U-shaped bend in the fatty acid. It straightens the fatty acid, making a shape similar to that observed in the saturated fats, which have no double bond. Humans cannot synthesize the *trans* geometry.

4. Fatty acids are classified by dependence on dietary sources. If the fatty acid is required for human health and cannot be synthesized by the body, it is referred to as essential. In other words, it is a vitamin. Both α-linolenic acid and linoleic acid are considered essential fats. Dietary fats high in α-linolenic acid are flax and walnut oils. Large amounts of linoleic acid are found in unrefined sunflower, corn, and soybean oils.

Under certain metabolic conditions, fats in addition to α-linolenic acid and linoleic acid become essential. Examples of conditionally essential fats are gamma-linolenic acid (GLA), eicosapentenoic acid (EPA), and docosahexenoic acid (DHA), shown in Figure 4.2 and Figure 4.3. Synthesis of these three fats requires the same rate-limiting enzyme, Δ-6-desaturase.[4] The activity of Δ-6-desaturase depends on zinc, B6, and magnesium.[5,6] Suboptimal levels reduce Δ-6-desaturase activity. The enzyme activity is impaired by high levels of insulin, such as that which occurs in type II diabetes and metabolic syndrome. High levels of saturated fats and monounsaturated fats interfere with the enzyme activity. Polyunsaturated *trans* fats compete for binding sites on Δ-6-desaturase. However, the metabolic by-products of the *trans* fats do not have the diverse functions shown in Figure 4.2 and Figure 4.3.[7]

OVERVIEW OF FOOD PREPARATION

The same principles established in the biochemistry laboratory are meaningful in the kitchen when using food fats such as those listed in Table 4.1. As also

Omega-3 pathway

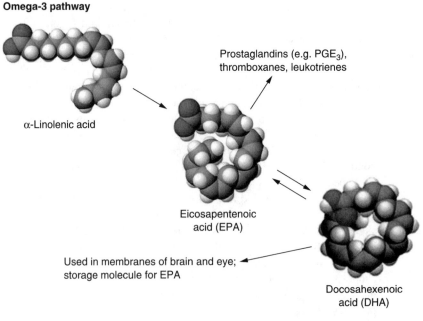

α-Linolenic acid

Prostaglandins (e.g. PGE$_3$), thromboxanes, leukotrienes

Eicosapentenoic acid (EPA)

Used in membranes of brain and eye; storage molecule for EPA

Docosahexenoic acid (DHA)

Mary G. Enig, Ph.D., Enig Associates, Inc., marye@enig.com

FIGURE 4.2 Omega-3 metabolic pathway.

indicated in Table 1, fats that are solid at room temperature are called "fats" and those that are liquid at room temperature are generally called "oils." A partial exception is coconut oil, which is solid at ambient temperature in temperate climates, but liquid in tropical climates where it is cultivated.

Figure 4.4 categorizes fats and oils by the degree of saturation. Naturally occurring fats and oils are not composed of all saturated or all unsaturated fatty acids. Rather they are mixtures of different amounts of various fatty acids. More than half of the fatty acids in saturated animal fats are unsaturated. For example, beef fat is 54% unsaturated, lard is 60% unsaturated, and chicken fat is about 70% unsaturated. When fats are totally saturated they are usually as hard as wax and they are not digested. When fats are almost totally unsaturated they are well digested, but they are very uncommon in the natural food supply.

Saturated fats and *trans* fats are generally solid at room temperature and unsaturated fats are generally oils. Saturated and *trans* fats have a straight shape, which allows for more dense packing. The *cis* double bond confers a bent irregular shape, which makes the fatty acids less densely packed liquids.

Cis double bonds are biochemically reactive with oxygen. Therefore, a fat with more double bonds is more prone to oxidation, generally described as stale, rancid, or fishy smelling. Saturated fats and *trans* fats have a long shelf life and can be exposed to high heat such as grilling and deep frying. Monounsaturated

Omega-6 pathway

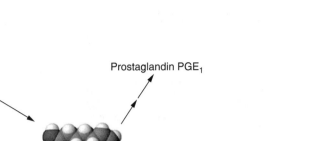

Linoleic acid

Prostaglandin PGE$_1$

γ-Linolenic acid

Prostaglandins (e.g. PGE$_2$),
thromboxanes, leukotrienes,
lipoxins

Arachidonic acid

Mary G. Enig, Ph.D., Enig Associates, Inc., marye@enig.com

FIGURE 4.3 Omega-6 metabolic pathway.

TABLE 4.1
Dietary fat sources

Food source	Examples
Animal adipose	Beef and lamb tallows, lard
Poultry adipose	Chicken, duck, goose fat
Fish adipose	Fish oils
Whole grains	Wheat germ oil
Seeds	Flax, pumpkin, sesame, grape, sunflower seed oils
Fruit	Olive, palm, avocado oils
Nuts	Coconut, palm kernel, macadamia, hazelnut, almond oils
Legumes	Peanut, soybean oil

fats have a shorter half-life and can be used for cooking, but not for deep frying. Sesame, hazelnut, olive, and canola oils are recommended for cooking because they are predominately monounsaturated. Polyunsaturated fats have a short shelf life and should be refrigerated or even stored in the freezer. Polyunsaturated fats should be used on salads and as toppings, since cooking with polyunsaturated fats

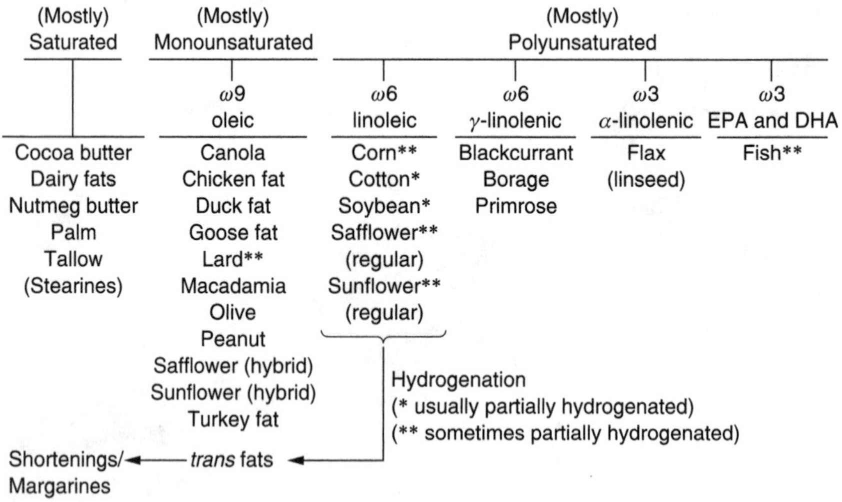

(Mostly) Saturated	(Mostly) Monounsaturated	(Mostly) Polyunsaturated				
	$\omega9$ oleic	$\omega6$ linoleic	$\omega6$ γ-linolenic	$\omega3$ α-linolenic	$\omega3$ EPA and DHA	
Cocoa butter	Canola	Corn**	Blackcurrant	Flax	Fish**
Dairy fats	Chicken fat	Cotton*	Borage	(linseed)	
Nutmeg butter	Duck fat	Soybean*	Primrose		
Palm	Goose fat	Safflower**			
Tallow	Lard**	(regular)			
(Stearines)	Macadamia	Sunflower**			
	Olive	(regular)			
	Peanut				
	Safflower (hybrid)				
	Sunflower (hybrid)	Hydrogenation			
	Turkey fat	(* usually partially hydrogenated)			
		(** sometimes partially hydrogenated)			
Shortenings/ ◄——— trans fats ◄					
Margarines					

FIGURE 4.4 Classification of fats and oils by long-chain fatty acids C14 to C22. (From Enig, M., *Know Your Fats: The Complete Primer for Understanding the Nutrition of Fats, Oils and Cholesterol*, Bethesda Press, Silver Spring, MD, 2000.)

induces oxidation. The gummy residue in salad bowls, filterless coffee machines, and frying pans is due to the polymers that are formed when polyunsaturates oxidize.

The more readily oxidizable oils have historically been consumed as nuts, seeds, and plants, where various antioxidants protect the oils from oxidation. Unrefined oils retain many of the natural fatty vitamins and antioxidants. Those fats and oils that are oxidized are not available either for use as energy or for structural purposes, because they are either in a polymerized unusable form or they contain toxic components. Breakdown products include oxidized fatty acids, oxidized sterols, peroxides, acrolein, hydrocarbons, and aromatic compounds. Natural antioxidants usually found in the seed oils are lost when these seed oils are extracted with solvents. Pesticides are predominantly fat soluble and therefore can be concentrated in fats and oils, and have been shown to contribute to the oxidative process of fats. The effects of refinement and pesticides on oils are in addition to the direct adverse effects of nutrient removal and xenobiotic exposure on human health.

The food industry has developed a processing method called partial hydrogenation to avoid rancidity and change the physical properties of oils into solid fats. By straightening the double bonds, a liquid vegetable oil can be converted into a viscous oil or solid fat, such as butter-like spreads, margarine, and Crisco®. Furthermore, distorting the double bond's geometry decreases its ability to react with oxygen, which in turn prevents fats from going stale or requiring refrigeration.

The third great benefit partial hydrogenation provides the food industry is a greatly expanded market for American-grown crops. The disadvantages of partial hydrogenation are its adverse health effects, most notably the synthesis of *trans* fats.

Trans fats currently comprise approximately 15% of U.S. fat intake. Avoiding *trans* fats and exploring less harmful methods of food processing are critical to public health. It is possible to make margarine without partially hydrogenating the oil. There are also several spreads made with emulsifiers that use unhydrogenated liquid oils and a process similar to the one used for making mayonnaise. Another technique used in Europe is making margarine from palm, palm kernel, or coconut oils that have triglycerides that crystallize satisfactorily. There are also methods of making soft margarines out of other unhydrogenated oils, using a process called interesterification. One such soft margarine, which was marketed in Canada, did not meet high consumer satisfaction and the health consequences are not fully explored.

For the consumer and patient, navigating through the labeling to select healthy cooking oils is challenging. Additionally, quality oils are sometimes difficult to find and generally cost double that of less healthful highly processed oils. Table 4.2 provides consumers with explanations for labeling claims.

OVERVIEW OF LIPIDS IN HUMAN PHYSIOLOGY AND DISEASE

GROWTH

Fat usually represents between 30 and 40 percent of the individual's diet in the Western world. This is in keeping with the range of fat that has been recommended in recent years: 30% for inactive people on moderate calories, 40% for active people on adequate calories, and 50% for infants and active, growing children. In summary, both total and proportional fat intake should increase with metabolic demands.

The most metabolically active times are in the womb and in infancy. Both maternal overnutrition and malnutrition have implications for the fetus and lactating infant, as discussed in Chapter 3. Approximately 50% of the caloric value of human milk is derived from fat. Human milk fat has a unique fatty acid composition. It is approximately 45 to 50% saturated, 35% monounsaturated, and 15 to 20% polyunsaturated. Of the saturated fatty acids made in the mammary gland, up to 18% can be fatty acids called lauric acid and capric acid. These two fatty acids have antimicrobial properties, which have been shown to confer the breast-fed infant protection against lipid-coated viruses, bacteria, and protozoa.[8]

Researchers in Europe questioned whether maternal consumption of *trans* fats interfered with the precise ratio of fats required by breast-fed infants. *Trans* fatty acids consumed by the lactating mother go directly into her milk at levels up to 18% of the total milk fat. In 1992 Koletzko demonstrated that maternal consumption of partially hydrogenated vegetable fats and oils is a risk factor in

TABLE 4.2
Glossary of terms used in labeling oils

Term	Significance
Cold pressed	Solvents were not used to extract oil from seeds or nuts
Expeller pressed	Solvents were not used to extract oil from seeds or nuts
Extra virgin	The first oil to be extracted
Natural	No significance
Organic	Meets federally established criteria for organic, which has been shown to contain less pesticide contamination
Partially hydrogenated oil	Contains *trans* fats; another way to suspect the presence of *trans* fats is when the sum of saturated, monounsaturated, and polyunsaturated fat content is less than the total fats
Toasted	Safe; seeds and nuts are roasted before extracting; this makes the oils taste more flavorful
Genetically modified organism (GMO)	GMO is not universally labeled; GMO may impose health risk depending on what was modified; GMO may reduce pesticide content
Unrefined	Unprocessed to help retain nutrients
Pesticide content	Not labeled, although organic has been shown to have less contamination with persistent organic pollutants
Oxidized material	Not labeled; polyunsaturated oils should be refrigerated upon opening and the expiration date observed to avoid oxidation after purchase
Interesterification	A newer method of making plant oils, not yet indicated on the label
Fat free	Of course, cooking oil is fat; the label means that the portion size is small enough that the total fat falls below labeling criteria
Expiration date	Unsaturated oils should have a clearly marked expiration date; Rancidity occurs from oxidized fats and generally smells like stale potato chips

Note: The glossary is intended to help patients in selecting healthy oils.

low-birth-weight infants. Maternal consumption of *trans* fats was also shown to interfere with proper levels of the elongated omega-3 fat DHA in the brains of infants.[9,10] Later, the *trans* fatty acids in human milk were found to correlate significantly with decreased visual acuity in infants. This shows that *trans* fatty acid-containing products should be avoided by lactating women.[11–13]

Childhood growth includes proliferation of adipocytes to accommodate dietary excess. The role that *trans* fat may play in the acquisition and composition of adipocytes is not known. Human adipose tissue in the United States has been measured as 40% saturated fatty acids, 57% monounsaturated fatty acids, and 3% polyunsaturated fatty acids.[14]

Persons who become obese in adolescence develop more fat cells than healthy weight adolescents. Obesity developed in adulthood is associated with a more modest increase in fat cell number and a large increase in fat cell size (Table 4.3).

TABLE 4.3
Fat cell characterization among healthy weight, obese, and formerly obese persons

Adult weight category	Fat cell size (μg of lipid per cell)	Fat cell number ($\times 10^9$)	Fat weight (lb)
Normal BMI	0.7	26	38
Juvenile onset obesity	0.9	85	168
Adult onset obesity	1.0	62	134
Reduced weight, following adult onset obesity	0.5	62	72

Source: Linder, M., in *Nutritional Biochemistry with Clinical Applications*, Linder, M., Ed., Elsevier Science Publishing, 1985, pp. 38–39.

Weight reduction in adulthood is associated with a decrease in fat cell size rather than in fat cell number.[15]

In light of childhood obesity and its potentially lifelong consequences, the suggestion of a childhood low-fat diet is raised to reduce total calorie intake. Restricting fat intake exclusively is not effective, partly because dietary fat promotes satiety. Children given low-fat diets or low-saturated-fat diets develop growth and health problems.[16–18] Certain medical conditions associated with obesity, such as hepatic steatosis and hypertriglyceridemia, improve with a proportional increase in dietary fat. Some childhood seizures respond to a high-fat diet, which induces ketogenesis.[19] The high-fat ketogenic diet is associated with weight loss rather than weight gain in contrast to most neuroleptic medications. Growing children should in general be encouraged to consume the minimally processed fats described previously.

Dietary fats also play an integral role in bone formation. Diets with meat, poultry, and dairy products were long considered beneficial to growing children, partly because of the saturated fats.[20] Saturated fats and omega-3 polyunsaturated fats both have demonstrated benefits in childhood growth. Animal studies have identified the optimal ratio of unsaturated fats to saturated fats as 1.1. The U.S. diet is high in omega-6 and highly processed, partially hydrogenated vegetable oils, with a ratio of unsaturated fats to saturated fats as high as 5.4.[1,20] High intake of omega-6 fats has been shown to depress bone formation.[21] The underlying biochemistry has also been of demonstrated benefit in treating rheumatoid arthritis by administering 2.6 g of supplemental omega-3 fats daily.[22]

BODY COMPOSITION

Since dietary fats play established roles in growth and metabolic rate, the question is proposed whether specialized fats, taken in high concentrations, may enhance body composition. One such consideration has been supplementation with conjugated linoleic acids (CLAs), a collective term used to describe a mixture of isomers of linoleic acid with conjugated double bonds. CLAs contain a double bond with *trans* geometry synthesized by microorganisms in the stomachs of ruminant animals such as cows and sheep. Therefore, dietary sources are dairy products and the meat of ruminant animals. After the discovery of CLAs in the 1970s, research focused on potential anticarcinogenic properties and favorable alterations in body composition were observed in the research animals. Results in small, human studies have been mixed[23–26] and have not spurred a large clinical trial. Studies suggest that if used as part of a weight reduction program, CLAs should be consumed at approximately 3 g daily for at least 12 weeks. These naturally occurring *trans* fats have not been sufficiently studied for potential adverse health effects.

A safer and possibly more effective approach is to consume CLAs, by eating dairy products. Dairy consumption is associated with weight reduction and improvement in body composition.[27] Effects are primarily attributed to vitamin D, calcium, probiotics, balanced macronutrient composition, and substitution for less healthful food.

Medium-chain triglycerides (MCTs) have been shown to enhance body composition by inducing satiety and facilitating fat metabolism.[28,29] MCTs are saturated fats 6 to 12 carbons long, which transit rapidly through the intestinal tract and are absorbed directly into the portal vein without being attached to chylomicrons. MCTs can be transported into the inner mitochondria for ATP synthesis independent of carnitine. Dietary intake of MCTs favors fat metabolism and is of interest to both endurance athletes and dieters.[28,30] The limiting disadvantage is that MCTs when dosed above 30 g consistently cause gastrointestinal cramping and diarrhea, and even 30 g is intolerable to many persons.[31] Coconut oil is composed of 50% lauric acid, a saturated fat that is 12 carbons long and only partially transported on chylomicrons, thereby exhibiting some characteristics of the shorter MCTs.[32] Coconut oil is better tolerated and is available as an unrefined oil rich in antioxidants.

Omega-3 fats are supplemented to limit the glucocorticoid medications required to manage chronic conditions such as asthma, arthritis, and inflammatory bowel disease.[22,33,34] By reducing the amount of a medication known to adversely affect body composition, omega-3 fats improve body composition secondarily.

Omega-3 fats can also improve body composition directly, through several mechanisms, in persons deficient in EPA and DHA.[31] EPA or DHA deficiency is common because the ratio of omega-3 fats to omega-6 fats in the diet is low and Δ-6-desaturase impairment is common. Fish oil contains EPA and DHA, which are independent of Δ-6-desaturase. Optimal amounts of supplemental fish oil range from 2 to 12 g; dosage varies with diet, medical conditions, omega-3 content, environment, and Δ-6-desaturase function. Flax oil contains α-linolenic acid, which requires Δ-6-desaturase as the first and rate-limiting step. Since Δ-6-desaturase is also the first and rate-limiting step for the omega-6 linoleic acid, persons with diabetes in whom Δ-6-desaturase is impaired by insulin benefit from GLA supplementation.[35] Improving Δ-6-desaturase function by correcting deficiencies in magnesium, zinc, and B6 is also recommended.

Improving lipid profiles is associated with improvements in body composition and the potential avoidance of statin medications that can interfere with muscle metabolism. To improve lipid profiles and potentiate the lipid improvements associated with exercise, interest has focused on the use of plant sterols. Plants sterols and stanols are similar to cholesterol in structure and function. Plant sterols and stanols are placed in functional foods and supplemented to lower cholesterol. Results are varied and the recent observation of a potential increase in stroke calls supplement use into question.[36–40] Conversely, avoiding dietary intake of *trans* fats has been demonstrated to improve lipid profiles. Omega-3 fats can also improve lipid profiles, especially when associated with exercise.

Daily consumption of essential fats is important for maintaining a fat-burning metabolism. Essential fatty acids are generally used for phospholipids in cell membranes rather than converted into triglycerides for storage in adipose tissue. Metabolism of adipose stores is associated with the lower plasma levels of essential fats. Deficiency in essential fatty acids can accompany extensive weight reduction. Furthermore, without daily dietary fat the gallbladder is unable to empty and can form gallstones.

ENDURANCE ATHLETICS

Since endurance exercise depletes muscle glycogen stores, any dietary intervention that favors B-oxidation of fats (fat burning) potentially spares muscle glycogen and enhances endurance. Athletes who consume mixed long-chain triglycerides (LCTs) 1 to 4 hours before competition, did not demonstrate increased fat metabolism during exercise.[31] Conversely, MCTs can enhance B-oxidation in endurance athletes, although gastrointestinal intolerance limits use.

Polyunsaturated fats are preferentially incorporated into cell membranes and dietary intake of omega-3 polyunsaturates favorably alters membrane properties. Increasing omega-3 fats in red blood cell membranes improves oxygenation and in mitochondrial membranes of muscles, may improve energy production. Omega-3 fats have been shown to favorably modulate the inflammatory response, which improves healing from tissue microtrauma, which often results from intense exercise.[34,41] Omega-3 fats reduce exercise-induced asthma.[33] Since unsaturated double bonds can undergo aberrant oxidation *in vivo*, just as they can in the kitchen, it is important to couple intake of highly unsaturated fats with antioxidants to reduce lipid peroxidation, harmful oxidation triggered by physiologic stress such as exercise.[42,43]

Red blood cell and plasma levels of fatty acids can be assayed and used to guide dietary intake and supplementation.[6] Testing can be repeated in 3 months to assess the impact of dietary interventions.

TABLE 4.4
Efficacy of fats used in body composition and athletic endeavors

Fat category	Efficacy
Fat in general	Effective at creating satiety and maintaining metabolic rate
Trans fats	Harmful; adverse effects on lipid profile and cell membranes; especially important to avoid during pregnancy, lactation, and athletic performance
CLAs	Limited benefit at improving body composition; insufficient safety data for supplementation, especially since CLAs are *trans* fat; more benefit is likely from dairy products, which contain CLA and improve body composition
GLA	Omega-6 fat supplemented at 360 mg daily is effective for persons with inhibited Δ-6-desaturase
EPA and DHA	Omega-3 fats found in fish oil; fish oil taken at 12 g daily is effective at reducing exercise-induced asthma and tissue damage, improving membrane fluidity and red blood cell deformability, augmenting exercise-mediated improvements in lipid profiles, and enhancing fat metabolism; Western diets generally contain too little omega-3 compared to omega-6, with inadequate conversion of essential omega-3 into EPA and DHA; safe when taken with appropriate antioxidants
Flax oil	Source of the essential omega-3 fat, -linolenic acid; ineffective in persons with inhibited Δ-6-desaturase
MCTs	Effective at creating satiety and easily metabolized for fuel; use is limited by gastrointestinal symptoms; coconut oil contains lauric acid (C-12), which is a partial MCT
LCTs	Pre-exercise LCT ingestion is of no benefit
Unrefined oils	Retain plant antioxidants important for protecting unsaturated fats from lipid peroxidation during physiologic stress such as endurance athletics
Plant sterols and stanols	Limited benefit at improving lipid profiles; insufficient safety data for supplementation; athletes may want to avoid supplementing because of potential adverse effects on membrane fluidity

In summary, dietary fat from food and supplements alters metabolism. Body composition and athletic performance can be enhanced with nutritional interventions such as those presented in Table 4.4.

REFERENCES

1. Gurr, M.H. and Harwood, J.L., *Lipid Biochemistry, an Introduction*, 4th ed., Chapman & Hall, London, 1991.
2. Enig, M., *Know Your Fats: The Complete Primer for Understanding the Nutrition of Fats, Oils and Cholesterol*, Bethesda Press, Silver Spring, MD, 2000.
3. Willett, W.C. and Leibel, R.L., Dietary fat is not a major determinant of body fat, *Am. J. Med.*, 113 (Suppl. 9B), 47S–59S, 2002.

4. Nakamura, M.T. and Nara, T.Y., Essential fatty acid synthesis and its regulation in mammals, *Prostaglandins Leukot. Essent. Fatty Acids*, 68, 145–150, 2003.

5. Tsuge, H., Hotta, N., and Hayakawa, T., Effects of vitamin B-6 on (n-3) polyunsaturated fatty acid metabolism, *J. Nutr.*, 130 (Suppl. 2S), 333S–334S, 2000.

6. Bralley, J.A., and Lord, R.S., *Laboratory Evaluations in Molecular Medicine*, The Institute for Advances in Molecular Medicine, Norcross, GA, 2001, p. 365.

7. Koletzko, B., *trans* Fatty acids may impair biosynthesis of long-chain polyunsaturates and growth in man, *Acta Paediatr.*, 81, 302–306, 1992.

8. Jensen, R.G., Lipids in human milk, *Lipids*, 34, 1243–1271, 1999.

9. Koletzko, B., Thiel, I., and Abiodun, P.O., The fatty acid composition of human milk in Europe and Africa, *J. Pediatr.*, 120, S62–S70, 1992.

10. Koletzko, B., Thiel, I., and Springer, S., Lipids in human milk: a model for infant formulae? *Eur. J. Clin. Nutr.*, 46 (Suppl. 4), S45–S55, 1992.

11. Innis, S.M., Perinatal biochemistry and physiology of long-chain polyunsaturated fatty acids, *J. Pediatr.*, 143 (Suppl. 4), S1–S8, 2003.

12. Innis, S.M., Gilley, J., and Werker, J. Are human milk long-chain polyunsaturated fatty acids related to visual and neural development in breast-fed term infants? *J. Pediatr.*, 139, 532–538, 2001.

13. Innis, S.M. and King, D.J., *trans* Fatty acids in human milk are inversely associated with concentrations of essential all-*cis* n-6 and n-3 fatty acids and determine *trans*, but not n-6 and n-3, fatty acids in plasma lipids of breast-fed infants, *Am. J. Clin. Nutr.*, 70, 383–390, 1999.

14. Mead, J. et al., *Lipids, Chemistry, Biochemistry and Nutrition*, Plenum Press, New York, 1986.

15. Linder, M., Nutrition and metabolism of fats, in *Nutritional Biochemistry with Clinical Applications*, Linder, M., Ed., Elsevier Science Publishing, Amsterdam, 1985, pp. 38–39.

16. Lifshitz, F. and Tarim, O., Considerations about dietary fat restrictions for children, *J. Nutr.*, 126 (Suppl. 4), 1031S–1041S, 1996.

17. Olson, R.E., Is it wise to restrict fat in the diets of children? *J. Am. Diet. Assoc.*, 100, 28–32, 2000.

18. Zlotkin, S., Nutrient intakes by young children in a prospective randomized trial of a low-saturated fat, low-cholesterol diet, *Arch. Pediatr. Adolesc. Med.*, 151, 962–964, 1997.

19. Livingston, S., The ketogenic diet in the treatment of epilepsy in children, *Postgrad. Med.*, 10, 333–336, 1951.

20. Watkins, B.A. et al., Bioactive fatty acids: role in bone biology and bone cell function, *Prog. Lipid Res.*, 40, 125–148, 2001.

21. Watkins, B.A., Li, Y., and Seifert, M.F., Nutraceutical fatty acids as biochemical and molecular modulators of skeletal biology, *J. Am. Coll. Nutr.*, 20 (Suppl. 5), 410S–416S; discussion 417S–420S, 2001.

22. Geusens, P. et al., Long-term effect of omega-3 fatty acid supplementation in active rheumatoid arthritis. A 12-month, double-blind, controlled study, *Arthritis Rheum.*, 37, 824–829, 1994.

23. Blankson, H. et al., Conjugated linoleic acid reduces body fat mass in overweight and obese humans, *J. Nutr.*, 130, 2943–2948, 2000.

24. Zambell, K.L. et al., Conjugated linoleic acid supplementation in humans: effects on body composition and energy expenditure, *Lipids*, 35, 777–782, 2000.

25. Thom, E., Wadstein, J., and Gudmundsen, O., Conjugated linoleic acid reduces body fat in healthy exercising humans, *J. Int. Med. Res.*, 29, 392–396, 2001.

26. Kreider, R.B. et al., Effects of conjugated linoleic acid supplementation during resistance training on body composition, bone density, strength, and selected hematological markers, *J. Strength Cond. Res.*, 16, 325–334, 2002.

27. Zemel, M.B. et al., Dairy augmentation of total and central fat loss in obese subjects, *Int. J. Obes. Relat. Metab. Disord.*, 29, 391–397, 2005.

28. Papamandjaris, A.A. et al., Endogenous fat oxidation during medium chain versus long chain triglyceride feeding in healthy women, *Int. J. Obes. Relat. Metab. Disord.*, 24, 1158–1166, 2000.

29. St-Onge, M.P. and Jones, P.J., Physiological effects of medium-chain triglycerides: potential agents in the prevention of obesity, *J. Nutr.*, 132, 329–332, 2002.

30. Seaton, T.B. et al., Thermic effect of medium-chain and long-chain triglycerides in man, *Am. J. Clin. Nutr.*, 44, 630–634, 1986.

31. Jeukendrup, A.E. and Aldred, S., Fat supplementation, health, and endurance performance, *Nutrition*, 20, 678–688, 2004.

32. Feltrin, K.L. et al., Effects of intraduodenal fatty acids on appetite, antropyloroduodenal motility, and plasma CCK and GLP-1 in humans vary with their chain length, *Am. J. Physiol. Regul. Integr. Comp. Physiol.*, 287, R524–R533, 2004.

33. Mickleborough, T.D., Ionescu, A.A., and Rundell, K.W., Omega-3 fatty acids and airway hyperresponsiveness in asthma, *J. Altern. Complement. Med.*, 10, 1067–1075, 2004.

34. Hankenson, K.D. et al., Omega-3 fatty acids enhance ligament fibroblast collagen formation in association with changes in interleukin-6 production, *Proc. Soc. Exp. Biol. Med.*, 223, 88–95, 2000.

35. Coste, T.C. et al., Peripheral diabetic neuropathy and polyunsaturated fatty acid supplementations: natural sources or biotechnological needs? *Cell. Mol. Biol.* (Noisy-le-grand), 50, 845–853, 2004.

36. Ratnayake, W.M. et al., Vegetable oils high in phytosterols make erythrocytes less deformable and shorten the life span of stroke-prone spontaneously hypertensive rats, *J. Nutr.* 130, 1166–1178, 2000.

37. Chen, J.T. et al., Meta-analysis of natural therapies for hyperlipidemia: plant sterols and stanols versus policosanol, *Pharmacotherapy*, 25, 171–183, 2005.

38. Ketomaki, A., Gylling, H., and Miettinen, T.A., Non-cholesterol sterols in serum, lipoproteins, and red cells in statin-treated FH subjects off and on plant stanol and sterol ester spreads, *Clin. Chim. Acta*, 353, 75–86, 2005.

39. Ketomaki, A.M. et al., Red cell and plasma plant sterols are related during consumption of plant stanol and sterol ester spreads in children with hypercholesterolemia, *J. Pediatr.*, 142, 524–531, 2003.

40. Plat, J. and Mensink, R.P., Effects of plant sterols and stanols on lipid metabolism and cardiovascular risk, *Nutr. Metab. Cardiovasc. Dis.*, 11, 31–40, 2001.

41. Lippiello, L., Fienhold, M., and Grandjean, C., Metabolic and ultrastructural changes in articular cartilage of rats fed dietary supplements of omega-3 fatty acids, *Arthritis Rheum.*, 33, 1029–1036, 1990.

42. Hennig, B. et al., Nutritional implications in vascular endothelial cell metabolism, *J. Am. Coll. Nutr.*, 15, 345–358, 1996.

43. Oostenbrug, G.S. et al., Exercise performance, red blood cell deformability, and lipid peroxidation: effects of fish oil and vitamin E, *J. Appl. Physiol.*, 83, 746–752, 1997.

5 Carbohydrate

John D. Bagnulo, M.P.H., Ph.D.

CONTENTS

INTRODUCTION

Carbohydrate has numerous, critical physiological roles in muscular health and development. In fact, while protein and fat have often received the most attention with respect to their influence on muscular health, carbohydrate is the rate-limiting macronutrient with respect to muscle growth, repair, and maintenance. Carbohydrate has an essential role in energy production, even though body carbohydrate stores are scant compared to protein stores in muscle and fat stores in body fat. When the body has insufficient exogenous carbohydrate from diet, it mobilizes endogenous carbohydrate via glycolysis. When endogenous stores are depleted, carbohydrate is synthesized from protein. In addition to meeting energy needs, carbohydrate is used in the regulation of fat and protein metabolism, governing the activation of and sorting enzymes, identifying cell surfaces and transport channels, water absorption and retention, and the delivery of dietary antioxidants.

Carbohydrate constitutes approximately 70 to 80% of the calories consumed worldwide.[1] In the United States, however, it is estimated that only approximately 50% of the calories consumed are from carbohydrate.[2] It is recommended by the National Academy of Sciences Food and Nutrition Board's latest Dietary Reference Intakes for Americans (2005) that carbohydrate represent between 45% and 65% of the calories in the diet.[3] The carbohydrate calories in an individual's diet are most often displaced by higher quantities of dietary animal protein, as plant protein and plant-based fat are usually accompanied by significant quantities of carbohydrate.

REDUCED CARBOHYDRATE DIETS

In recent years, a large number of individuals interested in weight loss have significantly restricted their carbohydrate intake. While this approach to weight loss has proved to be moderately effective, many researchers question the long-term risks that might be associated with limited carbohydrate consumption.[4] Low-carbohydrate and carbohydrate-restricted diets require gluconeogenesis to generate sufficient glucose for normal brain and neurological activity. While this process allows for the use of amino acids to form glucose, gluconeogenesis also creates ketone bodies. These by-products can accumulate to significant levels, which leads to mild metabolic acidosis, mild neurotoxicity, and electrolyte disturbances such as potassium loss. How the body removes hydrogen ions to reduce metabolic acidosis is discussed in the chapters on protein and osteoporosis.

The most problematic skeletal–muscular effect of a low-carbohydrate diet is the catabolism of protein. Gluconeogenesis and the use of additional amino acids to create the carbon skeletons necessary to enter Kreb's cycle ultimately reduce an athlete's skeletal muscle mass and impair athletic performance. This is discussed in the chapter on protein. Additionally, individuals interested in losing body fat are susceptible to losing skeletal muscle as well, which decreases the metabolic rate. Since carbohydrates help the body draw on fat stores, inadequate blood sugar levels can suppress fat metabolism over time.

Restricting carbohydrate intake reduces the body's supply of antioxidant and phytonutrients, which have demonstrated a capacity to help prevent cancer, heart disease, and other diseases. This is elaborated in the chapter on antioxidants. Blood antioxidant levels fall in both human and animal studies with decreased inclusion of carbohydrate-rich foods.[5,6]

There is an abundance of evidence that high-carbohydrate diets offer protection against obesity and other diseases.[7–9] In fact, researchers have shown that populations consuming as much as 30% more calories than Americans, but at a higher total carbohydrate percentage, were at a significantly lower body mass index (BMI) and had lower blood lipid levels.[10,11]

Genes that predispose people to obesity and a variety of other musculoskeletal health challenges can be suppressed by diet. This is discussed extensively in the chapter on nutrigenomics. To set the stage for similar studies in humans, a recent rodent study demonstrated that agouti mice, which are genetically predisposed to obesity, are able to maintain a healthier body composition by consuming healthier carbohydrates.[12]

Editor's Note

Since carbohydrate has fewer calories per gram than fat, calorie-counting dieters are sometimes encouraged to eat proportionately more carbohydrate. However, low carbohydrate diets also reduce subcutaneous fat and improve blood tests. Therefore, the public and researchers alike are debating optimal carbohydrate intake. The question more important than, "How much carbohydrate?" may be "What type of carbohydrate?"

CARBOHYDRATE QUALITY

To reconcile the seeming contradictions in the percentage and quantity of dietary carbohydrate, one must examine the quality of the dietary carbohydrates. The statement that all carbohydrates are reduced to glucose is reductionistic and fraught with errors. The quality of the carbohydrate food source may likely have more power to confer musculoskeletal health than the proportion of carbohydrate in the diet. Such an approach also sheds light on the otherwise conflicting results of carbohydrate quantity.

The discussion on carbohydrate quality begins with a review of individual dietary carbohydrates.

SUGARS

All carbohydrates are essentially made up of carbon, hydrogen, and oxygen. Additionally, the carbons present in carbohydrates are always chiral, having four different groups attached and existing in two different spatial arrangements (D and L configurations). The D form is the naturally occurring configuration of each of the monomeric building units or monosaccharides that ultimately form all carbohydrates, with D-glucose being the most abundant organic compound in the world. The most common monosaccharides provided by the diet are D-glucose, D-fructose, and D-galactose (Table 5.1).

Other monosaccharides that are not significant sources of calories, such as ribose, mannose, and arabinose, are critical to numerous processes and the relationship between cellular concentrations of these sugars and an individual's risk for disease or decreased athletic performance is not commonly recognized by health practitioners. D-Ribose has been heavily investigated for its use in both the synthesis and the repair of genetic material as well as in the replacement of

TABLE 5.1

Carbohydrate classes and major food sources that contribute significant quantities of each

Class	Subclass	Examples	Food sources
Sugar	Monosaccharides	Glucose	Honey
		Fructose	Powdered fructose
		Galactose	
	Disaccharides	Sucrose	Cane sugar
		Lactose	Milk
		Maltose	Barley malt
	Oligosaccharides	Maltodextrin	Gu® and sports supplements
Simple starches: contain significant amounts of hydrolyzed amylopectin			White flour, white rice, thoroughly cooked potato
Resistant starches: contain significant amounts of amylase			Beans, whole grains, sweet potatoes, vegetables
Fiber	Soluble	Gums	Oats, seeds
		Pectins	Apples, most fruits
		Some hemicelluloses	Vegetables, fruits, nuts/seeds
	Insoluble	Cellulose	Bran, whole grains
		Lignins	Seeds, whole grains
		Some hemicelluloses	Whole grains, vegetables

degraded and lost adenosine. Adenosine triphosphate (ATP) formation in the skeletal muscle of athletes engaged in intense exercise and in the cardiac muscle of individuals who have suffered ischemia is often limited by the levels of available adenosine. Several studies have shown the use of supplemental D-ribose by these individuals to be considerably beneficial, demonstrating enhanced ATP recovery and increased DNA/RNA repair.[13–16]

D-Mannose and D-arabinose are necessary for the Golgi apparatus' sorting of enzymes and other endogenous proteins. These monosaccharides are identification markers on cell surfaces where they help govern both cellular recognition and cell transport. In theory, if individuals had deficiencies in one or more of these sugars it could limit the rate of protein synthesis and impair growth and cellular repair.

Previously, the sugar alcohols sorbitol and xylitol have predominantly been used as sweeteners in chewing gum, as neither promote tooth decay. Recent studies, however, have provided researchers a more comprehensive picture of the potential use of these sugars. Xylitol, in particular, has demonstrated anti-inflammatory effects. These carbohydrates, with minimal dietary sources identified to date, are often referred to as glyconutrients. The potential use and incorporation of these physiologically essential sugars as dietary supplements is the focus of current research.[17]

Most recently, scientists have discovered that a foreign form of the five-carbon sugar, sialic acid, may have adverse effects on human health. N-Glycolylneuraminic acid (Neu5Gc) is found on the surface of most mammalian cells with the exception of humans. Fossil evidence suggests that humans lost the ability to produce this form of sialic acid around 20,000 years ago. Neu5Gc is immunogenic and causes the formation of antibodies in response to its presence, specifically Hanganutziu–Deicher antibodies. This sugar is absorbed by humans from meat and dairy products and is incorporated into tissues. Future research is needed to further elucidate the impact of this dietary sugar on human health.[18–21]

The consumption of high-intensity sweeteners, generally known as artificial sugars, has increased dramatically since inception. Most notably, aspartame has displaced more dietary sugar than any other synthetically produced sweetener. While preliminary studies have suggested that its regular use may be safe, many researchers still question its long-term consumption and suggest possible interference with normal neuron function, serotonin production, and smooth muscle cell relaxation. Aspartame contains large amounts of the amino acid aspartate, one of the body's predominant excitatory neurotransmitters. The potential for high concentrations of aspartate to overstimulate neurons is a leading theory in the explanation of aspartame-withdrawal headaches.[22,23]

Another shift in the diet is increased consumption of high-fructose corn syrup, which increases the dietary proportion of fructose to glucose. While the digestion of all carbohydrates starts in the mouth by the action of salivary amylase, glucose and fructose absorption primarily takes place in the duodenum and jejunum, with smaller amounts potentially retrieved in the ileum. Fructose absorption is generally limited to 50 to 60% of that ingested and large amounts (20 to 50 g) can cause intestinal distress as the unabsorbed portion reaches the large intestine.[24] Interestingly, however, glucose ingested simultaneously with fructose dramatically increases the absorption of the fructose present, raising the tolerable amount of total fructose able to be absorbed without gastrointestinal distress.[25] Researchers theorize that this might explain the significant energy contributions made by high-fructose corn syrup in spite of fructose's limited absorption in isolated doses. It should also be noted that fructose, as an effective reducing agent, can significantly reduce the bioavailability of specific trace minerals that may also be present in the small intestine.[26,27]

Oligosaccharides are between 2 and 20 sugar units long. The most common oligosaccharides are the disaccharides sucrose, lactose, and maltose. Sucrose, often called table sugar, is a glucose and fructose molecule found predominantly in sugarcane. Lactose is a glucose and galactose molecule found in many dairy products. Maltose is a glucose-glucose molecule found in some grains and cereals.

Although these sugars do require specific digestive enzymes for the hydrolysis of their glycosidic bonds, the reaction takes place rapidly and there is very little difference in the rate at which they contribute energy to the bloodstream.

Lactose can potentially pose a digestive problem for adults. Without exposure to this milk sugar, most individuals begin losing the ability to digest lactose at age 6 years. Worldwide, many populations have adopted a variety of fermentation methods that have enabled them to consume dairy products. The bacteria involved in these processes partially predigest the lactose and other disaccharides initially present in milk.

Maltodextrin is a sugar that can range from 4 to 12 glucose units long, is easily digested, and has become an increasingly popular ingredient in sport beverages and energy bars. See the chapter on ergogenics.

SIMPLE STARCHES

Polysaccharides essentially make up the remainder of all other classes of carbohydrates and are most frequently found in the amylose and amylopectin starch subgroups. Amylose starch molecules are longer, more linear chains of sugar units, while amylopectin starch groups often have a large number of branching sugar side chains. Both amylose and amylopectin chains can be made up of one or more different types of sugar units. The difficulty with which the sugar units can be separated from these molecules helps differentiate between simple starches and resistant starches. Simple starches tend to be high-amylopectin-containing foods that have been processed by cooking or hydrolysis. Rich sources of these starches include thoroughly cooked potatoes, refined wheat flour products (white flour), thoroughly cooked white rice, and modified food starches. Simple starches are easily hydrolyzed into their individual sugar constituents. In fact, a thoroughly cooked white potato is digested so effectively that it raises blood glucose levels as rapidly as many foods and beverages with large amounts of added refined sugar.

RESISTANT STARCHES

Resistant starches are a category of carbohydrates that includes beans, most vegetables, partially cooked tuber and root vegetables, squashes, apples, whole grains, and pasta cooked *al dente*. Resistant starches get their name from their small surface area to volume ratio, which reduces their exposure to digestive enzymes and release of monosaccharides into the intestinal lumen. Since digestion requires more time and effort to completely hydrolyze glycosidic bonds, resistant starches produce smaller increases in blood sugar levels over longer periods of time. Resistant starches have a favorable glycemic index (GI), as described later in this chapter and in Table 5.2. Resistant starches can promote musculoskeletal health.

TABLE 5.2
The GI is a measure of the area under the glucose response curve from the ingestion of 50 g of a test food divided by the area under the glucose response curve for 50 g of glucose

Grains, cereals, and breads	GI (glucose = 100)	Fruits and vegetables	GI (glucose = 100)
Corn flakes	84	Dates	103
Pretzels	83	Potato, baked	93
Rice cakes	82	new/boiled	62
Cheerios	74	Carrots, boiled	90
Kelloggs Raisin Bran	73	raw	60
White rice	72	Pumpkin	75
English muffins	70	Beets	69
White bread	70	Pineapple	66
Taco shells	68	Cantaloupe	65
Shredded wheat	67	Raisins	56
Post Grapenuts	67	Banana	55
Whole wheat bread	67	Corn	55
Brown rice	55	Sweet potato	52
Stoneground whole wheat bread	53	Yam	50
Oatmeal	49	Green peas	48
White pasta	41	Grapes	46
Whole wheat pasta	37	Plum	39
Barley	25	Apple	36
		Grapefruit	25
		Cherries	22
		Blueberries	18
		Watermelon	7

Dairy products	GI (glucose = 100)	Sweeteners/beverages	GI (glucose = 100)
Ice cream	61	Maltose	85
Skim milk	34	Sucrose	65
Whole milk	23	Coke	63
Nonfat yogurt (plain)	30	Honey	58
Whole yogurt	12	Fructose	23

FIBER

While fiber is a carbohydrate, it is certainly unique from a metabolic perspective. Lacking the proper digestive flora, humans are unable to hydrolyze the glycosidic bonds of fiber and therefore fiber does not contribute calories to an individual's diet. Yet fiber is essential for health and may be one of the most useful indices for a general assessment of a population's dietary habits. Higher levels of fiber intake are positively associated with a lower BMI, successful and maintained weight loss, and reduced risk of cancer and heart disease.[28–32]

Soluble fiber forms a viscous gel when exposed to sufficient water. Categories of soluble fiber are gums, pectins, and certain hemicelluloses. Soluble fibers are able to bind bile acids, preventing their enterohepatic circulation. The liver then synthesizes new bile acids, which lowers the body's total cholesterol pool. In addition, flora of the large intestine is able to produce short-chain fatty acids, such as propionic, butyric, and caprylic acids, from soluble fiber. These short-chain fatty acids have been shown to increase the health of the epithelial cells that line the colon and may help prevent colon cancer.[33–35]

Soluble fiber significantly delays gastric emptying. A meal high in soluble fiber before exercise could result in discomfort and decreased athletic performance. Large amounts of soluble fiber immediately after exercise could prevent the release of carbohydrates into the small intestine for absorption and potential use by recovering muscles. Therefore, it is recommended that the soluble fiber content of meals taken close to training time be kept at moderate levels.

Insoluble fiber is generally referred to as roughage. It is composed of the subgroups cellulose, hemicellulose, and lignans. These fibers offer the intestines bulk and help decrease transit time. Some insoluble fibers are able to bind specific molecules that may act as carcinogens and eliminate them before becoming absorbed. The National Academy of Sciences Food and Nutrition Board has recommended 40 g of total fiber from whole foods each day, with roughly half coming from soluble types and the other half from insoluble fiber. The modern diet falls substantially short of the recommended intake, with most Americans ingesting only one quarter of this amount, i.e., 8 to 10 g.[36]

CARBOHYDRATE UPTAKE AND HORMONAL CONTROL

Traveling to the liver via the portal vein, hepatocytes utilize significant quantities of the digested and absorbed monosaccharides: glucose, fructose, and galactose. The liver's clearance of fructose and galactose is much greater than that of glucose. Aside from metabolic requirements, the liver stores a limited amount of glycogen (approximately 90 to 140 g depending on size) from these sugars. Glucose not needed by the liver circulates to the rest of the body. Skeletal muscle is a major destination for glucose. Skeletal muscle is the only major tissue to utilize GLUT4 transport proteins for the uptake of glucose. This transport protein is insulin dependent, unlike the independent transport proteins utilized by the liver, nervous system, kidneys, and other major organs.

Fructose uptake by cells is governed by GLUT5 transport proteins and is insulin independent. Additionally, fructose requires one less phosphorylation reaction and, consequently, the use of less cellular ATP to prime the molecule for glycolysis and the production of energy. These two features of fructose have historically made it a focus of sports nutrition research investigating its potential use for high-energy-demanding athletics. However, at high doses fructose is not well tolerated by the gastrointestinal tract and its use in athletics is thereby limited.

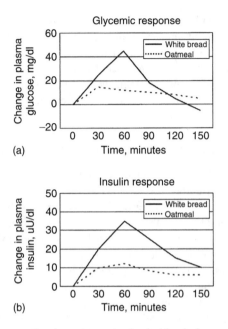

FIGURE 5.1 Insulin secretion in response to rise in blood glucose levels: (a) glycemic response after ingestion of 50 g of carbohydrate; (b) plasma insulin change after ingestion of 50 g of carbohydrate.

Insulin is secreted by the pancreas in response to any significant rise in blood glucose levels (Figure 5.1). Normal fasting blood glucose levels range from 60 to 90 mg/dl. In addition to facilitating the transport of glucose into the muscle cell, insulin also assists the uptake of amino acids, creatine, and other cellular proteins. A moderate carbohydrate supply and the subsequent release of insulin are important for muscle cell growth, repair, and structural integrity.

With the onset of exercise, there is the concomitant migration of GLUT4 transport proteins to the surface of muscle cells. This increase in the cell's ability to absorb is still insulin dependent. Excessive insulin released prior to or during exercise results in the rapid clearance of glucose from the bloodstream. Hypoglycemia or insufficient blood glucose dramatically impairs athletic performance and is often referred to as "bonking" or "hitting the wall." The increase in GLUT4 transport proteins and the activity of phosphofructokinase (the rate-limiting enzyme in glycolysis) lag briefly after exercise. As a result, the capacity for glycogen synthesis increases.[37]

As blood glucose levels decline, the hormone glucagon is released in an effort to maintain the relatively narrow acceptable physiological range. Glucagon increases the activity of phosphorylase (b), which acts primarily on hepatic glycogen stores, producing the necessary increases in available glucose. Epinephrine secretion increases with exercise and increases the activity of phosphorylase (a), which acts on both intramuscular and hepatic glycogen stores. With increased fitness, less glycogen is drawn upon at the onset of exercise, preserving these stores for exercise of higher intensity and longer duration. Carbohydrate consumption less than 150 g per day depletes total glycogen stores and can lead to further catabolism of skeletal muscle and other body proteins if sustained.

METABOLIC STORES OF CARBOHYDRATE

Glycogen synthesis and the maintenance of muscle glycogen stores have historically been the primary carbohydrate-related focus of athletes, coaches, and those interested in muscle development or performance. Previously, the scientific community placed the emphasis on the quantity and the timing of carbohydrate ingestion for glycogen repletion. This research has suggested that it might require carbohydrate consumption on the order of 10 g/kg of bodyweight daily and 60 to 70% of total calories to sufficiently replete glycogen.[38–40] Intramuscular glycogen stores provide the muscle cells with glucose and primarily determine a muscle group's capacity for high-intensity exercise.

Manipulating an athlete's carbohydrate consumption while simultaneously changing the intensity and duration of exercise can achieve significant increases in total body glycogen storage. While there are a variety of carbohydrate-loading or glycogen supercompensation plans employed by endurance athletes, most use a common glycogen depletion phase combined with carbohydrate restriction. This phase usually lasts 3 to 4 days, during which the body attempts to compensate by increasing its production of the enzyme necessary to store glycogen. This phase is followed by a 2 or 3 day period of high carbohydrate consumption. The result, on the day of competition, can be muscle glycogen levels at nearly 300% of what they would be otherwise.[41]

CARBOHYDRATES PROMOTE HYDRATION

Glycogen's hydrophilic nature enables each muscle sarcomere to retain more water, increasing the overall hydration within the muscle, allowing for greater contractile force. Intracellular water constitutes 53 and 65% of total body water and is responsible for each cell's ability to maintain electrolyte levels via simple or facilitated diffusion. It also enables muscle cells to eliminate metabolic waste products more effectively and to clear lactic acid during intense exercise. The synergistic effect of muscle flexibility and adequate intracellular hydration protects muscle groups from a wide variety of athletic injuries. Additionally, water absorption from the gastrointestinal tract is enhanced if there is a carbohydrate content to the beverage or gastric contents from which water is to be absorbed. A glucose content of 4 to 7% is of normal osmolarity, assuming it has minimal other ingredients. This range is optimal for increasing the rate of hydration.[42]

GLYCEMIC INDEX

The glycemic index (GI) is a measurement of how much glucose 50 g of a given food contributes to the average person's bloodstream over a period of time (Table 5.2). It is calculated by dividing the area under the glycemic curve by the area under the glycemic curve of a reference food. See Figure 5.1. The two most commonly used glycemic indices utilize white bread or glucose as references (GI = 100). The GI of a food is affected by numerous factors, including the protein, fat, fiber, water, and acid content of the meal, all of which delay gastric emptying. Foods containing large amounts of fat and sugar often have a lower GI than those that are mostly carbohydrate and have considerably fewer calories. Therefore, the GI should only be used in conjunction with other qualitative information in assessing a food's nutritional potential. The regular consumption of foods with a high GI promotes a number of deleterious changes in cellular and organ system physiology.[43] These changes seem to be the result of flooding the circulatory system with abnormally large concentrations of glucose.

As blood glucose levels rise, there is a proportionate decrease in lipolysis and the subsequent use of fatty acids for energy. Originally, researchers concluded that higher blood glucose levels and the accompanying rise in insulin secretion increased the synthesis of fatty acids for storage in the body. Studies demonstrate that elevations in blood glucose concentrations tend to spare the body's oxidation of fat, thereby inhibiting weight loss.[44]

GLYCOSYLATION

Under certain physiologic and food preparation conditions, carbohydrate strands attach themselves to proteins and nucleic acids in a process known as glycosylation. There is an abundance of scientific literature explaining the process of nongoverned glycosylation and its effects on protein health.[45–47] Also, refer to the chapter on protein. Unlike the glycosylation that takes place under the direction of the Golgi apparatus, nongoverned glycosylation is deleterious to the health of proteins. This glycosylation is the non-enzymatically controlled attachment of glucose to a peptide in a way that can seriously alter the functional capacity of certain enzymes and skeletal proteins and change the appearance of other proteins such as cell surface identification proteins. Advanced glysolylated end products (AGEs) are the biomarkers that indicate glycosylation has taken place. One AGE that is clinically monitored among persons with type II diabetes is glycosylated hemoglobin, often referred to as HbA1c. Elevated glycosylated hemoglobin is associated with lower elasticity of muscle fiber and connective tissue.

SUMMARY OF CLINICAL APPLICATIONS

Adequate carbohydrate can vary widely among adults, depending primarily on energy needs and variation in metabolism. Generally, adequate intake is between

55 and 70% of the calories consumed or between 6 and 10 g/kg of lean body mass. Therefore, a 180 lb (82 kg) individual at 15% body fat (69.7 kg) would require between 420 and 700 g of carbohydrate each day, depending on the activity level. Carbohydrate restriction has the disadvantages of loss of lean body mass, metabolic acidosis, and dehydration.

Not only carbohydrate quantity, but also carbohydrate quality influences musculoskeletal health. Individuals should be encouraged to include predominantly whole food sources of carbohydrates from fruits, vegetables, whole grains, and starchy root vegetables. Minimizing consumption of refined grains and grain products, foods with added sugars and sweeteners, and other sources of isolated sugars (i.e., fruit juice) reduces damage due to AGE formation and insulin resistance.

REFERENCES

1. Fennema, O.R., *Food Chemistry*, Marcel Dekker, New York, 1996.
2. CDC/National Center for Health Statistics, Trends in intake of energy and macronutrients, United States, 1971–2000, *Morb. Mortal. Wkly Rep.*, 53, 80–82, 2004.
3. National Academy of Sciences Food and Nutrition Board, Dietary Reference Intakes for Energy, Carbohydrate, Fiber, Fat, Fatty Acids, Cholesterol, Protein, and Amino Acids (Macronutrients), National Academy Press, Washington, DC, 2005.
4. Bravata, D. et al., Efficacy and safety of low-carbohydrate diets: a systemic review, *J. Am. Med. Assoc.*, 289, 1837–1850, 2003.
5. Record, I.R., Dreosti, I.E., and McInerney, J.K., Changes in plasma antioxidant status following consumption of diets high or low in fruits and vegetables or following dietary supplementation with an antioxidant mixture, *Br. J. Nutr.*, 85, 459–464, 2001.
6. Roberts, C.K., Barnard, R.J., Sindhu, R.K., Jurczak, M., Ehdaie, A., and Vaziri, N.D., A high-fat, refined-carbohydrate diet induces endothelial dysfunction and oxidant/antioxidant imbalance and depresses NOS protein expression, *J. Appl. Phys.*, 98, 203–210, 2005.
7. Astrup, A. et al., Low-fat diets and energy balance: how does the evidence stand in 2002? *Proc. Nutr. Soc.*, 61, 299–309, 2002.
8. Astrup, A., The role of dietary fat in the prevention and treatment of obesity. Efficacy and safety of low-fat diets., *Int. J. Obes. Relat. Metab. Disord.*, 25, 46s–50s, 2001.
9. Golay, A. and Bobbioni, E., The role of dietary fat in obesity, *Int. J. Obes. Metab. Disord.*, 21, 2s–11s, 1997.
10. Campbell, T.C. and Chen, J., Energy balance: interpretation of data from rural China, *Toxicol. Sci.*, 52, 87s–94s, 1999.
11. Lissner, L., Hetmann, B.L., and Bengtsson, C., Low-fat diets may prevent weight gain in sedentary women: prospective observations from the population study of women in Gothenburg, Sweden, *Obes. Res.*, 5, 43–48, 1997.
12. Morris, K.L. and Zemel, M.B., Effect of dietary carbohydrate source on the development of obesity in agouti transgenic mice, *Obes. Res.*, 13, 21–35, 2005.
13. Brault, J. and Terjung, R.L., Purine Salvage Rates Differ among Skeletal Muscle Fiber Types and are Limited by Ribose Supply, paper presented to American College of Sports Medicine, Jun. 1999.

14. Hellsten-Westing, Y., Norman, B., Balsom, P.D., and Sjodin, B., Decreased resting levels of adenine nucleotides in human skeletal muscle after high-intensity training, *J. Appl. Physiol.*, 74, 2523–2528, 1993.

15. Pasque, M.K. and Wechsler, A.S., Metabolic intervention to affect myocardial recovery following ischemia, *Ann. Surg.*, 200, 1–12, 1984.

16. Tullson, P.C. and Terjung, R.L., Adenine nucleotide synthesis in exercising and endurance-trained skeletal muscle, *Am. J. Physiol.*, 261, C342–C347, 1991.

17. Steinberg, L.M., Odusola, F., and Mandel, I.D., Remineralizing potential, antiplaque and antigingivitis effects of xylitol and sorbitol sweetened chewing gum, *Clin. Prev. Dent.*, 14, 31–34, 1992.

18. Tangvoranuntakul, P. et al., Human uptake and incorporation of an immunogenic nonhuman dietary sialic acid, *Proc. Natl. Acad. Sci. USA*, 100, 12045–12050, 2003.

19. Martin, M.J., Muorti, A., Gage, F., and Varki, A., Human embryonic stem cells express an immunogenic nonhuman sialic acid, *Nat. Med.*, 11, 228–232, 2005.

20. Bardor, M., Nguyen, D.H., Diaz, S., and Varki, A., Mechanism of uptake and incorporation of the non-human sialic acid N-glycolyneuraminic acid into human cells, *J. Biol. Chem.*, 280, 4228–4237, 2005.

21. Malykh, Y.N., Schauer, R., and Shaw, L. N-Glycolyneuraminic acid in human tumors, *Biochimie*, 83, 623–634, 2001.

22. Roberts, H.J., *Aspartame: Is It Safe?* Charles Press, Philadelphia, PA, 1990.

23. Blaylock, R.L., *Excitotoxins: The Taste That Kills*, Health Press, Santa Fe, NM, 1997.

24. Riby, J., Fujisawa, T., and Kretchmer, N., Fructose absorption, *Am. J. Clin. Nutr.*, 58, 748s–53s, 1993.

25. Truswell, A.S., Seach, J.M., and Thorburn, A.W., Incomplete absorption of pure fructose in healthy subjects and the facilitating effect of glucose, *Am. J. Clin. Nutr.*, 48, 1424–1430, 1988.

26. Ivaturi, R. and Kies, C., Mineral balances in humans as affected by fructose, high fructose corn syrup and sucrose, *Plant Foods Hum. Nutr.*, 42, 143–151, 1992.

27. Milne, D.B. and Nielsen, F.H., The interaction between dietary fructose and magnesium adversely affects macromineral homeostasis in men, *J. Am. Coll. Nutr.* 19, 31–37, 2000.

28. Jacobs, D.R., Meyer, K.A., Kushi, L.H., and Folsom, A.R., Whole-grain intake may reduce the risk of ischemic heart disease death in post-menopausal women: The Iowa Women's Health Study, *Am. J. Clin. Nutr.*, 68, 248–257, 1998.

29. Wolk, A. et al., Long-term intake of dietary fiber and decreased risk of coronary heart disease among women, *J. Am. Med. Assoc.*, 281, 1998–2004, 1999.

30. Klurfeld, D., Dietary fiber-mediated mechanisms in carcinogenesis, *Cancer Res.*, 52, 2055s–2059s, 1992.

31. Anderson, J. and Bryant, C., Dietary fiber: diabetes and obesity, *Am. J. Gastroenterol.*, 81, 898–906, 1986.

32. Kritchevsky, D., Dietary fiber, *Ann. Rev. Nutr.*, 8, 301–328, 1988.

33. Lupton, J. and Kurtz, P., Relationship of colonic luminal short chain fatty acids and pH to in vivo cell proliferation in rats, *J. Nutr.*, 123, 1522–1530, 1993.

34. McNeil, N., The contribution of the large intestine to energy supplies in man, *Am. J. Clin. Nutr.*, 39, 338–342, 1984.

35. Harris, P. and Ferguson, L., Dietary fiber: its composition and role in protection against colorectal cancer, *Mutat. Res.*, 290, 97–110, 1993.

36. Trock, B., Lanza, E., and Greenwald, P., Dietary fiber, vegetables, and colon cancer: critical review and meta-analyses of the epidemiologic evidence, *J. Natl. Cancer Inst.*, 82, 650–661, 1990.
37. Ivy, J.L., Muscle glycogen synthesis before and after exercise, *Sports Med.*, 11, 6, 1991.
38. Costhill, D.L., Carbohydrates for exercise: dietary demands for optimal performance, *Int. J. Sports Med.*, 9, 1, 1988.
39. Costhill, D.L., Sherman, W.M., Fink, W.J. et al., The role of dietary carbohydrates in muscle glycogen resynthesis after strenuous running, *Am. J. Clin. Nutr.*, 34, 1831–1836, 1981.
40. Sherman, W.M., Doyle, J.A., Lamb, D.R., and Strauss, R.H., Dietary carbohydrate, muscle glycogen, and exercise performance during 7 days of training, *Am. J. Clin. Nutr.*, 57, 27, 1993.
41. Sherman, W.M. et al., Effect of exercise–diet manipulation on muscle glycogen and its subsequent utilization during performance, *Int. J. Sports Med.*, 2, 114, 1981.
42. American College of Sports Medicine, Position stand on exercise and fluid replacement, *Med. Sci. Sports Exerc.*, 28, i–vii, 1996.
43. Ludwig, D.S., The glycemic index: physiological mechanisms relating to obesity, diabetes, and cardiovascular disease, *J. Am. Med. Assoc.*, 287, 2414–2421, 2002.
44. Hellerstein, M., Schwartz, J.-M., and Neese, R., Regulation of hepatic *de novo* lipogenesis in humans, *Annu. Rev. Nutr.*, 16, 523–557, 1996.
45. Yan, S.F., Ramasamy, R., Naka. Y., and Schmidt, A.M., Glycation, inflammation, and RAGE: a scaffold for the macrovascular complications of diabetes and beyond, *Circ. Res.*, 93, 1159–1169, 2003.
46. Newkirk, M.M. et al., Advanced glycation end-product (AGE)-damaged IgG and IgM autoantibodies to IgG-AGE in patients with early synovitis, *Arthritis Res. Ther.*, 5, R89–R90, 2003.
47. Kalousova, M., Skrha, J., and Zima, T., Advanced glycation end-products and advanced oxidation protein products in patients with diabetes mellitus, *Physiol. Res.*, 51, 597–604, 2002.

6 Protein

David I. Minkoff, M.D.

CONTENTS

INTRODUCTION

Musculoskeletal health depends on dietary protein. The word protein derives from the Greek word *proteos* meaning "primary — most important." Indeed the structure of the human body is built on a foundation of structural proteins, which are derived from dietary proteins. Each cell's genome codes for specific proteins that are used for the structure, regulation, and communication particles necessary for survival. These include muscle, enzymes, hormones, contractile proteins, immunoglobulins, neurotransmitters, bone structure proteins, oxygen, and carbon dioxide carrying molecules, to name a few. Almost half the total protein content in the body is present in just four proteins, myosin, actin, collagen, and hemoglobin.[1] Myosin and actin comprise muscle and collagen comprises bone and connective tissues. Protein is indeed *proteos* in the musculoskeletal system.

Most of the proteins ingested from the diet are not used for protein but as energy. The nitrogen-containing amine group is removed and the carbon skeleton is oxidized as substrate for adenosine triphosphate (ATP) production. The extra chemical steps in conversion of protein to carbohydrate make protein a low glycemic index food, a slow-release carbohydrate source.

Another role is in regional pH regulation. Because amino acids have amino groups and carboxylic acid groups they can function as buffers by accepting or donating hydrogen ions. Since there are many proteins in the vascular bed and interstitial spaces, they add a large pool of buffers to maintain acid base balance in addition to the phosphate and bicarbonate system buffers described by Dr. Brown in the chapter on bone nutrition.

PROTEIN AS A MACRONUTRIENT

What distinguishes protein from carbohydrates and fats, the other two macro-nutrients, is that only protein contains nitrogen. The ratio of protein in the diet varies among fad diets which have influenced our patients' food selection.

The "Atkins Diet"[2] with high protein, very low carbohydrate intakes, the Dr. Barry Sears "Zone Diet"[3] in which the recommended protein intake is 30% of total calories, to various low-protein high-carbohydrate diets such as the Ornish[4] or Pritikin Diets[5] where proteins may be only 10% of the total calorie intake. Others, including Wolcott,[6] have stated that an individual's protein needs are based on his or her genetic metabolic type. This type is determined by a long personal habits and likes/dislikes survey and blood chemistry measurements. Depending on the survey and lab results one type needs high protein, another moderate, and another low. Others including D'Adamo[7] have opined that each protein has a pre-dominant surface lectin type, and based on one's blood type an individual should eat only those proteins that have similar surface lectins as his or her ABO type. Also entering into this, in the athletic arena is the famous Tour de France winner Lance Armstrong's coach, Chris Carmichael,[8] who tailors an athlete's protein and carbohydrate amounts based on a seasonal training and racing schedule. Cordane and others have done extensive investigation into the protein rich diets of our Paleolithic ancestors. Their diets were mostly meat, fish, fowl, and the leaves, roots, and fruits of many plants. These "hunter" preagrarian types had healthier skeletons and musculature than later generations who ate grain-based diets.[9,10]

Is there an ideal protein source and amount for all people? History and current science would argue against this idea as individual needs and access are so unique. However, protein as an essential nutrient needs to be considered as part of a complex diet, lifestyle, and health status. This chapter will discuss protein metabolism, individualized protein requirements, and therapeutic uses of certain proteins and amino acids.

TABLE 6.1
The 20 amino acids used to build proteins

Alanine	Glutamic acid	Leucine*	Serine
Arginine	Glutamine	Lysine*	Threonine*
Asparagine	Glycine	Methionine*	Tryptophan*
Aspartic acid	Histidine	Phenylalanine*	Tyrosine
Cysteine	Isoleucine*	Proline	Valine*

*asterisk indicates that the amino acid is considered essential.

CLASSIFICATION OF AMINO ACIDS

The dietary proteins one consumes are digested and result in the absorption of single amino acids and occasionally short peptides. There is not a protein requirement per se. Rather, there is an amino acid requirement, since the body cannot make its own codes for proteins without an adequate supply of these essential nutrients.

Dietary protein provides 20 amino acids that are used to build body proteins. Eight of these amino acids are considered essential, which means they cannot be synthesized by the body. In Table 6.1, these eight are noted with an asterisk. The rest are considered nonessential amino acids, each of which can be synthesized either directly or indirectly from the essential ones.

DIGESTION AND ABSORPTION OF PROTEIN

Protein digestion is required for absorption of amino acids. For adequate digestion to occur, mastication must reduce the size of the food and increase surface area so that in the stomach, enzymatic digestion can begin. Here the excretion of hydrochloric acid creates a pH in the range of 1 to 2. The acid environment denatures (uncoils) the food proteins, which exposes their peptide bonds to pepsin. A pH of 2 is optimum for pepsin function.[11]

Protein digestion continues in the small intestine where the proteolytic enzymes such as enteropeptidases, trypsin, and chymotrypsin cleave peptide bonds that result in small peptide chains and single amino acids available for absorption. The intestinal cells have specialized transporter proteins in the cell membrane to bring the amino acids into and through the cells and released into the bloodstream. From here they are transported to individual organs for reassembly into required body proteins.[12,13]

PROTEIN QUALITY

All proteins are not equal in nutritional biological value. Biological value is the percentage of the ingested protein that the body is able to convert into body proteins as measured by net nitrogen retention. After a meal the ingested proteins are broken down into amino acids that are then absorbed. Depending on the ratio and amounts of these amino acids they may be used for anabolic activity in protein synthesis or catabolized into energy sources with resultant nitrogen waste. Whole egg has always been considered the food protein with the highest biological value. It has a net nitrogen retention value of 48%. This means that 48% of the egg protein is incorporated into body proteins (utilized nitrogen) and 52% of it is catabolized for energy with residual nitrogen waste. A unique amino acid formula that results in 99% net nitrogen usage has been discovered and formulated. This can be used as a standard to compare other proteins or amino acid blends to determine their biological value as measured by net nitrogen usage. High biological value proteins have better ratios and amounts of the eight essential amino acids and thus result in a better anabolic vs. catabolic ratio when consumed.[14]

Lower biological value proteins have deficient amounts of one or more essential amino acids. As a general rule, the animal-derived proteins such as eggs, meat, and fish, have higher biological value than vegetable-derived ones. Consumption of high biological value proteins is especially important when protein or calorie restriction is needed to ensure adequate protein intake.

Popular sources of protein supplementation today include both soy and whey. While both contain all eight essential amino acids, soy proteins are lower in cysteine and methionine but higher in glutamine and arginine compared to whey proteins. But effects on fitness and muscle development have not shown one to be more efficacious than the other. People with milk allergy or sensitivity are likely to use soy without crossover problems. Both soy and whey have unique other qualities, for example, whey contains glutathione which is an antioxidant and lactoferrins, which have bacteriostatic qualities, while soy contains genistein and diadzine, which have an adaptagenic effect on estrogen hormone regulation.

Editor's Note

Protein synthesis and repair is an ongoing 24-h a day process. A total of 1 to 4% of muscle protein is replaced daily. When intake of essential amino acids is insufficient, whether from binge eating, skipping breakfast, malabsorption, a poor quality diet, or intensive weight reduction, protein preventive maintenance declines and damaged proteins become more common.

NITROGEN BALANCE

Positive nitrogen balance is that condition where sufficient protein sources exist in the diet to add lean body mass and maintain repair processes. This is the normal anabolic state of the body from conception through puberty. This continues during periods of fitness training where lean muscle is added, or in healing associated with posttraumatic or surgical events.

The concept of negative nitrogen balance has traditionally meant the loss of more nitrogen (as a marker of protein stability) than one is taking in. This occurs drastically in catabolic states like postoperatively, following trauma, and during acute infections and illness. This increase in urinary nitrogen is due to the catabolism of visceral proteins and lean body mass to provide the essential amino acids that are not available in adequate amounts from dietary sources to carry on vital functions or needed as a source of energy in calorie-deprived diets.

Thus negative nitrogen balance is due to insufficient quantity and utilization of high biological protein. The needs may be greatly increased in metabolic states where high body demand exceeds intake such as post trauma, burns, postsurgery, or endurance exercise training. In addition to appropriate quantity and quality of protein consumed, sufficient calories must be consumed to meet the body's overall energy requirements.[15]

PROTEIN TURNOVER

Proteins in the body are not static and there is continuous breakdown and synthesis. When tissue proteins are broken down, the amino acids are reutilized for synthesis of new proteins. The rate of turnover of proteins varies widely. One factor in turnover rate parallels how closely a particular protein's concentration needs to be monitored. For example, enzymes and hormones have higher turnover rates because the concentration of these substances has to be regulated closely. Structural proteins such as collagen and myofibrils have relatively long lifetimes measured in months or years. In healthy persons, the total protein turnover is approximately 3% of all body proteins per day.[16]

A second factor in the turnover rate is availability of exogenous proteins to the body. Protein metabolism differs from carbohydrate and fat metabolism, in that the body does not store amino acids for future use. The amino acid "storehouse" is the tissue structure of the body itself or its circulating proteins, such as albumin. The body adapts to a protein deficient diet. If too few essential amino acids are available, the body will attempt to conserve its repair and rebuilding of proteins by slowing down the turnover rate of proteins. Proteins that normally have very rapid turnover have reduced turnover when the protein intake is below threshold levels. Skeletal muscle protein also decreases. Since muscle comprises a large portion of protein stores, declining turnover can be measured as decreased urinary nitrogen losses. The change is muscle mediated in part by thyroid hormone, as elaborated in Teitelbaum's chapter on fibromyalgia.

A third factor in protein turnover rate is the whole body state. A catabolic state of muscle breakdown is associated with high levels of endogenous glucocorticoids and other stress hormones. It is also associated with a low metabolic pH. Since amino acids are used as buffering agents and protein turnover can contribute to a metabolic acidosis, it is not surprising that protein turnover is slowed or stalled during the catabolic state.

Protein turnover is important because it is analogous to a car's preventive maintenance. Oil, filters, and fluids are replaced to preserve the car's precision parts and mechanical integrity. Similarly, the body replaces proteins before they have altered stereochemistry. Preventive maintenance is especially important for signaling proteins on cell surfaces and enzyme proteins and can be generalized to all body proteins. Two of the biochemical processes which cause road-wear are oxidation and glycation.[17,18] Our modern environment creates unprecedented opportunities for oxidative stress and glycated proteins, as elaborated in the carbohydrate chapter by Bagnulo, the antioxidant chapter by Harris, and the xenobiotics chapter by Jaffe. These are the markers of aging. Decreased protein turnover results in premature aging, immune deficiency, illness, and degenerative body changes in the structure and function of virtually all tissues.[18,19] For example, sarcopenia, which can be secondary to protein insufficiency, has been noted as an indicator of aging.[20,21] Refer to chapters by Bland and Short.

CLINICAL EVALUATION OF PROTEIN STATUS

The food diary of 3 to 7 days is a tool in assessing protein intakes. The diary tends to be revealing for both doctor and patient. Such items as nutritional supplements and medications should also be noted as they can effect protein digestion and assimilation. Protein assimilation also depends on bowel health, adequate sleep, and stress management. Protein nutrition can be observed on physical exam by noting such findings as tissue elasticity, amount of muscle tissue, hair and nail quality, and oral mucus membranes. Laboratory evaluations can also be helpful in looking at red cell mass, serum proteins and albumin, thyroid and sex hormone levels, and serum amino acid levels. Though none of these tests are specific, if low values are found, a protein deficiency may be the source.[22,23]

EXCESS PROTEIN INTAKE

For most people protein requirement is between 0.6 and 1.5 g of high biological protein/kg/d.[24,25] This is detailed in Table 6.2. In generally healthy persons who can excrete nitrogen waste, consuming levels of protein two to three times the recommended dietary allowance (RDA) is not harmful. Dietary protein consumed over and above physiologic needs, is not stored. The nitrogen-containing amine group is removed and the carbon skeleton is oxidized through pathways of glucose or fat metabolism, and burned for fuel or stored as glycogen or fat. The nitrogen waste generated is excreted in the urine as either urea or ammonia. A Finnish meta-review of the literature concluded that there is no evidence to suggest that in the absence of overt disease that renal function is impaired by high-protein diets or that bone density was worsened.[26] In one recent study of bodybuilders

TABLE 6.2
Meeting daily protein/amino acid requirements

Recommended dietary allowances (RDA) for dietary protein

Age (years)	RDA (g/d)	RDA (g/kg/d)
Males		
0–0.5	9.1	1.52
0.5–1	13.5	1.5
1–3	13	1.1
4–8	19	0.95
9–13	34	0.95
14–18	52	0.85
19–30	56	0.8
31–50	56	0.8
>50	56	0.8
Females		
0–0.5	9.1	1.52
0.5–1	13.5	1.5
1–3	13	1.1
4–8	19	0.95
9–13	34	0.95
14–18	46	0.85
19–30	46	0.8
31–50	46	0.8
>50	46	0.8
Pregnancy		
First trimester	71	1.1
Second trimester	71	1.1
Third trimester	71	1.1
Lactation		
First 6 months	71	1.1
Second 6 months	71	1.1

Source: Adapted from the Dietary Reference Intakes Series, National Academies Press. Copyright 1997, 1998, 2000, 2001, 2002, 2004, by the National Academies of Sciences.

with normal renal and hepatic function, on high-protein diets, the data revealed that despite higher plasma concentration of uric acid and calcium, renal clearances of creatinine, urea, and albumin that were within the normal range. Their data concluded that protein intake under 2.8 g/kg did not impair renal function in well-trained athletes during the time of the study.[27,28]

Persons with health conditions which limit protein, including liver and kidney diseases, are not elaborated in this chapter. Obese persons seeking to reduce body weight need to reduce total calorie consumption and may therefore wish to reduce protein calories. Catabolized protein has a caloric value of 4 cal/g, which is similar to that of carbohydrate. Of prime concern is that diets high in protein may also contain high saturated fat, low fiber, and high acid load. These concerns have sometimes been overshadowed by the main point that people are more likely to get too little protein than too much.

PROTEIN DEFICIENCIES — UNDERLYING CAUSES

There are many factors that can lead to protein deficiency. Lack of knowledge on the part of the patient as to what constitutes a protein, and how much is needed to meet daily requirements, is probably the first factor to consider. In addition, high-quality proteins can be expensive. One recent article about the Atkins and South Beach[29] high-protein diets called attention to this fact by asking "Are you rich enough to be thin?"

A third factor is that people with poor dentition or poor protein (or fat) digestion self-select to eat less protein. Such things as dental issues that prevent successful mastication will allow poorly chewed food to reach the stomach. Commonly, persons taking antacids, H2 blockers, and proton pump inhibitors have a functional achlorhydria, meaning stomach acid pHs will be in a near neutral range of 6 to 7. As the pH rises above 4, pepsin activity decreases or stops.[30] Hypochlorhydria and achlorhydria may also accompany aging, or may be due to inadequate nutrition or other chronic illness leading protein digestion problems. Clinically we see that once protein deficiency has occurred, the body's ability to make hydrochloric acid and or digestive enzymes may be compromised and a vicious circle could ensue starting with inadequate hydrochloric acid or enzymes leads to further inability to digest protein leads to inability to make hydrochloric acid.

As a further category, dieters who restrict protein intake or meals may also not provide sufficient protein. As a special category for the over a million individuals who have undergone bariatric surgery for extreme obesity, protein absorption is a lifelong challenge. Gastric stapling results in diminished stomach capacity, decreased volume of hydrochloric acid secretion, and drastically reduced calorie intakes.

In vegan or vegetarian patients, special attention should be taken to make sure protein requirements are being met. This is for several reasons. First, vegetable proteins have amino acid make ups that are much lower in biological value than animal proteins. Second, the quantity of protein per serving of vegetables is relatively low. When these two factors are combined, low quality and low concentration, care must be taken to ensure adequate protein intake. To overcome these potential deficiencies, Lappe in *Diet for a Small Planet*[31] suggests that by combining vegetable proteins that are complementary, the excesses and deficiencies of each can be overcome to arrive at a more quality protein blend. Though many cultures have had their intuitive solutions to this, such as combining beans and rice, or garbanzos and sesame, when calculations are done as to grams of protein consumed, many will fall short of the World Health Organization (WHO) suggested minimums. Prudence would suggest that vegetarians and vegans should be monitored using lab, performance and physical exam parameters to insure they meet protein requirements over the short and long term.[32]

In the hospital setting for patients with infection, surgery, or trauma, protein nutrition is extremely important to minimize morbidity and mortality. Protein is required for wound healing; hormone production to deal with stress from unfamiliar environment and the illness itself; immune function to prevent nosocomial illness and wound infections; prevention of bed sores; and muscle strength to prevent falls.

Lactation and pregnancy are states of increased protein requirements (Table 6.2). The protein content of breast milk is affected by the dietary protein intake of the mother. An inadequate protein intake by the mother may lead to impaired nutrition of the infant. Adequate amounts of essential proteins are necessary to provide quality nutrition for the developing infant.

Protein-losing enteropathies and compromised renal function are less common causes of protein deficiency that require special treatment. Significant loss of amino acids does not normally occur unless there is pathology in the kidney, skin, or intestine.[33]

PROTEIN AND EXERCISE REQUIREMENTS

While it is not possible to state categorically, exercise generally increases protein requirements. Endurance athletes on average have higher requirements than bodybuilders due to the catabolic losses of lean body mass following intense or prolonged aerobic exercise. Exercise also increases calorie expenditure and amino acids may be used as energy sources during prolonged exercise, especially if glucose needs are not met. This muscle catabolism may result in muscle soreness, atrophy of muscle tissue, poor healing, or chronic injury.[34]

Current research indicates that athletes participating in intense training, have protein requirements that are 1.5 to 2 times the RDA (of 0.8 g/kg/d) to maintain positive nitrogen balance. This represents 105 to 140 g of protein for a 70 kg athlete.[35] That is, three to four large chicken breasts or 17 to 22 eggs per day (Table 6.3). Those athletes who are training at high altitudes have an even higher demand for protein which is as much as 2.2 g/kg/d.[36]

Current consensus is that following intense exercise athletes should ingest a carbohydrate–protein mix (1 g/kg carbohydrate and 0.5 g/kg protein) within 30 min of completing exercise to accelerate glycogen and protein synthesis.[37]

PROTEIN AND SKELETAL MUSCLE

The body of a 70 kg male contains approximately 11 kg of protein. About 43% is present in skeletal muscle. The breakdown of the other tissues, is skin (at 15%),

TABLE 6.3
Dietary protein sources

Food	Protein (g)	Food	Protein (g)
Fish, meat, and poultry		*Legumes*	
Tuna, 3 oz drained	21.7	Tofu, 3 oz	6.9
Salmon, 3 oz	16.8	Black beans,* 1/2 cup	7.5
Ground beef,* 3 oz	25.7	Pinto beans,* 1/2 cup	7.0
Beef,* 3 oz	27.0	Garbanzo beans,* 1/2 cup	7.3
Chicken breast,* 3 oz	18.9	Nuts and seeds	
Chicken, dark meat,* 3 oz	22	Peanut butter, 2 tbl	8.1
Turkey breast,* 3 oz	25.7	Almonds, 1 oz	5.4
Turkey, dark meat,* 3 oz	24.3	Sesame seeds, 1 oz	7.5
		Fruits	
		Banana, 1 medium	1.2
Dairy		Apple, large	0
Skim milk, 1 cup	8.3	Orange, large	1.7
Whole milk, 1 cup	7.9	*Vegetables*	
Yogurt, low-fat, 1 cup	12.9	Corn,* 1/2 cup	2.2
Cottage cheese, 1 cup	28.0	Carrots,* 1/2 cup	0.8
American cheese, 1 oz	7.0	Green beans,* 1/2 cup	1.0
Egg,* 1 large	6.3	Green peas,* 1/2 cup	4.1
		Potatoes, white,* 1/2 cup	1.2
*Cooked			

blood (at 15%), liver and kidney (at 10%), and the other organs such as heart, lung, brain, and bone make up the rest.[38] In malnutrition, the collagen tends to be retained whereas the actin and myosin, that is, skeletal muscle is lost.[1] Therefore skeletal muscle, which comprises over 40% of protein mass of the healthy person is the largest contributor to protein loss.

PROTEIN AND BONE HEALTH

Issues in bone health, whether osteoporosis or healing fractures, are rarely thought of as a protein deficiency problem. But since approximately 50% of bone (by volume) is comprised of protein, sufficient dietary protein intake is mandatory to help maintain bone mass or regenerate new bone. This is discussed in detail by Brown in her chapter on bone nutrition.

PROTEIN AND IMMUNE FUNCTION

Immune function is very sensitive to a lack of protein intake because of the high cellular turnover rate of some immune cells and their messenger factors such as cytokines and antibodies. If the body's intake of protein is insufficient its immune cell posture can be altered and be compromised within days. Adequate amounts of high biological proteins are necessary to keep total immune function at optimal levels. Protein intake should be considered in athletes seeking to prevent viral illness after intense competition.

PROTEIN AND RED BLOOD CELL PRODUCTION

Red blood cell (RBC) production also requires adequate dietary protein/amino acid intake for cell structure and hemoglobin. Low RBC counts may be due not only to the lack of certain vitamins (B12, folate) and minerals (iron), but also to the lack of protein. Athletes and others with increased protein needs should evaluate protein intake to prevent anemia.

PROTEIN AND INJURIES

When tissue is injured, dietary protein requirements increase. The body requires extra proteins beyond normal daily requirements to optimize the recovery process. Inadequate dietary protein intake can impair the healing of strained ligaments, tendons, and muscle. Many athletes have greatly improved muscle strength and reduced recovery periods by paying attention to protein intake in their nutritional programs.

AMINO ACIDS AS THERAPEUTIC AGENTS

Sometimes when protein intake has been insufficient to meet physiologic needs, then individual amino acids or combinations of them have been used as therapeutic agents on a short-term basis to influence a specific metabolic pathway. The amounts required for such action are usually much more than for purely supplementation purposes. Here is an overview of some of the amino acids that have been used.

The amino acid tryptophan is a precursor to the sleep regulating hormone melatonin. Pharmacologic doses have been used as a sleep generating hypnotic. Tryptophan is also a precursor to serotonin and has been used in patients with depression. There are reports showing that tryptophan is equal to prescription selective serotonin reuptake inhibitors (SSRIs) in the treatment of depression.[39,40]

Another amino acid derivative is 5-hydroxytryptophan (5-HTP). It is the intermediate metabolite between tryptophan and serotonin. 5-HTP is well absorbed orally, even with food and can cross the blood–brain barrier and increase central nervous system (CNS) synthesis of serotonin. Serotonin regulation is tied to depression, anxiety, sleep, appetite, aggression, and sexual behavior. 5-HTP has been shown to be helpful for a variety of conditions, including depression, insomnia, headaches, and fibromyalgia.[41]

As an historical aside, in 1989, 37 Americans died and over 5000 others suffered severe disability with a painful blood disorder known as eosinophilia myalgia syndrome (EMS) after over-the-counter (OTC) tryptophan supplement use. The EMS was caused by a genetically engineered brand of tryptophan manufactured by Showa Denko, Japan's third largest chemical company. In 1988–1989 they began using a new process to genetically engineer the product using bacteria. During the process the product became contaminated. The contaminant was felt to be the cause of the EMS. Once discovered, all tryptophan was withdrawn from the market by the Food and Drug Administration (FDA). Due to these events, tryptophan now requires a physician's prescription.[42]

The branched chain amino acids (BCAAs) are leucine, isoleucine, and valine. These essential amino acids differ from other essential amino acids because they are mainly catabolized by the extrahepatic tissues, especially muscle. This allows them to be broken down quickly and used in the Krebs cycle for energy by muscle tissue. This may explain the muscle sparing effect associated with supplementation of these amino acids postexercise. Oral mixtures of BCAA have been used to improve post exercise recovery and reduce muscle catabolism postexercise and parenteral solutions have been used to improve nitrogen retention in postoperative and septic patients.[43,44]

Arginine has been shown to stimulate both growth hormone and insulin in human subjects, to reduce nitrogen loss in trauma and surgical patients, and improve lymphocyte function in healthy human volunteers. There is also some research showing that arginine will induce nitric oxide and be helpful in endothelial dysfunction seen in cardiovascular disease and hypertension. Arginine and lysine share the same intestinal and renal tubular transport proteins, so that if prolonged intake of high doses of lysine or arginine is given, a deficiency of the other could occur.[45,46]

Glutamine is the most highly concentrated amino acid in muscle cells and plasma. For this reason, glutamine supplementation has been associated with benefits that include muscle sparing after workouts and growth hormone stimulation. It may be helpful in sparing protein breakdown in postoperative and trauma patients. Glutamine is also the preferred energy source for stimulated lymphocytes and the rapidly turning over intestinal mucosal cells.[47–49]

Carnitine and acetyl-L-carnitine have also been studied. In a recent report, male aging was improved better with 2 g/d of acetyl-L-carnitine plus 2 g/d of propionyl-L-carnitine than testosterone undecanoate 160 mg/d or placebo at improving sexual function, mood, and fatigue in males age 60 to 74 years.[50,51]

N-Acetyl-cysteine (NAC) can induce glutathione production. Glutathione is one of the most important intracellular antioxidants. Whey protein is a rich source of NAC. It can be used as oral supplement to help prevent viral syndromes after marathon.[52]

Creatine has become a popular nutritional supplement among athletes. Over 500 research studies have studied its effects on muscle physiology and exercise capacity in diverse populations. Supplementing creatine short term (e.g., 20 g/d for 5 to 7 days) often increases total creatine content by 10 to 30% and phosphocreatine stores by 10 to 40%. Vegetarians have better responses than carnivores. A total of 70% of over 300 studies report statistically significant results as the ergogenic value of creatine. The other 30% show no effect. No studies showed ergolytic effects but muscle cramping can be a problem for some. The ergogenic effects include improvement in maximal power/strength (5 to 15%), work performed during sets of maximal effort muscle contractions (5 to 15%), single-effort sprint performance (1 to 5%), and work performed during repetitive sprint performance (5 to 15%). Creatine's effects are best seen in high-intensity exercise tasks rather than in endurance activities where they have not shown benefit.[53,54]

SUMMARY

From the pregnant woman nurturing the fetus, to childhood growth through full maturity, to the senior in the later stages of life, for the healthy, and for the injured, protein is a key nutrient for optimum health and longevity. By ensuring that the daily requirement of protein (and other essential nutrients) is met, the individual's body can in each stage of life, grow, maintain, and repair itself in the best manner possible.

REFERENCES

1. Picou, D., Halliday, D., and Garrow, J.S., Total body protein, collagen and non-collagen protein in infantile protein malnutrition, *Clin. Sci.*, 30, 345–351, 1966.
2. Atkins, R., *Dr. Atkins Diet Revolution*, Bantam Books, 1990.
3. Sears, B. and Lawren, B., *Enter the Zone: The Dietary Road Map to Lose Weight and More*, Harper Collins, 1996.
4. Ornish, D., *Dr. Dean Ornish Program for Reversing Heart Disease*, Ballantine Books, 1996.
5. Pritikin, R., *The New Pritikin Program*, Pocket Books, 1990.
6. Wolcott, W.L., *The Metabolic Typing Diet*, Random House, 2002.
7. D'Adamo, P., *Eat Right 4 Your Type*, Penguin Books, 1996.
8. Carmichael, C., *Chris Carmichael's Food for Fitness*, CTS, 2004.
9. Cordain, L., Eaton, S.B., Sebastian, A., Mann, N., Lindeberg, S., Watkins, B.A., O'Keefe, J.H., and Miller, J.B., Origins and evolution of the western diet: health implications for the 21st century, *Am. J. Clin. Nutr.*, 81, 341–354, 2005.
10. O'Keefe, J.H., Jr. and Cordain, L., Cardiovascular disease resulting from a diet and lifestyle at odds with our Paleolithic genome: how to become a 21st-century hunter-gatherer, *Mayo Clin. Proc.*, 79, 101–108, 2004.
11. Enzminger, A.H., Enzminger, M.G., Konlande, J.E., and Robson, J.R., *Foods and Nutrition Encyclopedia*, 2nd ed., vol. 2, CRC Press, 1994.

12. Chung, V.C., Young, S.K., Shaehehr, A., et al., Protein digestion and absorption in human small intestine, *Gastroenterology*, 76, 1415–1421, 1979.

13. Matthews, D.M., Intestinal absorption of peptides, *Physiol. Rev.*, 55, 537–608, 1975.

14. Luca-Moretti, M., A comparative double blind triple crossover net nitrogen utilization study confirms the discovery of the master amino acid pattern, *Ann. R. Natl. Acad. Med. Spain*, CXV, 1998.

15. Harper, A.E., McCollum and directions in the evaluation of protein quality, *J. Agric. Food. Chem.*, 29, 429–435, 1981.

16. Waterlow, J.C., Protein turnover with special reference to man, *Q. J. Exp. Physiol.*, 69, 409–438, 1984.

17. Short, K.R. and Nair, K.S., The effect of age on protein metabolism, *Curr. Opin. Clin. Nutr. Metab. Care*, 3, 39–44, 2000.

18. Ryazanov, A.G. and Nefsky, B.S., Protein turnover plays a key role in aging. *Mech. Ageing Dev.*, 123, 207–213, 2002.

19. Ramamurthy, B., Jones, A.D., and Larsson, L., Glutathione reverses early effects of glycation on myosin function, *Am. J. Physiol. Cell Physiol.*, 285, C419–C424, 2003.

20. de los Reyes, A.D., Bagchi, D., and Preuss, H.G., Overview of resistance training, diet, hormone replacement and nutritional supplements on age-related sarcopenia — a minireview, *Res. Commun. Mol. Pathol. Pharmacol.*, 113–114, 159–170, 2003.

21. Evans, W.J., Protein nutrition, exercise and aging, *J. Am. Coll. Nutr.*, 23(6 Suppl.): 601S–609S, 2004.

22. Pangborn, J., Amino acid analysis and therapy: opportunities and pitfills, in *Treatment Options in Energetic, Functional, Biologic Medicine*, Hank, J., Ed., Syllabus for the Great Lakes College of Clinical Medicine Symposium, Feb. 28–Mar. 2, Asheville, NC, 1997, p.7.

23. Pitkanen, H.T., Oja, S.S., Kemppainen, K., Seppa, J.M., and Mero, A.A., Serum amino acid concentrations in aging men and women, Department of Biology of Physical Activity, University of Jyvaskyla, Jyvaskyla, Finland.

24. Food and Nutrition Board, National Research Council, *Recommended Dietary Allowances*, 10th ed., National Academy Press, Washington, DC, 1989.

25. FAO/WHO, Energy and Protein Requirements, WHO Technical Report Series No. 522, WHO, Geneva, 1973.

26. Hamilton, A., Peak Performance #208, Jan. 2005.

27. Michaelsen, K.F., Are there negative effects of an excessive protein intake? *Pediatrics*, 106, 1293, 2000.

28. Poortmans, J.R. and Dellalieux, O., Do regular high protein diets have potential health risks on kidney function in athletes, *Int. J. Sport Nutr. Exerc. Metab.*, 10, 28–38, 2000.

29. Agatston, A., *The South Beach Diet*, St. Martins Press, 2003.

30. Campos, L.A. and Sancho, J., The active site of pepsin is formed in the intermediate conformation dominant at mildly acidic pH, *FEBS Lett.*, 538, 89–95, 2003.

31. Lappe', F.M., *Diet for a Small Planet*, Random House, 1971.

32. http://www.eatright.org/Public/GovernmentAffairs/92_17084.cfm.

33. Munro, H.N., Historical perspective on protein requirements: objectives for the future, in *Nutritional Adaptation in Man*, Blanter, K. and Waterlow, J.C., Eds., John Libbey, 1985, pp. 155–168.

34. Fielding, R.A. and Parkington, J., What are the dietary protein requirements of physically active individuals? New evidence on the effects of exercise on protein utilization during post-exercise recovery, *Nutr. Clin. Care*, 5, 191–196, 2002.
35. Sports Science #65, 1999. Available at: http://www.sportsci.org/jour/990/rbk/.html.
36. Butterfield, G., Amino acids and high protein diets, in *Perspectives in Exercise Science and Sports Medicine*, vol. 4, Ergogenics, Enhancement of Performance in Exercise and Sport, Lamb, D. and Williams, M., Eds., 1991, pp. 87–122.
37. Hamilton, A., Peak Performance #208, Jan. 2005.
38. Lentner, C., *Geigy Scientific Tables*, 8th ed., vol. 1, Units of Measurement, Body Fluids, Composition of the Body, Nutrition, Ciba-Geigy Corp., West Caldwell, NJ, 1981.
39. Maurizi, C.P., The therapeutic potential for tryptophan and melatonin: possible roles in depression, sleep, Alzheimer's disease and abnormal aging, *Med. Hypotheses*, 31, 233–242, 1990.
40. Shaw, K., Turner, J., and Del Mar, C., Tryptophan and 5-hydroxytryptophan for depression, Cochrane Database Syst Rev (England), 2002, (1) pCD003198.
41. Das, Y.T., Bagchi, M., Bagchi, D., et al., Safety of 5-hydroxy-L-tryptophan, *Toxicol. Lett.*, 150, 111–122, 2004.
42. Centers for Disease Control, Eosinophilia–myalgia syndrome associated with ingestion of L-tryptophan, United States, through August 24, 1990, J. Am. Med. Assoc., 264, 1655, 1990.
43. Mitch, W.E., Walsen, M., and Sapir, D.G., Nitrogen sparing induced by leucine compared with that inducted by its keto analogue, alpha-ketoisocaproate, in fasting obese man, *J. Clin. Invest.*, 67, 553–562, 1981.
44. Blackburn, G.L., Moldawer, L.L., Usui, S., Bothe, A., Jr., O'Keefe, S.J., Bistrian, B.R., Branched chain amino acid administration and metabolism during starvation, injury, and infection, *Surgery*, 86, 307, 1979.
45. Drexler, H., Zeiher, A.M., Meinzer, K., and Just, H., Correction of endothelial dysfunction in coronary microcirculation of hypercholesterolaemic patients by L-arginine, *Lancet*, 338, 1546–1550, 1991.
46. Azzara, A., Carulli, G., Sbrana, S., Rizzuti-Gullaci, A., Minnucci, S., Natale, M., et al. Effects of lysine-arginine association on immune functions in patients with recurrent infections, *Drugs Exp. Clin. Res.*, 21, 71–78, 1995.
47. Klimberg, V.S., Souba, W.W., Dolson, D.J., Salloum, R.M., Hautamaki, R.D., Plumley, D.A., et al. Prophylactic glutamine protects the intestinal mucosa from radiation injury, *Cancer*, 66, 62–68, 1990.
48. Buchman, A.L., Glutamine: is it a conditionally required nutrient for the human gastrointestinal system? *J. Am. Coll. Nutr.*, 15,199–205, 1996.
49. Souba, W.W., Klimberg, V.S., Plumley, D.A., Salloum, R.M., Flynn, T.C., Bland, K.I., and Copeland, E.M., The role of glutamine in maintaining a healthy gut and supporting the metabolic response to injury and infection, *J. Surg. Res.*, 48, 383–391, 1990.
50. Cavallini, G., Caracciolo, S., Vitali, G., Modenini, F., and Biagiotti, G., Carnitine versus androgen administration in the treatment of sexual dysfunction, depressed mood, and fatigue associated with male aging, *Urology*, 63, 641–646, 2004.
51. Kendler, B.S., Carnitine: an overview of its role in preventive medicine, *Prev. Med.*, 15, 373–390, 1986.
52. Lomaestro, B.M. and Malone, M., Glutathione in health and disease: pharmacotherapeutic issues, *Ann. Pharmocother.*, 29, 1263–1273, 1995.

53. Kreider, R.B., Effects of creatine supplementation on performance and training adaptations, *Mol. Cell. Biochem.*, 244, 89–94, 2003.

54. Branch, J.D., Effect of creatine supplementation on body composition and performance: a meta-analysis, *Int. J. Sport Nutr. Exerc. Metab.*, 13, 198–226, 2003.

55. Dietary Reference Intakes for Energy, Carbohydrate, Fiber, Fat, Fatty Acids, Cholesterol, Protein, and Amino Acids (Macronutrients), 2002, Food and Nutrition Board (FNB). Available at http://books.nap.edu/books/0309085373/html/465.html.

7 Antioxidants

Gabriel Keith Harris, Ph.D. and
David J. Baer, Ph.D.

CONTENTS

INTRODUCTION

What are antioxidants? What role do they play in musculoskeletal health? What is oxidative stress? How does it affect musculoskeletal health? In this chapter, we seek to address these questions and to provide the most up-to-date information on the subject of antioxidants and musculoskeletal health. This chapter is divided into three sections. The first section covers antioxidant biochemistry, dietary sources of antioxidants, and the detection of antioxidant compounds in humans. The second defines oxidative stress, discusses the dynamic balance between oxidation and reduction in the body, and describes methods for the measurement of oxidative stress. The third section discusses the known and potential effects of antioxidants on musculoskeletal health in relation to athletic performance, disease, obesity, and aging.

Editor's Note

Oxidation of human nucleic acids, proteins, and lipids might be compared to a more readily visible, nonhuman form of oxidation — rust. Food contains thousands of rust-fighting antioxidant nutrients and scientists continue to identify new antioxidant nutrients. Dietary antioxidants and antioxidants produced by the body itself create a complex network of protection against oxidative damage. A clinical trial of a diet high in antioxidants was shown to prolong survival.[*] Balanced calorie-restricted diets, which also prolong life, are associated with decreased oxidation. Antioxidant supplements used in known deficiency states and during intense oxidative stress may enhance athletic competition and protect against arthritis, obesity, osteoporosis, and muscle atrophy.

[*]de Lorgeril, M., et al., Mediterranean dietary pattern in a randomized trial: prolonged survival and possible reduced cancer rate, Arch. Intern. Med., 158, 1181-1187, 1998.

THE BIOCHEMISTRY OF ANTIOXIDANTS

Defined chemically, antioxidants prevent, inhibit, or terminate oxidation reactions, primarily those caused by free radicals. Free radicals are defined as molecules that possess unpaired electrons. Since thermodynamics favors the pairing of electrons, free radicals are highly reactive and tend to donate their odd electron to other molecules. The molecule receiving this electron becomes a radical and can continue the chain-reaction by passing its unpaired electron to other molecules. Free radicals react with and alter the structure of carbohydrates, lipids, and, most importantly, protein and DNA. These alterations in lipid and protein may result in a temporary reduction in the function of the organ in question and, in the case of DNA, permanent genetic damage. Free radical reactions may be caused by oxygen, nitrogen, or sulfur-containing molecules, also referred to as reactive oxygen, nitrogen, and sulfur species, respectively. Here we focus on reactive oxygen species (ROS). With regard to the musculoskeletal system, accumulated free radical damage could translate to a loss of muscle performance, a weakening of bone, and an increase in joint inflammation. Antioxidants serve to protect against this damage by preventing the formation of free radicals and other ROS or inactivating them after their formation. A helpful analogy would be to think of free radicals as fire, which is useful but potentially dangerous, and of antioxidants as flame retardants and fire extinguishers.

Free radical formation can be initiated by several mechanisms, including peroxide cleavage, radiation, metal catalysis, and enzymatic action. Free radicals are produced by or participate in numerous processes within the body, including energy production, immunity, cell signalling, eicosanoid formation, the oxidation of catecholamines, and the peroxidation of lipids. During the course of energy

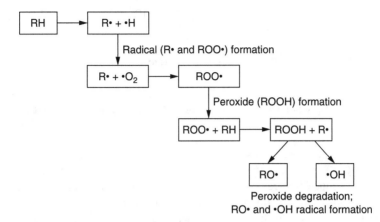

FIGURE 7.1 Lipid peroxidation and peroxide degradation.

production in the mitochondria, the ROS hydrogen peroxide and superoxide are formed. These ROS can "leak" out of the mitochondria and cause damage within the host cell or in adjacent cells. Immune cells, such as neutrophils and macrophages, are capable of producing superoxide, hydrogen peroxide, and nitric oxide, a form of reactive nitrogen, when responding to infection or inflammation. Cell signaling is partially reliant on reversible oxidations to carry information from the exterior to the interior of the cell. The formation of eicosanoids, such as prostaglandins and leukotrienes, results in the formation of the ROS superoxide. The oxidation of catecholamines, such as adrenaline, also contributes to the total burden of ROS in the body and may represent a link between stress (which is associated with high catecholamine levels) and disease.[1]

One of the most common forms of free radical-driven oxidation is lipid peroxidation. Lipid peroxidation can have dramatic destabilizing effects on cell membranes, which are composed largely of lipids. Alterations in the structural integrity of cell membranes, in turn, have a direct impact on the health and function of organ systems. Lipid peroxidation reactions proceed through three steps: initiation, propagation and termination. Figure 7.1 illustrates initiation and propagation reactions.

Initiation involves the formation of a lipid radical (R˙). The propagation step involves the reaction of a free radical with oxygen to form a peroxyl radical (ROO˙). This peroxyl radical can react with a lipid molecule (RH) to form a peroxide (ROOH) and another (R˙) lipid radical. Peroxides can be degraded to form additional free radical species. Since each radical can theoretically give rise to two others via the reactions outlined in Figure 7.1, the rate of lipid oxidation can increase logarithmically over time. The termination step is the reaction of free radicals with one another or with antioxidants to form unreactive products.

Antioxidants work through at least two basic mechanisms: the prevention of free radical formation and the inhibition or termination of free radical reactions.

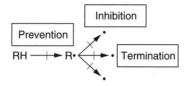

FIGURE 7.2 Ability of antioxidants to oppose free radical reactions at several stages.

As Figure 7.2 illustrates, some antioxidants prevent the initial formation of free radicals (R·). These preventive antioxidants include chelators, which bind the metals that induce free radical reactions, and enzymes that degrade peroxides, such as catalase and glutathione peroxidase. Other antioxidants inhibit free radical reactions by slowing them down or terminate them by stopping them altogether. Antioxidants that function in these ways do so by accepting radicals and becoming radicals themselves. Antioxidant radicals tend to be stable, and not pass on their unpaired electron. In this way, they effectively stop free radical chain reactions. The earlier free radical reactions are stopped, the lower the risk of tissue damage.

Any compound that acts as an antioxidant must be somewhat reactive. Due to this reactivity, antioxidants can switch roles and act as pro-oxidants if present at excessively high concentrations. Beta-carotene, which is responsible for the orange color of pumpkins and squash, has been shown to act as an antioxidant at low concentrations and as a prooxidant at high concentrations.[2] Thus, it is possible to have "too much of a good thing" as far as antioxidants are concerned. The key to preventing oxidative damage appears to be to have the right antioxidant present at the right time and place, and at the right concentration. The body is amazingly adept at doing just that.

EXOGENOUS AND ENDOGENOUS SOURCES OF ANTIOXIDANTS

The body relies on a wide variety of antioxidants to control free radical formation. There are two basic types of antioxidants, exogenous and endogenous. Exogenous antioxidants are those consumed as food or in supplement form. Endogenous antioxidants are those produced by the body itself. The blood levels of the endogenous antioxidants uric acid, ceruloplasmin, and albumin are approximately 10, 100, and 10,000 times greater, respectively, than those of the exogenous antioxidants vitamins C and E.[3] This observation has led some researchers to believe that exogenous antioxidants, aside from vitamins, are unimportant relative to their endogenous counterparts. Despite their relatively low levels, however, numerous studies have shown that the consumption of antioxidants in food or supplement form measurably affects urinary and blood markers of antioxidant status. This indicates that exogenous antioxidants serve important functions

TABLE 7.1
Common exogenous antioxidants

Type	Antioxidant	Primary food sources
Vitamins	Vitamin A	Liver
	Beta-carotene (previtamin A)	Orange and yellow vegetables
	Ascorbic acid	Fresh fruits
	Tocopherols and tocotrienols	Whole grains, plant oils
Phytochemicals	Carotenoids	Orange, red, and yellow vegetables
	Chlorophyll	Dark green vegetables
	Curcuminoids	Turmeric
	Flavonoids	Tea, onions, berries, chocolate, wine
	Lignan and lignin	Edible seeds
	Organic acids	Fruits
	Sterols	Plant oils
	Terpenes	Plant oils
Other	Coenzyme Q_{10}	Meat, nuts
	Glutathione	Meat, milk
	Lipoic acid	Organ meats, spinach
	N-Acetylcysteine	Meat, eggs, oats

even when present at very low concentrations. Currently, it is not clear what percentage of the burden of oxidative stress is shouldered by exogenous vs. endogenous antioxidants. What is clear is that foods high in antioxidant capacity are capable of reducing oxidative stress when consumed in appropriate amounts.

Exogenous antioxidants are a highly diverse group of compounds, the overwhelming majority of which come from plant sources. Since they come from plants, they are often referred to as phytochemicals. They include vitamins, flavonoids, carotenoids, and other compounds. Phytochemicals are often plant pigments. Anthocyanins, a class of flavonoids, are responsible for the red, blue and purple colors in strawberries, blueberries, and raspberries. Lycopene, a carotenoid, is responsible for the red color of tomatoes, watermelon, guava, and pink grapefruits. Over 4000 types of flavonoids and 500 types of carotenoids have been identified from fruits and vegetables.[4] Some nutraceutical supplements are concentrated exogenously obtained antioxidants which the body produces endogenously. Examples include glutathione and coenzyme Q_{10}. Table 7.1 lists exogenous antioxidants commonly found in the diet or consumed as supplements.

Since exogenous antioxidants must pass through the digestive tract, the degree of absorption and the metabolism of exogenous antioxidants before and after absorption affect their efficacy in the body. Diet has a profound effect on the absorption of antioxidants. For example, carotenoids are fat soluble. Eating carotenoids with fat generally increases their absorption. In many cases, only a small percentage of exogenous antioxidants consumed in foods or as supplements

TABLE 7.2
Endogenous antioxidants

Albumin	Glutathione
Billirubin	Glutathione peroxidase
Catalase	lLactoferrin
Ceruloplasmin	Superoxide dismutase
Coenzyme Q_{10}	Transferrin
Estradiol	Uric acid
Ferritin	

is absorbed. This may actually be beneficial since very high levels of any one antioxidant can be detrimental. Finally, absorption may not always be necessary to affect health. The presence of antioxidants in the digestive tract may benefit health by preventing the oxidation of food lipids as they pass through the digestive tract, even if the antioxidants themselves are not absorbed. Because exogenous antioxidants are metabolized extensively by gut bacteria, by intestinal cells, and by the liver, it may be just as important to study the antioxidant properties of phytochemical metabolites as those of the original compounds.

Endogenous antioxidants include small molecules such as glutathione, large proteins, such as albumin, and enzymes that degrade ROS, such as catalase. Table 7.2 lists major endogenous antioxidants. Because of differing chemical structures, antioxidants vary widely in solubility and other chemical properties. This, in turn, affects the final location of antioxidants in the body. Lipid-soluble antioxidants such as lipoic acid, coenzyme Q_{10}, and vitamin E associate with fat, cholesterol, and other lipids. Vitamin C, glutathione, and catechins are water soluble and are found in aqueous body compartments, such as blood plasma. Because of their distribution throughout the body, exogenous and endogenous antioxidants together form a protective network which is remarkably effective at preventing oxidative cell damage.

Regardless of the source of the antioxidant (food, supplements, endogenous production) several general principles apply to all of them. The first is that the effectiveness of antioxidants is directly related to the antioxidant to oxygen ratio. Some antioxidants, such as flavonoids, function well when the oxygen concentration is high. Others, such as carotenoids, function well when the oxygen concentration is low.[2,5] Oxygen concentration is, in turn, affected by the part of the body in question and the activity level of the individual. Organs such as the lungs are exposed to high oxygen concentrations due to their direct contact with air. Muscle, on the other hand, may be poorly supplied with oxygen if an individual is temporarily exercising beyond the body's capacity to replace oxygen. For this reason, it is important to consume a wide variety of antioxidants via the daily consumption of fruits and vegetables and the sensible use of supplements.

THE DYNAMIC BALANCE OF OXIDATION
AND REDUCTION

In order to remain alive, the human body must maintain a dynamic equilibrium between oxidation and reduction. This balance will always be slightly in favor of oxidation, since it is through oxidation that we derive energy. It is important to remember that just as antioxidants have their role in the human body, so do free radicals. Radicals such as nitric oxide deliver key signals that affect muscle contraction and blood pressure. Reversible oxidations involving hydrogen peroxide appear to activate important systems of intracellular communication known as mitogen-activated protein kinase, or MAPK pathways.

When oxygen levels are very high or very low, muscle performance is impaired and damage can result. Oxidative stress is an imbalance in oxidation and reduction reactions that favors oxidation; it results from an excess of free radical formation or a deficit of antioxidant protection. Oxidative stress has been shown to reduce several measures of muscle performance such as whole muscle contractility, myocyte calcium flux, and sarcomere shortening in mice.[6] Antioxidants were shown to lower muscle contractility in rats, although endurance was increased.[7] This reinforces the idea that a balance between oxidation and reduction must be maintained for maximal muscle function. It also suggests that the oxidative balance required for strength may be different than that required for endurance.

Oxidative stress can affect the long-term health of the musculoskeletal system because it can result in permanent genetic damage and can affect gene expression. Both the nucleus and the mitochondria, the energy-producing organelles of the cell, contain DNA. Damage to mitochondrial DNA can negatively impact energy production. Free radicals have the ability to increase the expression of genes related to inflammation, which, when manifested in diseases such as osteoarthritis, can affect the performance of the entire musculoskeletal system. It has estimated that 100,000 DNA strand breaks occur per cell per day, many of them related to oxidative damage.[8] Of these, the majority affect "renewable resources" such as sugars, proteins, lipids, or even RNA. Some cause easily repairable DNA damage. However, if even 0.1% of these events caused permanent DNA mutations, this would represent 100 mutations per cell per day. While large parts of the genome can be mutated without affecting cell function, mutation of key genes drastically affects not only organ function and performance, but chronic disease risk as well.

Because of the potential damage that can result from oxidative stress, the body has many systems in place to keep free radical formation in check. These systems are not perfect, however, and become less so as we age. In conditions of oxidative stress, the body upregulates the production of antioxidant enzymes and the blood levels of antioxidants such as uric acid and vitamin E increase. Interestingly, some evidence indicates that the intake of high levels of exogenous antioxidants may actually lower the levels of naturally occurring antioxidants in the blood. These changes in exogenous antioxidant levels appear to be an attempt to maintain homeostasis and suggest that the body may have an oxidative "set-point." ROS levels can vary dramatically, depending on activity level, dietary status, and general health.

ROS are constantly being formed as a result of normal metabolism. The formation of ROS increases rapidly under conditions such as hypoxia or aerobic exercise. If endogenous antioxidant levels or consumption of exogenous antioxidants are low, oxidative stress will result. In addition, lifestyle factors, such as smoking, excessive alcohol consumption, and intense exercise can also contribute to oxidative stress. Based on this information, it is possible that antioxidant supplements may be most effective in populations where oxidative status is compromised. Clinical applications are being investigated and are likely to include intense exercise, smoking, ischemia-related conditions, such as heart attacks and strokes, and advanced age.

QUANTIFYING OXIDATIVE STRESS

Because of the ephemeral nature of free radicals, with half-lives measured in seconds or even milliseconds, their direct detection is difficult. The measurement of oxidative stress in humans may be done in one of two ways: through the measurement of specific oxidation products or through global measures of oxidative stress. Table 7.3 lists common measures of oxidative stress. Specific measures allow researchers to track increases in the level of target compounds due to oxidative stress and decreases as a result of antioxidant treatment. Examples include the ferrous xylenol orange (FOX) assay, which measures peroxides, and 8-OHdG, a

TABLE 7.3
Methods of quantifying oxidative stress in humans

Assay type	Measures	Source[a]
Specific measure	4-Hydroxy-2-nonenal	P
	8-Hydroxy-2′-deoxyguanosine (8-OHdG)	BC, Sa, U
	Acetone, ethylene, ethane, isoprene, or pentane	G
	Isoprostane F_2-alpha	P, U
	LDL oxidation	P, S
	Peroxides: ferrous xylenol orange (FOX)	P
	Malondialdehyde	P, Sa, U
	Oxidized vs. reduced glutathione	BC
	Methionine and tyrosine oxidation products	P
Total antioxidant	Ferric reducing ability of plasma (FRAP)	P
	Oxygen radical absorbance capacity (ORAC)	P
	Total radical-trapping absorbance potential (TRAP)	P

[a]Sources of oxidative stress measures: S, serum; BC, blood cells; G, breath gases; P, plasma; Sa, saliva; U, urine.

measure of hydroxyl radical-induced DNA damage. Global measures, such as oxygen radical absorbance capacity (ORAC), ferric reducing ability of plasma (FRAP), or total radical-trapping absorbance potential (TRAP) are often referred to as measures of "total antioxidant capacity" because they do not measure specific oxidation products. They measure how resistant fluids such as blood and saliva are to oxidation over time. The antioxidant status of the human body can be determined by sampling whole blood, specific blood fractions or cell types, urine, saliva, and exhaled breath gases. Although blood-derived markers are often considered to be the "gold standard" for the measurement of oxidative stress, other measures that are more easily obtained have become increasingly popular. Thus, the effects of any free radical or oxidizing substance present are accounted for by "total antioxidant capacity" methods even though the specific ROS involved will not be identified. Regardless of the sample source, it is important to use several methods to quantify oxidative stress, because numerous factors can affect the performance of each assay. In the future, it may be possible to measure free radical formation real time in humans, but this technology is still under development. Until then, the state of the art will be the measurement of oxidation products.

ANTIOXIDANTS AND ATHLETIC PERFORMANCE

Can antioxidants counteract the oxidative stress caused by musculoskeletal injury or by exercise? What factors affect oxidative stress during exercise? Can a diet rich in antioxidants or antioxidant supplements improve athletic performance? Do antioxidants speed recovery from acute injury or from regular exercise? In this section, we will address these questions using the most current data available.

Both musculoskeletal injuries, a common result of contact sports, and exercise, which is itself a mild form of injury, can induce oxidative stress and inflammation. Injuries to muscle, ligament, or bone, cause free radical formation. Animal data indicate that ligament injury causes production of nitric oxide. Although nitric oxide is involved in the maintenance of a healthy vasculature, its overproduction can result in free radical damage and the apoptotic death of cartilage-producing chondrocytes, thus causing joint degradation.[9] The extent to which muscle is damaged by exercise is influenced by the type of exercise, as well as its duration and intensity. Aerobic exercise has been shown to increase circulating levels of lipid peroxides. Exercise also causes recruitment of immune cells: first neutrophils, then lymphocytes and macrophages to the exercising muscles. All of these cells are capable of producing free radicals and releasing inflammatory mediators. Figure 7.3 illustrates the interaction of the circulatory, immune, and muscular systems in the generation and inactivation of ROS in working muscle. These radicals may worsen the damage done by the original injury. In contrast, regular exercise increases free radical production, but also increases the levels of endogenous antioxidants such as glutathione and uric acid, potentially canceling negative effects.[10,11]

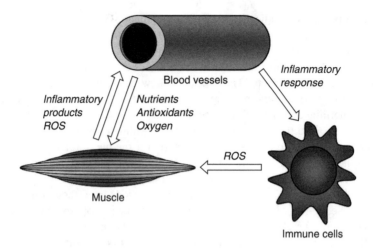

FIGURE 7.3 Interaction of the circulatory, immune and musculoskeletal systems in relation to ROS production.

Several factors, including exercise frequency and intensity, gender, and age affect exercise-induced oxidant stress. Regular exercise of moderate or vigorous intensity increases endogenous antioxidant defenses, but extremely intense exercise increases oxidative stress, especially for individuals who are overweight or sedentary. For this reason, persons who are sedentary during the week and engage in sports on the weekend may benefit from antioxidants.

Antioxidants supplements do not appear to improve athletic performance over the short term. Vitamin E supplementation for 2 months prior to the Kona Ironman Triathlon did not affect performance, but actually increased several measures of oxidative stress.[12] As noted earlier, antioxidants may have pro-oxidant activity when present at very high concentrations, as this example appears to demonstrate. The effects of gender on oxidant stress are controversial. Some authors suggest that due to the antioxidant effects of estrogen compounds, women have a greater resistance to oxidative stress than men.[13] Surprisingly, a study of Ironman triathletes found that men experienced greater reductions in oxidative stress postrace than women due to an increase in estradiol and a decrease in testosterone levels.[14] This indicates that the antioxidant needs of men and women involved in regular exercise programs are different, even after adjusting for differences in body weight. Irregular exercise appears to do more damage to the aged than to the young, but the aged are often less active, so it is difficult to separate the effects of aging per se from those of inactivity. In contrast, elderly persons engaging in regular resistance training show reductions in exercise-induced oxidative stress (lipid peroxides and malondialdehyde) and increases in endogenous antioxidant (glutathione) levels.[15]

If antioxidants do not enhance performance, do they benefit the athlete in any way? Maybe. Animal studies have shown that antioxidant pre-treatment can enhance exercise performance, but human studies have failed to do so, except in the most extreme conditions. One explanation for this inconsistency may be that humans have a superior system of endogenous antioxidants relative to the rodents typically used as test subjects, so that, in humans, no additional benefits are evident with supplementation above and beyond those observed for a healthy diet. Most human studies have found no enhancing effect of antioxidants on performance. Despite a lack of evidence for performance enhancement, there is limited evidence suggesting that antioxidants may enhance recovery and prevent minor damage caused by exercise.[16] By preventing or reducing repetitive damage to muscle, connective tissue and bone, antioxidants may reduce the risk of injuries and, possibly, lengthen athletic careers.

ANTIOXIDANTS AND OXIDATIVE STRESS IN MUSCULOSKELETAL DISEASE AND AGING

One of the most basic questions with regard to oxidative stress and disease is, "What comes first, the radical or the disease?" Often, but not always, the radical appears to come first. Free radicals and the oxidative stress they cause appear to play a part in the initiation of disease, and in the degenerative processes of aging. Musculoskeletal diseases associated with oxidative stress include muscular dystrophy, arthritis, and osteoporosis.[17–19] The disease process itself can result in the formation of additional free radical species, further increasing the possibility of oxidative damage.[4] Muscular dystrophy is associated with elevated measures of oxidative stress and with elevated levels of endogenous antioxidants. Elevated levels of lipid peroxides, malondialdehyde, and of the antioxidant ceruloplasmin have been observed in patients with hereditary muscular dystrophy.[20] In mice, vitamin E deficiency can induce muscular dystrophy, while mice afflicted with the disease display elevated expression of antioxidant enzymes, indicating that oxidative stress may play a role in its etiology. Unfortunately, attempts to slow or reverse the course of muscular dystrophy with antioxidants have so far been unsuccessful.

Of the approximately 100 inflammatory diseases grouped under the general term "arthritis," at least two types, osteoarthritis and rheumatoid arthritis have been linked to free radical damage. Osteoarthritis causes loss of connective tissue and an erosion of bone. High doses of vitamins C and E, as well as beta-carotene and selenium have been reported to improve the symptoms of this disease. Rheumatoid arthritis can result in debilitating joint stiffness and deformity and is characterized by the presence of immune cells in joint tissue, by elevated levels of nitric oxide, 8-OHdG, and by malondialdehyde. Some studies have indicated that antioxidants may prevent or inhibit rheumatoid arthritis, but more studies need to be conducted in order to confirm these observations. Exercise does not reduce oxidative stress in rheumatoid arthritis patients, suggesting that antioxidant supplementation may be beneficial in this case.[18] Despite increased markers of oxidative stress, such as 8-OHdG and malondialdehyde, rheumatoid arthritis patients also demonstrate elevated levels of plasma and salivary antioxidants, such as ceruloplasmin, indicating an attempt by the body to enhance antioxidant status.[21] See the chapter entitled "Osteoarthritis" for more information on the effects of nutrition on osteoarthritis.

Osteoporosis is a condition in which bone is progressively demineralized, decreasing bone strength and increasing the possibility of fractures. Free radical signaling is involved in the normal remodeling of bone, as well as in bone healing postfracture. Antioxidant status has been linked to a reduction in fractures, suggesting that while free radicals are necessary for bone metabolism, oxidative stress may accelerate osteoporosis. There is great interest in the effects of phytoestrogens, most of which are derived from soy products and some of which possess antioxidant activity, on osteoporosis. So far, soy studies have produced mixed results.[22] Although measures of oxidative stress were not significantly increased, the levels of exogenous and endogenous antioxidants are decreased in women suffering from osteoporosis.[23]

Two general models of aging have been proposed. One model suggests that aging results from the accumulation of damage over time. Based on this theory, maximum life span is achieved by avoiding oxidative stress and other DNA-damaging agents.[24] A second model of aging indicates that there is a genetically determined maximum lifespan and although lifestyle choices may shorten it, it cannot be lengthened.[25] Based on the most recent literature, it would appear that both theories have some validity. Calorie restriction, the only intervention consistently shown to lengthen lifespan in animal models, supports the free radical theory of aging because excessive calorie consumption increases ROS production and can cause oxidative stress.[26]

Can antioxidants extend life span? Animal models of lifetime antioxidant use generally show no affect on lifespan, but have shown effects on disease symptoms. This may indicate that antioxidants can increase the quality but not the quantity of life. In humans, measures of oxidative stress rise with age. At the same time, the blood levels of the endogenous antioxidants uric acid, endogenous antioxidant enzymes, and blood levels of vitamin E rise, in an apparent attempt by the body to counteract oxidative stress. These increases may continue up to age 80.[27,28] While the levels of some antioxidants increase with age, vitamin C levels do not change. The levels of other antioxidants, such as coenzyme Q_{10}, decline over time.[29] Although the system of antioxidants and DNA repair is never perfect and oxidative damage continually occurs at all ages, the rate of DNA and protein damage increase with time. Thus, it appears that at some point oxidative stress outpaces the ability of endogenous antioxidants to counteract it. The point at which this occurs may be influenced by lifestyle factors such as smoking, alcohol consumption, and the activity level of the individual. This may be the point at which antioxidant supplements could be utilized to prevent excessive damage to the musculoskeletal system.

ANTIOXIDANTS AND OXIDATIVE STRESS IN PRE- AND POSTOPERATIVE STATES

Operative procedures may call for a temporary interruption or reduction of blood flow (also known as ischemia) to particular areas of the body. When blood flow is restored (also known as reperfusion) reactive oxygen species are formed and oxidative stress results. It may seem paradoxical that a lack of oxygen results in oxidative stress, however, it appears that hypoxia primes tissue for oxidative stress by reducing the antioxidant defenses and increasing the activity of enzymes capable of producing free radicals. Pretreatment with antioxidants has been shown to reduce the damage associated with ischemia/reperfusion.[30]

ANTIOXIDANTS AND OXIDATIVE STRESS IN OBESITY

Although genes do play a role in obesity, chronic overconsumption of food and a sedentary lifestyle are important contributing factors. Both overeating and a lack of exercise have been shown to cause oxidative stress. Rats prevented from exercising showed decreases in total antioxidant capacity and in antioxidant enzyme levels, and increases in markers of oxidative stress.[31] Persons who are obese may not consume a diet containing sufficient antioxidants. Obesity is associated with low serum levels of the antioxidant vitamins A and E.[32] It is not clear if this is due to insufficient antioxidant intake, to increased oxidative stress, to a greater ability to store fat-soluble antioxidants, or to a combination of these factors.

Can antioxidants inhibit or prevent the damage associated with obesity? The answer appears to be yes. Antioxidants do appear to alleviate some of the oxidative stress associated with obesity. Studies of noninsulin dependent diabetics, who are often obese, indicate that the antioxidant lipoic acid alleviates both the oxidative stress and the symptoms associated with this disease.[33] Do antioxidants aid in weight loss or help to reduce percent body fat? Animal data indicate that this may be possible, but human data are lacking. Even if there are no direct effects on body fat, encouraging obese persons to consume more antioxidants by consuming more fruits and vegetables may reduce the caloric density of the diet, indirectly resulting in fat loss.

SUMMARY

In this chapter, we have discussed antioxidant biochemistry and sources, as well as the role antioxidants play in the musculoskeletal system in health and disease. Oxidative stress results from intense exercise, disease, surgical procedures, and obesity, and contributes to the physical "wear and tear" associated with aging. In response to these conditions, the body often upregulates the production of endogenous antioxidants. Antioxidants, whether dietary, supplemental, or endogenous, can dramatically reduce oxidative stress, potentially reducing long-term damage. Antioxidants show promise for the inhibition of exercise-induced muscle damage, the enhancement of postexercise recovery, the prevention of arthritis, the reduction of ischemia-induced tissue damage, and the prevention of oxidative damage induced by obesity. Finally, while antioxidants may not extend life span, they may be capable of increasing the quality of life by preventing injury and reducing the severity of age-related musculoskeletal diseases.

REFERENCES

1. Vanitallie, T.B., Stress: a risk factor for serious illness, Metabolism, 51, 40–45, 2002.
2. Zhang, P. and Omaye, S.T., Antioxidant and prooxidant roles for beta-carotene, alpha-tocopherol and ascorbic acid in human lung cells, Toxicol. In Vitro, 15, 13–24, 2001.
3. Beers, M.H. and Berkow, R., The Merck Manual of Diagnosis and Therapy, 17th ed., Merck and Company, Inc., 2004.
4. Hollman, P.C. and Katan, M.B., Dietary flavonoids: intake, health effects and bioavailability, Food Chem. Toxicol., 37, 937–942, 1999.
5. Zheng, Y., Wang, C.Y., Wang, S.Y., and Zheng, W., Effect of high-oxygen atmospheres on blueberry phenolics, anthocyanins, and antioxidant capacity. J. Agric. Food Chem., 51, 7162–7169, 2003.
6. Lawler, J.M. and Powers, S.K., Oxidative stress, antioxidant status, and the contracting diaphragm, Can. J. Appl. Physiol., 23, 23–55, 1998.
7. Khawli, F.A. and Reid, M.B., N-Acetylcysteine depresses contractile function and inhibits fatigue of diaphragm in vitro, J. Appl. Physiol., 77, 317–324, 1994.
8. Saul, R.L. and Ames, B.N., Background levels of DNA damage in the population, Basic Life Sci., 38, 529–535, 1986.
9. Hashimoto, S., Takahashi, K., Amiel, D., Coutts, R.D., and Lotz, M., Chondrocyte apoptosis and nitric oxide production during experimentally induced osteoarthritis, Arthritis Rheum., 41, 1266–1274, 1998.
10. Ohkuwa, T., Sato, Y., and Naoi, M., Glutathione status and reactive oxygen generation in tissues of young and old exercised rats, Acta Physiol. Scand., 159, 237–244, 1997.
11. Bailey, D.M., Young, I.S., McEneny, J., Lawrenson, L., Kim, J., Barden, J., and Richardson, R.S., Regulation of free radical outflow from an isolated muscle bed in exercising humans, Am. J. Physiol. Heart. Circ. Physiol., 287, H1689–H1699, 2004.
12. Nieman, D.C., Henson, D.A., McAnulty, S.R., McAnulty, L.S., Morrow, J.D., Ahmed, A., Heward, C.B., Vitamin E and immunity after the Kona Triathlon World Championship, Med. Sci. Sports Exerc., 36, 1328–1335, 2004.
13. Tiidus, P.M., Estrogen and gender effects on muscle damage, inflammation, and oxidative stress, Can. J. Appl. Physiol., 25, 274–287, 2000.
14. Ginsburg, G.S., O'Toole, M., Rimm, E., Douglas, P.S., and Rifai, N., Gender differences in exercise-induced changes in sex hormone levels and lipid peroxidation in athletes participating in the Hawaii Ironman triathlon. Ginsburg-gender and exercise-induced lipid peroxidation, Clin. Chim. Acta, 305, 131–139, 2001.

15. Vincent, K.R., Vincent, H.K., Braith, R.W., Lennon, S.L., Lowenthal, D.T., Resistance exercise training attenuates exercise-induced lipid peroxidation in the elderly, *Eur. J. Appl. Physiol.*, 87, 416–423, 2002.

16. Thompson, D., Williams, C., McGregor, S.J., Nicholas, C.W., McArdle, F., Jackson, M.J., Powell, J.R., Prolonged vitamin C supplementation and recovery from demanding exercise, *Int. J. Sport Nutr. Exerc. Metab.*, 11, 466–481, 2001.

17. Murphy, M.E. and Kehrer, J.P., Free radicals: a potential pathogenic mechanism in inherited muscular dystrophy, *Life Sci.*, 39, 2271–2278, 1986.

18. Rall, L.C., Roubenoff, R., Meydani, S.N., Han, S.N., and Meydani, M., Urinary 8-hydroxy-2′-deoxyguanosine (8-OHdG) as a marker of oxidative stress in rheumatoid arthritis and aging: effect of progressive resistance training, *J. Nutr. Biochem.*, 11, 581–584, 2000.

19. Basu, S., Michaelsson, K., Olofsson, H., Johansson, S., and Melhus, H., Association between oxidative stress and bone mineral density, *Biochem. Biophys. Res. Commun.*, 288, 275–279, 2001.

20. Hunter, M.I. and Mohamed, J.B., Plasma antioxidants and lipid peroxidation products in Duchenne muscular dystrophy, *Clin. Chim. Acta*, 155, 123–131, 1986.

21. Nagler, R.M., Salameh, F., Reznick, A.Z., Livshits, V., and Nahir, A.M., Salivary gland involvement in rheumatoid arthritis and its relationship to induced oxidative stress, *Rheumatology*, 42, 1234–1241, 2003.

22. Kreijkamp-Kaspers, S., Kok, L., Grobbee, D.E., de Haan, E.H.F., Aleman, A., Lampe, J.W., and van der Schouw, Y.T., Effect of soy protein containing isoflavones on cognitive function, bone mineral density, and plasma lipids in postmenopausal women: a randomized controlled trial, *J. Am. Med. Assoc.*, 292, 65–74, 2004.

23. Maggio, D., Barbani, M., Pierandrei, M., Polidori, M.C., Catani, M., Mecocci, P., Senin, U., Pacifici, R., and Cherubini, A., Marked decrease in plasma antioxidants in aged osteoporitic women: results of a cross-sectional study, *J. Clin. Endocrinol. Metab.*, 88, 1523–1527, 2003.

24. Gianni, P., Jan, K.J., Douglas, M.J., Stuart, P.M., and Tarnopolsky, M.A., Oxidative stress and the mitochondrial theory of aging in human skeletal muscle, *Exp. Gerontol.*, 39, 1391–1400, 2004.

25. Purdom, S. and Chen, Q.M., Linking oxidative stress and genetics of aging with p66Shc signaling and forkhead transcription factors, *Biogerontology*, 4, 181–191, 2003.

26. Meydani, M., Nutrition interventions in aging and age-associated disease, *Ann. N Y Acad. Sci.*, 928, 226–235, 2001.

27. Masafumi, K., Fujiko, A., Akihisa, I., and Hiroshi, S., Effect of aging on serum uric acid levels: longitudinal changes in a large Japanese population group, *J. Gerontol. A Biol. Sci. Med. Sci.*, 57, M660–M664, 2002.

28. Papas, A., *Antioxidant Status, Diet, Nutrition, and Health*, CRC Press, Washington, DC, 1999.

29. Lass, A., Kwong, L., and Sohal, R.S., Mitochondrial coenzyme Q content and aging, *Biofactors*, 9, 199–205, 1999.

30. Marczin, N., El-Habashi, N., Hoare, G.S., Bundy, R.E., and Yacoub, M., Antioxidants in myocardial ischemia-reperfusion injury: therapeutic potential and basic mechanisms, *Arch. Biochem. Biophys.*, 420, 222–236, 2003.

31. Lawler, J.M., Song, W., and Demaree, S.R., Hindlimb unloading increases oxidative stress and disrupts antioxidant capacity in skeletal muscle, *Free Radic. Biol. Med.*, 35, 9–16, 2003.

32. Viroonudomphol, D., Pongpaew, P., Tungtrongchitr, R., Changbumrung, S., Tungtrongchitr, A., Phonrat, B., Vudhivai, N., and Schelp, F.P., The relationships between anthropometric measurements, serum vitamin A and E concentrations and lipid profiles in overweight and obese subjects, *Asia Pac. J. Clin. Nutr.*, 12, 73–79, 2003.
33. Packer, L., Kraemer, K., and Rimbach, G., Molecular aspects of lipoic acid in the prevention of diabetes complications, *Nutrition*, 17, 888–895, 2001.

8 Water: A Driving Force in the Musculoskeletal System

Fereydoon Batmanghelidj†, M.D. and Ingrid Kohlstadt, M.D., M.P.H.

CONTENTS

Since the body is dependent on dietary intake of water, water is generally considered an essential nutrient. The amount of water consumed among individuals varies considerably, and the ideal amount of water intake for any given individual has not been scientifically established. Water has several physiologic functions: a solvent, a shape-friendly packing material, and a means of transport. Water may also have less characterized roles.

Generally, drinking water is a response to thirst. Thirst is induced by vasopressin release, which occurs in response to a 1% shift in osmolality, and thirst perception decreases with age.[1] As thirst perception declines, total water intake declines. Total body water declines with age: the human fetus is 80% water, the newborn child is 75% water and the healthy adult is 65% water. Possibly of more significance is that the ratio of water inside the cells to that outside the cells changes

---

† Dr. Fereydoon Batmanghelidj died on November 15, 2004, prior to completion of this manuscript. It is being published in his honor and in appreciation of his scientific contribution.

from 1.1 to 0.8, leading to intracellular dehydration.[2] Still unknown is under what circumstances, if any, drinking more water can forestall intracellular dehydration. This chapter probes possible associations between water consumption and musculoskeletal health and concludes with practical considerations on hydration.

Editor's Note

The 2003 Nobel Prize in chemistry was awarded to the physician–researcher Peter Agre for discovering and researching the water channel. Agre remarked that aquaporins had not been identified sooner because they were abundant. Certainly there is more about water that continues to elude us by sheer quantity.

HOW THE BODY MANAGES DROUGHT

Chapter 17 outlines the metabolic changes the body makes to maintain homeostasis and prioritize its most critical functions. Food restriction leads to a catabolic state. Similarly, in drought the body is forced to prioritize, placing thermoregulation and pH balance above healthy muscles and bones. Dr.Batmanghelidj proposes an interesting theory on drought management detailed in recent publications.[3,4]

HOW WATER TRANSPORT IS CHALLENGED IN THE OBESE STATE

Only 40 to 45% of ATP energy released in muscle contractions translates to mechanical work, and the remainder is converted to heat.[5] If this vast amount of heat from muscle contractions were to be left unused, it would denature the proteins contained in the muscle tissue. While some heat is used in further chemical reactions, excess heat is conducted away to maintain body temperature.

Obesity is allometric growth, the growth of fat disproportionate to muscle, as quantified in Chapter 1. Muscle is hydrated and is therefore a conductor. Conversely, fat is an insulator owing to its absence of water. This concept is the basis for body composition scales, which utilize impedance to distinguish fat from muscle. It also explains why an obese person comprises only 30 to 50% body water, in contrast to the 65% body water of nonobese adults. In the obese state, less water is available to dissipate heat. Additionally, adipose tissue between muscle and skin extends the distance heat is transported to be dissipated as sweat. Since thermoregulation is prioritized over healthy muscle maintenance, heat generating metabolic reactions may be slowed down. The scaling and resting metabolic rate calculations used for the allometric growth of obesity support this speculation.[6]

HOW WATER HELPS MAINTAIN CELLULAR HEALTH

Cells undergo a culling process, often called programmed cell death or apoptosis. Muscle atrophy results when many muscle cells undergo apoptosis. Diagnostic imaging studies demonstrate that in muscle atrophy, fat cells become space-holding interlopers where muscle once existed.

Hydration has been demonstrated to forestall apoptosis of cells other than muscle, and can be of benefit in acute muscle loss associated with rhabdomyolysis. Apoptosis is an important factor in the pathogenesis of radiocontrast nephropathy.[7] In 2005 Itoh and associates concluded: "At present, hydration is regarded as the only effective, though incomplete, prophylactic regimen for radiocontrast nephropathy."[7] Compression-induced degeneration of the intervertebral disk has also been shown to be the result of apoptosis and dehydration.[8] Hydration conceivably plays a role in preventing muscle atrophy. Muscle contains much of the body's water and muscle is also a reservoir for various nutrients, possibly water as well. Dr. Batmanghelidj proposes a theory by which muscle water stores may be mobilized:

The most efficient system for water to enter the cell is by direct diffusion at the rate of 10^{-3} cm/s. When the serum composition is more dilute and water can freely flow through the cell membrane between the hydrophilic heads of the phospholipid parts of the lipid bilayer, it also transiently holds these structures together. It seems that at the phospholipid separation seen in the cell membrane, water develops the same sticky properties that it has when it becomes ice.[9] This bonding property of water is a transient process for the water molecules flowing through the membrane and is replaced by the water molecules that follow.

When water diffuses through the cell membrane, it increases the membrane fluidity. It expands the bilayer membrane creating a suitable fluid microenvironment for easy lateral diffusion of the catalytic unit of the cyclase when it is activated by hormone–receptor coupling at the cell membrane. See Figure 8.1. The hydrophobic segment of the phospholipid structures that project into the bilayer begins to repel the water and generate a strong lateral diffusion pressure that facilitates the enzyme–substrate activity within the membrane.[10]

Adequate presence of water in the bilayer membrane is vital to the efficiency of all the feedback mechanisms that are a part of the cell functions in any organ of the body. It particularly applies to the well-integrated process of nerve stimulation, muscle contractions, and joint movements. In a dehydrated state cholesterol deposits in the cell membranes and renders it much more rigid and easily damageable; the "lateral diffusion pressure" in the bilayer is lost; the hydrophobic projections in the bilayer interlock and render such cells ineffective and candidates for apoptosis.

Segment of cell membrane
Cell membrane is a bilayer

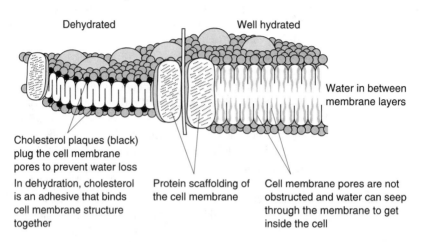

Dehydrated   Well hydrated

Water in between
membrane layers

Cholesterol plaques (black)
plug the cell membrane
pores to prevent water loss

In dehydration, cholesterol   Protein scaffolding of   Cell membrane pores are not
is an adhesive that binds   the cell membrane   obstructed and water can seep
cell membrane structure   through the membrane to get
together   inside the cell

FIGURE 8.1 The bilayer membrane in two different states, hydrated and dehydrated, demonstrating the separation of the two layers when water gets in between and establishes a lateral diffusion pressure that helps in the enzyme–substrate actions. In a dehydrated state this ability is compromised.

In early dehydration, the rate of water diffusion through the cell membrane diminishes. When the rate of direct diffusion of water into the cells of the body diminishes and becomes insufficient for adequate hydration of cells in the body, an alternate system is used. The backup mechanism depends on the delivery of water through special channels, called aquaporins. Aquaporins only allow water molecules to enter in a single file, without the ionic load. It resembles a reverse osmosis system.[11,12] Vasopressin has been shown to activate some of these water channels.[12] This suggests that by the time thirst is experienced, cellular hydration is already compromised.

HOW DEHYDRATION MAY CONTRIBUTE TO KNEE OSTEOARTHRITIS

Although the bone tissue is amply supplied with small blood vessels that are situated under the periosteum, the main circulation to the long bones of the body is restricted to only one medullary or nutrient artery. Accompanied by one or two veins, the artery passes through the foramen, mostly situated in the center of the shaft of the bones. Flat bones have more than one artery and vein that maintain blood circulation to the bone.

The cartilage tissue that is attached at its base to the bones within the joints of the body need to be fully hydrated to act as an effective shock absorber and to

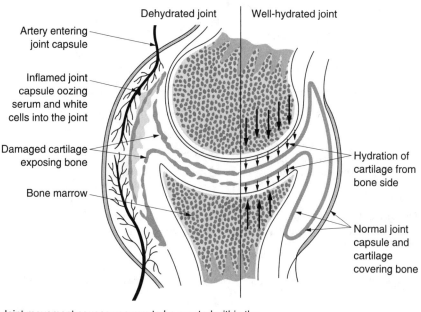

Dehydrated joint | Well-hydrated joint

Artery entering joint capsule

Inflamed joint capsule oozing serum and white cells into the joint

Damaged cartilage exposing bone

Bone marrow

Hydration of cartilage from bone side

Normal joint capsule and cartilage covering bone

Joint movement causes vacuum to be created within the joint space. Water will be pulled through the bone and the cartilage into the joint cavity, if it is freely available.

FIGURE 8.2 Model of a hydrated joint against a dehydrated joint; the direction of water and nutrient flow in the hydrated joint and the inflammatory capsule of a dehydrated joint when water and nutrient diffusion through the bone heads is reduced.

be able to facilitate low-friction movement of the joint. Cartilage receives nutrients by diffusion through the cancellous end of the bones they attach. See Figure 8.2. Serum diffusion to the cartilage and the joint is facilitated by the suction property of vacuum, and is instantly established when the joint is fully flexed or extended.

In a dehydrated state of the body and because of the restrictive cuff quality of the arterial foramen in the bone, the blood vessels are unable to dilate to facilitate the added rate of serum diffusion to the joint and its cartilaginous linings. As a means of indirect compensation, the blood vessels to the capsule of the joint dilate. An inflammatory process — with associated pain — establishes and some serum diffuses through the synovial membrane into the inflamed joint as shown in Figure 8.2.

The knee joint is particularly vulnerable to the inflammatory process associated with dehydration. Nutrient arteries are directed away from the knee; upward in the femur and downward in the tibia and fibula.[13] The reason for the development of the arteries pointing away from the knee joint is to service the earlier fusion of the epiphyses distal to the knee joint. This anatomic anomaly leaves the

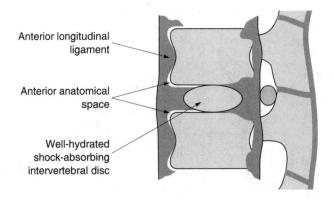

Anterior longitudinal
ligament

Anterior anatomical
space

Well-hydrated
shock-absorbing
intervertebral disc

FIGURE 8.3 The anatomical design of the vertebral column highlighting the anatomical space and its relationship to the intervertebral disc in the vertebral column.

knee joint most vulnerable in later years of life when gradual dehydration reduces the rate of blood flow to the bones.

HOW DEHYDRATION MAY EXACERBATE BACK PAIN

Vertebral discs support the weight of the upper body. Anatomically, the entire weight of the torso rests on the fifth lumbar disc, a common location for osteoarthritis. The discs are composed of the nucleus pulposus and the annulus fibrosis. The nucleus pulposus consists of 88% water and is held in position by the annulus fibrosis. The annulus is a very strong fibrous structure that attaches itself at the back to the edge of the vertebrae above and below and also the posterior longitudinal ligament. In front, it connects to the anterior longitudinal ligament that attaches to the center of the body of the vertebrae above and below. See Figure 8.3. By not attaching itself to the lip of the vertebrae in front, an anatomical space is created between the ligament, the disc, and the vertebrae above and below.

The role of this anatomical space in the design of the spinal column has not been fully explained in the medical literature. Most posit that the anatomical space vacuum-packs the entire structure of the column and all that it holds together. By creating vacuum when the spine moves into extension, water and its solutes are encouraged to diffuse into the space and hydrate the disc core and its fibrous attachments. When lubricated, the disc moves into the center of the cartilaginous endplates on the surface of the vertebrae above and below. The anatomical space increases the flexibility of the spine and gives it freedom of motion.

In dehydration, the discs begin to lose substance and become less effective as wedges between the vertebrae. Normally, they would keep the body upright with minimal muscle activity. But in their dehydrated state, the back muscles are forced to work constantly to stop the body from falling forward. The center of gravity of the body is normally in front, around the longitudinal arch of the foot. Thus, foot pain and back pain from the spasm of the back muscles might herald dehydration of the body in its spinal column. When patients are hydrated, exercises that create intermittent vacuum in the disc spaces augment treatment for low back pain.[3,14]

HOW WATER REDUCES FOOD INTAKE

Water adds volume to food without adding calories. Rolls demonstrated that the volume of liquid foods influences appetite more than does the food's energy density (calories).[15–17] When food is hydrated, fewer calories are required to satisfy subjective perceptions and stretch the gastrointestinal tract to release gut satiety peptides. The result is that foods with high water content are less likely to be overconsumed. Conversely, dried foods promote portion distortion.

Rolls' research additionally suggests the possibility that food is eaten, in part, to satisfy thirst. To further this speculation, it is interesting to note that hunger and satiety signals are colocated in the brain. The paraventricular nucleus, which is central to satiety signaling, also releases vasopressin to signal thirst.[18] Furthermore, Chapter 13 details how the neurotransmitters histamine and serotonin communicate hunger. Dr. Batmanghelidj theorizes similar roles for histamine and serotonin in the thirst mechanism.[3]

HOW TO PUT HYDRATION INTO PRACTICE

While much remains to be learned about water's diverse roles in human physiology, the practical applications are well demonstrated. Not only does adequate hydration prevent injuries, it also enhances performance.[19] Garite reasoned that research on hydration for sports performance could be applied to childbirth. He demonstrated that doubling the intravenous fluid rate reduced labor time and the need for oxytocin.[20]

The following are practical considerations for oral hydration. Filtered water is the recommended form of water. While boiling water can destroy microbes, metal toxins become concentrated as water evaporates with boiling. Bottled water can be a visual cue to drink before becoming thirsty. There are two disadvantages of bottled water. Plastic bottles can break down upon exposure to intense heat and release xenobiotics into the water. Bottled water is also a risk factor for campylobacter infection, a cause of infectious diarrhea.[21]

When appreciable amounts of water are lost from perspiration, such as during hot climates, athletic events, and sauna use, electrolytes should be replaced. Adding a pinch of sea salt to a glass of water reduces the risk of hyponatremia. Sodium is needed to absorb water from the gastrointestinal tract. Carbohydrate helps sodium cotransport water into cells. Only a little carbohydrate is needed.

A 15% carbohydrate solution had no added benefit on hydration over a 2% carbohydrate solution.[22] Rice powder may be a more effective carbohydrate than glucose in rehydration.[23] The amino acids glycine, alanine, and glutamine and various cereal powders can also promote rehydration, but not more effectively than glucose.[23] For athletes there is no advantage of intravenous hydration over oral hydration.[24] In extreme cold environments, loading the body with a hyperosmolar solution of glycerol may impart a hydration advantage.[25] A rationale for magnesium supplementation to replace sweat loss is presented by Dr. Burford-Mason in Chapter 9.

Overhydration can occur from inadequate sodium intake and intake of too much water, especially when cell membrane permeability is compromised. Hyponatremia can result in death in an otherwise healthy individual. Incidence of dilutional hyponatremia among athletes was underscored by a study conducted at the 2002 Boston Marathon, where 13% of studied participants had hyponatremia and 0.6% had a critically low serum sodium of 120 mmol/l or less.[26] Risk factors included a race time of more than 4 hours and body mass index extremes.

An individual's water needs vary with stress and with sweat, urinary, and respiratory losses. Cold climates, high altitude, and temperature-controlled indoor air generally increase water needs. Urine color can be a useful indicator, with pale, almost clear urine indicating adequate hydration. A urine dipstick can quantify osmolality. A summary message to convey to patients is, "Drink water before becoming thirsty."

REFERENCES

1. Phillips, P.A. et al., Reduced thirst after water deprivation in healthy elderly men, *N. Engl. J. Med.*, 311, 753–759, 1984.
2. Bruce, A. et al., Body composition. Prediction of normal body potassium, body water and body fat in adults on the basis of body height, body weight and age, *Scand. J. Clin. Lab. Invest.*, 40, 461–473, 1980.
3. Batmanghelidj, F., *Water for Health, for Healing, for Life*, Warner Books, New York, NY, 2003.
4. Batmanghelidj, F., *Your Body's Many Cries for Water*, Global Health Solutions, 1997.
5. Guyton, A., Contraction of skeletal muscle, in *Textbook of Physiology*, W.B. Saunders, Philadelphia, 1991, p. 68.
6. Livingston, E.H. and Kohlstadt, I., Simplified RMR predicting formulas for normal sized and obese individuals, *Obes. Res.*, 13 (7): 1255–62, 2005.
7. Itoh, Y. et al., Clinical and experimental evidence for prevention of acute renal failure induced by radiographic contrast media, *J. Pharmacol. Sci.*, 97, 473–488, 2005.
8. Lotz, J.C. et al., Compression-induced degeneration of the intervertebral disc: an in vivo mouse model and finite-element study, *Spine*, 23, 2493–506, 1998.
9. Watterson, J.G., The role of water in cell architecture, *Mol. Cell. Biochem.*, 79, 101–105, 1988.
10. Katchalski-Katzir, E., Conformational changes in biological macromolecules, *Biorheology*, 21, 57–74, 1984.

11. Agre, P. et al., Aquaporin water channels — from atomic structure to clinical medicine, *J. Physiol.*, 542 (Pt 1), 3–16, 2002.

12. Stoenoiu, M.S. et al., Corticosteroids induce expression of aquaporin-1 and increase transcellular water transport in rat peritoneum, *J. Am. Soc. Nephrol.*, 14, 555–565, 2003.

13. Gray, H. et al., *Gray's Anatomy*, 29th ed., Lea & Febiger, Philadelphia, pp. 276, 282.

14. Long, A., Donelson, R., and Fung, T., Does it matter which exercise? A randomized control trial of exercise for low back pain, *Spine*, 29, 2593–2602, 2004.

15. Bell, E.A., Roe, L.S., and Rolls, B.J., Sensory-specific satiety is affected more by volume than by energy content of a liquid food, *Physiol. Behav.*, 78, 593–600, 2003.

16. Rolls, B.J., Drewnowski, A., and Ledikwe, J.H., Changing the energy density of the diet as a strategy for weight management. *J. Am. Diet. Assoc.*, 105 (Pt 2), 98–103, 2005.

17. Kral, T.V. and Rolls, B.J., Energy density and portion size: their independent and combined effects on energy intake, *Physiol. Behav.*, 82, 131–138, 2004.

18. Phillips, P.A. et al., Osmotic thirst and vasopressin release in humans: a double-blind crossover study, *Am. J. Physiol.*, 248 (Pt 2), R645–R650, 1985.

19. Bilzon, J.L., Allsopp, A.J., and Williams, C. Short-term recovery from prolonged constant pace running in a warm environment: the effectiveness of a carbohydrate-electrolyte solution, *Eur. J. Appl. Physiol.*, 82, 305–312, 2000.

20. Garite, T.J. et al., A randomized controlled trial of the effect of increased intravenous hydration on the course of labor in nulliparous women, *Am. J. Obstet. Gynecol.*, 183, 1544–1548, 2000.

21. Evans, M.R., Ribeiro, C.D., and Salmon, R.L., Hazards of healthy living: bottled water and salad vegetables as risk factors for *Campylobacter* infection, *Emerg. Infect. Dis.*, 9, 1219–1225, 2003.

22. Galloway, S.D., Dehydration, rehydration, and exercise in the heat: rehydration strategies for athletic competition, *Can. J. Appl. Physiol.*, 24, 188–200, 1999.

23. Duggan, C. et al., Scientific rationale for a change in the composition of oral rehydration solution, *J. Am. Med. Assoc.*, 291, 2628–2631, 2004.

24. Casa, D.J. et al., Intravenous versus oral rehydration during a brief period: stress hormone responses to subsequent exhaustive exercise in the heat, *Int. J. Sport Nutr. Exerc. Metab.*, 10, 361–374, 2000.

25. O'Brien, C. et al., Glycerol hyperhydration: physiological responses during cold air exposure, *J. Appl. Physiol.*, 99 (2): 515–21, 2005.

26. Almond, C.S. et al., Hyponatremia among runners in the Boston Marathon, *N. Engl. J. Med.*, 352, 1550–1556, 2005.

9 Magnesium

Aileen P. Burford-Mason, Ph.D.

CONTENTS

INTRODUCTION

Magnesium is the fourth most abundant mineral in the body and, after potassium, the second most plentiful intracellular cation. Intimately involved in multiple aspects of metabolism, magnesium is a required cofactor for over 300 regulatory enzymes.[1] Besides its requirement for specific enzymes, magnesium is involved indirectly in all enzymatic processes, as adenosine triphosphate (ATP) must be complexed to magnesium to be metabolically available.[2] Magnesium is required for carbohydrate, fat, and protein ultilization.[3,4] During cell replication, magnesium is required to maintain an adequate supply of purine and pyrimidine nucleotides necessary for DNA and RNA production.[4] Virtually all hormonal reactions are magnesium dependent.[5] Through its association with sodium, potassium, and calcium, magnesium is closely involved in maintaining cellular electrolyte balance and adequate amounts of magnesium are needed to maintain normal levels of potassium.[5] It is required to maintain voltages across cell membranes and for the transfer of electrical impulses in neurons and muscle cells.[6]

MAGNESIUM REQUIREMENTS

Total body content of magnesium is about 25 g. Approximately 50 to 60% is found in bone, and 30 to 40% is intracellular, found mainly in muscle cells. Extracellular magnesium accounts for only about 1% of total body magnesium. Of the magnesium present in bone, one-half is exchangeable and serves as a reservoir from which magnesium can be withdrawn to maintain normal extracellular magnesium concentrations.[1] The remainder is tightly bound in the bone matrix.

The recommended daily allowance (RDA) for magnesium varies with age, pregnancy, and lactation.[1] For women over 30 years of age, the RDA is 320 mg, with pregnancy increasing the requirements to 400 mg, and lactation to 360 mg. The RDA for men older than 30 is 420 mg. However, some experts believe that the RDA underestimates daily needs and a range of 500 to 750 mg has been suggested as more realistic.[7] Magnesium-rich foods include nuts, beans, avocado, whole-grain cereals, cocoa, and seafood. Refining or processing of food generally results in reduced magnesium content, and as processed foods have risen in Western diets, daily intake of magnesium has dropped.[1]

Water has historically made an important but variable contribution to magnesium intake depending on the hardness of the water in a particular region.[1,2] In many urban areas, water is softened, thus removing magnesium as well as other minerals.[1,2] A recent estimate of magnesium intake in a national sample of U.S. adults has confirmed that both men and women generally fail to meet the recommended daily intake,[8] and large numbers of individuals are thought to be at risk for magnesium deficiency. In one study, 39% of American women between 15 and 50 years of age had magnesium intakes less than 70% of the RDA.[9]

Since magnesium regulates skeletal, cardiac, and smooth muscle contraction, magnesium depletion has been shown to result in hypertension, as well as coronary and cerebral vasospasm.[10] Because of its potential to inhibit calcium influx into cells, magnesium has been dubbed "nature's physiological calcium channel blocker."[11] Conditions where magnesium deficiency may be an important contributing factor include cardiovascular disease, diabetes, depression, migraine and tension headaches, eclampsia, and asthma.[1,2]

MAGNESIUM AND MUSCULOSKELETAL HEALTH

Owing to its regulatory role in energy production, in the biosynthesis of catecholamines and other neurotransmitters needed for neuromuscular activity, as well as neurological excitability, muscle relaxation after contraction, and bone metabolism, magnesium is considered to play a key role in musculoskeletal functioning and health.[12] Deficiency of magnesium results in hypocalcemia, primarily through impaired secretion of parathyroid hormone required for normal calcium homeostasis.[13] In animal studies, magnesium has been shown to affect bone characteristics, promoting bone formation, preventing bone resorption, and increasing the dynamic strength of the bone.[14] Deficiency has therefore been implicated in the development of osteoporosis.[13,15] Several population studies have demonstrated a positive association between magnesium intake and bone mineral density. Data from the Framingham Heart Study show that magnesium intake positively correlates with hip bone mineral density in both men and women.[15] Oral administration of magnesium as the sole treatment in postmenopausal osteoporosis has been shown to increase bone density.[16]

Poor magnesium status has been implicated in the arthralgias and the myalgias characteristic of conditions like fibromyalgia[17] and chronic fatigue syndrome.[18] The muscle pains, weakness, and cognitive impairment of fibromyalgia have been shown in human studies to associate with elevated levels of inflammatory cytokines, particularly those that promote hyperalgesia, fatigue, depression, and pain.[19] The expression of these inflammatory molecules is in turn thought to be due to an initial release of substance P, a neurotransmitter involved in the transmission of pain impulses from the peripheral receptors to the central nervous system.[19]

A central role for magnesium has been hypothesized in this cascade of events: when normal mice were fed a magnesium-deficient diet, an early (day 5) increase in substance P was observed. This was followed after 3 weeks by dramatically increased serum levels of several inflammatory cytokines, including interleukin-1, interleukin-6, and tumor necrosis factor-α.[20] Magnesium deficiency may therefore play a role in the initiation or perpetuation of musculoskeletal disorders like fibromyalgia or chronic fatigue. Patients with both the conditions have been shown to benefit from magnesium supplementation.[18,21]

Confirmation of an important role for magnesium in musculoskeletal functioning comes from studying patients with the genetic disorder Gitelman's syndrome (GS). GS is usually identified in children and is characterized by significant hypomagnesemia, low urinary output of calcium, and intermittent episodes of muscle weakness and tetany.[22] Although usually considered a mild disorder, studies have shown that a high proportion of adult patients with molecularly identified GS suffer from cramps, muscle aches, as well as fatigue, dizziness, and generalized weakness[22] — a clinical picture reminiscent of fibromyalgia.

MAGNESIUM HOMEOSTASIS

The concentration of magnesium in serum is maintained within a narrow range by the small intestine and the kidney. When dietary intake is high, excretion of magnesium via the kidneys increases. Conversely, when intake falls, the small intestine and kidney both increase their fractional magnesium absorption.[23] If magnesium depletion continues, bone stores help to maintain serum magnesium concentration by exchanging part of their content with extracellular fluid.[24]

This ability of the gastrointestinal tract and the kidneys to regulate magnesium homeostasis is affected by the health of both organs. Inflammatory bowel disease limits the capacity to absorb magnesium, resulting in lower body stores.[24] After surgical resection both urinary magnesium excretion and muscle magnesium content have been shown to decrease in parallel with increasing resection length, and muscle fatigue — an early sign of magnesium deficiency — has been shown to be associated with low muscle magnesium concentration not detected by determination of the serum magnesium.[25] Although a greater or a lesser effect on magnesium nutriture might be expected after bariatric surgery for morbid obesity, depending on the length of intestine that is bypassed, this possibility has received surprisingly little attention. But with the current increase in the number of bariatric procedures being performed complications related to hypomagnesemia are likely to emerge. There are reports of postbariatric surgery Wernicke's encephalopathy, a neurologic disorder of acute onset caused by a thiamine deficiency, which sometimes does not respond to thiamine administration.[26] Magnesium is required for the phosphorylation of thiamine to the coenzyme form thiamine pyrophosphate, which in turn is involved in the pentose–phosphate pathway (transketolase) and the tricarboxylic acid cycle. Wernicke's encephalopathy refractory to thiamine administration has been shown to respond to magnesium.[27]

Chronic diarrhea and vomiting may also result in magnesium deficiency.[24] Polyuria associated with poorly controlled diabetes causes depletion of magnesium stores, as does excessive alcohol intake.[28,29] Because calcium competes for absorption with magnesium, excessive calcium intake, either from foods or from supplements, can lead to magnesium deficiency.[30] An extensive range of commonly used medications have been shown to trigger magnesium depletion, including diuretics, birth control pills and hormone replacement, cancer chemotherapy, corticosteroids, some antibiotics, insulin, and painkillers.[1,23]

In animal studies, increased exposure to heavy metals, such as lead and cadmium, decreases blood and organ magnesium accumulation and increases urinary magnesium excretion. This observation has important implications for heavy-metal detoxification, since the reaction appears to be reversible: increasing animals' magnesium intake after exposure to lead and cadmium leads to increased urinary elimination of both metals.[31] In lead-intoxicated animals, high-dose oral magnesium supplementation was comparable to intravenous EDTA-chelation therapy.[32] In human studies, magnesium nutriture has been shown to modify the response of children to industrial pollution. Blood and urine levels of cadmium were compared in children from areas of high and low heavy-metal pollution, and found to be inversely correlated with urine magnesium rather than the level of pollution to which the children were exposed.[33]

DIET AND MAGNESIUM STATUS

Refining grains depletes them of magnesium. Although refined cereal products are frequently enriched with iron and calcium removed in processing, the magnesium content is not replenished. In the short term, a diet high in starchy or sugary foods alters the way the body handles magnesium, resulting in excessive urinary magnesium loss.[34] In the long term, such a diet predisposes to the development of insulin resistance. Insulin is required to shift magnesium from the extracellular to the intracellular space, and thus insulin resistance will result in a reduced capacity for tissue magnesium accretion and storage.[34]

Absorption of magnesium is dependent on several elements of diet other than magnesium content. Diets containing both less than 30 g of protein per day or more than 90 g/d appear to reduce intestinal magnesium absorption.[1] Magnesium forms insoluble soaps with fatty acids in the intestine, which, although beneficial in inhibiting the absorption of dietary fat, also decreases magnesium availability.[35] Phosphoric acid in carbonated beverages inhibits absorption by binding to magnesium in the bowel.[36] Nondigestible plant fibers significantly impact magnesium status: cereal and legumes are rich in phytates, which reduce absorption of minerals, including magnesium.[37] On the other hand, fermentable fibers from fruits and vegetables, such as fructo-oligosaccharides (FOS), can enhance magnesium absorption.[38] FOS appears to enhance magnesium absorption preferentially, while not consistently affecting absorption of the other minerals.[38]

NONDIETARY FACTORS AND MAGNESIUM STATUS

Exercise, particularly if it is intense or prolonged, may affect magnesium status.[39,40] During endurance exercise, serum and urinary magnesium concentrations decrease, although calcium status appears to be unaffected. This is thought to result from increased demand for magnesium by skeletal muscle under conditions of sustained exertion.[39,40] Sweat also has to be considered as a potential avenue for exercise-induced magnesium loss, especially when performed at high temperatures.[41] One study found that men subjected to controlled exercise in heat (8 h on ergocycles at 100°F) lost 15.2 to 17.8 mg/d in sweat, which represented 4 to 5% of total daily magnesium intake. Magnesium losses through exertion and sweat may contribute to the development of exercise-induced wheezing or asthma. In epidemiological studies, the general decline in respiratory function has been linked to declining intakes of magnesium as well as vitamin C.[42]

Intravenous magnesium sulfate is known to be effective and safe as an adjuvant treatment for acute brochocospasm in asthmatic patients.[43] A role for magnesium in the treatment and prevention of exercise-induced wheezing or asthma might therefore be implied. However, only a few studies have attempted to investigate magnesium status in this patient population. In one small study (13 children aged 6–13 years), the ability of inhaled magnesium sulfate to enhance the efficacy of salbutamol on exercise-induced asthma was studied.[44] Patients performed a 6 min running test on three separate days. In six of the 13 patients, pretreatment with magnesium prevented FEV1 decreases greater than 20%, with the combination of salbutamol and magnesium showing better protection than either agent used alone. The authors concluded that $MgSO_4$ inhalation could be a useful prophylaxis against exercise-induced bronchoconstriction. Stress, whether physical (i.e., exercise), medical (i.e., surgery and drugs), environmental (i.e., noise and pollution), or emotional (i.e., excitement and depression) changes magnesium homeostasis and increases urinary magnesium losses.[45,46] For example, even short-term exposure to excessive noise rapidly induces increased renal magnesium output, which is thought to contribute to the hearing loss associated with noise exposure.[47] Magnesium treatment has been shown to reduce both temporary and permanent noise-induced hearing loss.[48] In animal models, noise exposure has been shown to alter the magnesium content of myocardium, especially in animals with suboptimal magnesium intakes, suggesting that this may be an explanation for the known association between chronic noise exposure and cardiovascular disease.[49] The impact of hypomagnesemia on postoperative outcome is well established, and the use of magnesium therapy in the perioperative period is increasing because of its beneficial effects on cardiac function and rhythm, muscle strength, vascular tone, and the central nervous system. In older patients undergoing hip surgery magnesium depletion was associated with repetitive ventricular arrhythmias.[50] Table 9.1 shows the various types of stressors that have been shown to affect magnesium status.

Apart from GS, an autosomal recessive disorder, several other genetic magnesium-wasting syndromes have been identified.[61] Intestinal magnesium wasting is associated with the *TRPM6* gene, which encodes an apical epithelial magnesium-conducting channel expressed in the intestine and in the kidney. Intra- and extracellular magnesium levels are associated with the major histocompatibility

TABLE 9.1
Physical, medical, environmental, and psychological stressors known to affect magnesium status

	Stressor	Ref.
Physical	Exercise and exertion	39, 40
	Heat and cold	2, 51, 52
	Sleep deprivation	53, 54
	Pain	55
	Childbirth	56
Medical	Trauma	2, 57
	Burns	57, 58
	Surgery	2, 4
	Infection	57, 60
	Drugs	1, 23
Environmental	Noise	47–49
	Pollution	59
	Allergy	60
Psychological	Anxiety	45, 46
	Depression	45, 46
	Examination stress	54
	Excitement	45, 46

complex (HLA). Individuals possessing HLA B35 genes have higher red cell and plasma magnesium, and HLA-B38 positive individuals have lower levels compared to noncarriers of either gene.[62] In GS, multiple mutations in the *SLC12A3* gene, which encodes the thiazide-sensitive sodium chloride cotransporter, have been identified.[61]

CALCIUM AND MAGNESIUM BALANCE

An aspect of magnesium nutrition, which has received relatively little attention, and which is likely to be of significance not only for musculoskeletal health but also for other apparently unrelated health conditions, including heart disease and stroke, and respiratory health is the maintenance of the balance between calcium and magnesium. Intracellular calcium concentrations regulate muscle contraction, including skeletal, cardiac, and smooth muscle. Rising concentration of free calcium causes muscle fibers to contract, and removal of calcium back into intracellular storage sites (sarcoplasmic reticulum) or out of the cell is necessary for depolarization to occur and for the muscle to return to a relaxed phase.[63] This removal of calcium to the external cellular environment is a magnesium-dependent mechanism: high levels of ATP in the form of a magnesium complex (MgATP) are required.[1,2] Deficiency of magnesium relative to calcium may therefore result in sustained contraction of muscle cells, which may be central to the development of many of the signs and symptoms of magnesium deficiency.[63] In addition to its action on muscle fiber, magnesium deficiency will affect innervation of muscle, since increased intracellular calcium influx results in neuronal hyperexcitability, and therefore will contribute to muscle hypertonicity.[1,2]

This requirement for calcium and magnesium to be in balance may explain some of the anomalies seen with the intraoperative use of high-dose magnesium infusions. Although the use of supraphysiological magnesium infusions has been shown to decrease the incidence of ventricular fibrillation in surgical patients and in enclampsia, it is also associated with an excess of cardiogenic shock and heart failure.[6] However, an excess of magnesium beyond physiological requirements for efficient smooth muscle contraction and relaxation might be expected to cause problems, since magnesium acts as a calcium antagonist by inhibiting the cellular uptake of calcium. Calcium blockade by pharmaceutical agents has been shown to increase the risk of heart failure.[64] In the case of elective surgery, therefore, oral magnesium supplementation using the methods described later in this chapter may be an alternative and safer approach.

DIET AND CALCIUM–MAGNESIUM BALANCE

A dramatic shift in calcium to magnesium balance, with potential implications for musculoskeletal health, may be seen in modern diets. Although basic physiological needs for essential nutrients have remained largely unchanged since prehistoric times, diets have become progressively more divergent from the diets of our ancient ancestors, and health may have suffered in the transition.[65] Two modern dietary patterns have been identified.[66] One, the most common in Western societies, is high in red meat, fried potatoes, high-fat dairy products, refined grains, and sweets and desserts. The other is based mainly on vegetables, fish, fruit, poultry, and whole grains. Popularly referred to as the urban caveman diet, the latter most closely approximates to a hunter-gatherer or Paleolithic diet.[65] Large cohort studies have shown that the urban caveman diet offers greater protection from degenerative diseases compared with diets conforming to the current healthy eating dietary guidelines.[66] Table 9.2 shows the balance of calcium to magnesium in a prototype urban caveman diet compared to a more typical Western diet. As can be seen, there is a dramatic difference in the calcium to magnesium ratio between the two diets.

TABLE 9.2
Comparison of calcium to magnesium balance in two compendium diets

Diet 1: hunter-gatherer prototype	Calcium to magnesium ratio (mg/100 g food)	Diet 2: typical Western diet	Calcium to magnesium ratio (mg/100 g food)
Whole wheat	0.4:1.0	Bagel (white)	2.0:1.0
Oats	0.4:1.0	Pancakes	4.0:1.0
Wild rice	0.2:1.0	Doughnut	1.8:1.0
Blueberries	1.2:1.0	Cookies	13:1.0
Cranberries	1.4:1.0	Blueberry muffin	3.1:1.0
Apples	1.4:1.0	White rice	3.6:1.0
Hazelnuts	1.1:1.0	Macaroni	0.4:1.0
Walnuts	0.8:1.0	Eggs	4.6:1.0
Eggs	4.6:1.0	Chicken breast	0.5:1.0
Venison	0.3:1.0	Hamburger	0.5:1.0
Pheasant	0.6:1.0	French fries	0.2:1.0
Salmon	0.3:1.0	Onions	2.5:1.0
Trout	1.9:1.0	Orange juice	1.0:1.0
Oysters	0.8:1.0	Ice cream	4.0:1.0
Shrimp	1.4:1.0	Milk	7.0:1.0
Spinach	1.4:1	Yogurt (plain)	11.0:1.0
Turnip	2.0:1.0	Cheese (hard)	26.0:1.0
Average	1.3:1.0 Ca/Mg	Average	4.95:1 Ca/Mg

Note: Diet 1 represents a modern day version of a hunter-gatherer diet, high in lean protein, essential fats, and unrefined carbohydrates. It would achieve a calcium to magnesium balance of 1.3:1. Diet 2 represents a typical Western diet, high in refined food and dairy products and low in vegetables. There is a dramatic shift in the calcium to magnesium balance, which is approximately 5:1 calcium to magnesium.

Source: USDA food database, www.nal.usda.gov (accessed Jan. 2005).

One of the central benefits of a hunter-gatherer style diet may therefore be that it shifts the calcium to magnesium balance to one that is more compatible with cardiovascular and musculoskeletal physiology. The higher calcium to magnesium ratio observed in the Western diet would favor an elevation of intracellular free calcium and deficiency of intracellular free magnesium. This would increase the threshold for skeletal, cardiac, and vascular smooth muscle contractility.[67] In vascular smooth muscle, this has been shown to cause vasoconstriction and increase blood pressure, and in heart muscle it increases contractility, predisposing to left ventricular heart failure.[67] Deficiency of magnesium relative to calcium in skeletal muscle would predispose to symptoms similar to those seen in GS, such as tetany, muscle cramps, and painful spasms.[22] It may also manifest itself as fibromyalgia, chronic fatigue syndrome, and repetitive strain injury.

IDENTIFICATION OF MAGNESIUM DEFICITS

Because magnesium moves between compartments and across membranes, laboratory assessment of magnesium status is notoriously difficult.[68] A drop in serum magnesium is quickly normalized from bone or intracellular stores. Therefore, serum or plasma magnesium is not a reliable indicator of magnesium status. Depletion of muscle magnesium has been shown in the presence of normal plasma, red blood cell, or mononuclear blood cell magnesium concentrations.[68,69] Recently, intracellular ionized magnesium measured in sublingual epithelial cells has been promoted as a reliable marker of tissue magnesium stores.[70] Sublingual epithelial cells are thought to approximate tissue stores because of their rapid turnover time (<3 days), and are easy to access. In cardiac patients undergoing bypass surgery, magnesium was lower in such cells compared to healthy controls, where no difference in serum measurements was observed. Magnesium content of sublingual cells correlated well with atrial biopsy specimens taken from the same patients during surgery.[70] However, the test is not routinely available, and as yet there are no published data to support the reliability of the test in less seriously ill patients.

A functional approach, using clinical evidence of calcium–magnesium imbalance as an indicator of magnesium inadequacy is a simple way to assess magnesium nutrition in individual subjects. Musculoskeletal markers of calcium–magnesium imbalance include muscle cramps, spasms, fasciculations, and restless leg syndrome.[71] Confirmatory evidence of an imbalance can be ascertained from the evidence of cardiovascular and smooth muscle cell malfunctioning (Table 9.2). Correction of musculoskeletal and other symptomatology, such as constipation, by physiological oral magnesium supplementation is the best proof that magnesium deficiency was the cause of these symptoms.

MAGNESIUM SUPPLEMENTS

Dietary intake of magnesium can be addressed through the adoption of diet one (Table 9.1). However, where significant amounts of dairy products or calcium supplements are consumed, additional magnesium supplements are usually needed. Except in the case of overt renal failure, where they are contraindicated, oral supplementation with magnesium salts may be the most effective way to improve magnesium status.[71]

Although results from clinical trials have been variable, magnesium supplementation has been shown to benefit many conditions, where magnesium deficits are thought to play a role. It can reduce blood pressure in a dose-dependent manner.[72] It can also reduce leg cramping during pregnancy[73] and in nonpregnant chronic nocturnal cramp sufferers.[74] Even the muscle weakness, asthenia, leg cramps, and tetany associated with genetic magnesium wasting syndromes may respond positively to oral supplementation.[75] In patients with cardiovascular disease, 365 mg magnesium citrate daily for 6 months improved exercise tolerance, diminished exercise-induced chest pain, and improved the quality of life as measured by standard quality-of-life questionnaires.[76] In clinical trials not showing benefit, failure to control for variables such as diet, stress, medications, and supplemental calcium are thought to have confounded outcomes of the clinical trials, which show no benefit to supplemental magnesium.

Physiological oral magnesium supplementation of 5 mg/kg/day has been suggested as appropriate.[71] However, since magnesium needs vary considerably from one individual to another and even somewhat within the same individual depending on concomitant stress levels, diet and medication use, a standard dosing regime is not optimal. Magnesium dosage can be adjusted by titrating intake to bowel tolerance. Bowel tolerance draws on the observation that excess magnesium causes diarrhea and insufficient magnesium inhibits normal gastrointestinal peristalsis.[77] A very gradual increase in magnesium (every 3–4 days) and small incremental doses (50 mg magnesium glycinate/day) to generate 1–3 soft bowel movements daily gives the best results. It is important that the gastrointestinal capacity to absorb magnesium is not exceeded, as this will result in diarrhea which will in turn deplete magnesium stores. Evidence of adequate tissue stores is suggested by the absence of typical signs of calcium/magnesium imbalance suggested in Table 9.3.

Calcium and magnesium may be taken together, usually in divided daily doses at a 2:1 ratio. See Chapter 25. Additional magnesium may be supplemented to bowel tolerance.

The type of magnesium used is also important. Magnesium hydroxide has been used to treat constipation in geriatric patients with beneficial results, not only on bowel function but also on markers of lipid and carbohydrate metabolism, indicating a systemic as well as a laxative effect.[78] Magnesium oxide is also used for supplementation but, compared with the citrate salts of magnesium, is not well absorbed.[79] A major downside to magnesium citrate is that although well absorbed, it is rapidly eliminated by the kidney,[79] and may therefore not be the best form to use when tissue deficits need to be redressed. Recently, protein-bound forms of magnesium have been shown to be well absorbed and highly bioavailable.[80] Clinical experience suggests that amino acid chelates of

TABLE 9.3
Minor functional signs of magnesium deficits

System	Symptom
Musculoskeletal	Cramps
	Fasciculations
	Muscle tension
	Myalgias
	Restless leg syndrome
Cardiovascular	Arrhythmias
	Palpitations
Smooth muscle	Asthma or shortness of breath
	Constipation
	Frequency of urination
	Wheezing after exercise
	Vascular headache

Note: Such symptoms may be used to identify functional hypomagnemia and to monitor response to supplementation.

magnesium (glycinate, aspartate, and tartrate) offer the most consistent overall therapeutic effect.

CAUTION: EXCESS MAGNESIUM

No adverse effects have been reported for magnesium intakes from food.[1] Most reported adverse effects from nonfood sources have been with intravenous administration at supraphysiological doses, rather than physiological oral supplementation.[2,71] In patients with compromised renal function, however, oral supplements may result in hypermagnesemia, symptoms of which include lethargy, loss of deep tendon reflexes, difficulty in breathing, hypotension, bradycardia, and cardiac arrest.[81] Even in those with apparently normal kidney function, very large doses of magnesium-containing laxatives and antacids have occasionally been known to cause magnesium toxicity.[81] A case of hypermagnesemia has been reported in a 16-year-old girl after she decided to take an oral suspension of aluminum magnesia antacid every 2 h rather than as prescribed. After 3 days, she became unresponsive and lost deep tendon reflexes, but recovered after discontinuation of the antacid.[82] Excess magnesium and magnesium deficiency can be confused since both can cause mental status changes, nausea, and muscle weakness. Clinical symptoms of excess magnesium can be distinguished from those of magnesium deficiency by the accompanying diarrhea and abnormally low blood pressure.[77]

ACKNOWLEDGMENT

The author wishes to thank Linda Rapson, M.D., for helpful discussions in the preparation of this chapter.

REFERENCES

1. Dietary Reference Intakes, Calcium, Phosphorus, Magnesium, Vitamin D, and Fluoride, National Academy of Science, Institute of Medicine, Washington, DC, 1997.
2. Seelig, M. and Rosanoff, A., *The Magnesium Factor*, New York, Avery, 2003, pp. 153–175.
3. Garfinkel, L. and Garfinkel, D., Magnesium regulation of the glycolytic pathway and the enzymes involved, *Magnesium*, 4, 60–72, 1985.
4. Rubin, H., Central role for magnesium in coordinate control of metabolism and growth in animal cells, *Proc. Natl. Acad. Sci. USA*, 72, 3551–3555, 1975.
5. Gums, J.G., Magnesium in cardiovascular and other disorders, *Am. J. Health Syst. Pharm.*, 61, 1569–1576, 2004.
6. Perry, R.S. and Illsley, S.S. Basic cardiac electrophysiology and mechanisms of antiarrhythmic agents, *Am. J. Hosp. Pharm.*, 43, 957–974, 1986.
7. Littlefield, N.A. and Hass, B.S., Is the RDA for magnesium too low? *FDA Sci. Forum*, 1996 (Abstract # C-13).
8. Ford, E.S. and Mokdad, A.H. Dietary magnesium intake in a national sample of U.S. adults, *J. Nutr.*, 133, 2879–2882, 2003.
9. Sojka, J.E. and Weaver, C.M., Brief critical reviews: magnesium supplementation and osteoporosis, *Nutr. Rev.*, 53, 71–74, 1995.
10. Iannello, S. and Belfiore, F., Hypomagnesemia. A review of pathophysiological, clinical, and therapeutical aspects, *Panminerva Med.*, 43, 177–209, 2001.
11. Iseri, L.T. and French, J.H., Magnesium: nature's physiological calcium channel blocker, *Am. Heart J.*, 108, 188–193, 1984.
12. Laires, M.J., Monteiro, C.P., and Bicho, M., Role of cellular magnesium in health and human disease, *Front Biosci.*, 9, 262–276, 2004.
13. Rude, R.K., Magnesium deficiency: a cause of heterogeneous disease in humans, *J. Bone Miner. Res.*, 13, 749–758, 1998.
14. Stendig-Lindberg, G., Koeller, W., Bauer, A., and Rob, P.M., Prolonged magnesium deficiency causes osteoporosis in the rat, *J. Am. Coll. Nutr.*, 23, 704S–711S, 2004.
15. Tucker, K.L., Hannan, M.T., Chen, H., Cupples, L.A., Wilson, P.W., and Kiel, D.P., Potassium, magnesium, and fruit and vegetable intakes are associated with greater bone mineral density in elderly men and women, *Am. J. Clin. Nutr.*, 69, 727–736, 1999.
16. Sojka, J.E. and Weaver, C.M., Magnesium supplementation and osteoporosis, *Nutr. Rev.*, 53, 71–74, 1995.
17. Bates, D., Buchwald, D., and Dawson, D., Clinical laboratory test findings in chronic fatigue: red blood cell magnesium and chronic fatigue syndrome, *Lancet*, 337, 757–760, 1991.
18. Manuel y Keenoy, B., Moorkens, G., Vertommen, J., Noe, M., Neve, J., and De Leeuw, I., Magnesium status and parameters of the oxidant–antioxidant balance in

patients with chronic fatigue: effects of supplementation with magnesium, *J. Am. Coll. Nutr.*, 19, 374–382, 2000.

19. Wallace, D.J., Linker-Israeli, M., Hallegua, D., Silverman, S., Silver, D., and Weisman, M.H., Cytokines play an aetiopathogenetic role in fibromyalgia: a hypothesis and pilot study, *Rheumatology*, 40, 743–749, 2001.

20. Weglicki, W.B. and Phillips, T.M., Pathobiology of magnesium deficiency: a cytokine/neurogenic inflammation hypothesis, *Am. J. Physiol.*, 263, R734–R737, 1992.

21. Holdcraft, L.C., Assefi, N., and Buchwald, D., Complementary and alternative medicine in fibromyalgia and related syndromes, *Best Pract. Res. Clin. Rheumatol.*, 17, 667–683, 2003.

22. Cruz, D.N., Shaer, A.J., Bia, M.J., Lifton, R.P., and Simon, D.B., Gitelman's syndrome revisited: an evaluation of health-related problems and quality of life, *Kidney Int.*, 59, 710–717, 2001.

23. Pelton, R., Lavalle, J.B., Hawkins, E.B., and Krinsky, D., *Drug-induced nutrient depletion handbook*, 2nd ed., Lexi Comp Clinical Reference Library, San Diego, CA, 2001.

24. Rude, R.K., Magnesium deficiency: a cause of heterogeneous disease in humans, *J. Bone Miner. Res.*, 13, 749–758, 1998.

25. Hessov, I., Hasselblad, C., Fasth, S., and Hulten, L., Magnesium deficiency after ileal sesections for Crohn's disease, *Scand. J. Gastroenterol.*, 18, 643–669, 1983.

26. Salas-Salvado, J., Garcia-Lorda, P., Cuatrecasas, G., Bonada, A., Formiguera, X., Del Castillo, D., Hernandez, M., and Olive, J.M. Wernicke's syndrome after bariatric surgery, *Clin. Nutr.*, 19, 371–373, 2000.

27. Traviesa, D.C., Magnesium deficiency: a possible cause of thiamine refractoriness in Wernicke-Korsakoff encephalopathy, *J. Neurol. Neurosurg. Psychiatry*, 37, 959–962, 1974.

28. Papazachariou, I.M., Martinez-Isla, A., Efthimiou, E. et al., Magnesium deficiency in patients with chronic pancreatitis identified by an intravenous loading test, *Clin. Chim. Acta.*, 302, 145–154, 2000.

29. Campbell, R.K. and Nadler, J., Magnesium deficiency and diabetes, *Diab. Educ.*, 18, 17–19, 1992.

30. Celotti, F. and Bignamini, A., Dietary calcium and mineral/vitamin supplementation: a controversial problem, *J. Int. Med. Res.*, 27, 1–14, 1999.

31. Soldatovic, D., Matovic, V., Vujanovic, D., and Stojanovic, Z., Contribution to interaction between magnesium and toxic metals: the effect of prolonged cadmium intoxication on magnesium metabolism in rabbits, *Magnes. Res.*, 11, 283–288, 1998.

32. Soldatovic, D., Vujanovic, D., Matovic, V., and Plamenac, Z., Compared effects of high oral Mg supplements and of EDTA chelating agent on chronic lead intoxication in rabbits, *Magnes. Res.*, 10, 127–133, 1997.

33. Kobylec-Zamlynska, B., Zamlynski, J., Bodzek, P., Zmudzinska-Kitczak, J., and Binkiewicz, P., Environmental exposure to cadmium and level of magnesium in blood and urine of pre-school children from regions of different degree of pollution, *Ginekol. Pol.*, 69, 871–877, 1998 (in Polish; English summary).

34. Barbagallo, M., Dominguez, L.J., Galioto, A., Ferlisi, A., Cani, C., Malfa, L., Pineo, A., Busardo, A., and Paolisso, G., Role of magnesium in insulin action, diabetes, and cardio-metabolic syndrome X, *Mol. Aspects Med.*, 24, 39–52, 2003.

35. Vaskonen, T., Dietary minerals and modification of cardiovascular risk factors, *J. Nutr. Biochem.*, 14, 492–506, 2003.

36. Johnson, S., The multifaceted and widespread pathology of magnesium deficiency, *Med. Hypotheses*, 56, 163–170, 2001.

37. Hallberg, L., Brune, M., and Rossander, L., Iron absorption in man: ascorbic acid and dose-dependent inhibition by phytate, *Am. J. Clin. Nutr.*, 49, 140–144, 1989.

38. Coudray, C., Demigne, C., and Rayssiguier, Y., Effects of dietary fibers on magnesium absorption in animals and humans, *J. Nutr.*, 133, 1–4, 2003.

39. Bohl, C.H. and Volpe, S.L., Magnesium and exercise, *Crit. Rev. Food Sci. Nutr.*, 42, 533–563, 2002.

40. Buchman, A.L., Keen, C., Commisso, J., Killip, D., Ou, C.N., Rognerud, C.L., Dennis, K., and Dunn, J.K., The effect of a marathon run on plasma and urine mineral and metal concentrations, *J. Am. Coll. Nutr.*, 17, 124–127, 1998.

41. Consolazio, C.F., Nutrition and performance, in *Progress in Food and Nutrition Science*, Vol. 7, Johnson, R.E., Ed., Pergamon Press, Oxford, 1983, pp.1–187.

42. McKeever, T.M., Scrivener, S., Broadfield, E., Jones, Z., Britton, J., and Lewis, S.A., Prospective study of diet and decline in lung function in a general population, *Am. J. Respir. Crit. Care Med.*, 165, 1299–1303, 2002.

43. Alter, H.J., Koepsell, T.D., and Hilty, W.M., Intravenous magnesium as an adjuvant in acute bronchospasm: a meta-analysis, *Ann. Emerg. Med.*, 36, 191–197, 2000.

44. Manzke, H., Thiemeier, M., Elster, P., and Lemke, J., Magnesium sulfate as adjuvant in beta-2-sympathicomimetic inhalation therapy of bronchial asthma, *Pneumologie*, 44, 1190–1192, 1990 (in German; English summary).

45. Seelig, M.S., Consequences of magnesium deficiency on the enhancement of stress reactions; preventive and therapeutic implications (a review), *J. Am. Coll. Nutr.*, 13, 429–446, 1994.

46. Cernak, I., Savic, V., Kotur, J., Prokic, V., Kuljic, B., Grbovic, D., and Veljovic, M., Alterations in magnesium and oxidative status during chronic emotional stress, *Magnes. Res.*, 13, 29–36, 2000.

47. Attias, J., Sapir, S., Bresloff, I., Reshef-Haran, I., and Ising, H., Reduction in noise-induced temporary threshold shift in humans following oral magnesium intake, *Clin. Otolaryngol.*, 29, 635–641, 2004.

48. Nageris, B.I., Ulanovski, D., and Attias, J., Magnesium treatment for sudden hearing loss, *Ann. Otol. Rhinol. Laryngol.*, 113, 672–675, 2004.

49. Ising, H., Babisch, W., and Kruppa, B., Noise-induced endocrine effects and cardiovascular risk, *Noise Health*, 1, 37–48, 1999.

50. Zuccala, G., Pahor, M., Lattanzio, F., Vagnoni, S., Rodola, F., De Sole, P., Cittadini, A., Cocchi, A., and Bernabei, R., Detection of arrhythmogenic cellular magnesium depletion in hip surgery patients, *Br. J. Anaesth.*, 79, 776–781, 1997.

51. Stendig-Lindberg, G., Moran, D., and Shapiro, Y., How significant is magnesium in thermoregulation? *J. Basic. Clin. Physiol. Pharmacol.*, 9, 73–85, 1998.

52. Verde, T., Shephard, R.J., Corey, P., and Moore, R., Sweat composition in exercise and in heat, *J. Appl. Physiol.*, 53, 1540–1545, 1982.

53. Takase, B., Akima, T., Uehata, A., Ohsuzu, F., and Kurita, A., Effect of chronic stress and sleep deprivation on both flow-mediated dilation in the brachial artery and the intracellular magnesium level in humans, *Clin. Cardiol.*, 27, 223–227, 2004.

54. Takase, B., Akima, T., Uehata, A., Ohsuzu, F., and Kurita, A., Effect of chronic stress and sleep deprivation on both flow-mediated dilation in the brachial artery and the intracellular magnesium level in humans, *Clin. Cardiol.*, 27, 223–237, 2004.

55. Alloui, A., Begon, S., Chassaing, C., Eschalier, A., Gueux, E., Rayssiguier, Y., and Dubray, C., Does Mg2+ deficiency induce a long-term sensitization of the central nociceptive pathways? *Eur. J. Pharmacol.*, 469, 65–69, 2003.

56. Handwerker, S.M., Altura, B.T., Jones, K. et al. Maternal-fetal transfer of ionized serum magnesium during the stress of labor and delivery: a human study, *J. Am. Coll. Nutr.*, 1995, 14, 376–381.

57. Bergstrom, J.P., Larsson, J., Nordstrom, H. et al., Influence of injury and nutrition on muscle water and electrolytes: effects of severe injury, sepsis, and burns, Acta Chir. Scand., 153, 261–266, 1987.

58. Klein, G.L., Nicolai, M., Langman, C.B. et al., Dysregulation of calcium homeostasis after severe burn injury in children: possible role of magnesium depletion, *J. Pediatr.*, 131, 246–251, 1997.

59. Kobylec-Zamlynska, B., Zamlynski, J., Bodzek, P., Zmudzinska-Kitczak, J., and Binkiewicz, P., Environmental exposure to cadmium and level of magnesium in blood and urine of pre-school children form regions of different degree of pollution, *Ginekol. Pol.*, 69, 871–877, 1998 (in Polish; English summary).

60. Galland, L., Magnesium and immune function: an overview, *Magnesium*, 7, 290–299, 1988.

61. Knoers, N.V., deJong, J.C., Meij, I.C., Van Den Heuval, L.P., and Bindels, R.J., Genetic renal disorders with hypomagnesemia and hypocalcuria, *J. Nephrol.*, 16, 293–296, 2003.

62. Henrotte, J.G., Pla, M., and Dausset, J., HLA- and H-2-associated variations of intra- and extracellular magnesium content, *Proc. Natl. Acad. Sci. USA*, 87, 1894–1898, 1990.

63. Fauk, D., Fehlinger, R., Becker, R., Meyer, E., Kemnitz, C., Reichmuth, B., and Stephan, A., Transient cerebral ischaemic attacks and calcium-magnesium imbalance: clinical and paraclinical findings in 106 patients under 50 years of age, *Magnes. Res.*, 4: 53–58, 1991.

64. Opie, L.H., Calcium antagonists, ventricular arrhythmias, and sudden cardiac death: a major challenge for the future, *J. Cardiovasc. Pharmacol.*, 18, S81–S86, 1991.

65. O'Keefe, J.H., Jr. and Cordain, L., Cardiovascular disease resulting from a diet and lifestyle at odds with our Paleolithic genome: how to become a 21st-century hunter-gatherer, *Mayo. Clin. Proc.*, 79, 101–108, 2004.

66. McCullough, M.L., Feskanich, D., Stampfer, M.J., Giovannucci, E.L., Rimm, E.B., Hu, F.B., Spiegelman, D., Hunter, D.J., Colditz, G.A., and Willett, W.C., Diet quality and major chronic disease risk in men and women: moving toward improved dietary guidance, *Am. J. Clin. Nutr.*, 76, 1261–1271, 2002.

67. Resnick, L.M., Cellular calcium and magnesium metabolism in the pathophysiology and treatment of hypertension and related metabolic disorders, *Am. J. Med.*, 93, 11S–20S, 1992.

68. Dewitte, K., Stockl, D., Van de Velde, M., and Thienpont, L.M., Evaluation of intrinsic and routine quality of serum total magnesium measurement, *Clin. Chim. Acta.*, 292, 55–68, 2000.

69. Arnold, A., Tovey, J., Mangat, P., Penny, W., and Jacobs, S., Magnesium deficiency in critically ill patients, *Anaesthesia*, 50, 203–205, 1995.

70. Haigney, M.C., Silver, B., Tanglao, E., Silverman, H.S., Hill, J.D., Shapiro, E., Gerstenblith, G., and Schulman, S.P., Noninvasive measurement of tissue magnesium and correlation with cardiac levels, *Circulation*, 92, 2190–2197, 1995.

71. Durlach, J., Durlach, V., Bac, P., Mara, M., and Guiet-Bara, A., Magnesium and therapeutics, *Mages. Res.*, 7, 313–328, 1994.
72. Widman, L., Wester, P.O., Stegmayr, B.K., and Wirell, M., The dose-dependent reduction in blood pressure through administration of magnesium. A double blind placebo controlled cross-over study, *Am. J. Hypertens.*, 6, 41–45, 1993.
73. Young, G.L. and Jewell, D., Interventions for leg cramps in pregnancy, *Cochrane Database Syst. Rev.*, Vol. I, CD000121, 2002.
74. Roffe, C., Sills, S., Crome, P., and Jones, P., Randomised, cross-over, placebo controlled trial of magnesium citrate in the treatment of chronic persistent leg cramps, *Med. Sci. Monit.*, 8, CR326–CR330, 2002.
75. Puchades, M.J., Gonzalez Rico, M.A., Pons, S., Miguel, A., and Bonilla, B., Hypokalemic metabolic alkalosis: apropos of a case of Gitelman's syndrome, *Nefrologia*, 24, 72–75, 2004.
76. Shecter, M., Mertz, N.B., Stuehlinger, H.G., Slany, J., Pachinger, O., and Rabinowitz, B., Effects of oral magnesium therapy on exercise tolerance, exercise-induced chest pain, and quality of life in patients with coronary artery disease, *Am. J. Cardiol.*, 91, 517–521, 2003.
77. Whang, R., Clinical perturbations in magnesium metabolism — hypomegnesemia and hypermagnesemia, in *Magnesium and the Cell*, Birch, N.J., Ed., Academic Press, London, 1993, pp. 5–14.
78. Kinnunen, O. and Salokannel, J., Comparison of the effects of magnesium hydroxide and a bulk laxative on lipids, carbohydrates, vitamins A and E, and minerals in geriatric hospital patients in the treatment of constipation, *J. Int. Med. Res.*, 17, 442–454, 1989.
79. Lindberg, J.S., Zobitz, M.M., Poindexter, J.R., and Pak, C.Y., Magnesium bioavailability from magnesium citrate and magnesium oxide, *J. Am. Coll. Nutr.*, 9, 48–55, 1990.
80. Schuette, S.A., Lashner, B.A., and Janghorbani, M., Bioavailability of magnesium diglycinate vs magnesium oxide in patients with ileal resection, *J. Parenter. Enteral Nutr.*, 18, 430–435, 1994.
81. Xing, J.H. and Soffer, E.E., Adverse effects of laxatives, *Dis. Colon Rectum*, 44, 1201–1209, 2001.
82. Nordt, S., Williams, S.R., Turchen, S., Manoguerra, A., Smith, D., and Clark, R., Hypermagnesemia following an acute ingestion of Epsom salt in a patient with normal renal function, *J. Toxicol. Clin. Toxicol.*, 34, 735–739, 1996.

10 Vitamin D: Importance for Musculoskeletal Function and Health

Michael F. Holick, Ph.D., M.D.

CONTENTS

INTRODUCTION

Vitamin D is known as the sunshine vitamin because the major source of vitamin D is from exposure to sunlight. However, vitamin D is really a hormone. The reason is that once vitamin D is made in the skin or ingested from the diet it enters the bloodstream bound to a vitamin D binding protein (DBP). Vitamin D enters the liver, where it undergoes its first modification on carbon 25 where a hydroxyl group is introduced forming 25-hydroxyvitaminD (25(OH)D). 25(OH)D is the major circulating form of vitamin D that is used by physicians to determine a person's vitamin D status. However, 25(OH)D is biologically inert and must undergo an additional modification in the kidneys where a hydroxyl group is placed on carbon 1 to form 1,25-dihydroxyvitaminD (1,25(OH)$_2$D). 1,25(OH)$_2$D is considered to be the biologically active form of vitamin D responsible for carrying out all of the biological functions of vitamin D in the body. The fact that vitamin D undergoes these transformations in the body before it can carry out its biologic functions in distant target organs makes it a hormone.

HISTORY

Vitamin D is one of the oldest hormones/vitamins that has existed essentially unchanged for more than 500 million years.[1,2] Phytoplankton and zooplankton when exposed to sunlight in the oceans had the ability to photosynthesize vitamin D.[2] Although the function of vitamin D in these simple life-forms is not well understood, it has been suggested that because the precursor of vitamin D, provitamin D, and its photoproducts are able to absorb solar ultraviolet B (UVB) radiation they may have played a role as a natural sunscreen for these organisms.[2,3]

As life evolved in the oceans, it took advantage of the plentiful source of calcium and used this element for a wide variety of metabolic processes and as the major component of the exo- and endoskeletons of aquatic invertebrates and vertebrates. Calcium was also important for neuromuscular transmission and played a key role in the evolution of skeletal muscle function.

The life-forms that left the ocean environment for terra firma approximately 350 million years ago required calcium not only for maintenance of the vertebrate skeletons, but also for neuromuscular function and most metabolic processes. On land, the calcium was locked in the soil and was absorbed by the plants' root system into the plants' leaves. Life-forms needed an efficient method of absorbing dietary calcium. One mechanism was for these animals to be exposed to sunlight, which produces vitamin D in the skin, which is responsible for increasing the efficiency of intestinal absorption of dietary calcium. Thus, throughout evolution, vitamin D and calcium had an intimate role to play in the development of the vertebrate skeleton, the maintenance of neuromuscular function, and the overall health and well-being of most vertebrates including humans.

THE DAWN OF RICKETS

The importance of sunlight for human health became apparent with the industrial revolution in northern Europe. People began congregating in cities and lived in dwellings that were built in close proximity to each other. The burning of coal and wood polluted the atmosphere and as a result children living in these industrialized cities had little direct exposure to sunlight. Whistler, DeBoot, and Glissen recognized that children who lived in the inner cities in northern Europe often had severe growth retardation as well as skeletal deformities especially of the legs

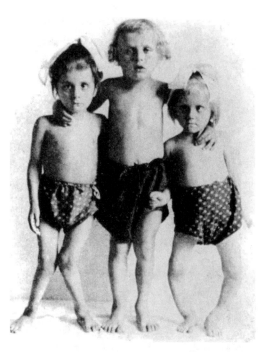

FIGURE 10.1 Typical presentation of rickets. The child in the middle does not have rickets; the children on either side have severe muscle weakness and bone deformities including bowed legs (right) or knock-knees (left). (Copyright Michael F. Holick, 2003. Used with permission.)

(Figure 10.1). It was also observed that these children were much weaker and often suffered from muscle weakness (Figure 10.2). The disease migrated to northeastern United States, where children in Boston and New York City who were raised in similar polluted sunless environments developed the same devastating bone deformities classic for rickets. By 1900, the disease was so prevalent, that upward of 80 to 90% of children in northeastern United States and northern Europe suffered from this debilitating disease.[1]

The Polish physician Snaidecki recognized in 1822 that his young patients in Warsaw often suffered from rickets whereas his pediatric patients living in the farms outside Warsaw were not afflicted with the disease.[4] He suggested that it was the lack of sun exposure that was the major cause of rickets. However, it took another 100 years before this insightful observation was finally proven when Huldschinsky exposed children with rickets to a mercury arc lamp and reported dramatic healing of rickets.[5] This was quickly followed by the observation by Hess and Unger[6] who reported that exposing children in New York City to sunlight on the roof of their hospital for several months had a curative effect on rickets.

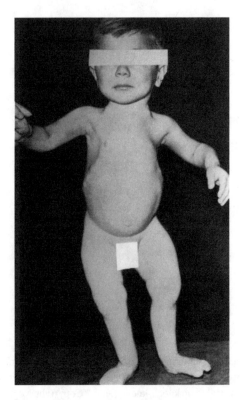

FIGURE 10.2 This child with rickets has severe muscle weakness and bony deformities including bowed legs and knob-like projects in the middle of his ribcage called the rachitic rosary. (From Fraser, D., Scriver, C.R., in *Endocrinology*, De Groot, L.J. et al., Eds., Grune and Stratton, New York, 1979, pp. 797–808. With permission.)

The realization that exposure to sunlight or artificial ultraviolet radiation resulted in treating rickets led Steenbock and Black[7] and Hess and Weinstock[8] to expose a wide variety of foods and vegetable oils to ultraviolet radiation. They demonstrated that this simple process imparted the antirachitic activity to all of these foods and oils. This prompted Steenbock to suggest that ultraviolet irradiation of milk and other foods could be a simple way to prevent rickets in children.[9] This ultimately led to the fortification of milk with vitamin D. Food manufacturers saw this as an opportunity to market their products with vitamin D and therefore bread, soda, hot dogs, custard, and even beer were fortified with vitamin D.[10] Today in the United States and Canada, milk, some cereals, breads, and yogurts are fortified with vitamin D. In Europe, however, most countries forbid the fortification of dairy products with vitamin D because of the unfortunate outbreak of neonatal vitamin D intoxication after World War II in Great Britain.[11]

PHOTOSYNTHESIS OF VITAMIN D AND FACTORS THAT INFLUENCE IT

When a person is exposed to sunlight if the sunlight contains UVB radiation with wavelengths between 290 and 315 nm, the radiation penetrates into the skin where it is absorbed by DNA, RNA, and proteins as well as 7-dehydrocholesterol. 7-Dehydrocholesterol (provitamin D_3) is the precursor of cholesterol and is present in the plasma membrane of both epidermal keratinocytes and dermal fibroblasts[12]. When the solar UVB radiation is absorbed by 7-dehydrocholesterol, the energy causes a splitting of the B-ring to form previtamin D_3 (Figure 10.3). Previtamin D_3 is thermally unstable and is rapidly converted to vitamin D_3. Once formed the vitamin D_3 leaves the skin and enters the circulation bound to the DBP.[13]

The major source of vitamin D for most humans is exposure to sunlight. There are a wide variety of factors that influence the production of vitamin D_3 in skin. Very little UVB radiation penetrates through the ozone layer to reach the earth's surface. Typically, no more than 0.1% of the total UV radiation that enters into the earth's atmosphere and reaches the earth's surface is the high-energy UVB radiation.

Since the stratospheric ozone layer is very efficient in absorbing UVB radiation any alteration in the sun's angle can have a dramatic influence on the total number of UVB photons reaching the earth's surface. This explains why during winter very few UVB photons are able to penetrate to the earth's surface at latitudes above 37°. Thus, people living north of Atlanta, GA, make very little vitamin D_3 in their skin during exposure to sunlight during the months of November through March.[1,14] At much higher latitudes in Canada and northern Europe this is extended to the months of October through April. Similarly, early and late in the day the zenith angle of the sun is increased and thus, very few UVB photons reach the earth's surface. The most efficient time to make vitamin D_3 in the skin is between the hours of 10:00 A.M. and 3:00 P.M. (Figure 10.4).[1,14,15]

Skin pigmentation is efficient in absorbing UVB radiation. Thus, increased skin pigmentation markedly reduces the ability of the skin to produce vitamin D. Deeply pigmented individuals require 5 to 10 times longer sunlight exposure to make the same amount of vitamin D as a light-skinned Caucasian (Figure 10.5).

Sunscreens are intended to efficiently absorb UVB radiation similar to melanin skin pigment. A sunscreen with a sun-protection factor (SPF) of 8 reduces the amount of UVB photons entering into the skin by 95%. Thus, the topical use of a sunscreen with an SPF of 8 reduces the capacity of the skin to produce vitamin D_3 by 95% (Figure 10.6).[16]

Aging decreases many metabolic processes and reduces the amount of 7-dehydrocholesterol in human skin.[17] There is approximately 25% as much 7-dehydrocholesterol in the skin of a 70-year-old compared to a 20-year-old. This is why the elderly are able to increase their blood level of vitamin D_3 to only 25% of a young adult after exposure to the same amount of UVB radiation (Figure 10.6).[18]

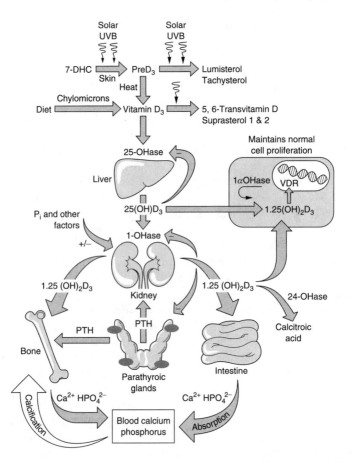

FIGURE 10.3 Schematic representation for cutaneous production of vitamin D and its metabolism and regulation for calcium homeostasis and cellular growth. During exposure to sunlight, 7-dehydrocholesterol (7-DHC) in the skin absorbs solar ultraviolet (UVB) radiation and is converted to previtamin D_3 (preD_3). Once formed, D_3 undergoes thermally induced transformation to vitamin D_3. Further, exposure to sunlight converts preD_3 and vitamin D_3 to biologically inert photoproducts. Vitamin D coming from the diet or from the skin enters the circulation and is metabolized in the liver by the vitamin D-25-hydroxylase (25-OHase) to 25-hydroxyvitamin D_3, 25(OH)D_3. 25(OH)D_3 re-enters the circulation and is converted in the kidney by the 25-hydroxyvitamin D_3-1α-hydroxylase (1-OHase) to 1,25-dihydroxyvitamin D_3, 1,25(OH)$_2D_3$. A variety of factors, including serum phosphorus (P_i) and parathyroid hormone (PTH) regulate the renal production of 1,25(OH)$_2$D. 1,25(OH)$_2$D regulates calcium metabolism through its interaction with its major target tissues, the bone and the intestine. 1,25(OH)$_2D_3$ also induces its own destruction by enhancing the expression of the 25-hydroxyvitamin D-24-hydroxylase (24-OHase). 25(OH)D is metabolized in other tissues for the purpose of regulation of cellular growth. (Copyright Michael F. Holick, 2003. Used with permission.)

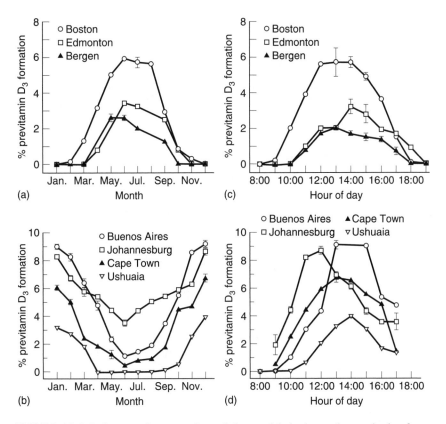

FIGURE 10.4 Influence of season, time of day, and latitude on the synthesis of pre-vitamin D_3 in the northern (a and c) and southern (b and d) hemispheres. The *x*-axis in C and D represents the end of the 1 h exposure time in July. (Adapted from Lu, Z., Chen, T., Kline, L. et al., in *Biologic Effects of Light, Proceedings*, Holick, M. and Kligman, A., Eds.,Walter De Gruyter, Berlin, 1992, pp. 48–51. With permission.)

The skin has a large capacity to produce vitamin D_3. An adult wearing a bathing suit and exposed to an amount of sunlight that causes a slight pinkness to the skin (1 minimal erythemal dose [MED]) produces an amount of vitamin D_3 in the skin comparable to taking an oral dose of between 10,000 and 25,000 inter-national units (IU) of vitamin D_2 (Figure 10.7).[1,19] Thus, it is easy to obtain an adequate amount of vitamin D_3 from either casual or sensible exposure to sun-light, i.e., typically no more than 25% of the time that it would take to cause 1 MED of arms and legs or hands, face, and arms two to three times a week during the spring, summer, and fall between 10 A.M. and 3:00 P.M.[1,15] The elderly benefit from exposure to sunlight and typically need to expose more skin to sunlight to make enough vitamin D_3 (Figure 10.6).[18]

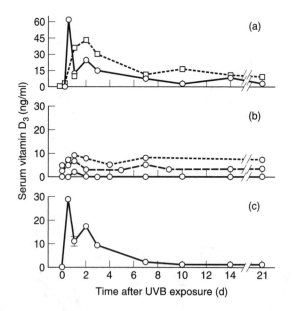

FIGURE 10.5 Serum concentrations of vitamin D in two lightly pigmented white (skin type II) (a) and three heavily pigmented black (skin type V) (b) subjects after total-body exposure to 54 mJ/cm² of UVB radiation (c) after re-exposure of one panel b subject to 320 mJ/cm² of UVB radiation. (From Clemens, T.L., Adams, J.S., Henderson, S.L., and Holick, M.F., *Lancet*, 1, 74–76, 1982. With permission.)

SOURCES OF VITAMIN D

As much as 95% of most humans' vitamin D requirement comes from casual exposure to sunlight. The diet is incapable of providing most humans with their vitamin D requirement.[20] The reason is that very few foods naturally contain vitamin D. These include oily fish such as salmon, mackerel, and herring and typically they contain about 400 to 500 IU (1 IU = 25 ng) of vitamin D_3 per a 3.5 ounce serving. Cod liver oil and sun-dried mushrooms also naturally contain vitamin D. Milk, some cereals, and some yogurts are fortified with vitamin D. Typically, there is 100 IU (2.5 μg) in an 8 oz. glass of milk and some orange juices.

The first vitamin D that was discovered was from the irradiation of yeast. This vitamin D, known as vitamin D_2, comes from the irradiation of ergosterol, which is a major sterol component in yeast extract. The difference between vitamin D_2 and vitamin D_3 is that there is a double bond between carbons 22 and 23 in the side chain and there is a methyl group on carbon 24 (Figure 10.8). Although vitamin D_2 is effective in preventing rickets and having all of the biologic functions of vitamin D_3, there is mounting evidence that vitamin D_2 is only about

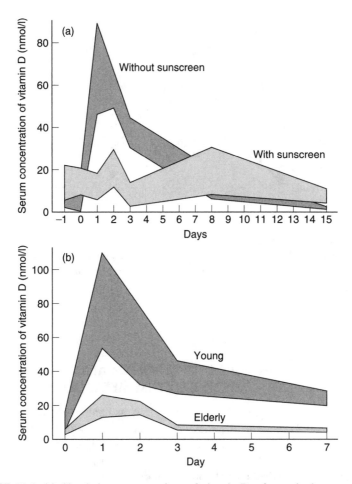

FIGURE 10.6 (a) Circulating concentrations of vitamin D_3 after a single exposure to 1 minimal erythemal dose of simulated sunlight with a sunscreen, with a sun protection factor of 8 (SPF-8), or a topical placebo cream. (b) Circulating concentrations of vitamin D in response to a whole-body exposure to 1 minimal erythemal dose in healthy young and elderly subjects. (From Holick, M.F., *Am. J. Clin. Nutr.*, 60, 619–630, 1994. With permission.)

10 to 40% as effective as vitamin D_3 in maintaining blood levels of 25(OH)D.[21,22] Despite this difference in activity, 1 IU of vitamin D_2 or vitamin D_3 is equal to 25 ng.

When vitamin D_3 is made in the skin it is bound to the DBP, which transports it to the liver. Both vitamin D_2 and vitamin D_3 (D represents D_2 and D_3) coming from the diet are incorporated in the chylomicrons and absorbed into the lymphatic system, which distributes the vitamin D into the venous circulation. It is bound to the DBP as well as lipoproteins and travels to the liver.

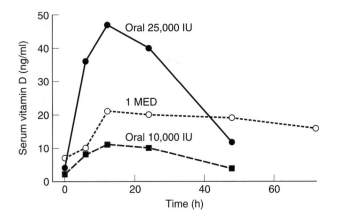

FIGURE 10.7 Comparison of serum vitamin D levels after a whole-body exposure to 1 minimal erythemal dose of simulated sunlight compared with a single oral dose of either 10,000 or 25,000 IU of vitamin D$_2$. (From Holick, M.F., *Curr. Opin. Endocrinol. Diabetes,* 9, 87–98, 2002. With permission.)

VITAMIN D METABOLISM AND FUNCTIONS ON CALCIUM METABOLISM

Vitamin D is metabolized sequentially in the liver and kidneys on carbons 25 and 1 to form 1,25(OH)$_2$D.[1] The major factors that regulate the kidney's production of 1,25(OH)$_2$D include parathyroid hormone (PTH), as well as serum calcium, and phosphorus (Figure 10.3).[1,23] PTH, low-serum phosphorus, and low-serum calcium all stimulate the kidney to produce more 1,25(OH)$_2$D. Once 1,25(OH)$_2$D has carried out its biologic functions it induces its own destruction by stimulating gene expression of the enzyme (25-hydroxyvitaminD-24-hydroxylase) cyp-24, which places a hydroxyl group on carbon 24 followed by a hydroxyl group on carbon 23 resulting in the oxidative cleavage of the 1,25(OH)$_2$D side chain to form the water-soluble and biologically inactive calcitroic acid.[1,23] 1,25(OH)$_2$D leaves the kidney bound to the DBP. Its major physiologic function is to maintain serum calcium in a normal physiologic range in order to maintain most body functions. It accomplishes this by interacting with its specific nuclear receptor, the vitamin D receptor (VDR).[23,24] When 1,25(OH)$_2$D interacts with the VDR in the small intestine, it signals the intestinal cells to increase the efficiency of the absorption of dietary calcium (Figure 10.3). In a vitamin D deficient state, the small intestine absorbs no more than 10 to 15% of dietary calcium. In a vitamin D sufficient state the small intestine absorbs 30 to 40% of the dietary calcium. During pregnancy, lactation and the growth spurt 1,25(OH)$_2$D can increase this efficiency up to 80%.[19,23]

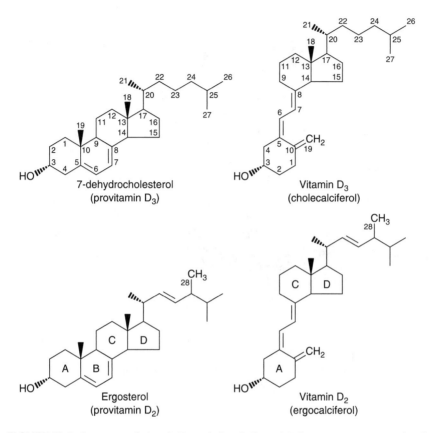

FIGURE 10.8 Structures of vitamin D_2 and vitamin D_3 and their precursors ergosterol and 7-dehydrocholesterol. (Copyright Michael F. Holick, 2003. Used with permission.)

1,25(OH)$_2$D is also responsible for increasing the efficiency of dietary phosphorus absorption. In a vitamin D deficient state approximately 60% of dietary phosphorus is absorbed while in a vitamin D sufficient state the intestine absorbs 80%.

When dietary calcium is inadequate to satisfy the body's requirement, 1,25(OH)$_2$D interacts with its VDR in the osteoblast, which is responsible for bone mineralization. However, the interaction of 1,25(OH)$_2$D with the osteoblast's VDR results in the expression of receptor activator of NFκB(RANK) ligand (RANKL) on the plasma membrane of osteoblasts.[1,25] This acts as a sentinel for the precursor of the osteoclast, which has the receptor RANK on its cell surface. The RANKL on the osteoblast signals the premature osteoclast to become a mature cell. Once mature, the osteoclast releases enzymes to destroy the bone matrix to release the precious calcium and phosphorus stores into the bloodstream (Figure 10.9).

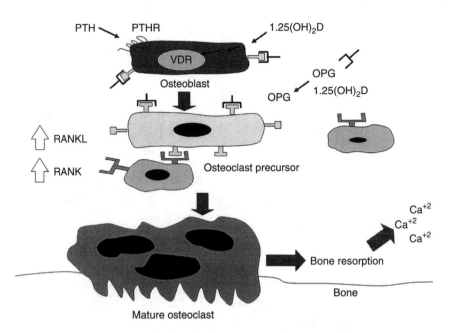

FIGURE 10.9 Both $1,25(OH)_2D$ and PTH stimulate the mobilization of calcium from the skeleton by interacting with their respective receptors on osteoblasts, which induce expression of receptor activator of NF_{kB} (RANK) ligand (RANKL). The RANK on the immature osteoclast binding to RANKL causes the osteoclast to mature. (Copyright Michael F. Holick, 2004. Used with permission.)

NONCALCIUM FUNCTIONS OF VITAMIN D

Almost every tissue and cell in the body possesses VDR, including the brain, heart, pancreas, stomach, skin, skeletal muscle, monocytes, and activated T and B lymphocytes.[26] One of the functions of $1,25(OH)_2D$ is to regulate cell growth and maturation. $1,25(OH)_2D$ is one of the most potent hormones that keep cellular growth in check.[1] This is the likely explanation for why vitamin D deficiency has been associated with increased risk of developing many common cancers including cancer of the colon, breast, prostate, and esophagus.[27–30]

$1,25(OH)_2D$ also increases insulin secretion and is a potent regulator of the immune system.[1,31] Evidence suggests that vitamin D deficiency increases risk of many common autoimmune diseases including type I diabetes, multiple sclerosis, rheumatoid arthritis, and Crohn's disease.[1,32–35]

$1,25(OH)_2D$ has also been demonstrated to regulate the production of the blood pressure hormone renin in the kidney.[36] This is the likely explanation for the observation that the people who live at higher latitudes and are more prone to vitamin D deficiency are at higher risk of cardiovascular heart disease and hypertension.[37–39]

ROLE OF VITAMIN D IN SKELETAL MUSCLE FUNCTION

Classically, vitamin D deficiency causes proximal muscle weakness, i.e., weakness in the muscles of the upper arms and upper legs. Typically, patients with proximal muscle weakness have difficulty in getting up from a sitting position. Signs of proximal muscle weakness can be seen in the children photographed in Figure 10.1 and Figure 10.2. Muscle weakness was also the primary symptom among Arab women in Denmark, who customarily covered themselves from the sun.[40] It had been assumed that the role of vitamin D on muscle function was by its indirect action on maintaining calcium and phosphorus homeostasis. It is now appreciated that vitamin D exerts direct effects on skeletal muscle function.

VDRs are present in human skeletal muscle.[41,42] Although the exact function of $1,25(OH)_2D_3$ interacting with the VDR in skeletal muscle is not yet well understood, there are a variety of studies that have shown that $1,25(OH)_2D_3$ is critically important for regulating skeletal muscle function. It is well known that aging is associated with decreased skeletal muscle function and weakness. It has been observed that the number of VDRs in skeletal muscle decreases with age. Thirty-two women aged 21 to 91 years who had undergone hip or spinal surgery had their skeletal muscle evaluated for the presence and number of VDRs. As can be seen in Figure 10.10, there was a significant decrease in the number of VDRs with increasing age.[43] The number of VDRs in a 90-year-old was approximately 30% of those in the skeletal muscle from a 20-year-old. Because the number of VDRs is important for the function of $1,25(OH)_2D_3$, these data suggest that the age-related decrease in VDRs may be responsible for the muscle weakness observed in older men and women.

One method to evaluate the importance of $1,25(OH)_2D$ and its receptor on skeletal muscle function is to develop a mouse model that does not have a VDR. Endo reported that mice that were unable to express the VDR had small and variable muscle fibers.[44]

It has been reported that the VDR genotype, i.e., polymorphism is associated with efficiency of intestinal calcium absorption and may play a role in increasing risk of osteoporosis.[45,46] When the VDR genotype was evaluated with muscle strength in nonobese older women, a 23% difference in quadricep strength and 7% difference in grip strength was observed between the VDR genotypes bb and BB of the VDR.[47] Further, confirmation of the importance of vitamin D in skeletal muscle function and strength was provided by Bischoff et al.[48] They evaluated the NHANES III database and correlated serum levels of 25(OH)D with lower-extremity strength in 4100 adults 60 years of age and older. As seen in Figure 10.11, both men and women who had a 25(OH)D of <10 ng/ml (<25 nmol/l) required at least 4 s to walk 8 ft. However, those adults who had a 25(OH)D of >30 ng/ml (>80 nmol/l), needed only approximately 3.7 s, 30% less time, to walk the same distance. A similar observation was made for adults who stood up from a sitting position. People with 25(OH)D levels of <10 ng/ml took approximately 15 s to stand up, and those with 25(OH)D levels greater that 30 ng/ml took approximately 14 s to rise from sitting.[48]

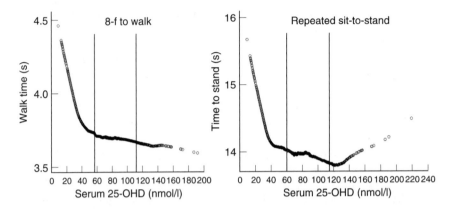

FIGURE 10.10 Regression plots of lower-extremity function on the 8-ft. (i.e., 2.4 m) walk test and the sit-to-stand test by 25-hydroxyvitamin D (25(OH)D) concentrations. Plots are adjusted for sex, age, race, or ethnicity, BMI, calcium intake, poverty–income ratio, number of medical comorbidities, self-reported arthritis, use of a walking device, month of assessment, activity level (inactive or active), and metabolic equivalents in the active elderly. The vertical lines denote the reference range for 25(OH)D. (From Bischoff, H.A., Dietrich, T. et al., *Am. J. Clin. Nutr.*, 80, 752–758, 2004. With permission.)

Ninety percent of hip fractures involve falls. Five percent of elderly persons fracture due to falls each year and 20 to 40% of these falls involve hip fracture. Pfeifer was one of the first to demonstrate that treatment of elderly ambulatory women with 800 IU of vitamin D_3 a day along with 1200 mg of calcium decreased body sway by 9%.[49]

Bischoff conducted a double-blind randomized controlled trial of 122 elderly women (mean age, 85.3 years; range 63 to 99 years) in a long-stay geriatric care facility.[50] The participants received 1200 mg of calcium plus 800 IU of vitamin D_3 a day. The control group received 1200 mg of calcium a day, but no vitamin D supplementation. The women were followed for the number of falls that they experienced over the next 12 weeks. Controlling for age, the number of falls in a 6 week pretreatment period and baseline 25(OH)D levels revealed that the mean number of falls per person per week was 0.034 in the calcium and vitamin D group compared to 0.076 in the calcium fortified group. This translated into a 49% reduction in falls. Fifty percent of the women had a 25(OH)D below 12 ng/ml and 90% were below 31 ng/ml. The women who received calcium and vitamin D had a 71% increase in 25(OH)D levels and an 8% increase in 1,25(OH)₂D compared to baseline values. The control group that only received calcium had no significant change in 25(OH)D levels. In addition, musculoskeletal function improved significantly in the group of women who received both calcium and vitamin D. Sixty-two of the women completed all of the muscle

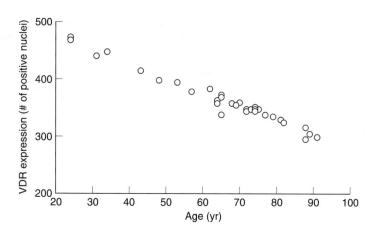

FIGURE 10.11 Nuclei positive for the vitamin D receptor (VDR) by age. The scatter plot gives the predicted number of VDR positive nuclei by age, controlling for biopsy location (gluteus medius or transversospinalis muscle) and 25-hydroxyvitamin D serum levels based on the linear regression model (age: β estimate $= -2.56$; $p = .047$). (From Bischoff, H.A., Borchers, M., Gudat, F. et al., *J. Bone Miner. Res.*, 19, 265, 2004. With permission.)

strength testing including grip strength, knee extensor and flexor strength, and timed up and go test. There was significant musculoskeletal function improvement in the calcium plus vitamin D group compared to the group that received calcium alone.

It is important to consider vitamin D status in the elderly for muscle function and strength in order to decrease risk of falling, and therefore, decrease the major cause of fractures in the elderly.

DETECTION OF VITAMIN D DEFICIENCY

Vitamin D deficiency is probably the most common endocrinopathy for children and adults. It has been estimated that more than 50% of adults over the age of 50 are vitamin D deficient.[51–53] Young adults who always wear sun protection or are working indoors during the time when the sun is able to make vitamin D_3 in the skin are also at risk of vitamin D deficiency. In Boston, it was reported that 32% of young adults aged 18 to 29 years were vitamin D deficient at the end of the winter.[54] Recently, Sullivan reported in young white Maine girls aged 9 to 11 years that 48% were vitamin D deficient at the end of the winter, and 17% who always wore sun protection remained vitamin D deficient at the end of the summer.[55] In Boston, Gordon[56] reported that 52% of African American and Hispanic adolescent boys and girls were vitamin D deficient throughout the year. This is not only a problem for people that live in more northern latitudes, but also is a global problem. Nesby-O'Dell[57] reported that 42% of African American women aged 15 to 49 years throughout the entire United States were vitamin D deficient at the end of the winter.

The best method to monitor vitamin D status is to measure circulating concentrations of 25(OH)D.[1] 25(OH)D has a half-life in the circulation of approximately 2 weeks and is the major circulating form of vitamin D. It is a barometer of vitamin D status that results from dietary intake and sun exposure. Circulating concentrations of 1,25(OH)$_2$D should not be measured to determine vitamin D status. The reasons for this are that 1,25(OH)$_2$D has a half-life of approximately 4 h in the circulation and circulates at 1000 times less concentration compared to 25(OH)D. Furthermore, as an individual becomes vitamin D deficient, there is a compensatory increase in PTH levels, which stimulates the kidneys to produce 1,25(OH)$_2$D. Thus, as a person is becoming vitamin D deficient, the 1,25(OH)$_2$D levels are typically either normal or mildly elevated.

Serum calcium concentrations are usually normal in vitamin D deficiency unless all of the calcium has either been mobilized from the skeleton or is unavailable for mobilization.

The assays that are used to measure 25(OH)D have been either radioim-muno-assays (RIA), or competitive protein binding assays (CPBA) using the DBP as the binder. However, since both the RIA and the CPBA assays typically are performed on serum without any chromatography, these assays often over-estimate the total 25(OH)D levels by as much as 20%.[58] High-performance liquid chromatography separates 25(OH)D$_2$ and 25(OH)D$_3$ from other vitamin D metabolites and will quantitate total concentrations of both of these 25 hydroxylated metabolites. However, this assay is often time-consuming and therefore, is not commercially available. Recently, the sensitivity of mass spectroscopy (MS) has been incorporated into the liquid chromatography (LC) system. The tandem combination of LC with the MS provides a very sensitive and efficient assay to measure 25(OH)D$_2$ and 25(OH)D$_3$. This recently became commercially available and is likely to be one of the methods of choice to quantify 25(OH)D$_2$ and 25(OH)D$_3$.

STRATEGIES TO TREAT VITAMIN D DEFICIENCY

The simplest and least expensive way to maintain a normal vitamin D status is to obtain sensible limited exposure to sunlight during the spring, summer, and fall.[1,15] Since vitamin D is fat soluble, if an adequate amount of vitamin D is produced during the spring, summer, and fall, it is stored in adipose tissue and released during winter.

With the recognition that vitamin D deficiency is epidemic in both the United States and Europe, it is not only important to detect this endocrinopathy, but also to aggressively treat it. It has been estimated that 1000 IU of vitamin D$_3$

a day is required to satisfy the body's requirement for vitamin D in the absence of any sun exposure.[59-61] However, with the vitamin D tank being empty, it is important to fill it before vitamin D supplementation of 1000 IU of vitamin D_3 a day is initiated. In the United States, only vitamin D_2 is available in pharmacologic doses. Typically, I treat patients with 50,000 units of vitamin D_2 once a week for 8 weeks. This often raises blood levels of 25(OH)D by more than 100% and raises the blood levels into the 30 to 40 ng/ml range.[53,62] I typically treat patients who are prone to vitamin D deficiency with 50,000 units of vitamin D_2 every other week after correcting their vitamin D deficiency. This often keeps the 25(OH)D in the range of 30 to 40 ng/ml, which is considered to be ideal for maximizing intestinal calcium absorption.[63] I check their 25(OH)D levels after the 8 weeks of vitamin D_2 therapy and once a year, ideally in November or December.

There are approximately 10 million Americans who suffer from some type of fat malabsorption syndrome. Often, they are unable to absorb dietary vitamin D. Vitamin D is no longer available for intramuscular injection mainly because it was not very bioavailable. Intravenous use of vitamin D does not work and therefore, is infrequently used. A simple method for correcting vitamin D deficiency in patients who are unable to absorb any vitamin D through the gastrointestinal tract is to have the patients exposed to UVB radiation either from a tanning bed or from a lamp source that emits this type of radiation. Typically, I recommend that patients who go to a tanning salon be exposed to 25% of the time recommended for maximized tanning. This will reduce the risk of skin damage, while maximizing vitamin D_3 production in the skin. We observed in a patient with Crohn's disease who had only 2 ft. of small intestine left, that when exposed to tanning bed radiation three times a week for 3 months, she had a 700% increase in her 25(OH)D levels and had complete resolution of her muscle aches and bone pains associated with vitamin D deficiency osteomalacia.[64]

VITAMIN D INTOXICATION

It is very difficult to cause vitamin D intoxication. Although the safe upper limit for vitamin D for adults is 2000 IU/day, Vieth reported that healthy men receiving 4000 to 10,000 IU of vitamin D a day demonstrated no signs of toxicity.[65] Typically, tens of thousands of units of vitamin D a day need to be ingested before vitamin D intoxication is observed.[65-67] The hallmark for vitamin D intoxication is hypercalcemia and hyperphosphatemia associated with a 25(OH)D level of greater than 100 ng/ml.

CONCLUSION

The expanded roles of vitamin D are illustrated in Figure 10.12. Since VDRs are present in almost all of the tissues in the body, more fundamentally important roles

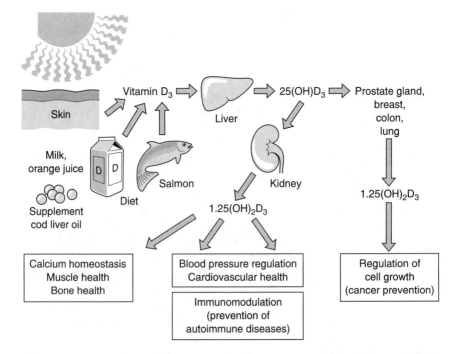

FIGURE 10.12 The biologic consequences of the metabolism of 25-hydroxyvitamin D_3 ($25(OH)D_3$) to 1 ^{25}dihydroxyvitamin D_3 ($1,25(OH)_2D_3$) in the kidney and other organs. (Copyright Michael F. Holick, 2004. Used with permission.)

of vitamin D are anticipated to emerge. Because vitamin D is so important for health, measurement of 25(OH)D once a year, preferably at the end of the fall season, is prudent and cost-effective in preventing and treating musculoskeletal conditions.

ACKNOWLEDGMENT

This work was supported in part by NIH grant M01RR00533 and the UV Foundation.

Editor's Note

Indoor activities, sunscreen, glass enclosures, low-fat diets, and south-to-north migration all contribute to the high prevalence of vitamin D deficiency. Obesity may also be a risk factor. At first this may seem counterintuitive since vitamin D is a fat-soluble vitamin stored in adipose tissue. However, recall that vitamin D synthesized from sunlight must travel through the skin to the liver to begin activation. Obese persons may saturate adipose tissue with vitamin D before sufficient amounts can reach the liver to begin activation.[67] Low-serum 25-OH-D has been found in obese persons with adequate adipose tissue levels. Furthermore, people who undergo malabsorptive-type bariatric surgery destroy their vitamin D as the fat is being mobilized, and therefore remain vitamin D deficient after the surgery.

REFERENCES

1. Holick, M.F., Sunlight and vitamin D for bone health and prevention of autoimmune diseases, cancers, and cardiovascular disease, *Am. J. Clin. Nutr.*, 80 (Suppl.), 1678S–1688S, 2004.
2. Holick, M.F., Phylogenetic and evolutionary aspects of vitamin D from phytoplankton to humans, in *Vertebrate Endocrinology: Fundamentals and Biomedical Implications*, Vol. 3, Pang, P.K.T. and Schreibman, M.P., Eds., Academic Press, Orlando, FL, 1989, pp. 7–43.
3. Holick, M.F., Vitamin D: A millennium perspective, *J. Cell. Biochem.*, 88, 296–307, 2003.
4. Sniadecki, J. Jerdrzej Sniadecki (1768–1838) on the cure of rickets, 1840; as cited in Mozolowski, W., *Nature*, 143, 121–124, 1939.
5. Huldschinsky, K., Heilung von Rachitis durch Kunstliche Hohensonne, *Dtsch. Med. Wochenschr.*, 45, 712–713, 1919.
6. Hess, A.F. and Unger, L.J., The cure of infantile rickets by sunlight, *J. Am. Med. Assoc.*, 77, 39–41, 1921.
7. Steenbock, H. and Black, A., The reduction of growth-promoting and calcifying properties in a ration by exposure to ultraviolet light, *J. Biol. Chem.*, 61, 408–422, 1924.
8. Hess, A.F. and Weinstock, M., Antirachitic properties imparted to inert fluids and to green vegetables by ultraviolet irradiation, *J. Biol. Chem.*, 62, 301–313, 1924.
9. Steenbock, H., The induction of growth-prompting and calcifying properties in a ration exposed to light, *Science*, 60, 224–225, 1924.
10. Holick, M.F., Biologic effects of light: historical and new perspectives, in *Proceedings, Symposium on the Biological Effects of Light, Switzerland*, M.F. Holick and E.G. Jung, Eds., Kluwer Academic Publishers, Dordrecht, 1998, pp. 11–32.
11. British Pediatric Association, Hypercalcemia in infants and vitamin D, *Br. Med. J.*, 2, 149–151, 1956.
12. MacLaughlin, J.A., Anderson, R.R., and Holick, M.F., Spectral character of sunlight modulates photosynthesis of previtamin D3 and its photoisomers in human skin, *Science*, 216, 1001–1003, 1982.
13. Holick, M.F., Tian, X.Q., and Allan, M., Evolutionary importance for the membrane enhancement of the production of vitamin D_3 in the skin of poikilothermic animals, *Proc. Natl. Acad. Sci.*, 92, 3124–3126, 1995.
14. Webb, A.R., Kline, L., Holick, M.F., Influence of season and latitude on the cutaneous synthesis of vitamin D_3: exposure to winter sunlight in Boston and Edmonton will not promote vitamin D_3 synthesis in human skin, *J. Clin. Endocrinol. Metab.*, 67, 373–378, 1988.

15. Holick, M.F., *The UV Advantage*, ibooks, New York, 2004.
16. Matsuoka, L.Y, Ide, L., Wortsman, J., MacLaughlin, J., and Holick, M.F., Sunscreens suppress cutaneous vitamin D_3 synthesis, *J. Clin. Endocrinol. Metab.* 64, 1165–1168, 1987.
17. MacLaughlin, J. and Holick, M.F., Aging decreases the capacity of human skin to produce vitamin D_3, *J. Clin. Invest.*, 76, 1536–1538, 1985.
18. Holick, M.F., Matsuoka, L.Y., and Wortsman, J., Age, Vitamin D, and solar ultraviolet, *Lancet*, 1104–1105, November 4, 1989.
19. Holick, M.F., Vitamin D: the underappreciated D-lightful hormone that is important for skeletal and cellular health, *Curr. Opin. Endocrinol. Diabetes*, 9, 87–98, 2002.
20. Moore, C., Murphy, M.M., Keast, D.R., and Holick, M.F., Vitamin D intake in the United States, *J. Am. Diet. Assoc.*, 104, 980–983, 2004.
21. Tang, H.M., Cole, D.E.C., Rubin, L.A., Pierratos, A., Siu, S., and Vieth, R., Evidence that vitamin D_3 increases serum 25-hydroxyvitamin D more efficiently than does vitamin D_2, *Am. J. Clin. Nutr.*, 68, 854–858, 1998.
22. Armas, L.A.G., Hollis, B., and Heaney, R.P., Vitamin D_2 is much less effective than vitamin D_3 in humans, *J. Clin. Endocrinol. Metab.*, 89, 5387–5391, 2004.
23. Holick, M.F., Vitamin D: photobiology, metabolism, mechanism of action, and clinical applications, in *Primer on the Metabolic Bone Diseases and Disorders of Mineral Metabolism*, 5th ed., Favus, M., Ed., American Society for Bone and Mineral Research, Washington, DC, 2003, chap. 20, pp. 129–137.
24. MacDonald, P., Molecular biology of the vitamin D receptor, in *Vitamin D — Physiology, Molecular Biology, and Clinical Applications*, Holick, M.F., Ed., Humana Press, Totowa, NJ, 1999, pp. 109–128.
25. Khosla, S., The OPG/RANKL/RANK system, *Endocrinology*, 142, 5050–5055, 2001.
26. Stumpf, W.E., Sar, M., Reid, F.A. et al., Target cells for 1,25-dihydroxyvitamin D3 in intestinal tract, stomach, kidney, skin, pituitary, and parathyroid, *Science*, 206, 1188–1190, 1979.
27. Garland, C.F., Garland, F.C., Shaw, E.K., Comstock, G.W., Helsing, K.J., and Gorham, E.D., Serum 25-hydroxyvitamin D and colon cancer: eight-year prospective study, *Lancet*, 18, 1176–1178, 1989.
28. Garland, F.C., Garland, C.F., Gorham, E.D., and Young, J.F., Geographic variation in breast cancer mortality in the United States: a hypothesis involving exposure to solar radiation, *Prev. Med.* 19, 614–622, 1990.
29. Hanchette, C.L. and Schwartz, G.G., Geographic patterns of prostate cancer mortality, *Cancer*, 70, 2861–2869, 1992.
30. Grant, W.B., An estimate of premature cancer mortality in the U.S. due to inadequate doses of solar ultraviolet-B radiation, *Cancer*, 70, 2861–2869, 2002.
31. Mathieu, C. and Adorini, L., The coming of age of 1,25-dihydroxyvitamin D_3 analogs as immunomodulatory agents, *Trends Mol. Med.*, 8, 174–179, 2002.
32. Hypponen, E., Laara, E., Jarvelin, M-R., and Virtanen, S.M., Intake of vitamin D and risk of type 1 diabetes: a birth-cohort study, *Lancet*, 358, 1500–1503, 2001.
33. van der Mei, I., Ponsonby, A-L., Dwyer, T., Blizzard, L., Simmons, R., and Taylor, B.V., Past exposure to sun, skin phenotype, and risk of multiple sclerosis: case–control study, *Br. Med. J.*, 327, 316–317, 2003.
34. Merlino, L.A., Curtis, J., Mikuls, T.R., Cerhan, J.R., Criswell, L.A., and Saag, K.G., Vitamin D intake is inversely associated with rheumatoid arthritis, *Arthritis Rheum.*, 50, 72–77, 2004.

35. Cantorna, M.T., Munsick, C., Bemiss, C., and Mahon, B.D., 1,25-Dihydroxychole-calciferol prevents and ameliorates symptoms of experimental murine inflammatory bowel disease, *J. Nutr.*, 130, 2648–2652, 2000.

36. Li, Y., Kong, J., Wei, M., Chen, Z.F., Liu, S., and Cao, L.P., 1,25-Dihydroxyvitamin D$_3$ is a negative endocrine regulator of the renin-angiotensin system, *J. Clin. Invest.*, 110, 229–238, 2002.

37. Rostand, S.G., Ultraviolet light may contribute to geographic and racial blood pressure differences, *Hypertension*, 30, 150–156, 1979.

38. Weishaar, R.E. and Simpson, R.U., The involvement of the endocrine system in regulating cardiovascular function: emphasis on vitamin D$_3$. *Endocr. Rev.*, 10, 1–15, 1989.

39. Holick, M.F., Sunlight and vitamin D: both good for cardiovascular health, *J. Gen. Intern. Med.*, 17, 733–735, 2002.

40. Glerup, H., Mikkelsen, K., Poulsen, L. et al., Commonly recommended daily intake of vitamin D is not sufficient if sunlight exposure is limited, *J. Intern. Med.*, 247, 260–268, 2000.

41. Bischoff, H.A., Borchers, M., Gudat, F. et al. *In situ* detection of 1,25-dihydroxy-vitamin D$_3$ receptor in human skeletal muscle tissue. *Histochem. J.*, 33, 19–24, 2001.

42. Boland, R., Role of vitamin D in skeletal muscle function, *Endocr. Rev.*, 7, 434–447, 1986.

43. Bischoff, H.A., Borchers, M., Gudat, F. et al., Vitamin D receptor expression in human muscle tissue decreases with age, *J. Bone Miner. Res.*, 19, 265, 2004.

44. Endo, I., Inoue, D., Mitsui, T., Umaki, Y., Akaike, M., and Yoshizawa, T., Deletion of vitamin D receptor gene in mice results in abnormal skeletal muscle development with deregulated expression of myoregulatory transcription factors, *Endocrinology*, 144, 5138–5144, 2003.

45. Krall, E.A., Parry, P., Lichter, J.B., and Dawson-Hughes, B., Vitamin D receptor alleles and rates of bone loss: influences of years since menopause and calcium intake, *J. Bone Miner. Res.*, 10, 978–984, 1995.

46. Kiel, D.P., Myers, R.H., Cupples, L.A. et al., The BsmI vitamin D receptor restriction fragment length polymorphism (bb) influences the effect of calcium intake on bone mineral density, *J. Bone Miner. Res.*, 12, 1049–1057, 1997.

47. Geusens, P., Vandevyver, C. et al., Quadriceps and grip strength are related to vitamin D receptor genotype in elderly nonobese women, *J. Bone Miner. Res.*, 12, 2082–2088, 1997.

48. Bischoff, H.A., Dietrich, T. et al., Higher 25-hydroxyvitamin D concentrations are associated with better lower-extremity function in both active and inactive persons ≥ 60 y, *Am. J. Clin. Nutr.*, 80, 752–758, 2004.

49. Pfeifer, M., Begerow, B., Minne, H.W., Abrams, C., Nachtigall, D., and Hansen, C., Effects of a short-term vitamin D and calcium supplementation on body sway and secondary hyperparathyroidism in elderly women, *J. Bone. Miner. Res.*, 15, 1113–1118, 2000.

50. Bischoff, H.A., Stahelin, H.N., Dick, W., Akos, R., Knecht, M., Salis, C., Nebiker, M., Theiler, R., Pfeifer, M., Begerow, B., Lew, R., and Conselmann, M., Effects of vitamin D and calcium supplementation on falls: a randomized controlled trial, *J. Bone Min. Res.*, 18, 343, 2003.

51. Lips, P., Duong, T., Oleksik, A., Black, D., Cummings, S., Cox, D. et al., A global study of vitamin D status and parathyroid function in postmenopausal women with

osteoporosis: baseline data from the multiple outcomes of Raloxifene evaluation clinical trial, *J. Clin. Endocrinol. Metab.*, 86, 1212–1221, 2001.

52. Dawson-Hughes, B., Harris, S.S., Krall, E.A., and Dallal, G.E., Effect of calcium and vitamin D supplementation on bone density in men and women 65 years of age or older, *N. Engl. J. Med.*, 337, 670–676, 1997.

53. Malabanan, A., Veronikis, I.E., and Holick, M.F., Redefining vitamin D insufficiency, *Lancet*, 351, 805–806, 1998.

54. Tangpricha, V., Pearce, E.N., Chen, T.C., and Holick, M.F., Vitamin D insufficiency among free-living healthy young adults, *Am. J. Med.*, 112, 659–662, 2002.

55. Sullivan, S.S., Rosen, C.J., Halteman, W.A., Chen, T.C., and Holick, M.F., Seasonal changes in serum 25(OH)D in adolescent girls in Maine, *J. Am. Diet Assoc.*, 105, 971–974, 2005.

56. Gordon, C.M., DePeter, K.C., Estherann, G., and Emans, S.J., Prevalance of vitamin D deficiency among healthy adolescents, Endo2003, Endocrine Society Meeting (Abstr.) OR21-2, 2003, p. 87.

57. Nesby-O'Dell, S., Scanlon, K.S., Cogswell, M.E., Gillespie, C., Hollis, B.W., and Looker, A.C., Hypovitaminosis D prevalence and determinants among African American and white women of reproductive age: third national health and nutrition examination survey, 1988–1994. *Am. J. Clin. Nutr.* 76, 187–192, 2002.

58. Binkley, N., Krueger, D. et al., Assay variation confounds the diagnosis of hypovitaminosis D: a call for standardization, *J. Clin. Endocrinol. Metabol.*, 89, 3152–3157, 2004.

59. Heaney, R.P., Barger-Lux, J., Dowell, M.S., Chen, T.C., and Holick, M.F., Calcium absorptive effects of vitamin D and its major metabolites, *J. Clin. Endocrinol. Metabol.*, 82, 4111–4116. 1997.

60. Tangpricha, V., Koutkia, P., Rieke, S.M., Chen, T.C., Perez, A.A., and Holick, M.F., Fortification of orange juice with vitamin D: a novel approach to enhance vitamin D nutritional health, *Am. J. Clin. Nutr.*, 77, 1478–1483, 2003.

61. Vieth, R., Vitamin D supplementation, 25-hydroxyvitamin D concentrations, and safety, *Am. J. Clin. Nutr.*, 69, 842–856, 1999.

62. Malabanan, A.O., Turner, A.K., and Holick, M.F., Severe generalized bone pain and osteoporosis in a premenopausal black female: effect of vitamin D replacement. *J. Clin. Densitom.*, 1, 201–204, 1998.

63. Heaney, R.P., Dowell, M.S., Hale, C.A., and Bendich, A., Calcium absorption varies within the reference range for serum 25-hydroxyvitamin D, *J. Am. Coll. Nutr.*, 22, 142–146, 2003.

64. Koutkia, P., Lu, Z., Chen, T.C., and Holick, M.F., Treatment of vitamin D deficiency due to Crohn's disease with tanning bed ultraviolet B radiation, *Gastroenterology*, 121, 1485–1488, 2001.

65. Vieth, R., Chan, P-C., and MacFarlane, G.D., Efficacy and safety of vitamin D3 intake exceeding the lowest observed adverse effect level 18, *Am. J. Clin. Nutr.*, 73, 288–294, 2001; Jacobus, C.H., Holick, M.F., Shao, Q. et al., Hypervitaminosis D associated with drinking milk, *N. Engl. J. Med.*, 326, 1173–1177, 1992.

66. Koutkia, P., Chen, T.C., and Holick, M.F., Vitamin D intoxication associated with an over-the-counter supplement, *N. Engl. J. Med.*, 345, 66–67, 2001.

67. Wortsman, J., Matsuoka, L.Y., Chen, T.C., Lu, Z., and Holick, M.F., Decreased bioavailability of vitamin D in obesity, Am. *J. Clin. Nutr.*, 72, 690–693, 2000.

11 Chromium: Roles in the Regulation of Lean Body Mass and Body Weight

Richard A. Anderson, Ph.D.

CONTENTS

CHROMIUM AND HUMAN HEALTH

Trivalent chromium (Cr) is essential to human health. The essentiality of Cr has been known since the late 1950s from animal studies, and conclusive documentation in humans was not provided until 1977, when it was reported that a lady on total parenteral nutrition developed severe signs and symptoms of diabetes that were refractory to insulin.[1] Addition of Cr to her total parenteral nutrition solution led to a normalization of the signs and symptoms of diabetes, and exogenous insulin was no longer required. This work has subsequently been verified in the literature on three separate occasions.[2-4] Since these studies, there have been numerous studies documenting the role of Cr in human and animal nutrition, and the reader is urged to consult recent reviews[5-7] as well as those that question the essentiality and safety of Cr.[8,9]

Human studies suggest the following:

1. Healthy normal subjects with good glucose tolerance do not respond to supplemental Cr. This is to be expected because Cr is a nutrient and not a therapeutic agent and will, therefore, only be of benefit to those who are showing signs of deficiency.
2. Studies of Cr use of 250 μg or less per day do not consistently show significant effects. The inconsistency of the data is likely a function of absorption, which varies considerably with different Cr forms. See Table 11.2.
3. Studies involving subjects with impaired glucose tolerance or diabetes and consuming more than 250 μg of Cr usually do show significant effects of supplemental Cr.

SIGNS AND SYMPTOMS OF CHROMIUM DEFICIENCY IN HUMANS

Obese rats consuming supplemental Cr picolinate displayed lower insulin levels, improved glucose control, and increased phosphoinositol-3-kinase activity.[10] An effect of Cr on phosphoinositol-3-kinase documents a specific effect of Cr in a key control site in the insulin signaling cascade, which is the system responsible for the overall control of the sugar, fat, and energy metabolism. These observations prompted scientists to examine Cr's role in insulin resistance and the closely related body composition in humans.[10,11]

The signs and symptoms of Cr deficiency reported for humans are shown in Table 11.1. Chromium deficiency leads to decreased insulin sensitivity, and therefore variables that are regulated by insulin are often altered by Cr deficiency. In the presence of Cr in a useable form, lower amounts of insulin are required. Several early studies have shown that supplemental Cr has beneficial effects on risk factors associated with cardiovascular disease including total cholesterol, triglycerides, and HDL cholesterol,[11-14] and blood Cr has also been shown to be inversely related to cardiovascular disease.[15,16] These older studies have been questioned because of analytical difficulties, but the basic premise that body Cr concentrations are inversely related to the incidence of cardiovascular diseases has been substantiated, and recent studies show that diabetic men with cardiovascular disease have lower toenail Cr than do healthy control subjects.[17] Chromium has also been shown recently to be beneficial in the treatment of depression and to be free of negative side effects.[18] Studies on rats show that Cr picolinate also affects brain serotonin and noradrenaline, which helps explain its effects on depression in humans.[19] There are also preliminary studies on the role of Cr in the reversal of polycystic ovarian syndrome, which is characterized by decreased insulin sensitivity, and new studies are also emerging on the

TABLE 11.1
Signs and symptoms of chromium deficiency observed in humans

Impaired glucose tolerance
Elevated circulating insulin
Decreased insulin binding
Decreased insulin receptor number
Glycosuria
Fasting hyperglycemia
Hypoglycemia
Elevated cholesterol
Decreased HDL cholesterol
Elevated triglycerides
Increased ocular eye pressure
Decreased lean body mass
Increased fat mass
Increased body weight
Gestational diabetes
Steroid-induced diabetes
Type 2 diabetes
Atypical depression
Peripheral neuropathy
Encephalopathy

Note: All these signs and symptoms except the last two have been observed in normal free-living subjects consuming their normal diets.

substantiation of earlier studies reporting the reversal of gestational diabetes with supplemental Cr.[20]

Chromium was shown to have highly significant effects on fasting and post-prandial glucose and insulin of 155 people with type 2 diabetes.[21] There was a dose–response effect over four months, with larger effects at 1000 µg of Cr per day as Cr picolinate than at 200 µg per day. In addition to improvements in glucose and insulin, hemoglobin A1C decreased from 8.5 ± 0.2% to 6.6 ± 0.1% in the group receiving 1000 µg of Cr as Cr picolinate (hemoglobin A1C values below 6.5% are in the upper range of normal for older subjects), while hemoglobin A1C values were intermediate (7.5 ± 0.2%) in the group receiving 200 µg daily. These results were confirmed recently in a double-blind placebo controlled study involving 50 subjects with type 2 diabetes.[22] Similar to the earlier study of Anderson et al.,[21] supplemental Cr (200 µg twice daily as Cr picolinate) led to significant improvements in fasting and postprandial glucose and hemoglobin A1C. As stated previously, not all studies have reported significant effects of supplemental Cr and the reader is urged to consult detailed reviews on the effects of supplemental Cr.[5,7,23]

CHROMIUM AND LEAN BODY MASS AND BODY WEIGHT

The fact that not all studies show beneficial effects of supplemental Cr on lean body mass[8,24,25] is consistent with the expected observations that not all people are marginally or overtly deficient in Cr. In addition to the selection of subjects, duration of study, and form of Cr, the effects of Cr on weight and lean body mass may be masked by poor diets and a sedentary lifestyle. Chromium should be considered as one factor that affects insulin sensitivity and related lean body mass but is certainly not, for most individuals, the dominant factor.

Recent meta-analysis showed that there was a significant reduction in body weight caused by Cr, but it was stated that "a body weight reduction of 1.1 to 1.2 kg during an intervention period of 10 to 13 weeks (i.e., 0.08 to 0.1 kg/week) seems too small to be clinically meaningful."[26] Improvements in this range, if sustained, could lead to loss or prevention of gain of roughly 4 kg or 8 lb per year, which certainly could lead to large changes over time. Improvements in insulin-related variables that affect body weight and lean body mass are because of changes in metabolism and should not be confused with those associated with changes in dietary intake and energy expenditure. Lasting changes in insulin sensitivity and changes in metabolism could lead to lasting changes in body weight and composition. However, the long-term lasting and cumulative effects of Cr have not been determined.

In a study involving 20 M and 20 F swimmers receiving 400 μg daily of Cr as Cr picolinate, Cr significantly increased LBM (3.3%), decreased fat mass (−4.6%), and decreased percent body fat (−6.4%) compared with the placebo group.[27] Females had a greater change for percent fat compared with males (−8.2 and −4.7%, respectively). Effects were not significant after 12 but only after 24 weeks. This study supports the concept that studies involving Cr supplementation and LBM should be longer than 12 weeks and involve 400 μg of supplemental Cr daily or more.[24]

In a study involving very low calorie diets (3.34 MJ/d), diets were supplemented daily with placebo, 200 μg of Cr as Cr picolinate, or 200 μg of Cr as Cr yeast for 6 months.[28] Subjects were on the 3.34 MJ/d diet for the first 8 weeks. Weight losses in all groups after the initial 8 weeks were similar. After an additional 16 weeks, LBM was lower except in the group consuming Cr picolinate, with an increase of 1.81 ± 2.7 kg ($p < .0001$). Therefore, Cr consumed during and after weight reduction induced by a low calorie diet increased lean body mass. This may decrease the "yo-yo dieting effects" because weight loss would lead to a relative preservation of lean body mass and preferential fat loss. Normally dieting is associated with loss of both muscle and fat, but when weight is regained, there is increased accumulation of fat and not lean body mass. Because muscle tissue burns three times more calories than fat tissue, there would be even greater weight gains caused by the consumption of the same number of calories as before the diet, when muscle mass was greater.

In a study involving 154 subjects consuming a protein and carbohydrate drink containing no added Cr or 200 or 400 μg of Cr as Cr picolinate, both groups consuming Cr displayed improved body composition after 72 days.[29] Subjects were free-living and were not provided with weight loss, dietary, or exercise guidance. Body composition was measured by using underwater weighing with residual lung volumes determined by helium dilution. There were no significant changes in the placebo group. Body composition changes tended to be greater in the older subjects and in those consuming the higher level of Cr.

These studies involving improved LBM due to supplemental Cr in humans are supported by animal studies conducted mainly using pigs. Chromium increases longissimus muscle area and decreases percent fat in pigs.[30,31] Some studies have reported that Cr has no effects on LBM, but this may be related to form of Cr used (see the section "Form of Chromium"). But following the original studies showing beneficial effects of Cr on lean body mass, pig producers started adding Cr to the feed of sows, which would also affect the Cr status of the young pigs.[32] Using a highly available form of supplemental Cr, Cr was shown recently to increase carcass lean percentage, increase longissimus muscle area, and decrease back fat thickness and carcass fat percentage in pigs.[33]

Recent studies involving goats have helped elucidate and substantiate the role of Cr in weight control. Goats fed a high-refined carbohydrate, low-Cr diet also show elevated blood glucose and insulin.[34,35] The increases in blood glucose after 20 months of a low-Cr diet were 33% and that of circulating insulin almost 200% in comparison with the control group. There were also large increases in weight gain in the animals consuming the low-Cr diet compared with those of the controls (Figure 11.1, lower panel), with corresponding increases in feed consumption (Figure 11.1, upper panel). The increases in weight gain are attributed to the antilipolytic effects of insulin leading to accumulation of triglycerides in the adipose tissue. Elevated insulin levels in the low-Cr animals would also lead to decreased glucagon. Because glucagon stimulates lipolysis, decreased glucagon may lead to decreased lipolysis and subsequent accumulation of body fat and weight gain.

There were no effects until after 28 weeks on the low-Cr diet of low nutritional quality. If it takes more than 28 weeks to detect significant changes in body weight in rapidly growing goats, it is not surprising that most of the human studies, which are usually 12 weeks or less in duration, also are unable to detect significant changes in people with conventional diets.

While there are numerous anecdotal reports of Cr changing cravings for sugar and effects on total caloric intake, the studies of Frank et al.[34,35] are the first to report increased dietary intake in the low-Cr animals. Studies involving pigs report increased feed efficiency on account of Cr in animals consuming diets of marginal nutritional quality as well as effects on lean body mass and litter size.[31]

Chromium decreases cortisol concentration in humans.[36] This becomes important regarding weight control because cortisol increases circulating insulin and increases fat accumulation.[37] Adrenalectomy of obese rats leads to a normalizing of insulin and decreased fat accumulation, and after glucocorticoid administration, there is a return to elevated insulin levels and accumulation of fat.[38]

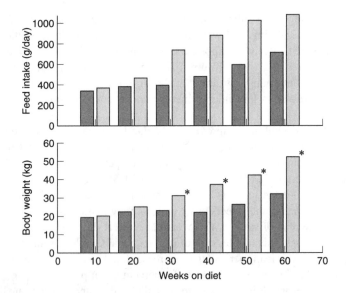

FIGURE 11.1 Feed intake and body weight of goats fed a low-Cr diet, gray bars, and diet supplemented with Cr, black bars. *Significant effect of Cr at $p < .05$; significance not given in original source for food intake.

Source: Adapted from Frank et al.[35]

CHROMIUM INTAKE AND REQUIREMENTS

The estimated safe and adequate daily dietary intake (ESADDI) for Cr for children 7 years old to adults of 50 to 200 µg/d was established by committees of the U.S. National Academy of Sciences in 1980 and affirmed in 1989. The ESADDI is similar to an RDA and is usually established before the RDA. The Food and Drug Administration proposed a reference dietary intake for Cr effective in 1997 of 120 µg/d. However, the new committee of the Institute of Medicine has proposed that the normal intake of Cr should serve as the adequate intake — 20 µg for women and 30 µg for men more than 50 years old and 25 µg for women and 35 µg for men 19 to 50 years old.[39] It is unclear why the adequate intake for Cr is lower for people more than 50 years old when one of the primary functions of Cr is to combat problems associated with the insulin and glucose metabolism, which increase with age.[40] Indices of Cr status such as the Cr content of hair, sweat, and urine were shown to decrease with age in a study involving more than 40,000 people.[41]

The proposed adequate intakes are nearly identical to the average of intakes reported in 1985 of 25 ± 1 µg for women and 33 ± 3 µg for men.[42] There have been more than 30 studies reporting beneficial effects of supplemental Cr for people with blood glucose values ranging from hypoglycemia to diabetes when consuming diets of similar Cr content.[5,7,23] In a controlled diet study, consumption of normal diets in the lowest quartile of normal Cr intakes but near the new adequate intakes led to detrimental effects on glucose[43] in subjects with marginally impaired glucose tolerance (90 min glucose between 5.5 and 11.1 mmol/l, (100 to 200 mg/dl) after an oral glucose load of 1 g/kg body weight. The average person of more than 25 years age has blood glucose in this range.[40] Consumption of the same diets by people with good glucose tolerance (90 min glucose less than 5.5 mmol/l) did not lead to changes in glucose and insulin variables. This is consistent with previous studies demonstrating that the requirement for Cr is related to the degree of glucose intolerance and demonstrates that an intake of 20 μg/d of Cr is not adequate for people with decreased insulin sensitivity such as people with marginally impaired glucose tolerance and certainly not for those with impaired glucose tolerance or diabetes.

The intake of Cr may also have decreased because of changes in methods of food preparation. Trace Cr is absorbed from the containers in which it is prepared. For example, Cr is present in beer in moderate concentrations. Initially this was attributed to the yeast used in brewing. More recently it has been appreciated to be the result of the metal containers with which beer comes in contact during brewing. Stainless steel is an amalgam generally containing 18% Cr. When foods with an acidic pH are prepared in stainless steel cookware, the Cr content of the food increases measurably. The shift from steel to cookware with nonstick coatings therefore reduces the population-wide Cr intake.

The metabolic need for chromium has increased. Previously adequate dietary intakes are likely to be suboptimal for insulin signaling in modern-day living. For example, foods high in refined carbohydrates enhance Cr losses.[44] States that increase cortisol levels also increase Cr loss. The studied examples include intense exercise, cold exposure, infection, burns, and trauma. Exogenous corticosteroid administration in treatment of various medical conditions also increases Cr losses and therefore Cr need.[45,46]

Both pregnancy and lactation increase demand for Cr as well as many other nutrients. During these physical states, gastrointestinal absorption of Cr has been shown to increase correspondingly.[47] However, the Cr demand exceeds absorption and may play a role in the breakdown of insulin signaling during pregnancy, often called gestational diabetes.[20]

Supplemental iron is used to enhance athletic performance. Iron is also taken, often unknowingly, in supplements or as fortified foods. Persons homozygous or heterozygous for hemochromatosis (approximately 2% of the population) absorb more of this dietary iron than is helpful, increasing body iron stores to the detriment of their metabolism. Iron competes with Cr for receptor binding sites, which functionally decreases Cr. Elevated iron stores lead to insulin resistance and bronze (skin color of patients with late stage disease) diabetes. Cr insufficiency is a contributing factor. Therefore Cr supplementation is likely to be beneficial in persons with increased body iron stores.

TRACE LEVELS OF CHROMIUM

The designation of Cr as a trace element comes from early studies in which the Cr concentrations of tissues and body fluids were too low to be accurately determined but in which it appeared that a "trace" amount was present. The amount of Cr in tissues and body fluids is in the parts per billion range (ng/g). To put this in perspective, this is less than one penny in ten million dollars! Normal Cr concentrations in the blood are usually in the range of 0.1 to 0.5 ng/g,[48] with similar concentrations in the urine[49] of people consuming normal diets without consuming Cr supplements. Supplemental Cr usually increases these values fivefold to 10-fold (see the section on Form of Chromium). There are no reliable data on the Cr concentrations in human tissues because human samples are often contaminated during the collection or storage of tissues in part because of the ubiquitous use of stainless steel (roughly 18% Cr) in the medical industry. Chromium concentrations in the tissues of rats are in the range of 1 to 10 ng/g on a wet weight basis, with the highest concentrations in the kidney.[50] Chromium supplementation leads to linear increases in Cr concentrations in the tissues, with the greatest concentrations in the kidneys.[50,51] Increases in tissue Cr remain linear at dietary intakes ranging from 5 to 100 mg of Cr/kg of diet.

FORM OF CHROMIUM

All ingested Cr found in the urine, except contaminating Cr, was absorbed. Therefore, because there is a rapid turnover of most of the absorbed Cr, urinary Cr losses in response to a Cr load can be used as a measure of Cr absorption.[52] Chromium chloride alone increases urinary Cr losses more than twofold (Table 11.2). The Cr nicotinate complexes appeared to be poorly absorbed, and the urinary losses were not significantly greater than those for days when additional Cr was not consumed. The Cr pidolate complex, which improved the antioxidant variables of subjects with type 2 diabetes mellitus (DM),[53] was absorbed in a manner similar to that of Cr chloride. The Cr nicotinate–glycinate–cysteinate–glutamate complex was poorly absorbed, in contrast to what was observed in rat studies.[50] Chromium methionate, a supplement which is often used in animal studies,[54] was not absorbed as efficiently as the Cr picolinate complexes. Complexes containing histidine were absorbed the best among the Cr complexes tested. Addition of histidine to the amino acid complexes tested increased Cr absorption, and the complexes with the highest Cr absorption were the Cr complexes synthesized with histidine (Table 11.2).

Starch, has been shown to increase Cr absorption when added to the diet of rats but was shown to strongly inhibit Cr absorption in humans when added to several forms of Cr before the Cr capsules were made.[52] Chromium added to a popular multivitamin and multimineral complex was also shown to be not absorbed (unpublished observation). Therefore, there should be some measure of

TABLE 11.2
Urinary chromium losses of human subjects after consumption of designated chromium compounds

Form of chromium	Urinary Cr losses (ng/g)
Basal losses	256 ± 48^d
+Cr chloride	655 ± 74^c
+Cr nicotinate	262 ± 69^d
+Cr nicotinate (commercial)	160 ± 60^d
+Cr-NA-GLY-CYS-GLU[a]	300 ± 92^{cd}
+Cr pidolate	643 ± 131^c
+Cr methionate	1065 ± 199^{bcd}
+Cr picolinate	2082 ± 201^b
+Cr picolinate (commercial)	2048 ± 327^b
+Cr glycinate–glutamate–histidinate	2188 ± 169^b
+Cr histidinate	

Notes: 1. Subjects consumed 200 µg of Cr of each of the forms, and urine was collected the day of consuming the Cr and the following day (data are for the two days combined). Urinary Cr losses are a measure of Cr absorption because all Cr in urine (except contaminating Cr) has been absorbed.

2. Values with different superscripts are significantly different at $p < .05$.

[a]Chromium nicotinate–glycinate–cysteinate–glutamate complex.

Source: Anderson et al.[52]

Cr absorption in studies involving Cr supplementation to ensure that the form of Cr, under the conditions used, is being absorbed.

SAFETY OF CHROMIUM

There is no clinical evidence of Cr toxicity in humans. Some isolated anecdotes of poor health outcomes in persons taking supplemental Cr have been reported in the literature, and each of these has an alternate explanation for the adverse outcome.

Trivalent Cr, the form of Cr found in foods and nutrient supplements, is considered one of the least toxic nutrients. The reference dose established by the U.S. Environmental Protection Agency for Cr is more than 2000 times the new adequate intakes. The reference dose (RfD) is defined as "an estimate (with uncertainty spanning perhaps an order of magnitude) of a daily exposure to the human population, including sensitive subgroups, that is likely to be without an appreciable risk of deleterious effects over a lifetime."[55] This conservative estimate of a safe intake has a much larger safety factor for trivalent Cr than almost any other nutrient. The ratio of the RfD to the adequate intake or RDA is 2000 or more for Cr, compared with less than 2 for other trace elements such as zinc, roughly 2 for manganese, and 5 to 7 for selenium. Anderson et al.[51] demonstrated a lack of toxicity of Cr chloride and Cr picolinate in rats at levels more than 2000 times the upper limit of the adequate daily dietary intake for humans (based on body weight). There have been no documented toxic effects at oral intakes of Cr of 10 to 50 times the normal intakes, and most of the studies report beneficial effects.

Physiology allows variable absorption of Cr, based on needs. The chromium absorption from foods is inversely related to the dietary intake.[42] At daily intakes of roughly 10 μg, absorption is 2% and decreases to 0.5% at 40 μg.

There are several studies reporting toxic effects of injected Cr in animals or in cell culture systems where there are minimal normal protective measures. The largest protective mechanism for Cr is the gastrointestinal tract, which allows usually less than 2% of the Cr to be absorbed. Not even studies with oral Cr intakes far outside the normal supplemental intake ranges show signs of toxicity for trivalent Cr, and the committee of the Institute of Medicine involved with setting recommended intakes as well as upper limits of intake was not able to set an upper limit for Cr because there were no adequate studies reporting signs of Cr toxicity when Cr was consumed by the normal means.[39] Toxicity studies conducted with injected Cr should not be confused with those involving oral intakes because not only is the absorption of Cr low (usually less than 2%) but toxic forms of Cr may be changed in the absorption process. For example, low levels of toxic hexavalent Cr can be converted to the relatively nontoxic trivalent form in the normal processes associated with absorption.

Chromium picolinate, the most popular form in nutritional supplements, has been reported to have toxic effects under nonphysiological conditions in cell cultures, in fruit flies, and after injection in rats (see review in reference 8). With these studies in mind, even higher levels than those used in the study of Anderson et al.[51] were fed to rats and mice to monitor toxicity at levels thousands of times those that would normally be found under conditions of supplementation.[56] Chromium was added to the diet because the oral route would more closely mimic the effects associated with high levels of Cr supplementation. Rats and mice were fed up to 50,000 ug of Cr picolinate monohydrate for 13 weeks with no effects on body weights, organ weights, survival, clinical chemistry parameters, hematology, or histopathology. The amount of Cr picolinate administered to the animals was sufficient to turn the feces of the animals red on account of the red color of the Cr picolinate, but still no toxicity was detected.[56] These results obviously do not suggest that there are no conditions where Cr ingested orally would not be toxic, but the levels are far outside the range of normal intake associated with supplemental Cr. Chromium picolinate has been reviewed under the demanding requirements of a Generally Recognized as Safe (GRAS) determination and has been found to be safe at exposures to Cr (as Cr picolinate) at least as high as 900 μg/d.[57]

Editor's note

Chromium (Cr) is an essential trace mineral present in human tissues at concentrations less than 1/100th that of iron. These are concentrations so small that only recent technologic advances have made measurements possible. Cr influences specific enzymes in the insulin signaling pathway that lead to increased insulin sensitivity. Insufficient Cr is associated with insulin resistance, resulting in gradual, unfavorable changes in body composition. There is evidence that whereas Cr intake may have only decreased slightly in the recent decades, the body's demand has increased appreciably because of modern-day stressors and refined carbohydrates, which increase Cr losses. Patients on prednisone, persons with insulin resistance, and persons experiencing physical stress have demonstrated benefits from additional Cr intake.

SUMMARY

Dietary intakes of Cr are often suboptimal, based upon the fact that there are numerous peer-reviewed studies documenting beneficial effects of Cr on insulin sensitivity, body composition, and related variables. At suboptimal levels of Cr, higher levels of insulin are required. The response to Cr is dependent upon the Cr intake and status, degree of glucose intolerance, stage and duration of diabetes, age, and lean body mass of the subjects. Obviously there are many factors that alter insulin sensitivity and body composition, and Cr is only one of these factors and therefore will only be of benefit to those whose insulin resistance is caused by suboptimal dietary Cr. Chromium is safe at all of the levels tested for oral intakes and therefore may be a safe and inexpensive aid to improved glucose and insulin metabolism and body composition.

REFERENCES

1. Jeejeebhoy, K.N., Chu, R.C., Marliss, E.B., Greenberg, G.R., and Bruce-Robertson, A., Chromium deficiency, glucose intolerance, and neuropathy reversed by chromium supplementation, in a patient receiving long-term total parenteral nutrition, *Am. J. Clin. Nutr.,* 30, 531–538, 1977.
2. Freund, H., Atamian, S., and Fischer, J.E., Chromium deficiency during total parenteral nutrition, *JAMA*, 241, 496–498, 1979.
3. Brown, R.O., Forloines-Lynn, S., Cross, R.E., and Heizer, W.D., Chromium deficiency after long-term total parenteral nutrition, *Dig. Dis. Sci.,* 31, 661–664, 1986.
4. Anderson, R.A. Essentiality of chromium in humans, *Sci. Total Environ.,* 86, 75–81, 1989.
5. Anderson, R.A. Chromium, glucose intolerance and diabetes, *J. Am. Coll. Nutr.,* 17, 548–555, 1998.

6. Anderson, R.A, Chromium and insulin sensitivity, *Nutr. Res. Rev.*, 16267–16275, 2003.

7. Cefalu, W.T., and Hu, F.B., Role of chromium in human health and in diabetes, *Diabetes Care*, 27, 2741–2751, 2004.

8. Vincent, J.B., The potential value and toxicity of chromium picolinate as a nutritional supplement, weight loss agent and muscle development agent, *Sports Med.*, 33, 213–230, 2003.

9. Vincent, J.B, The biochemistry of chromium, *J. Nutr.*, 130, 715–718, 2000.

10. Cefalu, W.T., Wang, Z.Q., Zhang, X.H., Baldor, L.C., and Russell, J.C., Oral chromium picolinate improves carbohydrate and lipid metabolism and enhances skeletal muscle Glut-4 translocation in obese, hyperinsulinemic (JCR-LA corpulent) rats, *J. Nutr.*, 132, 1107–1114, 2002.

11. Riales, R., and Albrink, M.J., Effect of chromium chloride supplementation on glucose tolerance and serum lipids including high-density lipoprotein of adult men, *Am. J. Clin. Nutr.*, 34, 2670–2678, 1981.

12. Abraham, A.S., Brooks, B.A., and Eylath, U., The effects of chromium supplementation on serum glucose and lipids in patients with and without non-insulin-dependent diabetes, *Metabolism*, 41, 768–771, 1992.

13. Roeback, J.R.J., Hla, K.M., Chambless, L.E., and Fletcher, R.H., Effects of chromium supplementation on serum high-density lipoprotein cholesterol levels in men taking beta-blockers. A randomized, controlled trial [see comments], *Ann. Intern. Med.*, 115, 917–924, 1991.

14. Rabinovitz, H., Friedensohn, A., Leibovitz, A., Gabay, G., Rocas, C., and Habot, B., Effect of chromium supplementation on blood glucose and lipid levels in type 2 diabetes mellitus elderly patients, *Int. J. Vitam. Nutr. Res.*, 74, 178–182, 2004.

15. Newman, H.A.I., Leighton, R.F., Lanese, R.R., and Freedland, N.A., Serum chromium and angiographically determined coronary artery disease, *Clin. Chem.*, 24541–24544, 1978.

16. Simonoff, M., Chromium deficiency and cardiovascular risk, *Cardiovasc. Res.*, 18, 591–596, 1984.

17. Rajpathak, S., Rimm, E.B., Li, T., Morris, J.S., Stampfer, M.J., Willett, W.C., and Hu, F.B., Lower toenail chromium in men with diabetes and cardiovascular disease compared with healthy men, *Diabetes Care*, 27, 2211–2216, 2004.

18. Davidson, J.R., Abraham, K., Connor, K.M., and McLeod, M.N., Effectiveness of chromium in atypical depression: a placebo-controlled trial, *Biol. Psychiatry*, 53, 261–264, 2003.

19. Franklin, M., and Odontiadis, J., Effects of treatment with chromium picolinate on peripheral amino acid availability and brain monoamine function in the rat, *Pharmacopsychiatry*, 36, 176–180, 2003.

20. Jovanovic, L., Gutierrez, M., and Peterson, C.M., Chromium supplementation for women with gestational diabetes mellitus, *J. Trace Elem. Exp. Med.*, 1291–1298, 1999.

21. Anderson, R.A., Cheng, N., Bryden, N.A., Polansky, M.M., Chi, J., and Feng, J., Elevated intakes of supplemental chromium improve glucose and insulin variables in individuals with type 2 diabetes, *Diabetes*, 46, 1786–1791, 1997.

22. Bahijri, S.M., and Mufti, A.M., Beneficial effects of chromium in people with type 2 diabetes, and urinary chromium response to glucose load as a possible indicator of status, *Biol. Trace Elem. Res.*, 85, 97–109, 2002.

23. Althuis, M.D., Jordan, N.E., Ludington, E.A., and Wittes, J.T., Glucose and insulin responses to dietary chromium supplements: a meta-analysis, *Am. J. Clin. Nutr.,* 76, 148–155, 2002.

24. Anderson, R.A., Effects of chromium on body composition and weight loss, *Nutr. Rev.,* 56, 266–270, 1998.

25. Kobla, H.V., and Volpe, S.L., Chromium, exercise, and body composition, *Crit. Rev. Food Sci. Nutr.,* 40, 291–308, 2000.

26. Pittler, M.H., Stevinson, C., and Ernst, E., Chromium picolinate for reducing body weight: meta-analysis of randomized trials, *Int. J. Obes. Relat. Metab. Disord.,* 27, 522–529, 2003.

27. Bulbulian, R., Pringle, D.D., and Liddy, M.S., Chromium picolinate supplementation in male and female swimmers, *Med. Sci. Sports Exerc.,* 28511, 1996.

28. Bahadori, B., Wallner, S., Schneider, H., Wascher, T.C., and Toplak, H., Effect of chromium yeast and chromium picolinate on body composition of obese, non-diabetic patients during and after a formula diet, *Acta Med. Austriaca,* 24, 185–187, 1997.

29. Kaats, G.R., Blum, K., Fisher, J.A., and Adelman, J.A., Effects of chromium picolinate supplementation on body composition: a randomized double-masked placebo-controlled study, *Curr. Ther. Res.,* 57747–57756, 1996.

30. Page, T.G., Southern, L.L., Ward, T.L., and Thompson, D.L.J., Effect of chromium picolinate on growth and serum and carcass traits of growing-finishing pigs, *J. Anim. Sci.,* 71, 656–662, 1993.

31. Lindemann, M.D., Wood, C.M., Harper, A.F., Kornegay, E.T., and Anderson, R.A., Dietary chromium picolinate additions improve gain: feed and carcass characteristics in growing-finishing pigs and increase litter size in reproducing sows, *J. Anim. Sci.,* 73, 457–465, 1995.

32. Mooney, K.W., and Cromwell, G.L., Efficacy of chromium picolinate and chromium chloride as potential carcass modifiers in swine, *J. Anim. Sci.,* 75, 2661–2671, 1997.

33. Wang, M.Q., and Xu, Z.R., Effect of chromium nanoparticles on growth performance, carcass characteristics, pork quality and tissue chromium in finishing pigs, *Asian–Aust. J. Anim. Sci.,* 17, 1118–1122. 2004.

34. Frank, A., Danielsson, R., and Jones, B., Experimental copper and chromium deficiency and additional molybdenum supplementation in goats. II. Concentrations of trace and minor elements in liver, kidneys and ribs: haematology and clinical chemistry, *Sci. Total Environ.,* 249, 143–170, 2000.

35. Frank, A., Anke, M., and Danielsson, R., Experimental copper and chromium deficiency and additional molybdenum supplementation in goats. I. Feed consumption and weight development, *Sci. Total Environ.,* 249, 133–142, 2000.

36. Anderson, R.A., Insulin, glucose intolerance and diabetes: recent data regarding the chromium connection, in *Trace Elements and Nutritional Health Disorders, Proceedings of the First International Bio-minerals Symposium,* Institut Rosell-The Americas, Montreal, QC, 2002, pp. 179–186.

37. Freedman, M.R., Horwitz, B.A., and Stern, J.S., Effect of adrenalectomy and glucocorticoid replacement on development of obesity, *Am. J. Physiol.,* 250(4 Pt. 2), R595–R607, 1986.

38. Strack, A.M., Sebastian, R.J., Schwartz, M.W., and Dallman, M.F., Glucocorticoids and insulin: reciprocal signals for energy balance, *Am. J. Physiol.,* 268(1 Pt. 2), R142–R149, 1995.

39. Anonymous, *Dietary Reference Intakes for Vitamin A, Vitamin K, Arsenic, Boron, Chromium, Copper, Iodine, Iron, Manganese, Molybdenum, Nickel, Silicon, Vanadium and Zinc,* National Academy Press, Washington, DC, 2001, pp. 197–223.

40. Harris, M.I., Noninsulin-dependent diabetes mellitus in black and white Americans, *Diabetes Metab. Rev.,* 671–690, 1990.

41. Davies, S., McLaren, H.J., Hunnisett, A., and Howard, M., Age-related decreases in chromium levels in 51,665 hair, sweat, and serum samples from 40,872 patients — implications for the prevention of cardiovascular disease and type II diabetes mellitus, *Metabolism,* 46, 469–473, 1997.

42. Anderson, R.A., and Kozlovsky, A.S., Chromium intake, absorption and excretion of subjects consuming self-selected diets, *Am. J. Clin. Nutr.,* 41, 1177–1183, 1985.

43. Anderson, R.A., Polansky, M.M., Bryden, N.A., and Canary, J.J., Supplemental-chromium effects on glucose, insulin, glucagon, and urinary chromium losses in subjects consuming controlled low-chromium diets, *Am. J. Clin. Nutr.,* 54, 909–916, 1991.

44. Kozlovsky, A.S., Moser, P.B., Reiser, S., and Anderson, R.A., Effects of diets high in simple sugars on urinary chromium losses, *Metabolism,* 35, 515–518, 1986.

45. Ravina, A., Slezak, L., Mirsky, N., and Anderson, R.A., Control of steroid-induced diabetes with supplemental chromium, *J. Trace Elem. Exp. Med.,* 12375–12378, 1999.

46. Ravina, A., Slezak, L., Mirsky, N., Bryden, N.A., and Anderson, R.A., Reversal of corticosteroid-induced diabetes mellitus with supplemental chromium, *Diabetes Med.,* 16, 164–167, 1999.

47. Anderson, R.A., Stress effects on chromium nutrition of humans and farm animals, in *Proceedings of Alltech's Tenth Symposium on Biotechnology in the Feed Industry,* Lyons, T.P. and Jacques, K.A., Eds., University Press, Nottingham, U.K., 1994, pp. 267–274.

48. Anderson, R.A., Bryden, N.A., and Polansky, M.M., Serum chromium of human subjects: effects of chromium supplementation and glucose, *Am. J. Clin. Nutr.,* 41, 571–577, 1985.

49. Anderson, R.A., Polansky, M.M., Bryden, N.A., Patterson, K.Y., Veillon, C., and Glinsmann, W.H., Effects of chromium supplementation on urinary Cr excretion of human subjects and correlation of Cr excretion with selected clinical parameters, *J. Nutr.,* 113, 276–281, 1983.

50. Anderson, R.A., Bryden, N.A., Polansky, M.M., and Gautschi, K., Dietary chromium effects on tissue chromium concentrations and chromium absorption in rats, *J. Trace Elem. Exp. Med.,* 911–925, 1996.

51. Anderson, R.A., Bryden, N.A., and Polansky, M.M., Lack of toxicity of chromium chloride and chromium picolinate in rats, *J. Am. Coll. Nutr.,* 16, 273–279, 1997.

52. Anderson, R.A., Polansky, M.M., and Bryden, N.A., Stability and absorption of chromium and absorption of chromium histidinate complexes by humans, *Biol. Trace Elem. Res.,* 101, 211–218, 2004.

53. Anderson, R.A., Roussel, A.M., Zouari, N., Mahjoub, S., Matheau, J.M., and Kerkeni, A., Potential antioxidant effects of zinc and chromium supplementation in people with type 2 diabetes mellitus, *J. Am. Coll. Nutr.,* 20, 212–218, 2001.

54. Kegley, E.B., Galloway, D.L., and Fakler, T.M., Effect of dietary chromium-L-methionine on glucose metabolism of beef steers, *J. Anim. Sci.,* 78, 3177–3183, 2000.

55. Mertz, W., Abernathy, C.O., and Olin, S.S., *Risk Assessment of Essential Elements,* ILSI Press, Washington, DC, 1994.

56. Rhodes, M.C., Hebert, C.D., Herbert, R.A., Morinello, E.J., Roycroft, J.H., Travlos, G.S., and Abdo, K.M., Absence of toxic effects in F344/N rats and B6C3F1 mice following subchronic administration of chromium picolinate monohydrate, *Food Chem. Toxicol.,* 43, 21–29, 2005.

57. Heimbach, J.T., and Anderson, R.A., Chromium: recent studies regarding nutritional roles and safety, *Nutr. Today,* 2005 (in press).

Section III

Fat Tissue

12 Energy Balance

Wayne C. Miller, Ph.D.

CONTENTS

METABOLIC RATE

THERMIC EFFECT OF FOOD

The 24-h energy expenditure can be broken down into three components, the thermic effect of food, the resting metabolic rate, and the energy cost of physical activity (Figure 12.1). The thermic effect of food is defined as the amount of

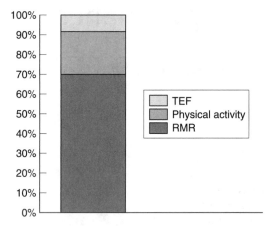

FIGURE 12.1 Relative contributions of resting metabolic rate (RMR), thermic effect of food (TEF), and physical activity to 24-h energy expenditure.

energy required to digest, absorb, and further process the energy-yielding nutrients in food (i.e., fat, protein, carbohydrate). These energy-expending processes for preparing food prior to its use in intermediary metabolism generate heat, and are therefore collectively called the *thermic* effect of food (TEF) or, alternatively, diet-induced *thermogenesis*. The contribution of the TEF to the 24-h energy expenditure is minimal, and ranges from 5 to 10%. Given a daily energy expenditure of 2500 kcal (10.46 MJ), the TEF would be between 125 and 250 kcal (523 and 1046 kJ).

The metabolic pathways for storing excess dietary fat in the body are more efficient than converting excess carbohydrate and protein into their storage forms, glycogen and fat. Consequently, the TEF for a high-protein or high-carbohydrate meal is greater than that for a high-fat meal. However, the TEF can only be increased by about 50 kcal (209 kJ) per day by altering the macronutrient composition of the diet. In addition, large meals produce higher values for TEF than the same amount of food consumed over several hours. Possible mechanisms to explain the elevated TEF with a large meal include increased central nervous system activity, greater production and release of hormones, greater enzyme activity, and an increased rate of absorption of nutrients. Nonetheless, variance in the TEF does not seem to make a difference in body fat stores within or among individuals.

RESTING METABOLIC RATE

The minimal amount of energy expended to sustain the basic body functions is called the resting metabolic rate (RMR). The RMR amounts to about 1 kcal kg^{-1}

(4 kJ) of body weight per hour or roughly 1800 kcal (7.53 MJ) per day for the average 75-kg man. The RMR accounts for approximately 60 to 75% of the total daily energy expenditure, and, therefore, anything that alters the RMR has the potential to significantly impact body fat stores. Factors that have been implicated in the variance found for RMR within and among individuals are body composition, gender, race, restrictive dieting, and exercise. Some of these factors are interrelated, some are subject to behavior modification, and yet some are nonmodifiable.

Body Composition

Individual differences in lean body mass account for most of the 25 to 30% variation in RMR among individuals. Persons with greater amounts of lean body mass have higher RMRs than those with less lean body mass. Fat mass adds relatively little to the RMR (Table 12.1). In fact, the RMR of obese individuals is strongly related to their lean body mass, not their fat mass. Variation in RMR within an individual is predominantly attributed to fluctuations in lean body mass. When an overweight or obese person loses weight, his or her RMR decreases in proportion to the amount of lean body mass that is lost. If RMR is expressed in absolute terms (kcal d^{-1}), obese individuals generally have values that are higher than nonobese persons, because the obese most often carry additional lean body mass with their added adiposity. If an individual gains muscle mass through athletic training, his or her RMR increases in proportion to the lean mass gained.

Muscles, organs, bone, and fluids make up most of the lean body mass. The tissues and organs that contribute most to the RMR are the liver, skeletal muscles, brain, heart, and kidneys (Table 12.1). The size of each of these is directly related to body size. The size of the skeletal muscle mass is also related to body type, muscle development, and age.

Maintaining muscular fitness through aging can help slow the loss of lean tissue and maintain the RMR (Chapter 18). However, declining lean body mass and decreased muscularity in older adults do not fully account for the reduction in

TABLE 12.1
Relative contributions of the tissues and organs to the RMR

Organ/tissue	kcal d^{-1}	Relative contribution (% RMR)
Liver	476	28
Brain	323	19
Heart	153	9
Kidneys	136	8
Muscle mass	306	18
Fat mass	34	2
Reminder	272	16

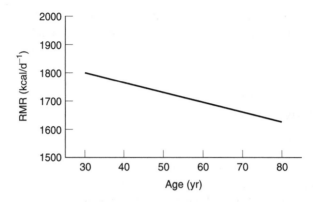

FIGURE 12.2 Average resting metabolic rate with age.

RMR of about 2% per decade after the age of 30 (Figure 12.2). It is hypothesized that the organs themselves become less active metabolically, and that this contributes to the decline in RMR with age.

Gender and Race

Many researchers have reported differences in RMR between men and women over a wide range in age and body weights. The consensus is that women have an RMR that is 5 to 10% lower than men. However, this does not necessarily reflect a true gender difference in the metabolic rates of individual tissues or organs. More likely, it reflects a difference in body composition between the genders. A woman generally possesses more body fat and less muscle mass than a man of a comparable weight and size. Since adipose tissue is metabolically less active than muscle tissue, the RMR of women is proportionately reduced when compared to men because of women's increased adiposity.

African-American men and women have a lower RMR than Caucasians and the magnitude of difference between the races is similar for both men and women.[1,2] These reports have measured the RMR for African-Americans to be anywhere from 5 to 20% below that of Caucasians. The difference in the RMR over a 24-h period ranges from 80 to 200 kcal (335 to 837 kJ). This metabolic discrepancy cannot be attributed to differences in age, body mass index, body composition, daily activity levels, menstrual cycle phase, or fitness level. The mechanism underlying this metabolic discrepancy has not yet been identified, and it is still controversial as to whether this difference in RMR between races is the cause of the higher prevalence of obesity in African-Americans.

Depressed RMR has been associated with high levels of obesity in southwestern American Indians.[3] The estimated risk of gaining more than 7.5 kg was four times greater for persons with an RMR that was 200 kcal d^{-1} (837 kJ) lower than predicted as compared to individuals with an RMR 200 kcal d^{-1} (837 kJ) above predicted values. Furthermore, a low RMR was found to be predictive of weight gain over a 4-year period in the same southwestern American Indians. Finally, values for RMR aggregated in families, with an intraclass correlation of 0.48 between RMR and magnitude of obesity. Although the mechanistic causes have not been elucidated, the data from these studies show that RMR differs among the races.

Calorie-Restricted Diets

Although logic seems to dictate that energy-restricted diets should assist weight control efforts by creating a negative energy balance, data now show that severe calorie restriction may actually hinder attempts at weight control. Bray was the first to demonstrate that a reduction in energy intake results in a decline in RMR. Later, he found that this decrease in RMR was about 15% when subjects were removed from a maintenance diet of 3500 kcal d^{-1} (14.64 MJ) and placed on a very-low-calorie diet of 450 kcal d^{-1} (1883 kJ).[4]

Although RMR drops while a person is on a very-low-calorie diet, most authors agree that when energy intake is restored to predieting levels, the RMR also returns to predieting levels, unless there is a decrease in lean body mass. In which case, the postdiet RMR per lean body mass ratio (RMR–LBM) would be equivalent to predieting levels. However, an early research paper contests that severe energy restriction lowers RMR–LBM significantly.[5] During this study, obese women were placed on a very-low-calorie diet for 3 weeks. The RMR–LBM declined to 94, 91, and 82% of the original value on days 3, 5, and 21, respectively (Figure 12.3). More research needs to be conducted in order to determine the long-term effects of energy-restricted diets on RMR, both for the chronic dieter as well as the person with anorexia.

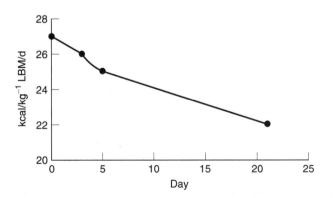

FIGURE 12.3 Resting metabolic rate per unit of lean body mass, during 21 days of very-low-calorie dieting.

Exercise

Even though less than 20% of the RMR is attributed to skeletal muscle,[6] the most dramatic effect on metabolic rate is strenuous exercise. During strenuous exercise, the total energy expenditure of the body may increase 15–25 times above resting levels.[6] This enormous elevation in the body's metabolic rate is the result of a 200-fold increase in the energy requirement of exercising muscles.[6]

Exercise physiologists have contended for years that aerobic exercise training increases RMR. More recent investigations, however, infer that aerobic exercise training does not automatically increase RMR significantly. For example, Wilmore[7] showed that RMR remained unchanged following 20 weeks of aerobic exercise training in men and women of all ages, in spite of a large increase of 18% $\dot{V}O_{2max}$.

Nonetheless, aerobic exercise may prevent the common age-related decline in RMR.[8] Endurance-trained, middle-aged, and older women presented a 10% higher RMR than sedentary women when RMR was adjusted for body composition. Although descriptive in nature, these data suggest that exercise may help prevent the age-related weight gain seen in sedentary women, and that the protective mechanism may be an altered RMR.

Because it is well accepted that strength training can increase muscle mass, and that muscle mass is very active metabolically, Byrne and Wilmore[9] have recently examined how strength training may differentially affect RMR in comparison to aerobic exercise training. This cross-sectional study found that there was no significant difference in RMR among strength-trained, aerobically trained, and untrained women. In a randomized controlled clinical trial, moderately obese men and women were assigned to one of three groups; diet plus strength training, diet plus aerobic training, or diet only.[10] The exercise protocols were designed to be isoenergetic. The mean weight loss among groups did not differ significantly after 8 weeks, but the strength-trained group lost less lean tissue mass than the other two groups. The RMR declined significantly in each group, with no difference among groups. These data indicate that neither strength training nor aerobic exercise training prevent the decline in RMR caused by restrictive dieting.[10]

Diet and Exercise Interactions

The implication for when an overweight individual attempts to lose weight by energy-restrictive dieting and exercise is that two opposing metabolic forces are working against each other that result in a hindrance of the weight loss process. This dilemma is illustrated in a series of metabolic measurements taken during treadmill exercise in mildly overweight (26% body fat) women who were cyclical dieters and healthy weight (21% body fat) nondieting controls.[11] Regardless of the workload examined, relative exercise energy expenditure was significantly lower in the dieters than the nondieters. These results demonstrate an increased efficiency of food utilization during exercise in chronic energy-restricting dieters.

Although the long-term effects of energy-restricted dieting on RMR are not currently known, daily exercise continued over a long period of time may reverse the detrimental effects of energy-restricted dieting on RMR. Early work revealed that daily aerobic exercise at 60% $\dot{V}O_{2max}$, initiated 2 weeks after a very-low-calorie diet (500 kcal d^{-1}, 2092 kJ d^{-1}), normalized the diet-induced dip in RMR and attenuated the diet-induced loss in lean body mass.[12] A later study found that when aerobic exercise was initiated simultaneously with a severely restricted diet, RMR was maintained, but the diet-induced loss in lean tissue was not safeguarded.[13] Other studies, in which a very-low-calorie diet and exercise were initiated simultaneously, have shown that exercise neither minimized the loss of lean tissue nor maintained RMR.[14,15]

The benchmark review of the effect of exercise on RMR, during restricted energy intake, is a meta-analysis by Ballor and Poehlman.[16] When diet-induced reductions in RMR were corrected for changes in body weight, RMR was reduced by less than 2%. These meta-analytical data indicate that exercise training does not differentially affect RMR during weight loss, nor enhance RMR during weight loss, and that reductions in RMR normally seen during weight loss are proportional to the loss of the metabolically active tissue.[16]

The relationship between diet, exercise, and metabolism is complex. Severely restrictive diets generally result in a transient decrease in metabolic rate, but whether this decrease is sustained has not been clearly shown. It may be that the variability in the metabolic response to diet restriction and exercise among individuals is influenced by the type of obesity (gluteal–femoral or abdominal), the cellular expression of obesity (hypertrophic or hyperplastic), or the genotype of obesity.[16] Some of the variation in the literature with respect to the effects of exercise training on RMR may also be related to the length of time between the last exercise training session and measurement of RMR. Herring et al.[17] reported that RMR was elevated immediately following an exercise session, but that within 39 h of the cessation of exercise the RMR had dropped 8%. Achieving an exercise-induced elevation in RMR is likely to require that the exercise stimulus be repeated daily or several times per week. Accordingly, the incremental effects of the energy cost of exercise itself combined with the incremental effects of the temporary postexercise elevations in metabolic rate may act synergistically to enhance weight loss success and long-term reduced weight maintenance.

Although the data are not consistently clear, the American College of Sports Medicine attests that exercise helps maintain the RMR and slows the rate of fat-free tissue loss that occurs when a person loses weight by severe energy restriction.[6] Whether exercise completely offsets the diet-induced reduction or only partially offsets the diet-induced reduction in RMR may depend on the severity and duration of the diet restrictions; type, duration, and intensity of exercise; and the magnitude of changes in body composition. Additional research is necessary to determine how the interactions of diet and exercise affect metabolic rate over prolonged periods of time, how long a regimen of diet and exercise can safely be employed, and what mechanisms are responsible for the diet and exercise effects on metabolism.

EXERCISE ENERGY EXPENDITURE

Energy Costs of Exercise

As heavy exercise can increase metabolic rate 20 times above resting levels, even short bouts of daily exercise may have a profound effect on body fat stores. In terms of measurement, the RMR of a 70-kg human is approximately 1.2 kcal min^{-1} (5.0 kJ), whereas the energy cost during strenuous exercise can be 18 to 30 kcal min^{-1} (75 to 125 kJ).[6] At first glance, these numbers look promising for weight loss; in that the energy cost of a 60-min exercise bout would be from 1080 to 1800 kcal (4518 to 7531 kJ). This translates into an exercise-induced weight loss of about one third to one half pound a day. However, theoretical estimates of energy expenditure during exercise, such as those previously described, are not realistic for the overweight or obese individual for several reasons. First, an intense exercise bout lasting 60 min is beyond the reach of most overweight people,[18] since the functional capacity of the overweight person is generally much less than the normal weight individual. Overweight people, who have a history of inactivity, generally can only increase their total energy expenditure by about eightfold during maximal exercise exertion,[18,19] and most of these people find it very difficult to sustain an exercise intensity of 75% maximal effort for 20 min.[18] Therefore, the best initial expectation for the overweight person would be to exercise for 20 min at an intensity that is six times the RMR (6 METS or 6 metabolic equivalents). Under these conditions (20 min at 6 METS), the predicted energy expenditure of the exercise session would only be about 150 kcal (628 kJ).

Although it may seem that the absolute contribution of the energy cost of activity to offset the daily energy balance during weight loss treatment is small, the relative contribution of exercise to the 24-h energy expenditure is important. The 20-min exercise bout described above may account for 10% or more of the daily energy expenditure for an obese person. Furthermore, exercise may have a metabolic effect beyond that which is accounted for during the actual exercise session itself.

Postexercise Energy Costs

It is well established that metabolic rate, measured as oxygen consumption, remains elevated for some period of time following exercise. This phenomenon has been termed excess postexercise oxygen consumption (EPOC). Studies have shown that the magnitude of EPOC is linearly related to the duration and intensity of exercise, and that EPOC following a moderate intensity exercise bout (70% $\dot{V}O_{2max}$.) accounts for about 15% of the total energy cost of the exercise.[20] The time for metabolism to return to baseline following an acute exercise session can vary from as little as 20 min to 12 h, depending on the duration and intensity of exercise. Increments of EPOC may play a significant role in the energy balance of the body. Unfortunately, the EPOC is insufficiently predictable as a measurable variable in exercise prescription for weight control.

Several factors have been identified as contributing to EPOC.[21] Intermediary substrates, such as lactate and free fatty acids, continue to be oxidized at an elevated rate following an exercise bout. The cost of replenishing glycogen stores also adds to the EPOC. Circulatory levels of catecholamines and other hormones, which stimulate metabolism, remain elevated postexercise. Increased respiration and elevated heart rate also add to the metabolic rate following exercise. Body temperature can remain elevated for as long as 2 h after exercise, raising energy expenditure slightly.

DETERMINING ENERGY INTAKE AND EXPENDITURE

Either reducing intake relative to expenditure or increasing expenditure relative to intake can disrupt the energy balance equation. When intake exceeds expenditure, a positive energy balance occurs and weight gain ensues. When expenditure exceeds intake, a negative energy balance occurs and weight loss follows. Regardless of whether the desired outcome is a negative energy balance or a positive energy balance, the measurement of energy intake and expenditure becomes critical to the success of the intervention.

The mean daily energy balance can be measured directly or estimated from prediction equations that are derived from behavioral, physiological, and biochemical parameters. Long-term energy balance values are almost always estimated from data derived from direct short-term measures, short-term predictions, or an average of the two. The accuracy of the long-term estimate is dependent, therefore, upon the accuracy of the short-term measure or prediction.

ASSESSING ENERGY INTAKE

Energy intake is most accurately determined by directly measuring food consumption. Regardless of the specific setting, direct measures of food consumption are obtained by weighing known quantities of food before and after an individual eats. In addition to knowing the quantity of food one eats, the exact composition of each food item must be known before an accurate assessment of intake can be obtained. Assuming there are no errors in physical measuring and calculations, there is only one real source for error in obtaining short-term measures of food consumption — behavior.

Direct measures of food intake require that the patient be monitored closely throughout the eating experience. The source for error in extrapolating direct measures to behavioral outcomes occurs when a patient behaves differently under observation than in the freely living condition. Hence, anything the clinician can do to mimic the freely living condition, while the patient is being observed, will enhance the probability of obtaining an accurate measure of food intake.

It is very expensive and time consuming to measure food consumption directly. Therefore, a majority of food intake assessments are done by recording a patient's eating behavior, and using this record to estimate mean nutrient intake. Two techniques are used to record a patient's food intake — dietary recalls and food frequency questionnaires. Dietary recalls require that the patient record or recall every food and beverage he or she consumed over a predetermined period of time. The length of time the food diary is kept can range from several days to several months.[22] Three days seem to be the shortest amount of time that is necessary to obtain accurate estimates of energy intake, whereas longer periods of time are necessary to estimate micronutrient intakes.[22] The weakness in 3-day records is that they may not accurately reflect long-term food consumption, particularly if an individual does not vary his or her eating patterns over the 3-day period.

Food frequency questionnaires are often used because they address longer nutrient intake patterns than 3-day records. This is particularly important for foods eaten less regularly than daily or weekly. Food frequency questionnaires are not actual records of food consumed at specific times, but estimates of patterns of food consumption. For example, a person may respond to an item on the food frequency questionnaire by indicating he or she eats a medium-size orange three times a month. The 3-day food diary will not show that this individual consumes oranges, if no oranges were eaten during the 3-day recording period. On the other hand, the same individual may indicate on the food frequency questionnaire that he or she drinks two cups of skim milk each day. The 3-day food diary may show a more accurate measure of 2.5 cups of milk each day.

The question of whether food diaries or food frequency questionnaires are more accurate has been debated often over the past 20 years. Both methods correlate well with actual measures of food intake. When compared to each other, the data generally show that food frequency questionnaires tend to overestimate consumption of total energy, carbohydrate, protein, and some of the vitamins and minerals when compared to food diaries. The overestimates obtained with food frequency questionnaires may result from subjects' overestimation of foods eaten, particularly for those foods that are consumed less frequently. Many researchers and clinicians use both food diaries and food frequency questionnaires with their patients and average the data from the two tools to get an estimation of energy intake.

Assessing Energy Expenditure

Heat is released in the process of cellular respiration as the energy-yielding nutrients fat, protein, and carbohydrate are metabolized to produce the energy necessary for biological functions. Heat is the by-product of this metabolism. The process of measuring this metabolic heat release is termed calorimetry. It is important to observe that since the rate of heat release is directly proportional to the rate of metabolism, metabolic rate can be determined by measuring heat release.

DIRECT CALORIMETRY

Direct calorimetry is the measurement of the heat emission from a person enclosed in a chamber. Because the change in temperature is measured directly, the technique is referred to as direct calorimetry. This change in temperature is measured in units with which we are all familiar, calories. The machines for measuring body heat loss are therefore called calorimeters. Several types of direct calorimeters have been utilized in studying human metabolism; room-sized chambers, booth or closet-sized chambers, and suit calorimeters. Room-sized direct calorimeters allow for the study of energy expenditure in "freely living" subjects. However, the room measurements are that of a small bedroom (3 × 3 m, 9 × 9 ft), and it is debatable whether a person is truly "freely living" in a room this confined. Closet-sized or suit calorimeters further confine the movement of a person, and therefore can only be used to estimate the individual's RMR.

Current-day direct calorimetry methods (room, closet, or suit) are used to study thermal equilibrium and heat exposure, heat regulation during exercise and sleep, the thermic effect of food, and energy substrate (fat, protein, and carbohydrate) oxidation rates. However, a complicating factor in research using direct calorimetry and "freely living" subjects is the need to control other sources of heat besides that which the subject is producing. For example, if the subject is performing treadmill or cycle ergometer exercise inside a room-sized direct calorimeter, the treadmill or ergometer generates heat. This heat produced from exercise equipment, largely as a result of friction, though small, may need to be accounted for in determining the total heat production of the individual.

INDIRECT CALORIMETRY

The heat liberated from the body is the result of the metabolism of food substrate in mitochondrial respiration (energy nutrients + O_2 → heat + CO_2 + H_2O). Therefore, oxygen consumption ($\dot{V}O_2$) and energy expenditure (heat release) are directly related. That is, as energy expenditure increases, $\dot{V}O_2$. increases as well. Most laboratories do not measure energy expenditure (heat production) directly, since the direct calorimetry equipment is not universally available and is very expensive. Therefore, a technique called indirect respiratory calorimetry is more commonly employed in exercise physiology laboratories or in clinical programs to measure O_2 consumption and estimate energy expenditure during resting and exercise conditions. This form of calorimetry directly measures the O_2 consumed in metabolism through the measurement of respiratory gases. The $\dot{V}O_2$ data are then converted to an equivalent energy cost in kilocalories. The indirect calorimetry technique, which provides energy expenditure data via the direct measurement of O_2 consumption, yields results comparable to direct methods. That is, when results from direct and indirect calorimetry are compared, there is no significant difference in the measured energy expenditure.

Heat production is derived indirectly in respiratory calorimetry by first measuring the metabolic consumption of O_2 and converting this value to energy expenditure. This is possible because the O_2 consumed can be converted to heat equivalents when the type of nutrients undergoing metabolism is known. The energy liberated when only fat is oxidized is 4.7 kcal$\cdot l^{-1}$ O_2 consumed, and 5.05 kcal$\cdot l^{-1}$ O_2 when only carbohydrate is consumed. Because a metabolized substrate is generally a combination of fat and carbohydrate, an average caloric expenditure is usually estimated as 5 kcal$\cdot l^{-1}$ O_2 consumed. For example, if a person exercises at an O_2 cost of 1.0 l$\cdot min^{-1}$, the approximate energy expenditure equals 5 kcal$\cdot min^{-1}$.

Indirect respiratory calorimetry may be performed by either closed-circuit spirometry or open-circuit spirometry. Closed-circuit systems have the patient breathing 100% O_2 from a prefilled spirometer connected to a recording apparatus to account for the O_2 removed from the spirometer and the CO_2 produced and collected by an absorbing material. By calculating the ratio of the volume of O_2 consumed and the CO_2 produced, a more exact caloric value for $\dot{V}O_2$ can be determined, rather than using an average of 5 kcal$\cdot l^{-1}$ O_2. This method is most commonly used to measure RMR in clinical laboratories. Its usefulness during exercise conditions is limited because of the resistance to breathing offered by the closed circuit and the large volumes of O_2 consumed during exercise.

To accommodate the exercising subject, the open-circuit technique is most commonly used. In this method, the patient inspires air directly from the atmosphere and measurements of the fractional amounts of O_2 inspired and O_2 expired are made. The respiratory volume is also measured. By knowing the percentage of inspired atmospheric air that is O_2, the percentage of expired air that is O_2, and the respiratory volume, the amount of O_2 consumed can be determined. For example, at a respiratory volume of 80 l$\cdot min^{-1}$, an inspiratory O_2 concentration of 20.93% (0.2093), and an expiratory O_2 concentration of 18.73% (0.1873), $\dot{V}O_2$ is 1.76 l$\cdot min^{-1}$ ($\dot{V}O_2$ = 80 l$\cdot min^{-1}$ × 0.022 or 1.76 l$\cdot min^{-1}$). At an average energy expenditure of 5 kcal$\cdot l^{-1}$ O_2, the exercise energy expenditure would be 8.8 kcal$\cdot min^{-1}$ (1.76 × 5 = 8.8).

The doubly labeled water method of indirect calorimetry works on a similar principle as indirect respiratory calorimetry — gas exchange. However, with doubly labeled water, CO_2 production is calculated rather than O_2 consumption. An oral dose of the stable isotopes of ^2H and ^{18}O is taken. The ^2H labels the body water pool, while the ^{18}O labels both the body water pool and the bicarbonate pool. The disappearance rates of the two isotopes measure the turnover of water and the turnover of water plus CO_2. Carbon dioxide production is calculated by the difference. Since CO_2 production and O_2 consumption are directly related, energy expenditure can be calculated by the same calorimetric equations as used for indirect respiratory calorimetry.

TABLE 12.2
Common prediction equations for RMR

$RMR = 73.3 \times BM^{0.74}$
$RMR = 13.75 \times BM + 500.3 \times H - 6.78 \times age + 66.5$ (men)
$RMR = 9.56 \times BM + 185.0 \times H - 4.68 \times age + 655.1$ (women)

Notes: RMR, kcal·d^{-1}; BM, body mass in kg; H, height in m.

Predicting Resting Energy Expenditure

Direct and indirect calorimetry methods for measuring energy expenditure are too complex, time consuming, and expensive for most settings. Therefore, major efforts have been made to derive prediction equations. The most common prediction equations derived are that of Klieber[23] and Harris and Benedict.[24] Both of these methods are based on the relationship between body mass (BM) and metabolic rate. Klieber demonstrated that RMR, relative to BM raised to the exponent of 0.74, was consistent for mature mammals, ranging in size from rats to steers (Table 12.2). Harris and Benedict included variables other than BM in their equation, namely height and age (Table 12.2). These equations are less predictive among obese persons.

The prediction equations mentioned above were developed from measures taken on subjects who were studied in the early 20th century, and were leaner, less physically active, ate a lower fat diet, weighed less, and had a shorter life span than people today. Furthermore, these equations were derived on a Caucasian population. Consequently, many clinicians report deviations between RMR predicted by the Klieber and Harris–Benedict equations and those measured in their patients. This observation has prompted the development of alternative equations, more suited for specific populations (e.g., African-Americans). These population-specific equations have limited universality and emphasize the need to create new generalized RMR prediction formulas using modern sampling, measurement, and statistical methodologies.

Predicting Exercise Energy Expenditure

During the middle of the 20th century, much research was performed to determine the energy cost of various activities. Tables and charts were published that gave caloric values for activities of daily living, work activities, recreational activities, and sport activities. The accuracy of these predictors of physical activity energy expenditure is similar to measuring RMR. Some generalized energy-expenditure prediction equations are made available by the American College of Sports Medicine for use in clinical populations.[25]

Editor's Note

Energy balance — calories in vs. calories out — does not fully explain body weight. Nevertheless, assessing energy balance is an important component of any weight reduction program. Furthermore, since meals (calories in) and exercise (calories out) influence metabolism at any given moment, strategic timing and dosing of diet and exercise can facilitate weight reduction and enhance body composition.

EXERCISE ENERGY NEEDS FOR THE PREVIOUSLY OBESE PATIENT

Several reviews have been written on exercise and weight control, and each concludes that exercise is a key factor in reduced weight maintenance. A consistent finding is that the more exercise, the better the maintenance of weight loss. Patients who expend at least 1500 to 2500 kcal (6.3 to 10.5 MJ) a week are more likely to maintain their full end-of-treatment weight loss.[26–28] Similar findings have been reported from the National Weight Control Registry, which includes a total of 784 males and females who have maintained an average weight loss of 30 kg for an average of 5.6 years.[29] Participants in the National Registry reported expending approximately 2830 kcal week^{-1} (11.8 MJ), or the equivalent of walking about 28 miles week^{-1}.

More exact estimates of exercise energy expenditure required for maintaining reduced weight come from Schoeller and colleagues,[30] who used doubly labeled water to estimate the metabolic cost of an exercise program needed to maintain weight loss in previously obese women. Metabolic measurements revealed that the women were exercising 700 kcal d^{-1} (2930 kJ d^{-1}) to maintain their reduced body weight. This translates into 80 min d^{-1} of moderate physical activity, 35 min d^{-1} of vigorous activity, or walking about 7 miles d^{-1}. This amount of exercise is almost unobtainable for most previously obese individuals, and is beyond what is recommended by the American College of Sports Medicine, the Centers for Disease Control and Prevention, and the Surgeon General for achievement and preservation of health.

EXERCISE ENERGY NEEDS FOR THE ANOREXIC PATIENT

A large proportion of anorexic patients couple their restrictive dieting behaviors with exercise, in an effort to enhance or maintain weight loss. Exercise recommendations for the anorexic patient focus on maintaining a positive energy balance and are summarized in Table 12.3. By following preset guidelines, the anorexic patient can safely participate in an exercise program.

TABLE 12.3
Exercise recommendations for the patient with anorexia nervosa

- The patient agrees to perform only the prescribed exercises in the facility, and will not exercise at home, at school, or anywhere else without approval

- The patient checks in with a staff member at the beginning of each exercise session

- The patient brings a nondiet sport drink (100 to 150 kcal) to every workout. The sport drink is consumed at the facility in the presence of a staff member

- The program consists of 20 to 30 min of flexibility and strength training

- The patient is not allowed to participate in an aerobic exercise program because aerobic conditioning will likely cause additional weight loss

- Aerobic exercise can be negotiated as the patient regains body weight

SUMMARY

Energy balance is fundamental to the human body. Interventions that target creating either a negative or positive energy balance are often part of medical treatments. Regardless of the treatment objective, the quantification of energy intake and expenditure is prerequisite to manipulating the energy balance equation to the direction desired. Energy balance in the body can be quantified through direct, indirect, and predictive measures.

REFERENCES

1. Forman, J.N., Miller, W.C., Szymanski, L.M., and Fernhall, B., Differences in resting metabolic rates of inactive obese African-American and Caucasian women, *Int. J. Obes.*, 22, 215–221, 1998.
2. Sharp, T.A., Bell, M.L., Grunwald, G.K., Schmitz, K.H., Sidney, S., Lewis, C.E., Tolan, K., and Hill, J.O., Differences in resting metabolic rate between White and African-American young adults, *Obes. Res.*, 10, 726–732, 2002.
3. Ravussin, E., Lillioja, S., Knowler, W.C., Christin, L., Freymond, D., Abbott, W.G.H., Boyce, V., Howard, B.V., and Bogardus, C., Reduced rate of energy expenditure as a risk factor for body-weight gain, *N. Engl. J. Med.*, 318, 467–472, 1988.
4. Bray, G.A., The energetics of obesity, *Med. Sci. Sports Exerc.*, 15, 32–40, 1983.
5. Fricker, J., Rozen, R., Melchior, J.-C., and Apfelbaum, M., Energy-metabolism adaptation in obese adults on a very-low-calorie diet, *Am. J. Clin. Nutr.*, 53, 826–830, 1991.
6. American College of Sports Medicine, *ACSM's Resource Manual for Guidelines for Exercise Testing and Prescription*, 4th edn, Lippincott Williams & Wilkins, Philadelphia, PA, 2001, pp. 17, 277–307, 499–512.

7. Wilmore, J.H., Stanforth, P.R., Hudspeth, L.A., Gagnon, J., Daw, E.W., Leon, A.S., Rao, D.C., Skinner, J.S., and Bouchard, C., Alterations in resting metabolic rate as a consequence of 20 weeks of endurance training: the HERITAGE Family Study, *Am. J. Clin. Nutr.*, 68, 66–71, 1998.

8. Van Pelt, R.E., Jones, P.P., Davy, K.P., Desouza, C.A., Tanaka, H., Davy, B.M., and Seals, D.R., Regular exercise and the age-related decline in resting metabolic rate in women, *J. Clin. Endocrinol. Metab.*, 10, 3208–3212, 1997.

9. Byrne, H.K. and Wilmore, J.H., The relationship of mode and intensity of training on resting metabolic rate in women, *Int. J. Sport Nutr. Exerc. Metab.*, 11, 1–14, 2001.

10. Geliebter, A., Maher, M.M., Gerace, L., Bernard, G., Heymsfield, S.B., and Hashim, S.A., Effects of strength or aerobic training on body composition, resting metabolic rate, and peak oxygen consumption in obese dieting subjects, *Am. J. Clin. Nutr.*, 66, 557–563, 1997.

11. Manore, M.M., Berry, T.E., Skinner, J.S., and Carroll, S.S., Energy expenditure at rest and during exercise in nonobese female cyclical dieters and in nondieting control subjects, *Am. J. Clin. Nutr.*, 54, 41–46, 1991.

12. Mole, P.A., Stern, J.S., Schulze, C.L., Bernauer, E.M., and Holcomb, B.J., Exercise reverses depressed metabolic rate produced by severe caloric restriction, *Med. Sci. Sports Exerc.*, 21, 29–33, 1989.

13. Mole, P.A., Daily exercise enhances fat utilization and maintains metabolic rate during severe energy restriction in humans, *Sports Med. Training Rehab.*, 7, 39–48, 1996.

14. Phinney, S.D., LaGrange, B.M., O'Connel, M., and Danforth, E., Jr., Effects of aerobic exercise on energy expenditure and nitrogen balance during very low calorie dieting, *Metabolism*, 37, 758–764, 1988.

15. VanDale, D., Saris, W.H.M., Schoffelen, P.F.M., and Hoor, F., Does exercise give an additional effect in weight reduction regimens? *Int. J. Obes.*, 11, 367–375, 1987.

16. Ballor, D.L. and Poehlman, E.T., A meta-analysis of the effects of exercise and/or dietary restriction on resting metabolic rate, *Eur. J. Appl. Physiol.*, 71, 535–542, 1995.

17. Herring, J.L., Mole, P.A., Meredith, C.N., and Stern, J.S., Effect of suspending exercise training on resting metabolic rate in women, *Med. Sci. Sports Exerc.*, 24, 59–65, 1992.

18. Granat-Steffan, H., Elliott, W., Miller, W.C., and Fernhall, B., Substrate utilization during submaximal exercise in obese and normal-weight women, *Eur. J. Appl. Physiol.*, 80, 233–239, 1999.

19. Miller, W.C., Wallace, J.P., and Eggert, K.E., Predicting max HR and the HR- $\dot{V}O_2$. relationship for exercise in obesity, *Med. Sci. Sports Exerc.*, 25, 1077–1081, 1993.

20. Bahr, R., Hansson, P., and Sejersted, O.M., Effect of duration of exercise on excess postexercise O_2 consumption, *J. Appl. Physiol.*, 62, 485–490, 1987.

21. Gaesser, G. and Brooks, G.A., Metabolic basis of excess postexercise oxygen consumption: a review, *Med. Sci. Sports Exerc.*, 16, 29–43, 1984.

22. Basiotis, P.P., Welsh, S.O., Cronin, F.J., Kelsay, J., and Mertz, W., Number of days of food intake records required to estimate individual and group nutrient intakes with defined confidence, *J. Nutr.*, 117, 1638–1641, 1987.

23. Kleiber, M., Body size and metabolism, *Hilgardia*, 6, 315–353, 1932.

24. Harris, J.A. and Benedict, F.G., *A Biometric Study of Basal Metabolism in Man*, Publication No. 279, Carnegie Institute of Washington, Washington, DC, 1919.

25. American College of Sports Medicine, *ACSM's Guidelines for Exercise Testing and Prescription,* 6th edn, Lippincott Williams & Wilkins, Philadelphia, PA, 2000, pp. 137–164, 302–303.

26. Hartmann, W.M., Stroud, M., Sweet, D.M., and Saxton, J., Long-term maintenance of weight loss following supplemented fasting, *Int. J. Eating Disorders*, 14, 87–93, 1993.

27. Jakicic, J., Wing, R., and Winters, C., Effects of intermittent exercise and use of home exercise equipment on adherence, weight loss, and fitness in overweight women, *JAMA,* 282, 1554–1560, 1999.

28. Jeffrey, R.W., Wing, R.R., Thorson, C., and Burton, L.R., Use of personal trainers and financial incentives to increase exercise in a behavioral weight loss program, *J. Consult. Clin. Psychol.,* 66, 777–783, 1998.

29. Klem, M.L., Wing, R.R., McGuire, M.T., Seagle, H.M., and Hill, J.O., A descriptive study of individuals successful at long-term maintenance of substantial weight loss, *Am. J. Clin. Nutr.,* 66, 239–246, 1997.

30. Schoeller, D.A., Shay, K., and Kushner, R.F., How much physical activity is needed to minimize weight gain in previously obese women? *Am. J. Clin. Nutr.,* 66, 551–556, 1997.

13 Neuroendocrine Regulation of Appetite

Carlo Contoreggi, M.D. and
Ingrid Kohlstadt, M.D., M.P.H

CONTENTS

INTRODUCTION

Appetite is generally considered the body's ability to regulate food intake. What is less well recognized is appetite's exactness. Food intake, absorption, and energy expenditure is amazingly precise. The average adult gains approximately 0.45 kg/year from ages 25 through 55.[1] When combined with a decrease in lean body mass of approximately 0.23 kg/year, this represents a 0.7 kg annual net increase of body fat. The energy imbalance of 5,250 kcal/year reflects a net surplus of fewer than 15 kcal/day, or the equivalent of two extra potato chips. The energy regulation is precise beyond the current limits of experimental measures. Short-term dysregulation usually goes unnoticed. However, when appetite is not checked by satiety over a longer period of time, body fat increases. Dysregulation of appetite is the primary pathway to obesity. Early identification and treatment of appetite dysregulation can prevent obesity.

CONTROL CENTERS

Mapping the appetite centers in the brain dates back to the early 1900s. Obesity was recognized as a syndrome more complex than dietary indiscretion and was thought to represent pituitary dysfunction. Patients with severe obesity occasionally were noted to have reduced gonadal function, abnormalities in water metabolism such as the syndrome of inappropriate antidiuretic hormone secretion, diabetes insipidus, and emotional disorders such as inappropriate sexual behavior or aggression.[2]

Today, the hypothalamus is the brain locus thought to exert the most control over appetite, analogous to a computer's central processing unit. Hypothalamic lesions were first identified in obese patients in the 1920s, when it was observed that lesions of the ventromedial nucleus (VMN) cause hyperphagia, while lesions of the lateral nucleus induce satiety.[3–8]

Systematic study of rodents has provided great detail and information about the central control of feeding and nutrient ingestion. Hypothalamic circuitry is highly redundant and strongly biased to increase feeding and maintain body energy stores. Rodent studies show that lesions of the VMN, arcuate nucleus, dorsal medial nucleus, and paraventricular nucleus (PVN) fail to permanently subdue the drive to eat. Anorexigenic sites, which curb feeding, integrate and overlap anatomically with orexigenic areas, which stimulate feeding. There is neurochemical colocalization of both orexigenic and anorexigenic mediators on single and closely associated neuronal groups. Neurochemical adaptations in the hypothalamus are dynamic; amplification and diminishment molecular signaling change in response to both internal (homeostatic) and external (environmental) stimuli. Internal stimuli include input from vagal afferent nerves, circadian and circannual hormone changes, and cues about satiety. External stimuli are as diverse as recent food intake, time of day, aromas, mood, sunlight, seasons, objects, and events that recall memories of food. The hypothalamus as the feeding control center is extensively connected to other regions of the central nervous system (CNS).

Meal composition and the frequency and timing of nutrient intake appear to be "hard wired" in the hypothalamic feeding centers. Hunger occurs with minimal input from the evolutionarily newer neocortex, leaving the higher cognitive parts of the brain little opportunity to "veto" food cravings. Some speculate that the evolutionary stress until this point in time has been that of inadequate nutrition. Therefore, the plasticity of neurochemical signaling and the redundant neuroanatomy of the hypothalamus speak to the complexity of chemical interactions all leaning to promote hyperphagia, body weight gain, and obesity.

NEUROENDOCRINE MESSENGERS

Understanding of the neuropeptides, neurotransmitters, and central actions of peripheral hormones is accelerating rapidly. A summary of these molecules is shown in Table 13.1. The following discussion of neurochemical messengers

TABLE 13.1
Neuroendocrine messengers of appetite regulation

	Increase appetite, promote weight gain	Decrease appetite, promote weight loss
Neuropeptides	Neuropeptide Y (NPY)	Bombesin
	Galanin	Enterostatin (central action)
		Corticotrophin-releasing hormone (CRH)
		Melanocyte-stimulating hormone
		Peptide analogs and antagonists (under development)
Neurotransmitters	Serotonin antagonists	Serotonin agonists and reuptake inhibitors
	Dopamine antagonists	Dopamine agonists and reuptake inhibitors
	Mu- and kappa-opioids	Mu- and kappa-opioid antagonists (under development)
	Gamma amino butyric acid (GABA)	Histamine H1 receptor agonists
	Histamine H1 antagonists	Norepinephrine β receptor agonists
	Norepinephrine α receptor agonists	
Central action of peripheral hormones	Insulin	Glucagon-like peptide-1
	Ghrelin (potentiating role)	Leptin
	Glucocorticoids	Cholecystokinin (CCK)
	Adipocytokines (other than adiponectin)	Adiponection
	Androgens (Chapter 20)	Estrogen (Chapter 14)
	Progestins (Chapter 14)	

provides a framework by which one can understand future therapeutic interventions and the importance of using multiple interventions for weight reduction.

NEUROPEPTIDES

Neuropeptides are potent CNS messengers. Nanogram changes in neuropeptide concentrations signal CNS events which regulate appetite and satiety. Since peptides do not readily cross the blood–brain barrier (BBB), peripheral administration has limited clinical utility. One area of drug development is to create nonpeptide analogs that modulate and decrease appetite and overeating. Nonpeptide analogs and antagonists have been developed to efficiently cross into the CNS and some of these neuropeptide analogs are under development to treat obesity. Molecular targets include neuropeptide Y (NPY), galanin, and bombesin.[9–15] Other neuropeptides such as somatostatin, enterostatin, thyrotropin-releasing hormone, gastrin, pancreatic polypeptide, alpha-melanocyte-stimulating hormone (αMSH), glucagon-like peptide-1, and vasoactive inhibitory peptide, are important though somewhat less well characterized.[16–18]

An important neuropeptide is corticotrophin-releasing hormone (CRH). First recognized as the hypothalamic regulator of the hypothalamic–pituitary–adrenal (HPA) axis, CRH stimulates release of adrenocorticotrophic hormone from the pituitary. CRH is a primary mediator of stress in the CNS. Acute stress will decrease food intake and release both stored glycogen and fat. Chronic HPA activation increases appetite and raises insulin through excess cortisol secretion. Obesity is a cardinal feature of Cushing's disease and Cushing's syndrome. In nonadrenal mediated obesity there are higher circulating cortisol levels, which in some will cause a higher threshold point for inhibition of the HPA axis. CRH mediates feeding through type 1 and type 2 receptor subtypes.[19–21]

NEUROTRANSMITTERS

Neuropeptides influence the release of neurotransmitters, which are not as potent, but exist in higher concentrations.

Opiates

Opioids are widely spread in multiple neural networks that regulate ingestive behavior; intake of palatable foods is rewarding and these foods may result in a change in opioid circuitry, either at the peptide or receptor level. Evidence supports opioids in reward-driven food ingestion; with endogenous opioids effecting nutrient consumption and preference.[22–24] Feeding rodents palatable diets (chocolate and high sucrose solutions) increases mu-opiate binding in reward centers. Mu-opioid antagonists used to treat alcohol and heroin dependence also decrease food intake in the short term. Opioid antagonists are used to treat bulimia and modestly decrease the frequency and intensity of binging episodes. However, in double-blind trials, the mu-opiate antagonist naltrexone failed to induce substantial long-term weight loss in obese patients.[25,26] The opiate system is highly complex with several classes of endogenous molecules effecting feeding. Kappa-opioid agonists increase and antagonists inhibit intake of calorie dense meals.[27–29] Several kappa-specific compounds are under investigation and are available for trials in substance-abusing patients; future applications will likely include obesity.

Serotonin

Serotonin (5-HT) is a neurotransmitter, which may suppress appetite. Anorectic effects are mediated through 1b and 2 receptor subtypes, but 1a receptors stimulate feeding. Regional serotonin receptor subtype density impacts the effect of serotonin on feeding. Serotonin-specific reuptake inhibitors (SSRIs) treat depression and other psychiatric disorders by increasing synaptic 5-HT. SSRIs also stimulate central postsynaptic 1b and 2 receptors with the overall effect to diminish appetite early in therapy.[30,31] Fenfluramine (racemic mixture, Pondimin®) and d-fenfluramine (Redux®) release 5-HT from the presynaptic nerve terminal, block reuptake, and stimulate central postsynaptic 1b and 2 receptors. This effect decreases appetite and induces satiety resulting in weight loss.[32] Serotonin antagonists both increase appetite and weight. Cyproheptadine, a mixed 5-HT 2a and histamine type-1 antagonist, stimulates appetite with weight gain in malignant and inflammatory cachexic conditions[33,34] and increases growth in children. Ketanserin is an antihypertensive medication with serotonin antagonist pharmacology that stimulates appetite and weight gain.[35,36]

Norepinephrine

Norepinephrine is implicated in arousal, sleep, and mood regulation. The response to norepinephrine depends on which receptor types and subtypes are stimulated. Norepinephrine stimulates appetite through α-adrenergic receptors and it inhibits food intake through β-adrenergic receptors. Stimulation of the β1-adrenergic receptor in the CNS will decrease food intake. The β2-adrenergic receptor agonists stimulate protein synthesis, which increases muscle mass. The β3-adrenergic receptor in the periphery enhances metabolic rate through the stimulation of lipolysis and thermogenesis in muscle. Therefore, noradrenergic agonists and antagonists influence appetite and weight variably, because of both specific pharmacology of the agents and variation in host response.

Agents with mixed actions and NE-specific α-agonists are also associated with increased appetite and weight gain.[37–40] Tricyclic antidepressants, which may have a complete or partial NE agonist effect, commonly increased appetite and weight.[41–43] Many noradrenergic antihypertensive agents affect appetite depending on CNS penetration. Propranolol, which readily crosses the BBB, induces weight gain. Atenolol does not readily cross the BBB and has less effect.

Ephedrine, a mixed α- and β-agonist, is highly effective in reducing appetite and body weight. Fatalities from its use prompted its removal from the market.[44,45]

Dopamine

Dopamine has a wide variety of functions in the CNS. It also has significant effects on weight and appetite as mentioned previously. Limbic dopamine pathways modulate motivational behaviors, and play a critical role in compulsive addictive and compulsive behaviors as well as eating disorders.

Generally, stimulating dopaminergic pathways decreases appetite and dopamine inhibition with antagonists diminishes satiety signals, increasing appetite and weight gain. Mixed dopamine agonists, including the antidepressant bupropion will decrease appetite and weight.[46] Mazindol, a dopamine reuptake inhibitor, is a highly effective anorexant.[47]

Dopamine antagonists are used to treat schizophrenia and psychosis. First-generation antipsychotics such as haloperidol act principally at the D2 receptor site, though these medications also may have pronounced antihistaminic properties. The indole derivative molindone is a dopamine antagonist that causes less appetite stimulation; this is possibly because of its chemical similarity and agonist-like activity to the indolamine, serotonin.[48] Many dopamine antagonist medications are available; most increase appetite with weight gain being a frequent side effect.[49–51] New antipsychotic medications are now available: clozapine, olanzapine, quetiapine, and zotepin are a few of the second-generation, atypical antipsychotic (AAP) drugs. Though these agents have a variety of pharmacologic effects, efficacy is principally associated with their serotonin 2A and dopamine 2 receptor antagonist actions. These receptors act independently to increase appetite and reduce satiety; when these actions are combined they have a supra-additive effect and have been shown to cause pronounced weight gain.[52–54] In addition to the central effects of the AAP drugs, these agents have been shown to have detrimental peripheral metabolic effects. These drugs may increase both insulin secretion and promote insulin resistance independent of their effects on appetite.[55–58]

Gamma Amino Butyric Acid

Gamma amino butyric acid (GABA) is a neurochemical, which can have a profound inhibitory effect on other neurotransmitter systems. Increased levels of GABA may dampen the satiety effects of serotonin and dopamine, resulting in increased appetite and weight gain. Specific pharmacologic sites of action are presently unknown. GABA activators are most often used as anxiolytics and anticonvulsants. Many anxiolytics, such as diazepam, are GABA agonists and thus stimulate appetite. Anticonvulsants, such as valproate, also stimulate GABA systems. Weight gain is a common side effect of this class of medication.[59–65]

Histamine

Histamine is widely expressed in the CNS of both rodents and primates, where it mediates anorexigenic effects. Histamine receptors are densely localized at both satiety and feeding areas, especially in the hypothalamic VMN and PVN. Several peptidergic neurons including neuropeptide Y and bombesin express histamine receptors.[66-68] Clinical observations point to histaminergic antagonists which stimulate appetite. Histamine type 1 (H$_1$) receptor antagonists, generally known as antihistamines, control allergic symptoms. Many antidepressant and antipsychotic medications are H$_1$ receptor antagonists as well. Pharmacologic effects of antihistamine medications on appetite are related to CNS penetration. Antihistamines with poor CNS penetration, such as astemizole, stimulate appetite less.[69-71] Cyproheptadine, which is both a serotonin (5HT$_{2a}$) and an H$_1$ antagonist, potently stimulates appetite.[72] Several lines of evidence suggest that histamine decreases food intake via H$_1$ receptors in the VMN or the PVN. Mutant mice lacking H$_1$ demonstrated leptin-induced suppression of food intake. However, the question remains as to why the circadian variation in the level of histamine is inversely correlated to the pattern of feeding.[73]

The action of histamine type 2 (H$_2$) antagonists on appetite and weight loss is unknown. Both central and peripheral effects may be involved. H$_2$ blockade reduces gastric acid secretion. Initial reports suggest that pre-prandial administration of the H2 receptor antagonist, cimetidine, improved weight loss. These finding have not been replicated in double blind trials.

PERIPHERAL HORMONES

Insulin

Insulin can regulate appetite centrally. To do so insulin crosses the BBB, even though it is a large protein. Insulin enters the brain by cell-mediated pinocytosis.[74-76] Insulin receptors are found in hypothalamic nuclei and other subcortical areas. These sites have been implicated in controlling feeding and nutrient intake. The concentration and sensitivity of the body to insulin regulation is effected by total body adiposity. Elevations of cerebrospinal fluid insulin have been reported in obese individuals.[77]

Insulin concentration varies with the nutritional status of the individual with postprandial states associated with higher insulin concentrations than after a prolonged fast. Exogenous insulin and medications which stimulate insulin promote weight gain and appetite. Acutely plasma glucose levels are inversely related to hunger and food intake, however with prolonged fasting both insulin and glucose concentrations drop and individuals report decreased appetite. Starvation is a profound catabolic state characterized by low glucose and insulin levels. During periods of starvation, patients report no appetite and an actual aversion to food.

Numerous medications principally used to control diabetes mellitus regulate insulin secretion or its actions. While these medications act primarily in the periphery, one assumes that concentrations of central insulin are also influenced. First and second generation sulfonylureas are available to treat type II diabetes. These drugs stimulate insulin secretion and promote weight gain.[78–81] Other medications potentiate cellular insulin, resulting in more effective insulin action. They may decrease insulin secretion reducing insulin resistance. Metformin reduces hepatic glucose production (gluconeogenesis) and stimulates glucose uptake into muscle tissue, reducing the endogenous or exogenous insulin necessary for glucose control.[82,83] Rosiglitazone and pioglitazone are thiazolidinediones, another medication class which decreases hepatic gluconeogenesis and increases skeletal muscle glucose uptake. Thiazolidinediones enhance hormone action at the insulin receptor, reduce insulin requirements and improve cellular insulin sensitivity. These medications are effective treatments for slowing the progression to type II diabetes in patients with obesity, metabolic syndrome, and polycystic ovarian syndrome.

Some medications improve glycemic control by slowing gastrointestinal (GI) absorption. Acarbose, an alpha-glucosidase inhibitor, slows carbohydrate absorption from the intestinal lumen. Slowed glucose absorption (i.e., reduced glycemic index) reduces the amount of insulin necessary to control plasma glucose. Orlistat® inhibits pancreatic and gastric lipases to decrease GI fat absorption by about 30% without effecting glucose absorption.

Glucagon-like Peptide-1

Glucagon-like peptide-1 (GLP-1) is a peripheral hormone released from the ileum in response to a meal. GLP-1 shows potent anorectic effects, with peripheral actions that are better delineated than its central effects. GLP-1 crosses the blood-brain barrier. Its receptors are expressed in the hypothalamus and brainstem, sites which regulate both ingestion and autonomic functions, though its precise CNS actions is unclear.[84] GLP-1 slows intestinal motility and gastric emptying, both of which contribute to peripheral satiety signaling.[85] Weight loss through ileal transposition is accompanied by increased ileal hormone secretion and synthesis in rats.[86–88]

Bariatric surgery increases GLP-1 secretion due to early arrival of nutrients to the ileum and surgery also enhances sensitivity to GLP-1. Parenteral infusion of GLP-1 and its synthetic analog, Exendin-4, both enhances satiety and diminishes hunger in diabetic patients. Exendin-4 shows considerable homology with GLP-1 and receptor affinity with a similar pharmacology. GLP-1 is not stable *in vivo*, which has lead to clinical investigations with Exendin-4.[86] An orally available, non-peptide agonist of GLP-1 could be of therapeutic benefit in weight management.[87]

Ghrelin

Ghrelin is a 28 amino acid peptide hormone discovered in 1999. Principally found in the stomach fundus, it is released in advance of and in response to feeding. Plasma ghrelin concentration increases twofold before a meal and decreases to basal concentrations within 1 hour after eating. The physiology of release is complex but involves central activation through sympathetic and parasympathetic peripheral afferents. Gut stimulation also appears critical for ghrelin release and inhibition, as intravenous nutrition does not decrease ghrelin secretion.

Ghrelin is also a potent endocrine hormone. Ghrelin receptors are found in the pituitary and hypothalamus and it acts as a secretagogue of growth hormone. The physiology and relevance of these interactions remain unknown at this time. Serum ghrelin concentrations can reflect nutritional status; inanition is associated with enhanced release, being a potent stimulus for eating.[89] Obesity and anorexia nervosa after dietary intervention show opposite effects suggesting that ghrelin is a good marker of nutritional status.[90] Ghrelin is reduced in obesity, metabolic syndrome, and type II diabetes. This may reflect a homeostatic shift to reduced caloric intake and hyperglycemia to maintain body weight.

Ghrelin response after surgical interventions for obesity may provide insights into the potent effects of ghrelin in the efficacy of these procedures. Gastric restrictive procedures cause an increase in ghrelin levels in contrast to bypass surgeries, which reduce circulating concentrations.[91–94]

Adrenal Steroid Hormones

The medical literature is replete with reports of glucocorticoids (GCs) causing increases in appetite and weight gain independent of the primary disease being treated.[95,96] Chronic administration of pharmacologic doses of GCs results in increased visceral fat deposition, insulin resistance, decreased muscle mass, hyperlipidemia (mainly as elevation in triglyceride concentration), and other metabolic derangements. GCs also influence the CNS directly. GCs inhibits leptin in the hypothalamus, possibly through stimulating NPY and inhibiting CRH secretion. Studies show glucocorticoids potentiate NPY-stimulated carbohydrate ingestion.[97–99] The adverse effects on appetite and metabolism are most evident when GCs are used at high doses.

Cholecystokinin

Cholecystokinin (CCK) is synthesized in the GI tract and enhances gastric emptying, gallbladder contraction, and release of pancreatic enzymes. CCK may induce satiety through activation of peripheral CCK receptors in the gut. Clinical trials with Ceruletide, a short-acting CCK analog, have failed to show a consistent effect on appetite. Activation of intestinal CCK receptors stimulates vagal nerve afferent signaling through the brain stem, to the hypothalamus, amygdala and other CNS sites. Whether gut-produced CCK crosses the BBB and relays significant control to satiety centers is unclear.[100,101]

Gastric banding surgery increases the peak and the slope of CCK secretion potentially increasing satiety signals. However, roux-en-Y (RYGB) gastric bypass procedures may not increase CCK.[102–105]

Leptin

Once thought to be inert, it is now known that adipose tissue secretes and responds to multiple endocrine mediators of metabolism, inflammation, and neurochemistry. Leptin is a peptide hormone synthesized in the periphery, specifically by fat cells. Adipose tissue production of leptin is effected by plasma insulin, glucose, adrenal steroids as well as food intake. Although it is produced in the periphery, leptin exerts its action centrally as a neuropeptide. In this way, leptin forms a feedback loop from adipocytes to the brain and contributes to long-term weight regulation.[106–109]

Leptin is rarely used clinically. An absolute leptin deficiency has been linked to a rare genetic defect. Low circulating leptin may predispose to obesity in the Pima Indians and other Native Americans. Since common obesity is not associated with leptin deficiency, simple administration of leptin or a leptin agonist does not benefit most obese individuals. Leptin levels are increased in most obese patients, suggesting that obese individuals likely have either an inherited or an acquired resistance to leptin satiety signals. The neurochemistry of leptin action in the CNS is complex. Leptin impacts many neurochemical systems which regulate hypothalamic appetite centers as well as molecular targets influencing motivation and reward systems. Leptin represents an appetite regulator with considerable redundancy. Fat storage regulation has direct input into neuroendocrine systems including the hypothalamic–pituitary–gonadal, hypothalamic–pituitary–thyroid, and HPA axis with clinically apparent effects when the leptin system is disrupted to the extreme.

Adipocytokines

Fat tissue secretes a number of inflammatory molecules including IL6, TNF-alpha, IL8, and IL10. Production increases with increased body fat stores and insulin resistance. They signal internally (autocrine) to modulate cellular responsiveness to nutrient load and the changing hormonal milieu; locally (paracrine) to adjacent fat cells to regulate fat mass expansion and contraction; and distantly (endocrine) to modulate other organs systems.

Adiponectin is a recently identified endocrine adipocytokine, produced exclusively by fat cells and secreted into the serum. In contrast to other cytokines, low levels are associated with insulin resistance.[110] Combined antiretroviral therapies can increase the expression and secretion of proinflammatory cytokines and decrease adiponectin. Antiviral medications can induce changes in fat cell physiology in a condition known as lipodystrophy.[111,112]

NUTRITIONAL MODIFIERS

Trace metals are nutritional cofactors in neuroendocrine pathways. Deficiency can precipitate alterations in food selection and caloric intake. For example, iron deficiency can result in cravings for nonfood substances such as clay and paper.

The cravings called pica resolve with iron supplementation and may recur with relapse of iron deficiency.[113] The neural pathway by which pica is mediated remains unknown. Chromium enhances insulin's action. Deficiency states are associated with increased gastric binding, competitive absorption and mineral corticoids which increase urinary excretion.[114] Zinc deficiency is anorexigenic, as described by Dweck in Chapter 17. Zinc impairs NPY release from the hypothalamic PVN.[115] Although most zinc in the brain is tightly bound to the metalloproteins for which it is the cofactor, some zinc is found in the vesicular pools located in the nerve terminals.[116] Zinc is concentrated in the olfactory bulb, where it plays a poorly characterized role in smell and taste. Zinc deficiency decreases taste intensity and alters taste selectivity. Taste is restored with oral zinc supplementation.

Excess minerals and the presence of heavy metal toxins can create mineral imbalances, which interfere with neuroendocrine regulation. For example, manganese excess interferes with the neurotransmitters glutamate and GABA.[117] Iron supplementation without chromium leads to chromium deficiency over time. Similarly, zinc supplementation without copper can induce a relative copper deficiency. Toxic metals such as lead, mercury, and cadmium compete with minerals for absorption and receptor binding sites, thereby altering the availability of minerals.

One well-studied foreign metal is lithium, administered therapeutically as a mood stabilizer. A well-known side effect of lithium therapy is weight gain. Lithium is thought to increase weight in several ways, acting both centrally, by reducing neurotransmission, and peripherally, by interfering with adipocyte intracellular signaling. Lithium competitively inhibits thyroid iodine uptake, which may result in chemical and clinical hypothyroidism. Lithium also reduces absorption of chemically similar trace minerals, thereby creating chronic mineral deficiencies which exacerbate appetite dysregulation and extracellular fluid retention.

Similar to minerals, B vitamins are enzyme cofactors. Low availability of various B vitamins has been shown to influence neurotransmitter activity. Vitamin D also has a recently identified role in enhancing insulin sensitivity, possibly both centrally and peripherally (see Chapter 10).

Water is another nutrient that modulates neuroendocrine response, as appetite and thirst are intertwined. A direct influence of water on histamine and corticotrophin releasing factors has been proposed.[118]

Dietary fat, more so than carbohydrate and protein, influences gut peptides to signal satiety. Chapter 4 discusses the unique characteristics of various dietary fats which are incorporated into cellular structures, where they modify receptor conformation, the kinetics of neuroendocrine signaling and as of yet unquantifiable effects on neuroendocrine pathways.

NEUROENDOCRINE SYNCHRONICITY

Food supply is obtained intermittently. Nutrient demand is continuous. One way the body balances supply and demand is by pulsatile secretion of neuroendocrine regulators. The predictable rises and falls throughout a 24 hour period can be altered by shift-work, travel across time zones, and lack of daytime sunlight exposure. Situations which disturb circadian rhythms increase the risk of obesity. Demonstrated shifts in neuroendocrine secretions may underlie the behaviors associated with circadian rhythm disturbances.[119,120]

SUMMARY

ADJUSTING A REDUNDANT SYSTEM

The neuroendocrine regulation of appetite has multiple overlapping controls and is therefore called a redundant system. The redundancy creates a strong bias to maintain energy intake and energy stores. As a result, efforts to reduce appetite and weight are confounded. Early medical management for weight reduction included triiodothyronine, human chorionic gonadotropin, and ephedrine. Such treatments raised metabolic rate and facilitated weight loss for only a very short term, because the redundant system compensated for the change.

APPLYING COMBINATION THERAPY

Since single pharmacologic interventions result in tachyphylaxis, another strategy is to target multiple physiological pathways at once. The medication combination of phenteramine and fenfluramine targeted two systems at once. These drugs are both amphetamine analogs with low abuse potential. Phentermine is a potent neuronal releasers and reuptake inhibitors of dopamine. Fenfluramine is a potent neuronal releaser and reuptake inhibitor of serotonin. In the early 1990s it was found that the combination of these drugs had a supra-additive effect on suppressing appetite and inducing satiety. The combination of drugs resulted, in some cases, profound weight loss. The duration of the appetite and weight loss effect seemed more durable and longer lasting when compared with the use of either agent alone. While fenfluramine was removed from the market in 1997 due to an association with cardiac valve disease and pulmonary hypertension, its combination with phentermine demonstrated the synergistic effect of combination therapy.

BROADENING COMBINATION THERAPY

The strategy of combination therapy extends beyond medical therapy and includes nutritional balance and weight reduction surgery. Since any departure from homeostasis favors energy conservation, maintaining adequate hydration, essential fats, B vitamins, and minerals can improve neuroendocrine regulation of appetite. Mineral stores can be measured, imbalances predicted and diets adjusted. Nutrition can be used to treat other medical conditions which promote obesity, either directly or through medications with adverse side effects.

Surgical procedures for weight reduction as described in Chapter 16 are more successful than current medical interventions, in part because they are combination therapies. Bariatric surgery alters several appetite signals. Less invasive and reversible surgical interventions can be combined with nutritional and medical interventions to reset the redundant system of appetite and body weight.

REFERENCES

1. Kuczmarski, R.J., Flegal, K.M., Campbell, S.M., and Johnson, C.L., Increasing prevalence of overweight among US adults. The National Health and Nutrition Examination Surveys, 1960 to 1991, *J. Am. Med. Assoc.*, 272, 205–211, 1994.
2. Bray, G.A., Dahms, W.T., and Swerdloff, R.S., The Prader–Willi syndrome: a study of 40 patients and a review of the literature, 62, 59–80, 1983.
3. Grossman, S.P., Hypothalamic regulation: a re-evaluation, in *The Body Weight System: Normal and Disturbed Mechanisms*, Cioffi, L.A., et al., Eds., Raven Press, New York, 1981, pp. 11–17.
4. Rabin, B.M., Ventromedial hypothalamic control of food intake and satiety: a reappraisal, Brain Res., 43, 317–342, 1972.
5. White, L. and Hain, R.F., Anorexia in association with a destructive lesion of the hypothalamus, *AMA Arch. Pathol.*, 68, 275–281, 1959.
6. Hetherington, A.W. and Ranson, S.W., Experimental hypothalamic–hypophyseal obesity in the rat, *Proc. Soc. Exp. Biol. Med.*, 41, 465, 1939.
7. Bray, G.A. and Gallagher, T.F., Jr., Manifestations of hypothalamic obesity in man: a comprehensive investigation of eight patients and a review of the literature, *Medicine*, 54, 301–333, 1975.
8. Hunsinger, R.N. and Wilson, C., Anorectics and the set point theory for regulation of body weight, *Int. J. Obes.*, 10, 205–210, 1986.
9. McCarthy, H.D., Crowder, R.E., Dryden, S., and Williams, G., Megestrol acetate stimulates food and water intake in rats: effects on regional hypothalamic neuropeptide Y concentration. *Eur. J. Pharmacol.*, 265, 99–102, 1994.
10. Lewis, D., Shellard, L., Koeslag, D.G., et al., Intense exercise and food restriction cause similar hypothalamic neuropeptide Y increase in rats, *Am. J. Physiol.*, 264(2 Pt 1), E279–E284, 1993.
11. Stephens, T.W., Basinski, M., Bristow, P.K., et al., The role of neuropeptide Y in the antiobesity action of the obese gene product, *Nature*, 377, 530–532, 1995.
12. Lambert, P.D., Wilding, J.P.H., Al-Dokhayel, A.A.M., et al., A role for neuropeptide-Y, dynorphin and noradrenaline in the central control of food intake after food deprivation, *Endocrinology*, 133, 29–32, 1993.
13. Tempel, D.L. and Liebowitz, S.F., Glucocorticoid receptors in PVN: interactions with NE, NYP, Gal in relation to feeding, *Am. J. Physiol.*, 265, E794–E800, 1993.
14. Tempel, D.L., Liebowitz, K.J., and Liebowitz, S.F., Effect of PVN galanin on macronutrient selection, *Peptides*, 9, 309–314, 1988.
15. Ohki-Hamazaki, H., Watase, K., Yamamoto, K., Ogura, H., Yamano, M., Yamada, K., Maeno, H., Imaki, J., Kikuyama, S., Wada, E., and Wada, K., Mice lacking bombesin receptor subtype-3 develop metabolic defects and obesity, *Nature*, 390, 165–169, 1997.

16. Vijayan, E. and McCann, S.M., Suppression of feeding and drinking activity in rats following intraventricular injection of thyrotropin releasing hormone (TRH), *Endocrinology*, 100, 1727–1730, 1977.

17. Clark, J.T., Kalra, P.S., Crowley, W.R., and Kalra, S.P., Neuropeptide Y and human pancreatic polypeptide stimulate feeding behavior in rats, *Endocrinology*, 115, 427–429, 1984.

18. Turton, M.D., O'Shea, D., Gunn, I., et al., A role for glucagon-like peptide-1 in the central regulation of feeding, *Nature*, 379, 69–72, 1996.

19. McCarthy, H.D., McKibbin, P.E., Perkins, A.V., Linton, E.A., and Williams, G., Alterations in hypothalamic NPY and CRF in anorexic tumor-bearing rats, *Am. J. Physiol.*, 264(4 Pt 1), E638–E643, 1993.

20. Spina, M., Merlo-Pich, E., Chan, R.K.W., Basso, A.M., Rivier, J., Vale, W., and Koob, G.F., Appetite-suppressing effects of urocortin, a CRF-related peptide, *Science*, 273, 1561–1564, 1996.

21. Morley, J.E., Neuropeptide regulation of appetite and weight, *Endocr. Rev.*, 8, 256–287, 1987.

22. Morley, J.E., Arcaini, L., Levine, A.S., Yi, G.K., and Lowy, M.T., Opioid modulation of appetite, *Neurosci. Biobehav. Rev.*, 7, 281–305, 1983.

23. Genazzani, A.R., Faccinetti, F., Petraglia, F., Pintor, C., and Corda, R., Hyperendorphinemia in obese children and adolescents, *J. Clin. Endocrinol. Metab.*, 62, 36–40, 1993.

24. Sternbach, H.A., Annitto, W., Pottash, A.L.C., and Gold, M.S., Anorexic effects of naltrexone in man, *Lancet*, 1, 388–389, 1982.

25. Wolkowitz, O.M., Doran, A.R., Cohen, M.R., Cohen, R.M., Wise, T.N., and Pickar, D., Effect of naloxone on food consumption in obesity, *N. Engl. J. Med.*, 313, 327, 1985.

26. Atkinson, R.L., Berke, L.K., Drake, C.R., Bibbs, M.L., Williams, F.L., and Kaiser, D.L., Effects of long-term therapy with naltrexone on body weight in obesity, *Clin. Pharmacol. Ther.*, 38, 419–422, 1985.

27. Cooper, S.J., Jackson, A., and Kirkham, T.C., Endorphins and food intake: kappa opioid receptor agonists and hyperphagia, *Pharmacol. Biochem. Behav.*, 23, 889–901, 1985.

28. Jewett, D.C., Grace, M.K., Jones, R.M., Billington, C.J., Portoghese, P.S., and Levine, A.S., The kappa-opioid antagonist GNTI reduces U50,488-, DAMGO-, and deprivation-induced feeding, but not butorphanol- and neuropeptide Y-induced feeding in rats, *Brain Res.*, 909, 75–80, 2001.

29. Levine, A.S., Grace, M., Billington, C.J., and Portoghese, P.S., Nor-binaltorphimine decreases deprivation and opioid-induced feeding, *Brain Res.*, 534, 60–64, 1990.

30. Leibowitz, S.F., Weiss, G.F., and Shor-Posner, G., Hypothalamic serotonin: pharmacologic, biochemical and behavioral analysis of its feeding-suppressive action, *Clin Neuropharmacol.*, 11, S51–S71, 1988.

31. Leibowitz, S.F. and Shor-Posner, G., Brain serotonin and eating behavior, *Appetite*, 7, 1–14, 1986.

32. Atkinson, R.L., Blank, R.C., Loper, J.F., Schumacher, D., and Lutes, R.A., Combined drug treatment of obesity, *Obes. Res.*, 3 (Suppl 4), 497S–500S, 1995.

33. Bergen, S.S., Appetite-stimulating properties of cyproheptadine, *Am. J. Dis. Child.*, 108, 270–73, 1964.

34. Kardinal, C.G., Loprinzi, C.L., Schaid, D.J., et al., A controlled trial of cyproheptadine in cancer patients with anorexia and/or cachexia, Cancer, 65, 2657–2662, 1990.

35. Woittiez, A.J., Wenting, G.J., van den Meiracker, A.H., et al., Chronic effect of ketanserin in mild to moderate essential hypertension, *Hypertension*, 8, 167–173, 1986.
36. Kenien, A.G., Zeidner, D.L., Pang, S.J., et al., The effect of cyproheptadine and human growth hormone on adrenocortical function in children with hypopituitarism, *J. Pediatr.*, 92, 491–494, 1978.
37. Cantú, T.G. and Korek, J.S., Monoamine oxidase inhibitors and weight gain, *Drug Intell. Clin. Pharm.*, 22, 755–759, 1988.
38. Paykel, E.S., Mueller, P.S., and De La Vergne, P.M., Amitriptyline, weight gain and carbohydrate craving: a side effect, *Br. J. Psychiatry*, 123, 501–507, 1973.
39. Fernstrom, M.H. and Kupfer, D.J., Antidepressant-induced weight gain: a comparison study of four medications, *Psychiatry Res.*, 26, 265–271, 1988.
40. Levitt, A.J., Joffe, R.T., Esche, I., and Sherret, D., The effect of disipramine on body weight in depressions, *J. Clin. Psychiatry*, 48, 27–28, 1987.
41. Davidson, J. and Turnbull, C., Loss of appetite and weight associated with the monoamine oxidase inhibitor isocarboxazid, *J. Clin. Psychopharmacol.*, 2, 263–266, 1982.
42. Walker, B.R., Deitch, M.W., Schneider, B.E., Hare, L.E., and Gold, J.A., Long-term therapy of hypertension with guanabenz, *Clin. Ther.*, 4, 217–227, 1981.
43. Nakra, B.R.S. and Grossberg, G.T., Carbohydrate craving and weight gain with maprotiline, *Psychosomatics*, 27, 376–381, 1986.
44. Griboff, S.I., Berman, R., and Silverman, H.I., A double-blind clinical evaluation of a phenylpropanolamine–caffeine–vitamin combination and a placebo in the treatment of exogenous obesity, *Curr. Ther. Res.*, 17, 535–543, 1975.
45. Altschuler, S., Conte, A., Sebok, M., Marlin, R.L., and Winick, C., Three controlled trials of weight loss with phenylpropanolamine, *Int. J. Obes.*, 6, 549–556, 1982.
46. Gardner, E.A., Effects of bupropion on weight in patients intolerant to previous antidepressants, *Curr. Ther. Res.*, 35, 188–199, 1984.
47. Maclay, W.P. and Wallace, M.G., A multi-centre general practice trial of mazindol in the treatment of obesity, *Practitioner*, 218, 431–434, 1977.
48. Doss, F.W., The effect of antipsychotic drugs on body weight: a retrospective review, *J. Clin. Psychiatry*, 40, 528–530, 1979.
49. Planansky, K. and Heilizer, F., Weight changes in relation to the characteristics of patients on chlorpromazine, *J. Clin. Exp. Psychopathol. Q. Rev. Psychiatry Neurol.*, 20(1), 53–7, 1959.
50. Klett, C.J. and Caffey, E.M., Jr., Weight changes during treatment with phenothiazine derivatives, *J. Neuropsychiatry*, 2, 102–108, 1960.
51. Vieweg, V., Godleski, L., Hundley, P., Harrington, D., and Yank, G., Antipsychotic drugs, lithium, carbamazepine, and abnormal diurnal weight gain in psychosis, *Neuropsychopharmacology*, 2, 39–43, 1989.
52. Rockwell, W.J.K., Ellinwood, E.H., and Trader, D.W., Psychotropic drugs promoting weight gain: health risks and treatment implications, *South. Med. J.*, 76, 1407–1412, 1983.
53. Cohen, S., Chiles, J., and MacNaughton, A., Weight gain associated with clozapine, *Am. J. Psychiatry*, 147, 4, 1990.
54. Gordon, H.L., Law, A., Hohman, K.E., and Groth, C., The problem of overweight in hospitalized psychotic patients, *Psychiatry Q.*, 34, 69–82, 1960.
56. Gallant, D.M. and Bishop, M.P., Molindone: a controlled evaluation in chronic schizophrenic patients, *Curr. Ther. Res.*, 10, 441–447, 1968.

57. Rice, D., Possible side effects of fluphenthixol decanoate, *Br. J. Psychiatry*, 123, 613, 1973.

58. Kellner, R., Rada, R.T., Egelman, A., and Macaluso, B., Long-term study of molindone hydrochloride in chronic schizophrenics, *Curr. Ther. Res.*, 20, 686–694, 1976.

59. Löscher, W. and Schimdt, D., Diazepam increases — aminobutyric acid in human cerebrospinal fluid, *J. Neurochem.*, 49, 152–157, 1987.

60. Frisbie, J.H. and Aguilera, E.J., Diazepam and body weight in myelopathy, *J. Spinal Cord Med.*, 18, 200–202, 1995.

61. Hanson, R.A. and Menkes, J.H., A new anticonvulsant in the management of minor motor seizures, *Dev. Med. Child Neurol.*, 14, 3–14, 1972.

62. Dreifuss, F.E., Penry, J.K., Rose, S.W., Kupferberg, H.J., Dyken, P., and Sato, S., Serum clonazepam concentrations in children with absence seizures, *Neurology*, 25, 255–258, 1975.

63. Chadwick, D., Gabapentin in partial epilepsy, *Lancet*, 335, 1114–1117, 1990.

64. Gardos, G. and Cole, J.O., Weight reduction in schizophrenics by molindone, *Am. J. Psychiatry*, 134, 302–304, 1977.

65. Lampl, Y., Eshel, Y., Rapaport, A., Sarova-Pinhas, I., Weight gain, increased appetite, and excessive food intake induced by carbamazepine, *Clin. Neuropharmacol.*, 14, 251–255, 1991.

66. Fukagawa, K., Sakata, T., Shiraishi, T., et al., Neuronal histamine modulates feeding behavior through H1-receptor in rat hypothalamus, *Am. J. Physiol.*, 256(3 Pt 2), R605–R611, 1989.

67. Sakata, T., Ookuma, K., Fukagawa, K., et al., Blockade of the histamine H1-receptor in the rat ventromedial hypothalmus and feeding excitation, *Brain Res.*, 441, 403–407, 1988.

68. Kang, M.K., Yoshimatu, H., Kurokawa, M., Oohara, A., and Sakata, T., Aminoglucose- induced feeding suppression is regulated by hypothalamic neuronal histamine in rats, *Brain Res.*, 631, 181–186, 1993.

69. Ellison, M.J., Horner, R.D., Lawler, F.H., and Jones, J.G., Lack of weight gain associated with short-term astemizole treatment. DICP, *Ann. Pharmacother.*, 24, 682–684, 1990.

70. Wilson, J.D. ad Hillas, J.L., Astemizole: a new long-acting antihistamine in the treatment of seasonal allergic rhinitis, *Clin. Allergy*, 12: 131–140, 1982.

71. Howarth, P.H., Emanuel, M.B., Holgate, S.T., Astemizole, a potent histamine H1-receptor antagonist: effect in allergic rhinoconjunctivitis, on antigen and histamine induced skin weal responses and relationship to serum levels, *Br. J. Clin. Pharmacol.*, 18, 1–8, 1984.

72. Drash, A., Elliott, J., Lags, H., Lavenstein, A.F., and Cooke, R.E., The effect of cyproheptadine on carbohydrate metabolism, *Clin. Pharmacol. Ther.*, 7, 340–346, 1966.

73. Masaki, T., Chiba, S., Yasuda, T., Noguchi, H., Kakuma, T., Watanabe, T., Sakata, T., and Yoshimatsu, H., Involvement of hypothalamic histamine H1 receptor in the regulation of feeding rhythm and obesity, *Diabetes*, 53, 2250–2260, 2004.

74. van Houten, M., Posner, B.I., Kopriwa, B.M., and Brawer, J.R., Insulin-binding sites localized to nerve terminal in rat median eminence and arcutae nucleus, *Science*, 207, 1081–1083, 1980.

75. van Houten, M., Posner, B.I., Kopriwa, B.M., and Brawer, J.R., Insulin-binding sites in the rat brain: in vivo localization to the circumventricular organs by quantitative radioautography, *Endocrinology*, 105, 666–673, 1979.

76. Polonsky, B.D., Given, E., and Carter, V., Twenty-four-hour profiles and pulsatile patterns of insulin secretion in normal and obese subjects, *J. Clin. Invest.*, 81, 442–448, 1988.

77. Woods, S.C., Lotter, E.C., McKay, L.D., and Porte, D., Jr., Chronic intracerebro-ventricular infusion of insulin reduces food intake and body weight of baboons, *Nature*, 282, 503–505, 1979.

78. Brogden, R.N., Heel, R.C., Pakes, G.E., Speight, T.M., and Avery, G.S., Glipizide: a review of its pharmacological properties and therapeutic use, *Drugs*, 18, 329–353, 1979.

79. Fowler, L.K., Glipizide in the treatment of maturity-onset diabetes: a multi-centre, out-patient study, *Curr. Med. Res. Opin.*, 5, 418–423, 1978.

80. Robb, G.H. and Lowe, S.M., Lack of weight gain with gliclazide treatment for 30 months in Type II diabetes, *Curr. Med. Res. Opin.*, 9, 7–9, 1984.

81. Holmes, B., Heel, R.C., Brogden, R.N., Speight, T.M., and Avery, G.S., Gliclazide: a preliminary review of its pharmacodyanmic properties and therapeutic efficacy in diabetes mellitus, *Drugs*, 27, 301–327, 1984.

82. Hermann, L.S., Scherstén, B., Bitzé, P.-O., Kjellstromöm, T., Lingärde, F., and Melander, A., Therapeutic comparison of metformin and sulfonylurea, alone and in various combinations. *Diabetes Care*, 17, 1100–1109, 1994.

83. Dagogo-Jack, S. and Santiago, J.V., Pathophysiology of type 2 diabetes and modes of action of therapeutic interventions, *Arch. Intern. Med.*, 157, 1802–1817, 1997.

84. Navarro, M., Rodriquez de Fonseca, F., Alvarez, E., Chowen, J.A., Zueco, J.A., Gomez, R., Eng, J., and Blazquez, E., Colocalization of glucagon-like peptide-1 (GLP-1) receptors, glucose transporter GLUT-2, and glucokinase mRNAs in rat hypothalamic cells: evidence for a role of GLP-1 receptor agonists as an inhibitory signal for food and water intake, *J. Neurochem.*, 67, 1982–1991, 1996.

85. Edwards, C.M., Stanley, S.A., Davis, R., Brynes, A.E., Frost, G.S., Seal, L.J., Ghatei, M.A., and Bloom, S.R., Exendin-4 reduces fasting and postprandial glucose and decreases energy intake in healthy volunteers, *Am. J. Physiol. Endocrinol. Metab.*, 281, E155–E161, 2001.

86. Strader, A.D., Vahl, T.P., Jandacek, R.J., Woods, S.C., D'Alessio, D.A., and Seeley, R.J., Weight loss through ileal transposition is accompanied by increased ileal hormone secretion and synthesis in rats, *Am. J. Physiol. Endocrinol. Metab.*, 288, E447–E453, 2005. Epub 2004 Sep. 28.

87. Vahl, T.P., Paty, B.W., Fuller, B.D., Prigeon, R.L., and D'Alessio, D.A., Effects of GLP-1-(7-36)NH2, GLP-1-(7-37), and GLP-1-(9-36)NH2 on intravenous glucose tolerance and glucose-induced insulin secretion in healthy humans, *J. Clin. Endocrinol. Metab.*, 88, 1772–1779, 2003.

88. Gutzwiller, J.P., Drewe, J., Goke, B., Schmidt, H., Rhorer, B., Lareida, J., and Beglinger, C., Glucagon-like peptides-1 promotes satiety and reduces food intake in patients with diabetes mellitus type 2, *Am. J. Physiol.*, 276, R1541–R1544, 1999.

89. Meier, U. and Gressner, A.M., Endocrine regulation of energy metabolism: review of pathobiochemical and clinical chemical aspects of leptin, ghrelin, adiponectin, and resistin, *Clin. Chem.*, 50, 1511–1525, 2004. Epub 2004, Jul. 20.

90. Nijhuis, J., van Dielen, F.M., Buurman, W.A., Greve, J.W., Ghrelin, leptin and insulin levels after restrictive surgery: a 2-year follow-up study, *Obes. Surg.*, 14, 783–787, 2004.

91. Fruhbeck, G., Diez-Caballero, A., Gil, M.J., Montero, I., Gomez-Ambrosi, J., Salvador. J., and Cienfuegos, J.A., The decrease in plasma ghrelin concentrations following bariatric surgery depends on the functional integrity of the fundus, *Obes. Surg.*, 14, 606–612, 2004.

92. Patriti, A., Facchiano, E., Sanna, A., Gulla, N., and Donini, A., The enteroinsular axis and the recovery from type 2 diabetes after bariatric surgery, *Obes. Surg.*, 14, 840–848, 2004.

93. Mason, E.E., Ileal [correction of ilial] transposition and enteroglucagon/GLP-1 in obesity (and diabetic?) surgery, *Obes. Surg.*, 9, 223–228, 1999.

94. Geloneze, B., Tambascia, M.A., Pilla, V.F., Geloneze, S.R., Repetto, E.M., and Pareja, J.C., Ghrelin: a gut–brain hormone: effect of gastric bypass surgery, *Obes. Surg.*, 13, 17-22, 2003.

95. Blanchette, V., Imbach, P., Andrew, M., et al., Randomised trial of intravenous immunoglobin G, intravenous anti-D and oral prednisone in childhood acute immune thrombocytopenic purpura, *Lancet*, 344, 703–707, 1994.

96. Loftus, J.K., Reeve, J., Hesp, R., David, J., Ansell, B.M., and Woo, P.M., Deflazacort in juvenile chronic arthritis, *J. Rheumatol. Suppl.*, 37, 40–42, 1993.

97. Tempel, D.L., McEwen, B.S., and Leibowitz, S.F., Adrenal steroid receptors in the PVN: studies with steroid antagonists in relation to macronutrient intake, Neuroendocrinology, 57, 1106–1113, 1993.

98. Tempel, D.L., Kim, T., and Leibowitz, S.F., The paraventricular nucleus is uniquely responsive to the feeding stimulatory effects of steroid hormones, *Brain Res.*, 614, 197–204, 1993.

99. Campfield, L.A., Smith, F.J., Guisez, Y., Devos, R., and Burn, P., Recombinant mouse OB protein: evidence for a peripheral signal linking adiposity and central neural networks, *Science*, 269, 546–548, 1995.

100. Melton, P.M., Kissileff, H.R., and Pi-Sunyer, F.X., Cholecystokinin (CCK-8) affects gastric pressure and ratings of hunger and fullness in women, *Am. J. Physiol.*, 263(2 Pt 2), R452–R456, 1992.

101. Kissileff, H.R., Pi-Sunyer, F.X., Thornton, J., and Smith, G.P., C-terminal octapeptide of cholecystokinin decreases food intake in man, *Am. J. Clin. Nutr.*, 34, 154–160, 1981.

102. Rubino, F., Gagner, M., Gentileschi, P., Kini, S., Fukuyama, S., Feng, J., and Diamond, E., The early effect of the Roux-en-Y gastric bypass on hormones involved in body weight regulation and glucose metabolism, *Ann. Surg.*, 240, 236–242, 2004.

103. Rieu, P.N., Jansen, J.B., Hopman, W.P., Joosten, H.J., and Lamers, C.B., Effect of partial gastrectomy with Billroth II or Roux-en-Y anastomosis on postprandial and cholecystokinin-stimulated gallbladder contraction and secretion of cholecystokinin and pancreatic polypeptide. *Dig. Dis. Sci.*, 35, 1066–1072, 1990.

104. Geary, N., Kissileff, H.R., Pi-Sunyner, F.X., and Hinton, V., Individual, but not simultaneous, glucagon and cholecystokinin infusions inhibit feeding in men, *Am. J. Physiol.*, 262(6 Pt 2), R975–R980, 1992.

105. Cavagnini, F., Magella, A., Danesi, L., et al. Ineffectiveness of ceruletide to reduce food intake and body eight in obese women hospitalized for weight reduction and treated with a restricted diet. A double-blind study, *Peptides*, 8, 455–459, 1987.

106. Jang, M., Mistry, A., Swick, A.G., and Romsos, D.R., Leptin rapidly inhibits hypothalamic neuropeptide Y secretion and stimulates corticotropin-releasing hormone secretion in adrenalectomized mice, *J. Nutr.*, 130, 2813–2820, 2000.

107. Montague, C.T., Faroogi, I.S., Whitehead, J.P., Soos, M.A., Rau, H., Wareham, N.J., Sewter, C.P., Digby, J.E., Mohammaed, S.N., Hurst, J.A., Cheetham, C.H., Earley, A.R., Barnett, A.H., Prins, A.H., and O'Rahilly, S., Congential leptin deficiency is associated with severe early-onset obesity in humans, *Nature*, 387, 903–908, 1997.

108. Ravussin, E., Pratley, R.E., Maffei, M., Wang, H., Freidman, J., Bennett, P.H., Bogardus, C., Relatively low plasma leptin concentrations precede weight gain in Pima Indians, *Nat. Med.*, 3, 238–240, 1997.

109. Constidine, R.V., Sinha, M.K., Heiman, M.L., et al., Serum immunoreactive-leptin concentrations in normal weight and obese humans, *N. Engl. J. Med.*, 334, 292–295, 1996.

110. Tagami, T., et al., Adiponectin in anorexia nervosa and bulimia nervosa, *J. Clin. Endocrinol. Metab.*, 89, 1833–1837, 2004.

111. Lagathu, C., Kim, M., Maachi, M., Vigouroux, C., Cervera, P., Capeau, J., Caron, M., and Bastard, J.P., HIV antiretroviral treatment alters adipokine expression and insulin sensitivity of adipose tissue in vitro and in vivo, *Biochimie*, 87, 65–71, 2005.

112. Nolan, D., Metabolic complications associated with HIV protease inhibitor therapy, *Drugs*, 63, 2555–2574, 2003.

113. Munoz, J.A., et al., Iron deficiency and pica, *Sangre*, 43, 31–34, 1998.

114. Beard, J.L., Boerl, M.J., and Derr, J., Impaired thermoregulation and thyroid function in iron-deficiency anemia, *Am. J. Clin. Nutr.*, 52, 813–819, 1990.

115. Levenson, C.W., Zinc regulation of food intake: new insights on the role of neuropeptide Y, *Nutr. Rev.*, 61, 247–249, 2003.

116. Trombley, P.Q., Horning, M.S., and Blakemore, L.J., Interactions between carnosine and zinc and copper: implications for neuromodulation and neuroprotection, *Biochemistry*, 65, 807–816, 2000.

117. Erikson, K.M. and Aschner, M., Manganese neurotoxicity and glutamate-GABA interaction, *Neurochem. Int.*, 43, 475–480, 2003.

118. Batmanghelidj, F., *Water for Health, for Health, for Life*, Warner Books, 2003.

119. Stunkard, A.J., Grace, W.J. and Wolff, H.G., The night eating syndrome; a pattern of food intake among certain obese patients, *Am. J. Med.*, 19, 78–86, 1955.

120. O'Reardon, J.P., et al., Circadian eating syndrome and sleeping patterns in the night eating syndrome, *Obes. Res.*, 12, 1789–1796, 2004.

14 Estrogen's Role in the Regulation of Appetite and Body Fat

Paula J. Geiselman, Ph.D. and
Steven R. Smith, M.D.

CONTENTS

INTRODUCTION

Women have a greater percentage of body fat than do men. In addition, women and men store fat in somewhat different locations. Sexual dimorphism of adiposity is apparent before puberty, and is accentuated as sex hormone levels rise to adult values during puberty. The gender difference in estrogen concentration explains much of the gender differences in adiposity.

This chapter reviews the literature focused on unopposed estrogen and the combination of estrogen and progesterone in the control of food intake and the regulation of body mass. Estrogen modulates both peripheral and central mechanisms in the control of food intake, body weight, and adiposity. This chapter discusses variations in estrogen levels — menstrual cycle phases, racial differences, pregnancy, lactation, menopause, polycystic ovary syndrome (PCOS), hormonal contraception — and the possible implications for clinical weight management.

GENDER AND RACIAL CONSIDERATIONS IN OBESITY

Obesity is associated with the development of a wide range of adverse health consequences in both men and women: Type 2 diabetes mellitus, gallbladder disease, dyslipidemia, insulin resistance, breathlessness, sleep apnea, coronary heart disease, hypertension, osteoarthritis (knees), hyperuricemia and gout, and some cancers.[1] In addition, there are a number of obesity-related adverse health conditions that are specific to women: breast cancer in postmenopausal women, endometrial cancer, PCOS, impaired fertility, and reproductive hormone abnormalities.[1] Binge eating is also more common among women. Therefore, identifying physiologic, dietary, and behavioral factors that uniquely contribute to weight gain, overweight, and obesity in women can have great clinical benefits.

Women may be more susceptible than men to weight gain, overweight, and obesity.[1-4] Changes in eating habits, activity levels, and physiologic factors have been suggested to promote increased fat deposition during adolescence, and this is especially likely to occur in girls.[2,4] After puberty, although both young men and young women show an increase in appetite for fat, this increased fat appetite is significantly greater and occurs much earlier in women than it does in men.[1,3] Also, in a 10 year National Health and Nutrition Examination Survey (NHANES) follow-up study, Williamson et al.[5] found that, in comparison with men, adult women have twice the incidence of major weight gain, thus further accumulating body fat. Women continue to experience an increase in adiposity with age, and at any body mass index (BMI), women average a greater percentage of body fat than do men. Indeed, the normal range of body fat in men is 12 to 20%, whereas the normal range for women is 20 to 30% body fat.[6]

Although overweight and obesity have become common conditions among women across various ethnic backgrounds in this country, the burden of weight gain, overweight, and obesity is disproportionate among some minority populations of women, especially African–American women. At ages 30 to 55 years, the incidence of major weight gain has been found to be 11.7% in Caucasian women and 17.3% in African–American women.[7] As reported from the NHANES III database, the prevalence of overweight and obesity is substantially greater in

African–American and Hispanic women than it is in either Caucasian women or in men.[8,9] In the African–American population, the percentage of obese women is 80% greater than the percentage of obese men; and it has also been reported that the prevalence of obesity in Hispanic women is considerably greater than in Hispanic men.[9]

ESTROGEN AND FOOD INTAKE

Women may be especially vulnerable to hyperphagia (overeating), weight gain, and obesity owing to fluctuations in the female sex hormones. In contrast to the stable patterns of daily food intake observed in males of many species, in females of many species caloric intake and body weight are cyclic and correlate with phases of the menstrual or estrous cycle. When estrogen is elevated and progesterone is low, females across species show a significant decrease in caloric intake and body weight.[10–25] Further, it has been reported in female rodent models that physiologic levels of estrogen within the estrus phase are inversely related to food intake.[10,26,27] Exogenous estrogen administration has also been shown to produce a significant decrease in food intake in female rodents.[27–29] Perhaps even more importantly, it has been demonstrated that the estrogenic inhibition of food intake observed in rodents is due entirely to a decrease in meal size rather than any other change that could occur in meal patterns.[26,30,31] This is noteworthy because meal size is considered to be the predominant determinant of total food intake.

Women experience the hypophagic effect of estrogen in the late follicular and periovulatory phases of the menstrual cycle when estrogen levels are elevated and progesterone concentrations are low. Conversely, during the luteal phase, when progesterone is elevated in opposition to estrogen, women significantly increase their caloric intake and body weight.[13,15,23,24] See Figure 14.1.

Women who are not obese increase their caloric intake during the postovulatory luteal phase by approximately 10% and possibly as much as 500 kcal during the luteal phase.[24,32] Consistent with these data, our laboratory has recently demonstrated that women ingest significantly more calories and larger meals in an acute food intake test during the luteal phase, when progesterone is elevated, than they do in the late follicular phase, when estradiol is elevated and levels of progesterone are low.[33] Hence, the premenstrual increase in food intake is a robust effect that can be detected in a single meal in the laboratory. As the duration of the luteal phase is approximately 2 weeks in the standard, 28 day menstrual cycle, it is possible that a marked and sustained increase in food intake during this phase could lead to weight gain and accumulation of excess body fat. However, energy expenditure also increases in the luteal phase. Whether or not the increase in energy expenditure can compensate for the increase in energy intake during the luteal phase may be a determining factor in obesity among women. The clinical

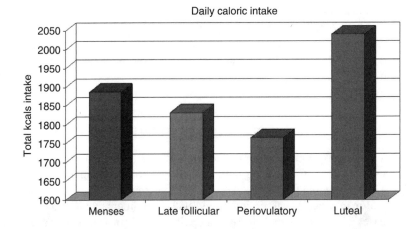

FIGURE 14.1 Daily caloric intake during phases of the menstrual cycle in women. Food intake during the late follicular and periovulatory phases is significantly less than food intake during the luteal phase. (Data are from Gong, E.J., Garrel, D., and Calloway, D.H., *Am. J. Clin. Nutr.*, 49, 252–258, 1989. Adapted with permission by the *American Journal of Clinical Nutrition.* Copyright Am J Clin Nutr: American Society for Clinical Nutrition.)

implications are many. As women are offered a scientific explanation of physiologic changes, they will be better equipped to control their weight.

ESTROGEN AND FOOD SELECTION

The next question is whether estrogen influences specific macronutrient (fat, carbohydrate, protein) intake. Young et al.[34] and Geiselman et al.[35] have demonstrated that the hypophagic response to estradiol observed in the rat has some specificity in decreasing fat intake. Consistent with these animal results, Tarasuk and Beaton[36] have reported that the greater caloric intake observed in the luteal phase in women is attributable to a significant increase in fat intake. Other investigators have ascribed the hyperphagia observed in the luteal phase to an increase in intake of both sweet and nonsweet, high-fat, high-carbohydrate foods.[37] Based on a number of studies using subjects' self-reports, one can conclude that women do tend to ingest at least slightly more dietary fat during the luteal phase as compared with the late follicular phase.[38–40] The above-cited, luteal-phase data were collected from women with endogenous levels of progesterone and estrogen. Women taking triphasic oral contraceptives, pharmacologic combinations of estrogenic compounds and progestin, eat proportionately more dietary fat than do women who are not taking oral contraceptives.[41]

Some contrasting reports conclude that the luteal phase is associated with "carbohydrate" craving or with a specific "sweet" appetite.[42–46] However, many of these reports were based on clinical experience only or on self-reports by women;

and there are alternative explanations as well. Typically, in these studies, the fat content of foods was disregarded, and foods such as chocolate, which is high in both fat and sugar content, were mislabeled as "sweets."

The relationship between the luteal phase and preference for dietary fat is of particular interest as high-fat foods and diets are associated with overeating. Rolls et al.[47] has found that women report significantly greater hunger 2 h after a high-fat/high-sugar confectionery snack, than 2 h after eating either a high-protein (chicken) or high-starch (pasta) snack. In addition, women's rating of pleasantness of the taste of the chicken and the pasta preloads decreased significantly from before to after each of these snacks, and pleasantness ratings for these foods decreased more than the ratings for uneaten foods with similar macronutrient content, thus showing sensory-specific satiety for the chicken and pasta snacks. However, there were no significant changes in pleasantness of taste following the high-fat/high-sugar confectionery, indicating no evidence of sensory-specific satiety for this snack. Two hours following consumption of each snack, the women in Rolls' study were offered a choice of foods. Analysis of energy intake in the meal revealed that women ate significantly more calories following the high-fat/high-sugar confectionery preload than they did following either the high-protein or the high-starch preload. In summary, women were hungrier after snacking on high-fat/high-sugar foods than after snacking on either high-protein or high-starch foods.

ESTROGEN AND THE ETHNIC GAP

There are striking ethnic differences in fat intake across the menstrual cycle, especially during the luteal phase. Our laboratory is investigating whether or not differences in fat intake during the luteal phase can help explain the ethnic difference in obesity among women. Using our Macronutrient Self-Selection Paradigm[©48] and our Food Preference Questionnaire[©,48] we are assessing fat and other specific macronutrient intake and fat preference in perimenopausal, menstruating African–American and Caucasian women in both the late follicular phase and the luteal phase of the menstrual cycle. We have obtained significant differences in fat and total caloric intake between these two groups of women, especially during the luteal phase. The perimenopausal African–American women selected and ingested significantly more fat and total calories across the menstrual cycle than did perimenopausal Caucasian women. This effect was greatest in the luteal phase when the African–American women's fat intake was 260 kcal (28.9 g) greater than fat intake in the Caucasian women in a single meal.[49] Hence, this pattern of macronutrient self-selection, which has been associated with hyperphagia and weight gain, demonstrates an ethnic difference in the perimenopausal African–American women in the risk for diet-induced hyperphagia, especially in the luteal phase. This pattern of macronutrient self-selection may be at least partially responsible for the fact that obesity rates are higher in African–American women than in Caucasian women.

Editor's Note

As part of a weight management strategy, women may wish to consciously decrease meal size during the luteal phase (when progesterone level is elevated in opposition to that of estrogen) of the menstrual cycle and also during menopause. Restoring age-appropriate physiologic levels of estrogen appears to be beneficial in weight management. Women who strive for a low-fat diet, should be aware of the recent study, which found that women using contraceptive pills consume a higher percentage of dietary fat than women who do not use hormonal contraception.

PREGNANCY, ESTROGEN, AND FOOD INTAKE

During pregnancy blood levels of estriol and estradiol increase significantly and continuously until close to parturition.[50,51] Concomitantly, plasma progesterone levels increase markedly during the first trimester and then continue to rise to significantly higher levels until the pregnancy is close to term. This hormonal characterization, with elevated levels of progesterone acting in opposition to the hypophagic effect of estrogen, would lead one to expect a significant increase in total caloric intake during pregnancy. Numerous animal studies show that appetite increases during pregnancy and that pregnancy produces significant increases in fat deposition and total body mass.[50]

Pregnant women are advised to increase calorie intake by 300 kcal/d to meet the increased energy demands. Appetite increases during pregnancy have not been easy to quantify. Data from some dietary surveys have indicated that pregnant women report puzzlingly small increases in caloric intake.[52,53] The studies used dietary self-reporting. Goldberg et al.[54] assessed energy expenditure in 12 pregnant women using the doubly labeled water, stable-isotope method. The dietary self-reports for 4 of the 12 pregnant women were implausible. These investigators, among others, have concluded that some subjects provide dietary self-reports that are biased toward underestimation.[54,55] However, even if food intake were measured objectively in pregnant women, data interpretation would still be problematic because physiologic changes during pregnancy would be confounded by changes due to nutritional advice.

LACTATION AND POSTPARTUM WEIGHT CONTROL

Lactating women are given the recommended dietary advice to increase their daily caloric intake by 500 kcal/d. Owing to the high energy demands of milk production, there is a common assumption that lactation helps women return to their normal body weight. However, as has been noted in the literature,[56–58] the vast majority of reports do not find an association between lactation and increased maternal weight loss in the postpartum condition.[56–58]

ESTROGEN DEFICIENCY AND THE LABORATORY RAT

Estrogen deficiency is well studied in rat models, in which deficiency is created by surgical removal of the ovaries. Following ovariectomy in rats, the cyclic patterns of food intake are eliminated,[14,59] and the animals show a dramatic increase in caloric consumption[27] and meal size.[60,61] The increase in meal size has been attributed to estradiol deficiency.[60,61] During the initial 3 to 5 weeks postovariectomy, the hyperphagic effect leads to a 20 to 25% increase in body weight,[26,28,62] which is primarily due to a specific increase in adiposity.[60,63–65] The hyperphagic response that leads to the increased adiposity following ovariectomy has been attributed to the elimination of the ovarian secretions of estradiol because physiologic replacement of this hormone reverses the hyperphagia.[21,28,62] It has also been demonstrated that a single injection of estradiol produces a significant decrease in food intake in ovariectomized monkeys.[21] Further, cyclic replacement of estradiol in ovariectomized rats both reverses the hyperphagia and produces a cyclic pattern of food intake.[60,66,67] However, administration of progesterone alone does not affect food intake in ovariectomized rats or monkeys,[21,60] but large doses of progesterone may antagonize estradiol.[14,59] Consistent with the above data showing that estrogen replacement reverses the hyperphagia in an estrogen-deficient animal, it has also been shown that pharmacologic replacement of estrogen to an estrogen-deficient animal decreases body weight; this effect is primarily due to a decrease in adiposity.[27,63–65]

LOSS OF OVARIAN FUNCTION

Studies on ovariectomized animals demonstrate the various benefits of estrogen replacement in abrupt loss of ovarian function. Women who have a sudden loss in ovarian function, usually due to surgical removal of the ovaries during the childbearing years, are given estrogen replacement. A remaining question is whether or not progesterone (bioidentical to the body's natural progesterone) replaced at physiologic concentrations can counteract estrogen's benefits in these women.

MENOPAUSE AND OBESITY

Menopause represents a gradual, life-stage appropriate, loss of ovarian function. Women may be especially vulnerable to overweight and obesity at menopause, which presents a weight-gain risk factor unique to women. Retrospective reports have indicated that weight gain is a common concern among women at menopause, and most investigators have reported a significant increase in body weight in menopausal women.[68]

It is not clear why women may be particularly at risk of rapid weight gain at the time of menopause.[69] It has been reported that physical activity during leisure time is decreased in menopausal women,[70] but other results are contradictory to this finding.[68,71] It has also been reported that menopausal women have a slightly decreased resting metabolic rate (RMR).[70] Both decrease in physical activity and slight decrease in RMR could contribute to a positive energy balance and weight gain in menopausal women. One would expect decreases in metabolic expenditure in menopausal women due to (1) loss of lean tissue mass and gain in fat mass and (2) loss of the luteal-phase increase in energy expenditure.[72]

The average woman gains an additional 1 to 2 kg at menopause, but it should be noted that increased health risks can occur with a relatively small increase in body weight.[1] Manson et al.[73] have reported that even mild to moderate obesity in middle-aged women significantly increases the risk of coronary disease. Moreover, some women have much greater weight gain at menopause, and a number of studies have suggested that menopause can present a high risk for the development of obesity in women.[74,75] Although it is not entirely clear to what extent changes in body weight may be due to menopause per se, independent of aging, it is clear that a progressive increase in weight gain does take place in women at the time of menopause.

Interestingly, Flegal et al.[75] have reported that for men, the prevalence of a BMI in the overweight range (25.0 to 29.9) was lowest in the 20 to 29 years age group, significantly increased in the 30 to 39 years age group, but not further significantly increased in older age groups.[75] On the contrary, in women the prevalence of a BMI in the overweight range increased substantially with each advancing age group.[75]

Although there is some controversy in the literature regarding the role of menopause per se on changes in adiposity, there are data suggesting that menopause may accelerate age-related changes in body composition, i.e., decreased lean tissue mass and increased fat tissue mass.[70,76,77] Furthermore, unlike premenopausal women who have sufficient estrogen levels to promote primarily lower body, gluteo-femoral, fat deposition, at menopause women have some specificity for an increase in their upper body, abdominal fat deposition.[17] This trend toward central obesity favors increased cardiovascular, cancer, and metabolic risks[78,79] in Caucasian menopausal women, but it is not yet clear whether African–American women experience these adverse effects to the same extent as Caucasian women.[80,81]

Several studies using x-ray imaging techniques have reported a shift toward abdominal fat distribution at menopause (which can occur even when there is no change in the waist:hip ratio). Dawson-Hughes and Harris[82] studied body composition changes across a 1 year period in 125 postmenopausal women and found an increase in trunk fat measured by dual-energy x-ray absorptiometry (DEXA). However, as there was no premenopausal comparison group in this study, it is not clear whether this change was due to menopause per se or merely aging. Ley et al.[83] also reported that postmenopausal women had more upper body fat, as measured by DEXA, than did premenopausal women. Svendsen et al.[84] statistically controlled for the effects of aging and still observed a significant independent effect of menopausal status on both total and abdominal fat percentage.

More recent studies have used computerized tomography (CT) scans as a direct measure of intra-abdominal fat in pre- and postmenopausal women and have consistently reported an increase in visceral abdominal fat with menopause. Enzi et al.[85] have reported that postmenopausal women have a decreased subcutaneous-to-visceral (*S/V*) fat ratio measured by CT scan as compared to age-matched premenopausal women. Similar findings were reported by Hunter et al.,[86] Kotani et al.,[87] and Zamboni et al.,[88] all of which suggest that menopause accelerates the accumulation of visceral fat. These findings are a matter of great concern because intra-abdominal visceral fat is the type of fat that is most highly associated with increased health risks.

As suggested above, estrogen deficiency at menopause has been implicated in the change in fat distribution occurring at this time. Estrogens appear to promote lower body, gluteo-femoral fat accumulation, whereas androgens have been associated with an upper body, abdominal fat distribution in premenopausal[89] and postmenopausal Caucasian women.[90] At menopause, there is a shift in the ratio of androgens to estrogens as ovarian estrogen production ceases while adrenal androgen production continues, which may be associated with the changes in fat distribution occurring at this time. The mechanism for this effect has been proposed by Rebuffe-Scrive and colleagues[91] to be related to alterations in lipoprotein lipase activity in different fat depots in premenopausal compared to postmenopausal women. See Figure 14.2, which illustrates the shift from "pear-shaped" to "apple-shaped" fat distribution, which can occur in women during menopause.

Few studies have investigated the effects of menopause on food intake.[68,70,77,92,93] The studies that have compared food intake in pre- and postmenopausal women have not found significant differences, but it should be noted that these studies have tended to rely on self-reports rather than directly measuring food intake. With the exception of a study of perimenopausal African–American and Caucasian women currently in progress in our laboratory, no studies have directly measured longitudinal changes across menopause in fat and other macronutrient intake in a validated and reliable paradigm using a wide spectrum of foods in which fat is commonly ingested by this population. The paucity of studies on food intake, and especially on fat and other macronutrient intake, in menopausal women is surprising in view of the evidence that dietary factors, especially highly palatable, high-fat, energy-dense diets, strongly influence the energy balance equation and are major modifiable factors that can promote weight gain and maintain overweight and obesity.[1]

Most symptoms and signs of menopause are due to decreased circulating estrogen levels, and this hormonal deficiency may also affect the control of food intake, especially fat appetite and intake, in menopausal women. Considered collectively, the above literature review suggests that the decrease in estradiol

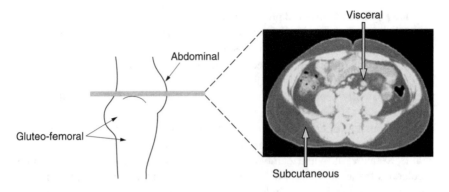

FIGURE 14.2 Abdominal and femoral–gluteal fat distribution. As estrogen levels decline during menopause, the body shifts weight from the femoral–gluteal region to the abdominal, visceral region — from "pear shape" to "apple shape." Concurrently, women's risk for cardiovascular disease and insulin resistance increases.

that occurs with menopause may promote an increase in energy intake, and specifically an increase in fat appetite and intake, thereby leading to an increase in body weight.

As there are differences in sex hormone levels in African–American and Caucasian women,[81] it is not known whether the decreased estrogen levels occurring at menopause would affect food and specific macronutrient intake in Caucasian and African–American women to the same extent. As noted above, no published studies have directly assessed changes in fat appetite and intake and other macronutrient intake across the menopausal transition in any racial group using a validated and reliable macronutrient self-selection paradigm.

REPLACING ESTROGEN DURING MENOPAUSE

Unopposed estrogen (conjugated equine estrogen [CEE]) administered to postmenopausal women produces a significantly smaller amount of weight gain than is observed in women given placebo.[69,94] However, results of studies that have administered CEE in combination with a progestational agent have not been consistent. For example, Espeland et al.[94] have reported that administration of CEE in combination with either medroxyprogesterone acetate (MPA, administered either continuously or cyclically) or micronized progesterone (administered cyclically) is as effective as CEE alone in suppressing weight gain. Other studies have reported that women administered CEE plus MPA gain as much weight as do control subjects.[93] Moreover, Aloia et al.[77] have reported that women administered CEE plus MPA gained significantly more weight than did women in the placebo group. A number of methodologic differences may account for the discrepancies in the results of studies in this literature.

CHOOSING ESTROGEN REPLACEMENT

Estrogens are a family of similarly structured steroid compounds that bind to the two estrogen receptors, alpha and beta, with differing affinities. Unfortunately, the literature is sparse on the relationship between the above-described sex or estrogen differences in food intake, body composition, and hormone replacement therapy (HRT), especially when conducted as randomized clinical trials (RCTs) to compare estrogens and progestins. The reasons for the lack of RCTs comparing HRT regimens on body composition is unclear but may be partially due to the lack of funding from HRT manufacturers. Certainly, the sparsity of this literature does not reflect the concerns expressed by women in the clinic. Both the type of estrogen (17beta vs. ethinyl estradiol) and the progestational agent can influence adipose tissue metabolism in a fashion predicted to influence fat patterning.[95] Several recent reports highlight the concerns surrounding the progestin component of HRT, especially with regard to insulin sensitivity.[96] Therefore, patients may wish to consider transdermal HRT available as creams or patches. Since the transdermal route avoids the pharmacologic challenges of oral administration, the bioidentical hormones can be used rather than hormonal metabolites.

ESTROGEN AS A NEUROENDOCRINE RESPONSE MODIFIER

Estrogen exerts its effects on the nexus of hormones that regulate energy balance. Leptin is one such hormone that is under the influence of estrogen. Leptin is an adipocyte-derived hormone that is secreted into the circulatory system, signaling levels of body fat and promoting negative energy balance and weight loss.[27,97] To exert its effects centrally, circulating leptin from the periphery is transported across the blood–brain barrier into the central nervous system (CNS),[98–102] where it acts by binding to receptors, especially in the hypothalamus, to alter the expression of a number of neuropeptides (neuropeptide Y [NPY], thyrotropin, corticotropin-releasing hormone, melanocyte-stimulating hormone, agouti-related protein, pro-opiomelanocortin, melanin-concentrating hormone, and cocaine- and amphetamine-regulated peptide)[27,103] that regulate neuroendocrine functioning and control energy intake and expenditure.[27,97,103]

Mystkowski and Schwartz[27] have published a thorough and insightful review of the common properties related to the control of food intake, body weight, and adiposity that estrogen shares with leptin. These authors have pointed out the reciprocal relationship between estrogen and leptin and have provided an extensive review of the effects of gonadal steroids and leptin on important hypothalamic neuropeptide systems involved in the control of food intake. It has been demonstrated, for example, that the serotonergic system (5-hydroxytryptamine [5-HT]), which is an important hypothalamic mechanism in the control of food intake, is modulated by estrogen.[61] This system is well documented in the selective suppression of fat intake[104–107] and, under some conditions, suppression of carbohydrate intake.[108] Insulin, which also has been shown to specifically reduce dietary fat intake,[109,110] is another CNS signal for adiposity and energy status that shares some common properties with estrogen.

In addition, estrogen attenuates mechanisms that increase food intake and body weight. NPY, which has an antagonistic relationship with 5-HT in the paraventricular nucleus of the hypothalamus, is one of the most potent stimuli for hyperphagia.[104,109] It has often been reported that the increase in food intake in response to NPY is due to a preferential increase in carbohydrate intake[104,111–113] and, to a lesser extent, to enhanced fat intake.[113,114] However, the macronutrient specificity of NPY may require further qualifications with respect to carbohydrate type, simple sugar vs. complex carbohydrate, and conditions of macronutrient availability. Mystkowski and Schwartz[27] have reviewed data indicating that estrogen may directly affect NPY production and suggesting a connection between estrogen, leptin, and NPY in the control of energy homeostasis.

Because eating behavior occurs in discrete episodes, i.e., meals, it is clear that meal size and/or meal frequency should be controlled to maintain energy balance.[60,66,67,115] However, it is meal size, not meal frequency, that is considered to be the major determinant of total caloric intake,[60,66,67] with the control of meal size being firmly coupled to signals of adiposity and changes in energy balance.[115] Notably, administration of leptin[116] or 5-HT[104,117–119] produces a significant decrease in meal size associated with the decrease in food intake, whereas animals treated with NPY show a delay in meal termination and thus ingest larger meal sizes, resulting in an increase in total caloric intake.[112]

As originally proposed by Gibbs et al. in 1973,[120] a number of peptides secreted by the gut during a meal signal satiation to the CNS, resulting in meal termination. For example, cholecystokinin (CCK), bombesin, gastrin-related peptide, neuromedin-B, glucagon, glucagon-like peptide-1, enterostatin, somato-statin, and apolipoprotein A-IV have been implicated in the control of meal size.[112] Among these peptides, CCK has been the best studied. As of 1992, it had been operationally proven that the release of CCK from the small intestine dur-ing a meal acted to physiologically decrease meal size in rats.[67,121] In humans it has also been demonstrated in double-blind studies that CCK infusion decreases meal size and does not disrupt the normal subjective experience of sati-ety.[60,66,67,121,122] No specific macronutrient intake effects of CCK have been estab-lished, but this peptide has been demonstrated to have a marked effect on both peripheral (enterostatin)[123,124] and CNS (5-HT)[104,125,126] effectors that are associ-ated with a selective inhibition of fat intake.

The estrogenic inhibition of food intake observed in rodents has been attrib-uted entirely to a decrease in meal size.[26,30,31] A considerable body of data has sug-gested that estradiol may partially exert this effect by potentiating the satiating effects of some of the gut peptides, especially CCK.

POLYCYSTIC OVARY SYNDROME

PCOS is a medical condition where estrogen levels are altered in relation to other hormones. The clinical characteristics of PCOS include polycystic ovaries, hyperandrogenism, obesity, menstrual disturbances, and hirsutism. The endocrine profile of women with PCOS is characterized by high plasma concentrations of ovarian and adrenal androgens, gonadotropin abnormalities, a relative increase in estrogen levels (especially estrone) derived from conversion of androgens, reduced levels of sex hormone binding globulin (SHBG), and often high levels of prolactin and insulin.[127] In the ovary, the cardinal feature is functional hyperandrogenism. Circulating concentrations of insulin and luteinizing hormone (LH) are almost always raised. The theca cells, which envelop the follicle and produce androgens for conversion in the ovary to estrogen, are overresponsive to this stimulation. They increase in size and overproduce androgens. The rise in LH levels is thought to be caused by the relatively high and unchanging concentrations of estrogens, which may alter the control of this hormone by the hypothalamic–pituitary axis.[128] This combination of raised levels of androgens, estrogen, insulin, and LH explains the classic PCOS presentation of hirsutism, anovulation or dysfunctional bleeding, and dysfunction of glucose metabolism.[129] Importantly, the elevated estrogen levels act to reverse the estrogen advantage, leading to increase in the risk of diabetes and cardiovascular disease.

The fundamental pathophysiologic defect of PCOS is poorly understood, but the primary defect may be insulin resistance, defined as the decreased ability of insulin to stimulate glucose disposal into target tissues, leading to hyperinsulinemia. Paradoxically, although the insulin regulatory molecules on the theca cells are responsive to insulin, those in the muscle and liver are resistant. Insulin resistance is a common characteristic of women with PCOS, occurring frequently with compensatory hyperinsulinemia and dyslipidemia.[130] There is complex interplay of the gonadal steroid abnormalities of PCOS and insulin resistance, with partial suppression of androgen levels improving the insulin resistance.[131] Thiazolidinedione treatment decreases both androgen and insulin levels.[132] Other approaches to improving insulin sensitivity, such as weight reduction and metformin, have also been shown to decrease androgen levels and restore ovulation.

Patients with PCOS are now recognized to have significant metabolic disturbances. Approximately 38% of women with PCOS demonstrate some degree of impaired glucose tolerance as a result of insulin resistance by the third or fourth decade of life.[133]

Obesity, a well-known risk factor for type 2 diabetes, is also a common characteristic of women with PCOS. Obesity has been reported to be present in 35 to 80% of women with PCOS.[133] Women with upper body obesity, which is the type most commonly seen in women with PCOS, have higher free androgen levels compared to those with lower body obesity[134] and exhibit significantly higher levels of insulin resistance.[135] The real question is whether the insulin resistance and obesity are causes or the result of the underlying pathophysiology of PCOS.

Weight loss is one of the simplest and most cost-effective approaches for improving insulin abnormalities and endocrine function. Weight reduction can improve insulin sensitivity, decrease circulating androgens, and increase SHBG, leading to improved ovulation in women with PCOS.[136,137] Although it is reasonable to recommend a weight-reducing diet and exercise as first-line therapy for all obese women with PCOS, those women with PCOS who are obese find it unusually difficult to lose weight.

CONCLUSION

Food intake and body weight are cyclic in women and correlate well with the phases of the menstrual or estrous cycle. When estrogen level is elevated and progesterone level is low, females across species show a significant decrease in caloric intake and body weight.[10–14] The hypophagic effect of estrogen is due to a decrease in meal size, which is the predominant determinant of total caloric intake.[30] Estrogen may function as a physiologic modulator of many neuroendocrine mechanisms that are major factors in energy homeostasis. Several of these neuroendocrine systems that estrogen modulates influence total caloric intake and macronutrient selection, particularly fat intake. Progesterone, which becomes elevated during the 2 week luteal phase in the standard 28 day cycle, acts antagonistically to the hypophagic effect of estrogen and promotes weight gain. Menopause, which is characterized by decreased circulating estrogen levels, also presents a weight-gain risk factor that is unique to women, and African–American women may be more vulnerable to weight gain at the time of this life transition than are Caucasian women.

ACKNOWLEDGMENTS

Paula J. Geiselman, Ph.D. is supported by NIH (NIA) grant R01 AG18239 ("Obesity prevention after smoking cessation in menopause") and an unrestricted grant from Bristol-Myers Squibb Foundation, Inc., Better Health for Women: A Global Health Program ("Prevention of lung cancer in women: development of an individually tailored, multidisciplinary, dietary and weight control, smoking cessation program for weight concerned women").

Steven R. Smith, M.D. is supported by USDA 2003-34323-14010, USDA Cooperative Agreement 58-6435-4-090, NIH ("Healthy transitions") R01DK50736-04, the Community Foundation of SE Michigan, and unrestricted educational grants from Takeda Pharmaceuticals, NA.

We would like to acknowledge the excellent administrative assistance of Mrs. Erin Wimberly and the critical comments of Dr. Karen Elkind-Hirsch, Ph.D.

REFERENCES

1. World Health Organization (WHO), Obesity: preventing and managing the global epidemic, in Report of a WHO Consultation on Obesity, Geneva, Switzerland, Jun. 3–5, 1997, published in 1998.

2. Wing, R., Changing diet and exercise behaviours in individuals at risk of weight gain, *Obes. Res.*, Suppl. 2, 277, 1995.

3. Leibowitz, S.F., Neurochemical-neuroendocrine systems in the brain controlling macronutrient intake and metabolism, *Trends Neurosci.*, 15, 491, 1992.

4. Dietz, W., Critical periods in childhood for the development of obesity, *Am. J. Clin. Nutr.*, 59, 955, 1994.

5. Williamson, D.F. et al., The 10-year incidence of overweight and major weight gain in US adults, *Arch. Intern. Med.*, 150, 665, 1990.

6. Bray, G.A., Contemporary diagnosis and management of obesity, in *Handbooks in Health Care Co.*, Newton, PA, 1998.

7. Williamson, D.F., Kahn, H.S., and Byers, T., The 10-y incidence of obesity and major weight gain in black and white US women aged 30–55 y, *Am. J. Clin. Nutr.*, 53, 1515S, 1991.

8. Clinical Guidelines on the Identification, Evaluation, and Treatment of Overweight and Obesity in Adults, http://www.nhlbi.nih.gov/guidelines/obesity/ob_home.htm.

9. Healthy People 2010, http://www.healthypeople.gov/.

10. Brobeck, K.R., Wheatland, M., and Strominger, J.L., Variations in regulation energy exchange associated with estrus, diestrus, and pseudopregnancy in rats, *Endocrinology*, 40, 65, 1947.

11. Wade, G.N., Gonadal hormones and behavioral regulation of body weight, *Physiol. Behav.*, 8, 523, 1972.

12. Czaja, J.A. and Goy, R.W., Ovarian hormones and food intake in female guinea pigs and rhesus monkeys, *Horm. Behav.*, 6, 329, 1975.

13. Morin, L.P. and Fleming, A.S., Variation of food intake and body weight with the estrous cycle, ovariectomy, and estradiol benzoate treatment in hamsters [*Merocricerus auratus*], *J. Comp. Physiol. Psychol.*, 92, 1, 1978.

14. Wade, G.N. and Schneider, J.E., Metabolic fuels and reproduction in female mammals, *Neurosci. Biobehav. Rev.*, 16, 235, 1992.

15. Gilbert, C. and Gillman, J., The changing pattern of food intake and appetite during the menstrual cycle of the baboon [*Papio ursinus*] with a consideration of some controlling endocrine factors, *S. Afr. J. Med. Sci.*, 21, 75, 1956.

16. Ota, K. and Yokoyama, A., Body weight and food consumption of lactating rats: effects of ovariectomy and of arrest and resumption of suckling, *J. Endocrinol.*, 38, 251, 1967.

17. Ota, K. and Yokoyama, A., Body weight and food consumption of lactating rats nursing various sizes of litters, *J. Endocrinol.*, 38, 263, 1967.

18. Yoshinaga, K., Hawkins, R.W., and Stocker, J.F., Estrogen secretion by the rat ovary *in vivo* during the estrous cycle and pregnancy, *Endocrinology*, 85, 103, 1969.

19. Tarttelin, M.F. and Gorski, R.A., The effects of ovarian steroids on food and water intake and body weight in the female rat, *Acta Endocrinol.*, 72, 551, 1973.

20. Ter Haar, M.B., Circadian and estrual rhythms in food intake in the rat, *Horm. Behav.*, 3, 213, 1972.

21. Wade, G.N., Sex hormones and behavioral regulation of body weight, *Adv. Stud. Behav.*, 6, 201, 1976.

22. Kanarek, R.B. and Beck, J.M., Role of gonadal hormones in diet selection and food utilization in female rats, *Physiol. Behav.*, 24, 381, 1980.

23. Dalvit, S.P., The effect of the menstrual cycle on patterns of food intake, *Am. J. Clin. Nutr.*, 34, 1811, 1981.

24. Pliner, P. and Fleming, A.S., Food intake, body weight, and sweetness preferences over the menstrual cycle in humans, *Physiol. Behav.*, 30, 663, 1983.

25. Kemnitz, J.W. et al., Changes in food intake during menstrual cycles and pregnancy of normal and diabetic rhesus monkeys, *Diabetelogia*, 26, 60, 1984.

26. Blaustein, J.D. and Wade, G.N., Ovarian influences on the meal patterns of female rats, *Physiol. Behav.*, 17, 201, 1976.

27. Mystkowski, P. and Schwartz, M.W., Gonadal steroids and energy homeostasis in the leptin era, *Nutrition*, 16, 937, 2000.

28. Wade, G.N., Some effects of ovarian hormones on food intake and body weight in female rats, *J. Comp. Physiol. Psychol.*, 88, 183, 1975.

29. Donohoe, T.P. et al., Effects of stereoisomers of estradiol on food intake, body weight and hoarding behavior in female rats, *Physiol. Behav.*, 32, 589, 1984.

30. Eckel, L.A., Houpt, T.A., and Geary, N., Spontaneous meal patterns in female rats with and without access to running wheels, *Physiol. Behav.*, 70, 397, 2000.

31. Drewett, R.F., The meal patterns of oestrous cycle and their motivational significance, *Q. J. Exp. Psychol.*, 26, 489, 1974.

32. Buffenstein, R. et al., Food intake and the menstrual cycle: a retrospective analysis, with implications for appetite research, *Physiol. Behav.*, 58, 1057, 1995.

33. Geiselman, P.J. et al., Relationship between the menstrual cycle and overeating in women, *Obes. Res.*, Suppl. 3, 329s, 1995.

34. Young, J.K., Nance, J.M., and Gorski, R.A., Dietary effects upon food and water intake and responsiveness to estrogen, 2-deoxy-glucose and glucose in female rats, *Physiol. Behav.*, 21, 395, 1978.

35. Geiselman, P.J. et al., Dietary self-selection in cycling and neonatally ovariectomized rats, *Appetite*, 2, 87, 1981.

36. Tarasuk, V. and Beaton, G.H., Menstrual-cycle patterns in energy and macronutrient intake, *Am. J. Clin. Nutr.*, 53, 442, 1991.

37. Jas, P. and Rogers, P.J., Menstrual Cycle Effects on Food Choice and Energy Intake, paper presented at the 11th International Congress on the Physiology of Food and Fluid Intake, Oxford University, Jul. 28–30, 1993.

38. Gallant, M.P. et al., Pyridoxine and magnesium status of women with premenstrual syndrome, *Nutr. Res.*, 7, 243, 1987.

39. Johnson, W.G. et al., Energy regulation over the menstrual cycle, *Physiol. Behav.*, 56, 523, 1994.

40. Barr, S.I., Janelle, K.C., and Prior, J.C., Energy intakes are higher during the luteal phase of ovulatory menstrual cycles, *Am. J. Clin. Nutr.*, 61, 39, 1995.

41. Eck, L.H. et al., Differences in macronutrient selection in users and nonusers of an oral contraceptive, *Am. J. Clin. Nutr.*, 65, 419, 1997.

42. Smith, S.L. and Sauder, C., Food cravings, depression, and premenstrual problems, *Psychocom. Med.*, 21, 281, 1969.

43. Abraham, G.E., Nutrition and the premenstrual tension syndromes, *J. Appl. Nutr.*, 36, 103, 1984.

44. Wurtman, R.J. and Wurtman, J.J., Carbohydrates and depression, *Sci. Am.*, 260, 68, 1989.

45. Bowen, D.J. and Grunberg, N.E., Variations in food preference and consumption across the menstrual cycle, *Physiol. Behav.*, 47, 287, 1990.

46. Brzezinski, A.A. et al., D-Fenfluramine suppresses the increased calorie and carbohydrate intakes and improves the mood of women with premenstrual depression, *Obstet. Gynecol.*, 76, 296, 1990.

47. Rolls, B.J., Hetherington, M., and Burley, V.J., The specificity of satiety: the influence of foods of different macronutrient content on the development of satiety, *Physiol. Behav.*, 43, 145, 1988.

48. Geiselman, P.J. et al., Reliability and validity of a macronutrient self-selection paradigm and a food preference questionnaire, *Physiol. Behav.*, 63, 919, 1998.

49. Geiselman, P.J. and Lovejoy, J.C., Ethnic differences in fat and other macronutrient intake and fat preferences across the menstrual cycle in perimenopausal, African–American and Caucasian women, in preparation.

50. Nelson, R.J. Parental behavior, in *An Introduction to Behavioral Endocrinology*, 2nd ed., Sinauer Associates, Inc., Sunderland, MA, 2000, chap. 7.

51. Parker, C.R. et al., Endocrine changes during pregnancy in a patient with homozygous familial hypobetalipoproteinemia, *N. Engl. J. Med.*, 314, 557, 1986.

52. Durnin, J.V.G.A., Is nutritional status endangered by virtually no extra intake during pregnancy? *Lancet*, 2, 823, 1985.

53. Committee on Medical Aspects of Food Policy, Dietary reference values for food energy and nutrients for the United Kingdom, in Report on Health and Social Subjects 41, Her Majesty's Stationery Office, London, 1991.

54. Goldberg, G.R. et al., Longitudinal assessment of energy expenditure in pregnancy by the doubly labeled water method, *Am. J. Clin. Nutr.*, 57, 494, 1993.

55. Schoeller, D.A. et al., Inaccuracies in self-reported intake identified by comparison with the doubly-labelled water method, *Can. J. Physiol. Pharmacol.*, 68, 941, 1990.

56. Newcombe, R.G., Development of obesity in parous women, *J. Epidemiol. Commun. Health*, 36, 306, 1982.

57. Rossner, S., Pregnancy, weight cycling and weight gain in obesity, *Int. J. Obes.*, 16, 145, 1992.

58. Lovejoy, J., The influence of sex hormones on obesity across the female life span, *J. Womens Health*, 7, 1247, 1998.

59. Wade, G.N. and Gray, J.M., Gonadal effects on food intake and adiposity: a metabolic hypothesis, *Physiol. Behav.*, 22, 583, 1979.

60. Geary, N., The effect of estrogen on appetite, *Medscape Womens Health*, 3, 3,1998, http://www.medscape.com/Medscape/WomensHealth/journal/1998/v03.../ pnt-wh3146.gear.htm.

61. Geary, N., The estrogenic inhibition of eating, in *Neurobiology of Food and Fluid Intake*, Stricker, E. and Woods, S., Eds., Plenum Publishers, New York, 2004, chap. 12.

62. Kakolewski, J., Cox, V., and Valenstein, E., Sex differences in body-weight changes following gonadectomy of rats, *Psychol. Rep.*, 22, 547, 1968.

63. Leshner, A.I. and Collier, G., The effects of gonadectomy on the sex differences in dietary self-selection patterns and carcass compositions of rats, *Physiol. Behav.*, 11, 671, 1973.

64. Gray, J.M. and Wade, G.N., Food intake, body weight, and adiposity in female rats: actions and interactions of progestins and antiestrogens, *Am. J. Physiol.*, 240, E474, 1981.

65. Sharp, J.C. et al., Analysis of ovariectomy and estrogen effects on body composition in rats by x-ray and magnetic resonance imaging techniques, *J. Bone. Miner. Res.*, 15, 138, 2000.

66. Geary, N., Estradiol and appetite, *Appetite*, 35, 273, 2000.

67. Geary, N., Estradiol, CCK and satiation, *Peptides*, 22, 1251, 2001.

68. Pasquali, R. et al., Body weight, fat distribution and the menopausal status in women, The VMH Collaborative Group, *Int. J. Obes. Relat. Metab. Disord.*, 18, 614, 1994.

69. The writing group for the PEPI trial, Effects of estrogen or estrogen/progestin regimens on heart disease risk factors in postmenopausal women: The Postmenopausal Estrogen/Progestin Interventions [PEPI] trial, *J. Am. Med. Assoc.*, 273, 199, 1995.

70. Poehlman, E.T., Toth, M.J., and Gardner, A.W., Changes in energy balance and body composition at menopause: a controlled longitudinal study, *Ann. Intern. Med.*, 126, 673, 1995.

71. Wing, R. et al., Weight gain at the time of menopause, *Arch. Intern. Med.*, 151, 97, 1991.

72. Solomon, S.J., Kurzer, M.S., and Calloway, D.H., Menstrual cycle and basal metabolic rate in women, *Am. J. Clin. Nutr.*, 36, 611, 1982.

73. Manson, J.E. et al., Body weight and longevity: a reassessment, *J. Am. Med. Assoc.*, 257, 353, 1987.

74. Heymsfield, S.B. et al., Menopausal changes in body composition and energy expenditure, *Exp. Gerontol.*, 29, 377, 1994.

75. Flegal, K.M. et al., Overweight and obesity in the United States: prevalence and trends, 1960–1994, *Int. J. Obes.*, 22, 39, 1998.

76. Wang, Q. et al., Total and regional body-composition changes in early postmenopausal women: age-related or menopause-related? *Am. J. Clin. Nutr.*, 60, 843, 1994.

77. Aloia, J.F. et al., The influence of menopause and hormonal replacement therapy on body cell mass and body fat mass, *Am. J. Obstet. Gynecol.*, 172, 896, 1995.

78. Bjorntorp, P., Visceral obesity: a "civilization syndrome," *Obes. Res.*, 1, 206, 1993.

79. Colombel, A. and Charbonnel, B., Weight gain and cardiovascular risk factors in the post-menopausal women, *Hum. Reprod.*, 12, 134, 1997.

80. Blair, D. et al., Evidence for an increased risk for hypertension with centrally located body fat and the effect of race and sex on this risk, *Am. J. Epidemiol.*, 119, 526, 1984.

81. Dowling, H.J. and Pi-Sunyer, F.X., Race-dependent health risks of upper body obesity, *Diabetes*, 42, 537, 1993.

82. Dawson-Hughes, B. and Harris, S., Regional changes in body composition by time of year in healthy postmenopausal women, *Am. J. Clin. Nutr.* 56, 307–313, 1992.

83. Ley, C.J., Lees, B., and Stevenson, J.C., Sex- and menopause-associated changes in body-fat distribution, *Am. J. Clin. Nutr.* 55, 950–954, 1992.

84. Svendsen, O.L., Hassager, C., and Christiansen, C., Age- and menopause-associated variations in body composition and fat distribution in healthy women as measured by dual-energy x-ray absorptiometry, *Metabolism*, 44, 369–373, 1995.

85. Enzi, G., Gasparo, M., Biondetti, P.R., Fiore, D., Semisa, M., and Zurlo, F., Subcutaneous and visceral fat distribution according to sex, age, and overweight, evaluated by computed tomography, *Am. J. Clin. Nutr.* 44, 739–746, 1986.

86. Hunter, G.R., Kekes-Szabo, T., Treuth, M.S., Williams, M.J., Goran, M., and Pichon, C., Intra-abdominal adipose tissue, physical activity and cardiovascular risk in pre- and post-menopausal women, *Int. J. Obes. Relat. Metab. Disord.* 20, 860–865, 1996.

87. Kotani, K., Tokunaga, K., Fujioka, S., Kobatake, T., Keno, Y., Yoshida, S., Shimomura, I., Tarui, S., and Matsuzawa, Y., Sexual dimorphism of age-related changes in whole-body fat distribution in the obese, *Int. J. Obes. Relat. Metab. Disord.* 18, 207–212, 1994.

88. Zamboni, M., Armellini, F., Milani, M.P., De Marchi, M., Todesco, T., Robbi, R., Bergamo-Andreis, I.A., and Bosello, O., Body fat distribution in pre- and post-menopausal women: metabolic and anthropometric variables and their inter-relationships, *Int. J. Obes. Relat. Metab. Disord.* 16, 495–504, 1992.

89. Pasquali, R., Casimirri, F., Cantobelli, S., Labate, A.M., Venturoli, S., Paradisi, R., and Zannarini, L., Insulin and androgen relationships with abdominal body fat distribution in women with and without hyperandrogenism, *Horm. Res.* 39, 179–187, 1993.

90. Kaye, S.A., Folsom, A.R., Soler, J.T., Prineas, R.J., and Potter, J.D., Associations of body mass and fat distribution with sex hormone concentrations in postmenopausal women, *Int. J. Epidemiol.* 20, 151–156, 1991.

91. Rebuffe-Scrive, M., Eldh, J., Hafstrom, L.O., and Bjorntorp, P., Metabolism of mammary, abdominal, and femoral adipocytes in women before and after menopause, *Metabolism* 35, 792–797, 1986.

92. Matthews, K.A. et al., Menopause and risk factors for coronary heart disease, *N. Engl. J. Med.*, 32, 641, 1989.

93. Reubinoff, B.E. et al., Effects of hormone replacement therapy on weight, body composition, fat distribution, and food intake in early postmenopausal women: a prospective study, *Fertil. Steril.*, 64, 963, 1995.

94. Espeland, M.A. et al., Effect of postmenopausal hormone therapy on body weight and waist and hip girths, *J. Clin. Endocrinol. Metab.*, 82, 1549, 1997.

95. Lindberg, U.B., Crona, N., Silfverstolpe, G., Bjorntorp, P., and Rebuffe-Scrive, M., Regional adipose tissue metabolism in postmenopausal women after treatment with exogenous sex steroids, *Horm. Metab. Res.* 22, 345–351, 1990.

96. Sites, C.K., L'Hommedieu, G.D., Toth, M.J., Brochu, M., Cooper, B.C., and Fairhurst, P.A., The effect of hormone replacement therapy on body composition, body fat distribution, and insulin sensitivity in menopausal women: a randomized, double blind, placebo-controlled trial, *J. Clin. Endocrinol. Metab.*, 2005.

97. Flier, J.S., What's in a name? In search of leptin's physiological role, *J. Clin. Endocrinol. Metab.*, 83, 1407, 1998.

98. Banks, W.A., Kastin, A.J., and Huang, W.E.A., Leptin enters the brain by a saturable system independent of insulin, *Peptides*, 17, 305, 1996.

99. Caro, J.F. et al., Decreased cerebrospinal-fluid/serum leptin ratio in obesity: a possible mechanism for leptin resistance, *Lancet*, 348, 159, 1996.

100. Golden, P.L., Maccagnan, T.J., and Pardridge, W.M., Human blood-brain barrier leptin receptor: binding and endocytosis in isolated human brain microvessels, *J. Clin. Invest.*, 99, 14, 1997.

101. Karonen, S.L. et al., Is brain uptake of leptin in vivo saturable and reduced by fasting? *Eur. J. Nucl. Med.*, 25, 607, 1998.

102. Woods, S.C. and Seeley, R.J., Adiposity signals and the control of energy homeostasis, *Nutr.*, 16, 894, 2000.

103. Mantzoros, C.S., The role of leptin in human obesity and disease: a review of current evidence, *Arch. Intern. Med.*, 130, 671, 1999.

104. Halford, J.C.G., Pharmacology of appetite suppression: implication for the treatment of obesity, *Curr. Drug Targets*, 2, 353, 2001.

105. Boeles, S. et al., Sumatriptan decreases food intake and increases plasma growth hormone in healthy women, *Psychopharmacology*, 129, 179, 1997.

106. Smith, B.K., York, D.A., and Bray, G.A., Chronic *d*-fenfluramine treatment reduces fat intake independent of macronutrient preference, *Pharmacol. Biochem. Behav.*, 60, 105, 1998.

107. York, D.A. et al., Enterstatin and 5HT: modulation of fat intake, in *Pennington Symposium Series, Nutrition, Genetics, and Obesity*, Louisiana State University Press, Baton Rouge, 1998, p. 246.

108. Leibowitz, S.F., Neurochemical-neuroendocrine systems in the brain controlling macronutrient intake and metabolism, *Trends Neurosci.*, 15, 491, 1992.

109. Woods, S.C., et al., Signals that regulate food intake and energy homeostasis, *Science*, 280, 1378, 1998.

110. Chavez, M. et al., Central insulin and macronutrient intake in the rat, *Am. J. Physiol.*, 271, R727, 1996.

111. Stanley, B.G. et al., Paraventricular nucleus injections of peptide YY and neuropeptide Y preferentially enhance carbohydrate ingestion, *Peptides*, 6, 1205, 1985.

112. Leibowitz, S.F. and Alexander, J.T., Analysis of neuropeptide Y-induced feeding: dissociation of Y1 and Y2 receptor effects on natural meal patterns, *Peptides*, 12, 1251, 1991.

113. Beck, B. et al., Chronic and continuous intracerebroventricular infusion of neuropeptide Y in Long-Evans rats mimics the feeing behavior of obese Zucker rats, *Int. J. Obes.*, 16, 295, 1992.

114. Stanley, B.G. et al., Repeated hypothalamic stimulation with neuropeptide Y increases daily carbohydrate and fat intake and body weight gain in female rats, *Physiol. Behav.*, 46, 173, 1989.

115. Schwartz, M.W. et al., Central nervous system control of food intake, *Nature*, 404, 61, 2000.

116. Flynn, M. et al., Mode of action of OB protein [leptin] on feeding, *Am. J. Physiol.*, 275, R174, 1998.

117. Blundell, J.E., Serotonin and the biology of feeding, *Am. J. Clin. Nutr.*, 55, 155S, 1992.

118. Blundell, J.E. and Halford, J.C.G., *CNS Drugs*, 9, 473, 1998.

119. Blundell, J.E., Is there a role for serotonin [5-hydroxytryptamine] in feeding?, *Int. J. Obes.*, 1, 15, 1977.

120. Gibbs, J., Young, R.C., and Smith, G.P., Cholecystokinin decreases food intake in rats. 1973., *Obes. Res.*, 5, 284, 1997.

121. Smith, G.P. and Gibbs, J., The development and proof of the CCK hypothesis of satiety, in *Multiple Cholecystokinin Receptors in the CNS*, Dourish, C.T., Cooper, S.J., and Iversen, S.D., Eds., Oxford University Press, Oxford, 1992, p. 166.

122. Beglinger, C. et al., A CCK-A receptor antagonist stimulates calorie intake and hunger feelings in humans, *Am. J. Physiol.*, 280, R1149, 2001.

123. Erlanson-Albertsson, C. et al., Pancreatic procolipase propeptide, enterostatin, specifically inhibits fat intake, *Physiol. Behav.*, 49, 1191, 1991.

124. Bowyer, M.J. et al., Identification of enterostatin, the pancreatic procolipase activation peptide in the intestine of rat: effect of CCK-8 and high-fat feeding, *Pancreas*, 4, 488, 1993.

125. Esfanhani, N. et al., *Pharmacol. Biochem. Behav.*, 51, 9, 1995.

126. Voigt, J.P., Sohr, R., and Fink, H., CCK-8S facilitates 5-HT release in the rat hypothalamus, *Pharmacol. Biochem. Behav.*, 59, 179, 1998.

127. Dunaif, A. and Thomas, A., Current concepts in the polycystic ovary syndrome, *Annu. Rev. Med.* 52, 401–419, 2001.
128. Norman, R.J., Wu, R., and Stankiewicz, M.T., 4: Polycystic ovary syndrome, *Med. J. Aust.* 180, 132–137, 2004.
129. Franks, S., Polycystic ovary syndrome, *N. Engl. J. Med.* 333, 853–861, 1995.
130. Nestler, J. E., Stovall, D., Akhter, N., Iuorno, M.J., and Jakubowicz, D.J., Strategies for the use of insulin-sensitizing drugs to treat infertility in women with polycystic ovary syndrome, *Fertil. Steril.* 77, 209–215, 2002.
131. Moghetti, P., Tosi, F., Castello, R., Magnani, C.M., Negri, C., Brun, E., Furlani, L., Caputo, M., and Muggeo, M., The insulin resistance in women with hyperandrogenism is partially reversed by antiandrogen treatment: evidence that androgens impair insulin action in women, *J. Clin. Endocrinol. Metab.* 81, 952–960, 1996.
132. Dunaif, A., Scott, D., Finegood, D., Quintana, B., and Whitcomb, R., The insulin-sensitizing agent troglitazone improves metabolic and reproductive abnormalities in the polycystic ovary syndrome, *J. Clin. Endocrinol. Metab.* 81, 3299–3306, 1996.
133. Marx, T.L. and Mehta, A.E., Polycystic ovary syndrome: pathogenesis and treatment over the short and long term, *Cleve Clin. J. Med.* 70, 31–3, 36–41, 45, 2003.
134. Kirschner, M.A., Samojlik, E., Drejka, M., Szmal, E., Schneider, G., and Ertel, N., Androgen–estrogen metabolism in women with upper body versus lower body obesity, *J. Clin. Endocrinol. Metab.* 70, 473–479, 1990.
135. Kissebah, A.H., Vydelingum, N., Murray, R., Evans, D.J., Hartz, A.J., Kalkhoff, R.K., and Adams, P.W., Relation of body fat distribution to metabolic complications of obesity, *J. Clin. Endocrinol. Metab.* 54, 254–260, 1982.
136. Pasquali, R., Antenucci, D., Casimirri, F., Venturoli, S., Paradisi, R., Fabbri, R., Balestra, V., Melchionda, N., and Barbara, L., Clinical and hormonal characteristics of obese amenorrheic hyperandrogenic women before and after weight loss, *J. Clin. Endocrinol. Metab.* 68, 173–179, 1989.
137. Harlass, F.E., Plymate, S.R., Fariss, B.L., and Belts, R.P., Weight loss is associated with correction of gonadotropin and sex steroid abnormalities in the obese anovulatory female, *Fertil. Steril.* 42, 649–652, 1984.
138. Gong, E.J., Garrel, D., and Calloway, D.H. Menstrual cycle and voluntary food intake, *Am. J. Clin. Nutr.*, 49, 252–258, 1989.

15 Childhood Obesity

Arline D. Salbe, Ph.D., R.D.,
Marlene B. Schwartz, Ph.D., and
Ingrid Kohlstadt, M.D., M.P.H.

CONTENTS

Editor's Note

Children are losing shape at the very time life should be taking shape! Obesity influences every aspect of a child's life. Not surprisingly, it also influences every component of the musculoskeletal system. A NIH scientist, a psychologist, and a medical doctor describe ways clinicians can make a difference.

PREVALENCE

Overweight affects one in ten children worldwide, reports the International Obesity Task Force to the World Health Organization.[1] The National Health and Nutrition Examination Surveys (NHANES) are U.S. population-representative cross-sectional studies that provide numbers for the epidemic curve of obesity in the United States. The NHANES III survey, conducted from 1988 to 1994, found that 11% of children and adolescents in the United States aged 6 to 17 years were overweight.[2] This represents almost a doubling of the prevalence rates reported in the previous NHANES II survey, which covered the period from 1974 to 1988.[3] Data from the most recent study, NHANES 1999 to 2002,[4] show that obesity rates in children have increased even further, to 16% of children and adolescents aged 6 to 19 years, a rate that is more than three times the target prevalence (5%) of overweight in children set for Healthy People 2010.[4] A disheartening statistic is that the heaviest children have become even heavier.[2]

CASE DEFINITION

Obesity in adults is defined by body mass index values (BMI, weight [kg]/height [m^2]).[5] Obesity in children is based on statistical definitions using reference populations.[6] In 2000, the Centers for Disease Control and Prevention published sex-specific BMI-for-age growth charts for girls and boys 2 to 19 years of age based on data from five national health examination studies covering the period from 1963 to 1994, thereby providing standards representative of the racial and ethnic diversity of the U.S. population.[6] "At risk of overweight" was defined as being at or above the 85th percentile, but less than the 95th percentile of the sex-specific BMI for age. "Overweight" was defined as being at or above the 95th percentile of the sex-specific BMI for age. The BMI charts are widely available (http://www.cdc.gov/growthcharts/) and currently recommended for regular use by pediatricians as part of the well-child visit. Assessment for overweight and at risk of overweight is obtained by plotting the child's BMI for age and sex, from which the BMI percentile ranking is derived.[7]

CRITICAL PERIODS

Dietz has described three critical periods in childhood when the risk of onset, complications, or persistence of obesity is increased.[8,9] These are the prenatal period, the period of "adiposity rebound," and adolescence.

PRENATAL

During the prenatal period, intrauterine growth can be affected by many factors. The Dutch famine study was the result of a natural experiment that presented an opportunity to study the effects of maternal nutrition on offspring later in life.[10]

In that study, it was found that growth retardation in the third trimester of pregnancy led to reduced height and weight, whereas growth retardation in the first and second trimesters resulted in increased prevalence of obesity among offspring at 18 years of age. Maternal diabetes, as type 1, type 2, or gestational diabetes, can also have significant effects on the offspring. The diabetic intrauterine milieu is characterized by increased concentrations of glucose, amino acids, and lipids in the maternal circulation, greater delivery of these nutrients to the fetus, elevated fetal insulin secretion, and accelerated fetal growth.[11,12] Because differentiation of adipose tissue and storage of triglycerides begins during the third trimester of pregnancy,[13] diabetes at this point in fetal development can hasten the accumulation of fat in the fetus and can result in infants that are both heavier and fatter than infants born to nondiabetic women.[14] The differences in weight found at later ages in offspring of women with diabetes may be because of what Dietz calls "entrainment" of appetite regulation or adipocyte number during the early intrauterine period, possibly as a consequence of the differentiation of the hypothalamic centers responsible for control of food intake.[8] Furthermore, a recent study has found that adult offspring of diabetic pregnancies are at higher risk of developing diabetes themselves. A decreased insulin secretory response is thought to be an underlying factor.[15]

Adiposity Rebound

The adiposity rebound (Figure 15.1) was described by Rolland-Cachera et al.[16] as the point of maximal leanness, defined using BMI, prior to the second period of rapid growth of body fat in children. The first period of rapid fat accumulation occurs during the first year of life and is characterized by fat cell hypertrophy. The second period, which starts at about 5 to 6 years of age, is thought to involve both hypertrophy and hyperplasia.[16,17] Fat deposition beginning at the point of the adiposity rebound is gradual and persists throughout life. In several studies, an early age at adiposity rebound was found to predict obesity in the teenage years as well as in adulthood.[17–19] Early age at adiposity rebound is associated with greater risk of glucose intolerance and diabetes in young adulthood.[20] Whether the age at adiposity rebound is genetically programmed and represents an inherited predisposition to obesity or is because of environmental influences has not been shown.[17] In summary, age 5 to 6 is a vulnerable period during which time physical inactivity and excess calorie intake should be addressed.

Adolescence

Adolescence is a period characterized by accretion of body fat in both boys and girls. Body fat as a percentage of body weight actually decreases in boys during adolescence. In girls, however, body fat as a percentage of body weight increases, a circumstance that can profoundly affect the quantity and persistence of obesity in females. Body fat deposition appears to be correlated to the timing

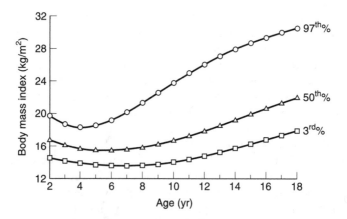

FIGURE 15.1 Changes in the percentiles of BMI among children and adolescents. Children with a BMI in the 97th percentile have an earlier rebound (4 years of age) compared to those in the 50th percentile (6 years of age) and those in the 3rd percentile (7 years of age). An earlier age at rebound is associated with a greater risk of obesity. (Adapted from Kuczmarksi, R.J., Ogden, C.L., Grummer-Strawn, L.M., Flegal, K.M., Guo, S.S., Wei, R., Mei, Z., Curtin, L.R., Roche, A.F., and Johnson, C.L., CDC growth charts: United States, *Advance Data*, 314, 1–28, 2000. With permission.)

of puberty, positively in boys but negatively in girls.[21] Moreover, sexual dimorphism in body fat distribution occurs during puberty, with fivefold greater central deposition of body fat in males compared to females.[22] Pubertal androgens can also affect the concentration of hormones such as leptin, which can in turn effect pubertal growth. In addition to the increased risk of adult obesity, adolescent obesity has been shown to independently increase adult mortality from cardiovascular disease, colorectal cancer, and ischemic heart disease.[23]

GENETICS AND THE EARLY ENVIRONMENT

The current increase in childhood obesity is most obvious among ethnic minority populations that may be more genetically susceptible to the interaction between genes and the environment (Figure 15.2); 24% of African-American and Hispanic children are above the 95th percentile of the sex-specific BMI for age.[4] Nowhere, however, is the trend in childhood obesity more apparent than in Native American communities, where overweight prevalence rates in children and adolescents range from 30 to 40%, much greater than in the overall population.[24–26] Minority groups also have a disproportionate amount of type II diabetes mellitus (T2DM). Over 40 years ago, Neel[27] proposed the thrifty genotype hypothesis to explain the enigma of diabetes, suggesting that diabetes is the expression of a thrifty gene that confers a survival advantage on people beset with alternating periods of abundant and limited food supplies, circumstances

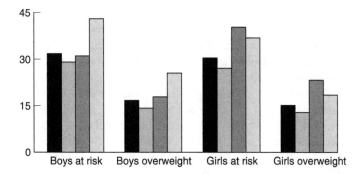

FIGURE 15.2 Prevalence of "at risk for overweight" and "overweight" in children 6 to 19 years of age by sex and racial/ethnic group; United States, 1999 to 2000. The prevalence of "at risk of overweight" ($\geq$85th percentile) in all children was 31.0% whereas the prevalence of overweight ($\geq$95th percentile) was 16.0%. All ethnicities (black bars), non-Hispanic white (light gray bars), non-Hispanic black (dark gray bars), Mexican Americans (white bars). (Adapted from data in Hedley, A.A., Ogden, C.L., Johnson, C.L., Carroll, M.D., Curtin, L.R., and Flegal, K.M., Prevalence of overweight and obesity among US children, adolescents, and adults, 1999–2000, *JAMA*, 291, 2847–2850, 2004. With permission.)

historically found among indigenous peoples. In addition, he hypothesized that individuals predisposed to diabetes differ metabolically from non-predisposed individuals starting from birth in that they have an increased efficiency in food intake or utilization and higher insulin secretion following food intake. The thrifty genotype is disadvantageous in modern times, however, when calories are abundant and a physically active lifestyle is unnecessary and it often results in obesity. Although a "thrifty" gene has yet to be uncovered, in Chapter 2, Bland discusses elements of Neel's hypothesis that are substantiated today.

Genetic and early environmental risk factors do not make obesity inevitable. This is illustrated by the genetic mutation that leads to Prader–Willi syndrome. Prader–Willi syndrome is associated with extraordinary hyperphagia and diet management is extreme. Even so, diagnosis before the age of 10 has a more favorable prognosis attributable to early initiation of diet management.[28]

POPULATION CASE STUDY OF CHILDHOOD OBESITY AND TYPE 2 DIABETES

Diabetes (T2DM) is highly prevalent among ethnic minority populations. The Pima Indians of Arizona are an indigenous, genetically homogeneous population that has undergone a very rapid lifestyle change in a relatively short period of time. The Pima Indians have the highest reported prevalence of T2DM in the world; by the age of 35 years, half the population has diabetes.[29] Furthermore, at each age, both the prevalence and incidence of T2DM in Pima Indians are higher now than in previous years, resulting in more people with diabetes at earlier ages, especially children.[30] As the age of onset of T2DM decreases, more women of childbearing age have diabetes or are at risk of developing gestational diabetes. The resulting offspring, who are heavier at birth and at risk of childhood obesity, are highly susceptible to developing T2DM themselves,[31] thus resulting in a cross-generational vicious cycle[32] whereby successive generations of women are at greater risk of already being obese and having T2DM at childbearing age than the preceding generation. A recent epidemiological study of this cohort concluded that *in utero* exposure to diabetes was responsible for 40% of the T2DM diagnosed in 5- to 19-year-old children from 1987 to 1996 and that more than 70% of those with prenatal exposure to diabetes developed the disease by 25 to 34 years of age.[33]

Since 1963, the Pima Indians of the Gila River Indian Community have participated in NIH-conducted studies aimed at identifying risk factors for obesity and T2DM. The studies have contributed to the definition of diabetes, the diagnostic criteria of the disease, clues to the development of T2DM, and much of our knowledge about the complications of T2DM. Pima volunteers have also participated in the Diabetes Prevention Program, which showed that a 7% decrease in body weight along with a daily 30-min walking regimen could delay the onset of T2DM in individuals at high risk of the disease.[34] Pima women who had diabetes during pregnancy and their offspring are now the focus of a number of studies designed to decrease the risks of obesity and diabetes in these high-risk children. For example, in a study to determine why offspring of diabetic pregnancies are heavier than their normoglycemic counterparts at a young age, we investigated the total energy expenditure in groups of 5-year-old children. Although we did not find differences in energy expenditure between these two groups,[35] we did find that both groups were similarly inactive (Figure 15.3). A study of food intake in children of diabetic vs. nondiabetic mothers is currently ongoing. It is our hope that these contributions by Pima Indian volunteers will have a significant impact on the health of their community and that of children worldwide.

MEDICAL CONSEQUENCES OF OBESITY

Eighty percent of obese children become obese adults, and obesity is more severe and the comorbidities appear earlier in adults who were obese as children.[36] Because of the increased risk of serious chronic diseases, obesity in childhood can reduce overall life expectancy.[37]

Childhood onset of T2DM and hypertension were previously rare. Prevalence is increasing with the obesity epidemic and therefore screening is now recommended.[38,39] Weight loss is the treatment of choice and can be more effective with early detection. The American Diabetes Association recommends screening for diabetes starting at 10 years of age (at puberty if earlier than 10 years) in children at risk of overweight ($\geq$85th percentile) who also have two of the following risk factors: (1) a family history of diabetes; (2) an ethnic background that includes

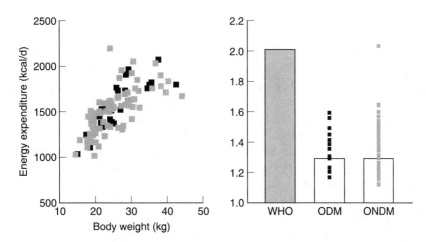

FIGURE 15.3 Total energy expenditure (left panel) and physical activity level (right panel) in 5-year-old offspring of women who were either diabetic or normoglycemic during the index pregnancy. There were no differences in total energy expenditure or physical activity level between the two groups of children. Both groups of children were similarly inactive as compared to the WHO recommendations.[42] (Adapted from Salbe, A.D., Fontvieille, A.M., Pettitt, D.J., and Ravussin, E., Maternal diabetes status does not influence energy expenditure or physical activity in 5-year old Pima Indian children, *Diabetologia*, 41, 1157–1162, 1998. With permission.)

American-Indian, African-American, Hispanic-American, or Pacific Islander heritage; or (3) signs of insulin resistance such as acanthosis nigricans, hypertension, dyslipidemia, or polycystic ovary syndrome.[40] Fasting plasma glucose concentrations measured every 2 years is the preferred screening regimen. Recommendations for screening, methods of assessment, and tables of established norms of blood pressure values for children have recently been published by the American Academy of Pediatrics.[41]

Overweight adolescents can develop fatty degeneration of the liver, known as hepatic steatosis.[42] Chemistry profiles show high concentrations of liver enzymes, which can normalize with weight reduction alone. Research suggests that the ratio of macronutrients in the diet influences the disease process; high fat is preferable to high refined carbohydrate (Chapter 5).[43] Hyperlipidemia, also common in overweight adolescents, may improve with weight reduction. Elevated triglycerides respond to reduction in refined carbohydrates and partially hydrogenated (*trans*) fats. Cholecystitis is more common with overweight in all ages, especially adolescence. Dieting without medical supervision, patterns such as skipping several meals and avoiding dietary fat, can prevent the gallbladder from emptying and lead to gallstone formation.

Sleep apnea occurs in approximately 7% of overweight children.[44] A related condition, obesity hypoventilation syndrome, also known as Pickwickian syndrome, requires specialized medical attention. Pseudotumor cerebri is a cause of headache from increased pressure in the skull. Although rare, it is associated with obesity and requires immediate attention.

Obesity affects the entire musculoskeletal system, often into adulthood. Overweight adolescents commonly experience early skeletal maturation. Early maturation is defined as a skeletal age more than 3 months in advance of chronologic age and is associated with increased body fat in adulthood. Glucose intolerance and T2DM create an adverse hormonal environment for muscle synthesis.

Obese children experience more traumatic injuries to anterior teeth, an observation authors attribute to a decrease in sports skillfulness.[45] Obese children experience more injuries of joints in the lower extremities and healing may take longer. For example, obese children are more likely to have persistent symptoms 6 months after an ankle sprain.[46] Overweight is associated with increased fracture risk. The increase in fracture risk is attributable to reduction in bone mineral density rather than to increased trauma.[47] Childhood obesity does not have a positive effect on bones. Overweight adolescents have low bone mineral levels for weight, which places excessive load on the immature femoral head.[48] The untoward biomechanical forces, combined with endocrinologic imbalances of low testosterone and growth hormone levels, predispose obese children to an otherwise rare condition, slipped capital femoral epiphysis (SCFE).[49] SCFE is a surgically corrected condition that often has an insidious onset of limping and hip pain. Early identification and treatment can prevent hip osteonecrosis and osteoarthritis.

BEHAVIORAL INTERVENTIONS

Overweight in childhood has psychosocial consequences. Often social discrimination leads to a negative self-image in adolescence that can persist.[50] Behavioral interventions for childhood obesity are best implemented with awareness of the child's psychosocial setting. The following is the approach developed and used by The Yale Center for Eating and Weight Disorders.

EMPATHIZE WITH PARENTS

Parents of overweight children are fighting against genetic, biological, psychological, and environmental forces. Medical professionals who take an empathic, supportive stance are most likely to be able to help these families. It is important to note that there is a very powerful societal stigma of obesity, and research suggests that health professionals — even those who specialize in obesity — have these negative implicit attitudes.[51,52] Overweight people are considered to have caused their condition by their behavior, and are therefore blamed and held personally responsible for making changes. In the case of childhood obesity, it is difficult to blame the child, so parents are blamed instead. Overweight parents may find it particularly difficult to ask for help from their child's doctor because they worry they will be judged for their own appearance. It is important to acknowledge the complex etiology of obesity and join with the parents in trying to identify strategies to help the child.

Cultivate Healthy Food Preferences

There is an informative body of research on how children develop food preferences, and this can guide interventions to address childhood obesity. Early in life, food preferences are strongly biologically driven. Children are born with a predisposition to prefer sweet tastes, dislike bitter and sour tastes, and they quickly develop a preference for salty tastes.[53,54] Further, there is evidence that children prefer energy-dense foods, which are typically high in fat.[55] The evolutionary function of this preference makes sense, as the problem during most of human history has been famine, not excess caloric intake. Our current culture compounds the strength of these preferences by repeatedly associating sweet energy-dense foods (e.g., cake, ice cream, cookies) with positive social situations and celebrations, which can increase a child's preference for those foods even further.

There is evidence, however, that children can learn to prefer the flavors that are most familiar. Sullivan and Birch[56] demonstrated that repeated exposure to a novel food that was sweetened, salty, or plain led to increased acceptance of that specific food. Further, at the end of the study, the children who were exposed to the plain food preferred it over the sweet and salty foods, and vice versa. This suggests that it is important for parents and others who feed children not to fall into the trap of sweetening foods (such as breakfast cereals) simply to gain immediate acceptance of that food — children will learn to prefer the unsweetened version of foods if they are continually exposed to them. Children are also reluctant to try new foods, unless those foods are so biologically appealing (i.e., sweet) that it overrides their neophobia.[57] Birch and colleagues[58] have demonstrated that approximately ten exposures of tasting food are adequate to establish acceptance in infants. This is an important message to share with parents, as some may not realize that rejection of new foods is an adaptive process, and successful food acceptance takes time. Parents should be encouraged to routinely give their children opportunities to taste new foods and foster an environment where noone is forced to eat anything, but "giving things a try" is expected.

Another important message to share with parents is to exercise caution when using food as a reward for good behavior. One study has found that children will increase their preference for foods that have been used as a reward,[59] and another retrospective study of adults found that people who recalled food being used as a reward, or withheld as a punishment, were more likely to struggle as adults with dietary restraint and binge eating.[60] Children are generally quite flexible, and will respond to all types of nonfood rewards, such as small toys, stickers, and the opportunity to spend time and play with a parent. Whenever possible, it is useful for the reward to be a natural outcome of the desired behavior. For example, if the child is cooperative and helps do the dishes, the parents will then have time to sit and play a game.

Discuss Safe Ways to Restrict Food Selection

One of the most controversial questions facing parents is whether or not to restrict less healthful foods from their overweight children. On the one hand, there is the "forbidden fruit" hypothesis — restrict a particular food and the child is going to want that food even more. There is a body of research that suggests that children will eat more when they believe their parents are not watching, and specifically, girls whose mothers restrict access to certain foods will eat more when given free access to those foods.[61–63] These authors suggest that when parents restrict access to high-sugar and high-fat foods, they may paradoxically increase their child's consumption of those foods when they are not around.

This interpretation assumes that the parents began restricting the foods, and the children's difficult self-regulation around those foods was a consequence. An alternative explanation is that there are children who innately have difficulty self-regulating their intake, and their parents' restrictive behavior is in response to that child's characteristic. There is support for this hypothesis in a study of mothers who have one overweight child and one lean child. They do not report different feeding practices for the two children; however, they do feel their overweight child has greater intake and more difficulty self-regulating than their slimmer child.[64]

In terms of what to recommend to parents, there is clinical support for the "out of sight, out of mind" position. A strategy called stimulus control is a standard component of every behavioral treatment for obesity and entails keeping the foods you do not want to eat out of your environment. Parents of overweight children sometimes report arguing with their children about how much of a certain food they should eat, or finding out their child is "sneaking" foods. The best way to handle this situation may be to prevent it and keep unhealthful foods out of the house entirely. The child can then make unrestricted food choices and still choose healthy food.

Reduce Advertising

One reaction to the rise in childhood obesity is to put more resources into educating parents and children so that concerns about health sway eating decisions away from the easy, convenient, and inexpensive options. The challenge is that any education campaign, such as the National Cancer Institute's "5 A Day" program or the Small Step program from the government's Department of Health and Human Services (www.smallstep.gov), is competing against the advertising messages from the food industry. An analysis of 1997 advertising dollars found that nearly seven times as much money was spent advertising confectionary and snacks (i.e., candy, gum, mints, cookies, crackers, nuts, chips, and other salty snacks) than was spent advertising fruits, vegetables, grains, and beans.[65] In that year, the USDA spent $333 million on nutrition education, while the food industry spent $7 billion promoting primarily unhealthy foods.[65]

Advertising to children has exploded in the past few decades, and concerns about this go beyond unhealthful foods.[66] Nonetheless, food is among the most commonly advertised products to children. It is estimated that the average child sees 10,000 food advertisements per year on television alone, and 95% of those are for candy, soft drinks, sugared cereals, and fast food.[51] From the parents' perspective, it means 9500 messages per year crafted specifically to make children want the very foods they need to limit. Even a parent who eats three meals a day, 365 days a year, with his or her child only has the opportunity to give 1095 competing nutritional messages. The food industry has a 9:1 lead. Further, parents' messages are far less attention grabbing, as they do not have movie tie-ins, favorite TV characters, and celebrities available to reinforce them.

Limit Television Time

Limiting television time has many benefits. First, it limits children's exposure to advertisements for unhealthful foods. Second, it is a completely sedentary activity. There is strong research evidence suggesting a link between the number of hours a child watches television and the risk of obesity, and reducing time in front of the television has been shown to have a beneficial impact.[67] Parents should limit television watching to no more than 1 h per day and make sure there is not a television in the child's bedroom. The rule needs to apply to the family. For example, all children should have their TV limited, not just the overweight child.

Eat Family Meals

Having meals as a family — not in front of the television — is highly recommended for several reasons. First, recent research found that adolescent girls who reported having frequent and pleasant family meals were less likely to engage in disordered eating.[68] Second, other research suggests that the meals children eat at home are healthier than the meals they eat at school, restaurants, or even other people's houses.[69] Third, a recent study suggests that family dinners are associated with a greater intake of fruits and vegetables among adolescents.[70] It is difficult for many families to find the time to eat together regularly during the week because of children's activity schedule and parent work schedules; however, physicians should strongly encourage parents to make it a priority to have meals together as often as possible.

Make Changes as a Family

It is important that any decisions about what foods to serve or what foods to limit are made for the entire family. Lean siblings may protest having potato chips or cookies no longer part of the weekly grocery list; however, the parents must explain that these changes are occurring for everyone's health and well-being. While childhood obesity is the reason that childhood nutrition is getting so much national attention, it is important to remember that it is just as undesirable for a thin child to eat a lunch of soda and ice cream as it is for an overweight child to do so.

Children are more likely to eat foods that are served at home and their parents are eating, and interestingly, they are also strongly influenced by what they see their peers eating.[71,72] This suggests that one of the most promising settings in which to increase healthful food acceptance may be schools. The hypothesis that children may be most likely to try new foods when they are introduced by peers at school is an important one to test in future research.

Keep Schools Accountable

Schools have become a battleground for issues linked to childhood obesity. In many communities, the vending machine and soft drink industries are fighting to maintain their presence in the schools and groups of parents, educators, and health professionals work to exclude them. In some cities and states, legislation has been proposed to change the foods available in schools. Another strategy used by some school districts is sending home "BMI report cards" to parents of overweight children, along with nutrition and health information.[73] This strategy is controversial, and its impact on weight has not been scientifically studied. It is possible that this procedure could stigmatize obesity even further, and the resources necessary for the program would be better spent improving the food environment or promoting physical activity. Research on the effectiveness of school interventions is needed, as legislators are eager to make changes.[71] Health professionals and parents have an important role to play in helping communities address these issues and making policy changes on the local level.

Alleviate Concerns about Eating Disorders

In addition to the health threats of childhood obesity, some are concerned that limiting access of certain foods to children may increase the likelihood of eating disorders. Popular press articles on childhood obesity in magazines such as *Newsweek* contain warnings to parents that if they are insensitive in how they talk with their child about losing weight, they risk creating "depression, anxiety, or a life-threatening eating disorder."[74] Even an editorial in the *New England Journal of Medicine* entitled "Losing weight — an ill-fated New Year's resolution" stated that losing weight is difficult, sustaining weight loss is almost impossible, and "the cure for obesity may be worse than the condition," and "countless numbers of our daughters and increasingly many of our sons are suffering immeasurable torment in fruitless weight-loss schemes and scams, and some are losing their lives."[75]

This concern is based on a misunderstanding of the appropriate public health messages. If the environment is improved so that healthful foods are readily available and unhealthful foods are out of sight, there is no reason to believe this will increase the likelihood of eating disorders. In fact, one could argue that the current environment promotes eating disorders because we send mixed messages to children; we glamorize an ultrathin body at the same time as we allow the food industry to heavily market and surround children with unhealthful foods. We set children up for the diet–binge cycle as they try to eat what is around them and lose weight at the same time.

A closer examination of the research on the etiology of eating disorders reveals that two of the best specific predictors of developing an eating disorder are childhood obesity and parental criticism of shape and weight.[76] This suggests that efforts to prevent childhood obesity may also help prevent eating disorders. Further, if part of the obesity prevention program also addresses stigma reduction, this may prevent eating disorders as well. One key goal in communicating with parents is to help them promote healthful behaviors, focus on well-being and fitness, and de-emphasize appearance.

KEEP A PUBLIC HEALTH PERSPECTIVE

While physicians can help their patients by educating them and their families, ultimately the locus of responsibility for childhood obesity needs to shift away from individuals and toward those who make public policy. Just as we as a society decided is was unacceptable for children to smoke on high school campuses, we must now examine the impact of allowing marketing and sales of soft drinks and snack foods in those same schools. The food industry has tried to frame the debate by saying that noone can prove that soft drinks or particular snack foods cause obesity, and therefore they are not the right target for change. This places the burden of proof on the wrong side. Parents and teachers should not have to prove something is harmful to get it out of schools — commercial industries should have to prove their products are healthful in order to have access to our children in schools.

SUMMARY

Clinicians can make a difference in childhood obesity. There are three critical periods in a child's development that have the largest impact on body composition. Clinicians may wish to concentrate efforts on obesity at that time. Genetic and early environmental predisposition to obesity is not a sentence to be obese. Lifestyle interventions have proven successful among two groups genetically predisposed to obesity — those with Prader–Willi syndrome and Pima Indians. Clinicians can diagnose and treat obesity-associated medical conditions, which can have a dramatic effect on the child's life-long health. Clinicians can incorporate behavioral interventions into their own treatment or refer patients for these interventions. Strategic nutrition interventions described throughout this textbook augment the treatment of obesity.

REFERENCES

1. Lobstein, T., Baur, L., and Uauy, R. for the IOTF Childhood Obesity Working Group, Obesity in children and young people: a crisis in public health, *Obes. Rev.*, 5 (Suppl. 1), 4–85, 2004.

2. Troiano, R.P. and Flegal, K.M., Overweight children and adolescents: description, epidemiology, and demographics, *Pediatrics*, 101, 497–504, 1998.

3. Ogden, C.L., Flegal, K.M., Carroll, M.D., and Johnson, C.L., Prevalence and trends in overweight among US children and adolescents, 1999–2000, *JAMA*, 288, 1728–1732, 2002.

4. Hedley, A.A., Ogden, C.L., Johnson, C.L., Carroll, M.D., Curtin, L.R., Flegal, and K.M., Prevalence of overweight and obesity among US children, adolescents, and adults, 1999–2000, *JAMA*, 291, 2847–2850, 2004.

5. National Heart, Lung and Blood Institute, *Clinical Guidelines on the Identification, Evaluation and Treatment of Overweight and Obesity in Adults: The Evidence Report*, National Institutes of Health, Bethesda, MD, 1998, NIH publication no. 98-408.

6. Kuczmarksi, R.J., Ogden, C.L., Grummer-Strawn, L.M., Flegal, K.M., Guo, S.S., Wei, R., Mei, Z., Curtin, L.R., Roche, A.F., and Johnson, C.L., CDC growth charts: United States, *Advance Data* 314, 1–28, 2000.

7. National Center for Chronic Disease Prevention and Health Promotion, *Use and Interpretation of the CDC Growth Charts*, 2001, http://www.cdc.gov/nccdphp/dnpa/growthcharts/guide_intro.html

8. Dietz, W.H., Critical periods in childhood for the development of obesity, *Am. J. Clin. Nutr.*, 59, 955–959, 1994.

9. Dietz, W.H., Overweight in childhood and adolescence, *N. Engl. J. Med.*, 350, 855–857, 2004.

10. Ravelli, G.-P., Stein, Z.A., and Susser, M.W., Obesity in young men after famine exposure in utero and early infancy, *N. Engl. J. Med.*, 295, 349–353, 1976.

11. Hollingsworth, D.R., Alterations of maternal metabolism in normal and diabetic pregnancies: differences in insulin-dependent, non-insulin-dependent, and gestational diabetes, *Am. J. Obstet. Gynecol.*, 146, 417–429, 1983.

12. Buchanan, T.A., Effects of maternal diabetes on intrauterine development, in *Diabetes Mellitus. A Fundamental and Clinical Text*, LeRoith, D., Taylor, S.I., and Olefsky, J.M., Eds., Lippincott-Raven, Philadelphia, PA, 1996, pp. 685–695.

13. Gellis, S.S. and Hsia, D.Y.Y., The infant of the diabetic mother, *Am. J. Dis. Child.*, 97, 1–41, 1959.

14. Plagemann, A., Harder, T., Kohlhoff, R., Rohde, W., and Dorner, G., Overweight and obesity in infants of mothers with long-term insulin dependent diabetes or gestational diabetes, *Int. J. Obes. Relat. Metab. Dis.*, 21, 451–456, 1997.

15. Sobngwi, E., Boudou, P., Mauvais-Jarvis, F., Leblanc, H., Velho, G., Vexiau, P., Porcher, R., Hadjadj, S., Pratley, R., Tataranni, P.A., Calvo, F., and Gautier, J.F., Effect of a diabetic environment in utero on predisposition to type 2 diabetes, *Lancet*, 361, 1861–1865, 2003.

16. Rolland-Cachera, M.F., Deheeger, M., Bellisle, F., Sempe, M., Guilloud-Bataille, M., and Patois, E., Adiposity rebound in children: a simple indicator for predicting obesity, *Am. J. Clin. Nutr.*, 39, 129–135, 1984.

17. Whitaker, R.C., Pepe, M.S., Wright, J.A., Seidel, K.D., and Dietz, W.H., Early adiposity rebound and the risk of adult obesity, *Pediatrics*, 101(3), 1998.

18. Siervogel, R.M., Roche, A.F., Guo, S., Mukherjee, D., and Chumlea, W.C., Patterns of change in weight/stature from 2 to 18 years: findings from long-term serial data for children in the Fels Longitudinal Study, *Int. J. Obes.*, 15, 479–485, 1991.

19. Williams, S., Davis, G., and Lam, F., Predicting BMI in young adults from childhood data using two approaches to modelling adiposity rebound, *Int. J. Obes. Relat. Metab. Disord.*, 23, 348–354, 1999.

20. Bhargava, S.K., Sachdev, H.S., Fall, C.H.D., Osmond, C., Lakshmy, R., Barker, D.J.P., Dey Biswas, S.K., Ramji, S., Prabhakaran, D., and Reddy, K.S., Relation of serial changes in childhood body-mass index to impaired glucose tolerance in young adulthood, *N. Engl. J. Med.*, 350, 865–875, 2004.

21. Wang, Y., Is obesity associated with early sexual maturation? A comparison of the association in American boys versus American girls, *Pediatrics*, 110, 903–910, 2002.

22. Dietz, W.H., Periods in childhood for the development of adult obesity — what do we need to learn? *J. Nutr.*, 127, 1884S–1886S, 1997.

23. Must, A., Jacques, P.F., Dallal, G.E., Bajema, C.J., and Dietz, W.H., Long-term morbidity and mortality of overweight adolescents, *N. Engl. J. Med.*, 327, 1350–1355, 1992.

24. Eisenmann, J.C., Katzmarzyk, P.T., Arnall, D.A., Kanuho, V., Interpreter, C., and Malina, R.M., Growth and overweight of Navajo youth: secular changes from 1955 to 1997, *Int. J. Obes. Relat. Metab. Disord.*, 24, 211–218, 2000.

25. Zephier, E., Himes, J.H., and Story, M., Prevalence of overweight and obesity in American Indian school children and adolescents in the Aberdeen area: a population study, *Int. J. Obes. Relat. Metab. Disord.*, 23, S28–S30, 1999.

26. Broussard, B.A., Johnson, A., Himes, J.H., Story, M., Fichtner, R., Hauck, F., Backman-Carter, K., Hayes, J., Gray, N., Valway, S., and Gohdes, D., Prevalence of obesity in American Indians and Alaska Natives, *Am. J. Clin. Nutr.*, 53, S1535–S1542, 1991.

27. Neel, J.V., Diabetes mellitus: a "thrifty" genotype rendered detrimental by progress? *Am. J. Hum. Genet.*, 14, 353–362, 1962.

28. Vogels, A. and Fryns, J.P., Age at diagnosis, body mass index and physical morbidity in children and adults with the Prader–Willi syndrome, *Genet. Couns.*, 15, 397–404, 2004.

29. Knowler, W.C., Pettitt, D.J., Saad, M.F., and Bennett, P.H., Diabetes mellitus in the Pima Indians: incidence, risk factors and pathogenesis, *Diabetes Metab. Rev.*, 6, 1–27, 1990.

30. Dabelea, D., Hanson, R.L., Bennett, P.H., Roumain, J., Knowler, W.C., Pettitt, D.J., Increasing prevalence of type II diabetes in American Indian children, *Diabetologia*, 41, 904–910, 1998.

31. Pettitt, D.J., Baird, H.R., Aleck, K.A., Bennett, P.H., and Knowler, W.C., Excessive obesity in offspring of Pima Indian women with diabetes during pregnancy, *N. Engl. J. Med.*, 308, 242–245, 1983.

32. Pettitt, D.J. and Knowler, W.C., Diabetes and obesity in the Pima Indians: a cross-generational vicious cycle, *J. Obes. Weight Regul.*, 7, 61–75, 1988.

33. Dabelea, D., Knowler, W.C., and Pettitt, D.J., Effect of diabetes in pregnancy on offspring: follow-up research in the Pima Indians, *J. Matern. Fetal Neonatal Med.*, 9, 83–88, 2000.

34. Knowler, W.C., Barrett-Connor, E., Fowler, S.E., Hamman, R.F., Lachin, J.M., Walker, E.A., Nathan, D.M., Diabetes Prevention Program Research Group, Reduction in the incidence of type 2 diabetes with lifestyle intervention or metformin, *N. Engl. J. Med.*, 346, 393–403, 2002.

35. Salbe, A.D., Fontvieille, A.M., Pettitt, D.J., and Ravussin, E., Maternal diabetes status does not influence energy expenditure or physical activity in 5-year old Pima Indian children, *Diabetologia*, 41, 1157–1162, 1998.

36. Must, A. and Strauss, R.S., Risks and consequences of childhood and adolescent obesity, *Int. J. Obes. Relat. Metab. Disord.*, 23, S2–S11, 1999.

37. Koplan, J.P., Liverman, C.T., Kraak, V.A., Eds., *Preventing Childhood Obesity: Health in the Balance*, National Academy Press, Washington, DC, 2004.

38. Fagot-Campagna, A., Emergence of type 2 diabetes mellitus in children: epidemiological evidence, *J. Pediatr. Endocrinol. Metab.*, 13 (Suppl. 6), 1395–1402, 2000.

39. Sorof, J.M., Lai, D., Turner, J., Poffenbager, T., and Portman, R.J., Overweight, ethnicity and the prevalence of hypertension in school-aged children, *Pediatrics*, 113, 475–482, 2004.

40. American Diabetes Association, Type 2 diabetes in children and adolescents, *Diabetes Care,* 23, 381–389, 2000.

41. American Academy of Pediatrics, The fourth report on the diagnosis, evaluation, and treatment of high blood pressure in children and adolescents, *Pediatrics*, 114 (Suppl.), 555–576, 2004.

42. Kinugasa, A., Tsunamoto, K., and Furukawa, N., Fatty liver and its fibrous changes found in simple obesity of children, *J. Pediatr. Gastroenterol. Nutr.*, 3, 408–414, 1984.

43. Solga, A. et al., Dietary composition and nonalcoholic fatty liver disease, *Dig. Dis. Sci.*, 49, 1578–1583, 2004.

44. Mallory, G.B., Jr., Fiser, D.H., and Jackson, R., Sleep-associated breathing disorders in morbidly obese children and adolescents, *J. Pediatr.*, 115, 892–897, 1989.

45. Petti, S., Cairella, G., and Tarsitani, G., Childhood obesity: a risk factor for traumatic injuries to anterior teeth, *Endod. Dent. Traumatol.*, 13, 285–288, 1997.

46. Timm, N.L. et al., Chronic ankle morbidity in obese children following an acute ankle injury, *Arch. Pediatr. Adolesc. Med.*, 159, 33–36, 2005.

47. Whiting, S.J., Obesity is not protective for bones in childhood and adolescence, *Nutr Rev,* 1, 60, 27–30, 2002.

48. Jingushi, S. and Suenaga, E., Slipped capital femoral epiphysis: etiology and treatment, *J. Orthop. Sci.*, 9, 214–219, 2004.

49. Wilcox, P.G., Weiner, D.S., and Leighley, B., Maturation factors in slipped capital femoral epiphysis, *J. Pediatr. Orthop.*, 8, 196–200, 1988.

50. Stunkard, A. and Burt, V., Obesity and body image II, *Am. J. Psychiatry*, 123, 1443–1447, 1967.

51. Puhl, R. and Brownell, K.D., Bias, discrimination, and obesity, *Obes. Res.*, 9, 788–804, 2001.

52. Schwartz, M.B., Chambliss, H.O., Brownell, K.D., Blair, S.N., and Billington, C., Weight bias among health professionals specializing in obesity, *Obes. Res.*, 11, 1033–1039, 2003.

53. Cowart, B., Development of taste perception in humans: sensitivity and preference throughout the lifespan, *Psychiatry Bull.*, 90, 43–73, 1981.

54. Cowart, B. and Beauchamp, G.K., Factors affecting acceptance of salt by human infants and children. In: Kare, M.R. and Brand, J.G. (eds) *Interaction of the Chemical Senses with Nutrition*. Academic Press: San Diego, 1986, 25–44.

55. Birch, L.L. and Fisher, J.O., Development of eating behaviors among children and adolescents, *Pediatrics,* 101, 539–549, 1998.

56. Sullivan, S.A. and Birch, L.L., Infant dietary experience and acceptance of solid foods, *Pediatrics*, 93, 271–277, 1994.

57. Birch, L.L. and Fisher, J.O., The role of experience in the development of children's eating behavior, in *Why We Eat What We Eat: The Psychology of Eating*, Capaldi, E.D., Ed., American Psychological Association, Washington, DC, 1996, pp. 113–141.

58. Birch, L.L., McPhee, L., Shoba, B.C., Pirok, E., and Steinberg, L., What kind of exposure reduces children's food neophobia? *Appetite*, 9, 171–178, 1987.

59. Newman, J. and Taylor, A., Effect of a means: end contingency on young children's food preferences, *J. Exp. Child Psychol.*, 21, 20–26, 1992.

60. Puhl, R. and Schwartz, M.B., If you are good you can have a cookie: how memories of childhood food rules link to adult eating behaviors, *Eating Behav.*, 4, 283–293, 2003.

61. Birch, L.L. and Fisher, J.O., Mothers' child-feeding practices influence daughters' eating and weight, *Am. J. Clin. Nutr.*, 71, 1054–1061, 2000.

62. Fisher, J.O. and Birch, L.L., Restricting access to foods and children's eating, *Appetite*, 32, 405–419, 1999.

63. Klesges, R.C., Stein, R.J., Eck, L.H., Isbell, T.R., and Klesges, L.M., Parental influence on food selection in young children and it's relationship to childhood obesity, *Am. J. Clin. Nutr.*, 53, 859–864, 1991.

64. Saelens, B.E., Ernst, M.M., and Epstein, L.H., Maternal child feeding practices and obesity: a discordant sibling analysis, *Int. J. Eat. Disord.*, 27, 459–463, 2000.

65. Gallo, A.E., Food Advertising in the United States. America's Eating Habits: Changes and Consequences, Food and Rural Economics Division, Economic Research Service, U.S. Department of Agriculture, http://www.ers.usda.gov/publications/aib750/aib750i.pdf

66. Linn, S., *Consuming Kids: The Hostile Takeover of Childhood*, New Press, New York, 2004.

67. Robinson, T.N., Reducing children's television viewing to prevent obesity: a randomized controlled trial, *JAMA*, 282, 1561–1567, 1999.

68. Neumark-Sztainer, D., Wall, M., Story, M., and Fulkerson, J.A., Are family meal patterns associated with disordered eating behaviors among adolescents? *J. Adolesc. Health*, 35, 350–359, 2004.

69. Biing-Hwan, L., Guthrie, J., and Frazao, E., American children's diets not making the grade, *Food Rev.*, 24, 8–17, 2001, http://www.ers.usda.gov/publications/Food Review/May2001/FRV24I2b.pdf

70. Granner, M.L., Individual, social, and environmental factors associated with fruit and vegetable intake among adolescents: a study of social cognitive and behavioral choice theories, *Dissertation Abstracts International: Section B: The Sciences and Engineering*, 64, 3222, 2004, University Microfilms International, U.S.A.

71. Jarvis, J., Bill would track children's weight, *Fort Worth Star-Telegram*, January 25, 2005.

72. Schwartz, M.B. and Puhl, R., Childhood obesity: a societal problem to solve, *Obes. Rev.*, 4, 57–71, 2003.

73. Chomitz, V.R., Collins, J., Kim, J., Kramer, E., and McGowan, R., Promoting healthy weight among elementary school children via a health report card approach, *Arch. Pediatr. Adolesc. Med.*, 157, 765–772, 2003.

74. Begely, S., What families should do, *Newsweek*, 136, 44–47, July 3, 2000.

75. Kassirer, J.P. and Angell, M., Losing weight — an ill fated New Year's resolution, *New Engl. J. Med.*, 338, 52–54, 1998.

76. Fairburn, C.G., Doll, H.A., Welch, S.L., Hay, P.J., Davies, B.A., and O'Connor, M.E., Risk factors for binge eating disorder: a community-based, case controlled study, *Arch. Gen. Psychiatry* 55, 425–432, 1998.

16 Bariatric Surgery: More Effective with Nutrition

Ingrid Kohlstadt, M.D., M.P.H.

CONTENTS

SURGERY REDUCES WEIGHT

Surgery is an effective treatment for obesity. The Swedish Obese Subjects Study (SOSS) followed 1268 obese persons for 10 years after nonrandom placement into medical or surgical management. The medically-managed group experienced a net weight gain of 1.6% in 10 years. In contrast, the surgical group receiving gastric bypass surgery maintained a 25% weight reduction 10 years postsurgery, and the groups receiving vertical banded gastroplasty and banding experienced 16.5 and 13.2% weight reduction, respectively.[1] Similarly, data for the U.S. Preventive Services Task Force indicates that surgical interventions sustain an average 19 kg weight reduction over 10 years, in contrast to 2 and 4 kg weight reductions for behavioral and pharmacologic interventions, respectively.[2]

Obesity decreases life expectancy and surgery is successful in reducing weight. Therefore, one might infer that weight reduction surgery extends life. However, this has not yet been demonstrated. Mortality data from the SOSS and other surgical databases may provide that link. Reasons to be cautious include the following: First, surgery itself carries a mortality risk of 0.5 to 2%. Second, surgery is associated with suboptimal levels of various nutrients even years later and the nutrient deficiencies may exacerbate the underlying medical conditions. Third, the surgery does not always achieve the stated goal of 50% of excess fat-weight reduction in one year and some weight recidivism is common, thereby minimizing the benefits of surgery. This chapter focuses on how strategic nutrition can make surgery safer and more effective.

MECHANISMS BY WHICH SURGERY REDUCES WEIGHT

As humans we have a long evolutionary heritage of "derth" control — famine, drought, illness, nutrient-specific deficiencies — and little experience in girth control. Weight control is an evolutionarily ancient system, hardwired by hundreds of thousands of generations of mammals before the newer cognitive reasoning centers of the brain existed. In summary, eating is largely a gut reaction.

The gut is precisely the target of weight loss surgery. Surgical interventions have been traditionally classified as restrictive or malabsorptive. Restrictive procedures significantly restrict the size of the reconstructed stomach pouch and its outlet lumen so that even with very little food, gut peptides such as neuropeptide Y (NPY), cholecystokinin (CCK), ghrelin, and glucagons-like peptide 1 (GLP-1) communicate the sensation of satiety to the hypothalamus and hindbrain.[3] The restrictive pouch also makes eating in excess result in nausea, vomiting, and sometimes pain. Restrictive procedures include vertical banded gastroplasty, adjustable banded gastroplasty, and roux-en y gastric bypass. Malabsorptive procedures shorten and bypass much of the absorptive potential of the small intestine, thereby decreasing the calories taken into the body. Malabsorptive procedures include biliopancreatic diversion, roux-en y gastric bypass (both restrictive and malabsorptive), and historically, jejuno-ileal bypass.

Since stomach sensation is partly controlled by stomach muscle tone, compliance, and rate of emptying, an intra-gastric balloon has been used to alter gastric motor function and storage capability.[4] The balloon is inflated in the gastric lumen for up to 6 months and can produce modest weight reduction.[5] It is used to treat early obesity and to reduce weight in the extremely obese prior to gastric surgery. However, it has not gained widespread clinical acceptance.

Implantable gastric stimulation involves surgically inserting a pacemaker-like device to slow gastric motility and thereby delay gastric emptying and create satiety. The device has been clinically tested with results demonstrating relatively low amounts of weight reduction, but concomitant improvements in hypertension and gastroesophageal reflux disease.[6,7] Both direct pyloric stimulation and antral stimulation have been shown to decrease CCK and other gut messengers (Chapter 13).[8,9] Since CCK is associated with vagal afferents, direct vagal stimulation is being studied in animal models.

Since adipose tissue is an endocrine organ and abdominal visceral fat is highly hormonally active, removing visceral fat during surgery may provide additional benefit. Intraoperative removal of the omentum, the fatty apron covering the vital organs, may improve insulin sensitivity two- to threefold compared to surgical interventions where the omentum was not removed.[10] The efficacy of this procedure has not been tested in controlled trials.

Editor's Note

With more than 5 million Americans having extreme obesity and the growing number of surgical interventions, clinicians of all specialties will care for patients with surgically treated obesity.

The current criteria for bariatric surgery are largely based on body mass index (BMI). Bariatric surgery is generally indicated in persons with a BMI of 40 or greater, and a BMI of 35 with severe comorbid conditions.[11] Exclusion criteria include substance abuse, pregnancy, uncontrolled hyperphagia, and mental disability.[11] Gastric balloon placement and antral pacing are less invasive forms of bariatric surgery and may be considered when obesity is less severe. Associated medical conditions in persons considering surgery as part of a comprehensive obesity management plan are reviewed in Table 16.1.

METHODS BY WHICH NUTRITION CAN AUGMENT OBESITY SURGERY

Dieticians counsel patients on dietary guidelines following bariatric surgery.[31] Patients are advised to eat slowly, taking at least 20 min per meal and chewing thoroughly. Hypohydration can occur following any of the procedures; patients should ingest liquids between meals, rather than during meals. Eating protein before carbohydrates and fats facilitates its ingestion and, hence, absorption. A chewable vitamin/mineral supplement is recommended. Peri-surgical dietary recommendations are an introduction to the lifelong nutritional considerations posed by obesity, weight reduction, and a surgically altered gastrointestinal tract.

Medical management, surgery, and nutrition are entwined. Table 28.3 in Chapter 28, presents a framework of ten nutritional interventions for surgical

TABLE 16.1

Conditions associated with extreme obesity and how those comorbidities respond to surgery and nutritional adjunctive treatment

Comorbidity	Effectiveness of surgery
Hepatic steatosis	Highly effective; nonsurgical management with carbohydrate reduction and nutrient supplementation also has demonstrated effectiveness[12,13]
Sleep apnea and obesity hypoventilation syndrome	Highly effective; conditions increase surgical risk, therefore presurgical treatment with a gastric balloon may be recommended; hypoventilation improves as intra-abdominal pressure normalizes[14]
Type II diabetes	Highly effective; omentectomy may provide additional benefit,[10] as do numerous nutritional interventions
Pseudotumor cerebri	Highly effective;[15] dramatic improvement following surgery suggests etiology is linked to increased intra-abdominal pressure[14]
Hypertriglyceridemia	Highly effective; other components of lipid profile are less responsive; low-carbohydrate diets and carnitine supplementation may be adjunctive[16,17]
Urinary incontinence	Highly effective; improves with normalizing intra-abdominal pressure[14]
Hypertension	Effective; improves with normalizing intra-abdominal pressure;[14] improved or resolved in three-quarters of bariatric surgery patients;[18] nonsignificant improvement over controls;[1] optimizing magnesium, alpha lipoic acid, arginine may enhance effectiveness;[19,20] hypertension increases risk of perioperative mortality[21]
Obesity-related cardiomyopathy	Effective; ventricular compliance improves with surgery[22] and adjunctive carnitine supplementation[23,24]
Degenerative joint disease	Effective; improves with weight reduction; nutrition should be optimized to minimize collagen loss; see Dr. Mischley's chapter on osteoarthritis
Infertility	Effective; patients are discouraged from conceiving the first year following surgery, because of undue risks to mother and offspring;[25] an adjustable band can allow for the additional caloric needs during pregnancy and lactation; optimize nutrients prior to conception
Proteinuria	Effective; reduces proteinuria associated with increased intra-abdominal pressure;[14] alpha lipoic acid can reduce damage from oxidative stress[26]
Polycystic ovary syndrome	Effective at reducing free androgens, insulin, and neck circumference[27]
Venous stasis disease	Effective; improves as intra-abdominal pressure normalizes[14]
Gastroesophageal reflux	Somewhat effective; restrictive procedures can exacerbate and gastric pacing may benefit
Peripheral neuropathy	Only effective to the extent that surgery improves diabetes; surgery exacerbates, primarily due to malnutrition;[28] antioxidants can ameliorate[29]
Gallstones	Ineffective; exacerbated by weight reduction[30]

patients. The current chapter applies these principles to bariatric surgery, especially preoperatively and during the first postoperative year of rapid weight loss.

ANTIOXIDANTS

Endogenous need for antioxidants increases with the physiologic stress of surgery. Obesity may place the body under additional inflammatory and oxidative stress, as evidenced by the direct association between obesity and serum levels of C-reactive protein.[32] Exogenous antioxidants are limited by decreased total food intake with consumption of fewer antioxidant-rich fresh fruits and vegetables. Additionally, in surgery with a malabsorptive component, there is reduced absorption of fat-soluble vitamins including the antioxidants beta-carotene, vitamin E, coenzyme Q 10, alpha lipoic acid, and essential fats. Collagen breakdown associated with weight reduction may be exacerbated by suboptimal vitamin C, which may occur due to increased demand.

In addition to a standard multivitamin prescribed postsurgically, patients may wish to consider supplementing with antioxidant preparations. Various antioxidants that may be of benefit include grape seed extract, olive leaf extract, quercetin, and turmeric. The antioxidant nutrient alpha lipoic acid may become conditionally essential following surgery, suggesting benefit in oral supplementation with 600 mg twice daily. Clinical trials have demonstrated alpha lipoic acid to be effective in conditions associated with oxidative stress such as diabetic neuropathy, nephropathy, hypertension, and hepatitis.[28,29] Alpha lipoic acid may also be of benefit in averting cardiac and skeletal muscle breakdown. Vitamin C should be optimized. A home urine assay for vitamin C status is described in Chapter 25.

ALKALINIZING FOODS

While the postsurgical diet tends to be low in highly alkalinizing (Chapter 25) whole fruits and vegetables, it is beneficially low in highly acidifying simple sugars, which can cause dumping syndrome. Dumping syndrome occurs when sugar passes rapidly through the stomach and is dumped into the jejunum, creating an osmotic load. Water is drawn from the vasculature to the intestine, leading to bowel distention, cramping, diarrhea, and hypovolemia. Insulin levels may become disproportionate to the available glucose, creating symptoms of hypoglycemia in some patients.

AMINO ACIDS

As discussed in the chapters on protein and sarcopenia, adequate dietary protein is needed to spare muscle particularly during the active phase of post-operative weight loss. The proportion of lean muscle mass lost with weight reduction is proportionately equal between those receiving medication and undergoing surgery for weight control purposes. However, the total amount of weight lost following surgery is significantly more, and loss of skeletal muscle and cardiac muscle is measurable on imaging studies.[33]

BONE NUTRIENTS

Obesity has been thought to be protective of bone density because of the estrogenic effect of adipose tissue and the day-to-day weight-bearing exercise that obesity imposes. The low threshold for suspicion can delay diagnosis of low bone mineral density, which can be associated with bariatric surgery. Calcium absorption is decreased in restrictive procedures because of increased gastric transit time, and in malabsorptive procedures because of the exclusion of the duodenum. Bariatric surgery decreases absorption of several other bone-building nutrients. Weight reduction without surgery also leads to bone loss in postmenopausal women, in which case calcium supplementation is only partially protective.[34] Therefore, a more comprehensive approach to bone health as outlined by Dr. Brown in Chapter 25 is recommended.

BIOTICS

Bariatric surgery presents additional reasons to administer probiotics. Healthy flora synthesize vitamins and curb the effects of invasive organisms. The role of microorganisms in carbohydrate digestion is currently under investigation for potential weight-reduction benefits.[35]

Another advantage of probiotics is their ability to metabolize lactose. Probiotics in yogurt contain the enzyme lactase. Yogurt can therefore be digested by many persons who otherwise experience lactose intolerance following bariatric surgery. Consumption of organic low-fat yogurt has also been shown to improve body composition.[36,37]

CORRECT DEFICIENCIES

Treatment for the period of weight reduction should minimize the consequences of intended calorie restriction. Several symptoms commonly experienced with significant weight reduction resemble the consequences of malnutrition outlined in Chapter 17: Alopecia, dry skin, osteopenia, loss of lean tissue including cardiac muscle, edema, thiamine deficiency, electrolyte disturbances, mineral imbalances, risk of refeeding syndrome (with total parenteral nutrition [TPN]), decrease (normalization in this case) in estrogen, and hepatic steatosis associated with carbohydrate intake.

B vitamin status is compromised. Table 28.4 of Chapter 28 outlines common medications that can contribute to B vitamin deficiencies. Thiamine deficiency is associated with malnutrition in general and is exacerbated by vomiting, that may occur following restrictive bariatric surgery. Vitamin B12 absorption is also diminished in restrictive procedures because the vitamin does not separate from protein foods and adequate intrinsic factor is not present for absorption. Folate deficiency results from inadequate dietary intake and some reduction in absorption in malabsorptive bariatric surgery.

Treating symptoms of B vitamin deficiency is a late-stage intervention. Preemptive B vitamin supplementation is the current standard of care for several reasons. B vitamins are cofactors in energy metabolism. Suboptimal amounts may increase catabolism and patients may feel unnecessarily tired. Adequate dosages of several B vitamins lower the cardiovascular disease risk factor homocysteine. In addition to its other attributes, folate supplementation can prevent congenital birth defects; up to 80% of patients having bariatric surgery are women of child-bearing age.[11] B12 deficiency can lead to irreversible nerve damage, and may do so more rapidly than the classical reports of this deficiency that usually takes years to develop in non-weight loss surgery patients. Peripheral neuropathy is common following bariatric surgery and most cases have been attributed to malnutrition.[28] B12 supplemented by mouth at 350 μg/d is generally adequate to maintain serum cobalamine levels; however, serum cobalamine levels should be measured.[38] Some persons may need parenteral administration. Forty-one percent of women in one study reported not taking a multivitamin long-term postbariatric surgery.[25] The literature documents that an exclusively breast-fed infant had B12 deficiency, and the mother who had undergone gastric bypass was asymptomatic.[39]

Magnesium is essential to fat metabolism (Chapter 4) and should be optimized; hypomagnesemia is common in the postoperative period. Since both dietary intake of magnesium-rich foods and absorption of magnesium decrease following bariatric surgery, suboptimal magnesium levels are likely to continue. In Chapter 9 Dr. Burford-Mason describes how persistent thiamine deficiency observed following bariatric surgery may be responsive to magnesium. The SOSS determined that the improvement in blood pressure 10 years after bariatric surgery was not statistically different from blood pressure in the nonsurgically treated controls in whom weight reduction was not retained.[1] In the same cohort, 2 years postsurgery, hypertension was significantly lower than in controls.[40] This prompts an interesting question of whether insidious nutrient deficiencies more prevalent among the surgical patients may counteract the beneficial effects of weight reduction on hypertension many years later. Low magnesium could be a contributing factor.

The daily multiple vitamin prescribed following bariatric surgery contains iron at the level generally required to maintain iron stores. In menstruating women and patients with anemia despite vitamin supplementation, additional iron supplementation is recommended. However, this practice fails to consider three important concerns. In persons homozygous or even heterozygous for hemochromatosis, the iron in the multiple vitamin is probably excessive and can have untoward metabolic effects. Iron causes gastrointestinal symptoms and may reduce adherence to a supplement regiment.[25] Iron supplementation further reduces chromium stores through competitive absorption. The association between chromium deficiency and muscle atrophy is explained in detail by Dr. Anderson (Chapter 11). Zinc deficiency has adverse metabolic effects on several pathways including inflammation and metabolism of fatty acids. Given these considerations, an assessment of mineral stores such as the provoked urine test described by Dr. Jaffe (Chapter 29) is appropriate for guiding mineral supplementation.

Along with suboptimal zinc and protein, essential fatty acid deficiency contributes to the copious hair loss that ensues 3 to 6 months following surgery.[30] Avoidance of trans fats and supplementation with the appropriate omega-3 and omega-6 fats described in Chapter 4 have been shown to improve fat metabolism and reduce hair loss, inflammation, risk of gallstones, and peripheral neuropathy.[30,41,42] Patients undergoing bariatric surgery are also at lifelong risk of fat-soluble vitamin deficiencies and benefit from annual screening.[30]

COMORBIDITIES

The U.S. Department of Agriculture Human Nutrition Research Center reports, "Obesity-related diseases are often undiagnosed before weight loss surgery, putting patients at increased risk for complications and/or early mortality."[43] Diagnosis and management are also important postsurgically, since weight recidivism is associated with the recurrence of comorbid conditions. For example, sleep apnea, which resolved following bariatric surgery, can unpredictably recur as weight returns. Sleep apnea contributes to insulin resistance and weight regain. Medical history can help intercept the sleep apnea–weight recidivism cycle. Table 16.1 reviews comorbidities of obesity and the efficacy of bariatric surgery in treating the conditions. Strategic nutrients of demonstrated benefit are also described in Table 16.1.

The macronutrient ratio most suitable for weight reduction is a popular discussion topic. While low-fat and low-carbohydrate diets appear similarly effective for the population at large, specific considerations can be made for the extremely obese.[16] Nonalcoholic fatty liver disease is associated with the metabolic syndrome and is common among bariatric surgical candidates. Solga and associates conducted a study to assess the effect of diet composition on liver histology prior to bariatric surgery.[12] High carbohydrate intake and low fat intake were associated with inflammation on intraoperative liver biopsy. The study supports advice that among the extremely obese, a low-fat diet is unnecessary and may even be ill advised.[44,45] The observation is consistent with physiologic shifts during food restriction and is clinically observed in refeeding following malnutrition. A low-carbohydrate diet has been shown to improve lipid profiles, especially triglyceride reduction, during nonsurgical weight loss.[16] The diminished absorption of fat and protein following surgery and the potential for dumping syndrome with carbohydrate ingestion are additional reasons to favor a low-carbohydrate diet.

CARNITINE

Carnitine supplemented at 2 grams daily has been demonstrated to have protein sparing effects on both cardiac and skeletal muscle.[23,24,46] Furthermore, it has been shown to improve endothelial dysfunction in obese individuals.[47] Since demands for carnitine increase disproportionately during pregnancy and lactation, carnitine supplementation would appear wise for women considering pregnancy following bariatric surgery.

DETOXIFICATION

Obese persons undergoing weight reduction are thought to be at elevated risk of persistent organic pollutant and heavy metal exposures. Toxins are lost through sweat and the obese have diminished sweat response. Organic pollutants are fat-soluble compounds stored preferentially in the adipose tissue. When fat stores are mobilized with weight reduction, the organic pollutants are also released into the circulation. Iron deficiency, which is common following bariatric surgery, has been shown to increase the absorption of heavy metal toxins. The presence of heavy metals can be assayed by the provoked urine test outlined by Dr. Jaffe in Chapter 29.

DEHYDROEPIANDROSTERONE AND SEX STEROIDS

Obtaining sex steroid profiles in persons with a history of bariatric surgery can identify persistent polycystic ovary syndrome and hormones below age-appropriate levels. Since adipose is an endocrine organ that modulates sex hormones and their ratios, hormone levels are expected to change with weight loss. Whether the lean-tissue sparing benefit of dehydroepiandrosterone (DHEA) applies to obesity as well as frailty has not been established. Therefore, DHEA could only be recommended to normalize low serum levels or low tissue levels measured by saliva testing.

Using serum and salivary testing to identify and then correct sex hormone imbalances is a potential adjunct to surgical management not yet studied in association with bariatric surgery. What has been demonstrated is that hormonal contraception can create hormonal imbalances, which can impair weight reduction following surgery. Hormonal contraception can alter food selection[48] and some formulations increase the risk of weight gain.[49] Hormonal contraception and obesity both increase the risk of thromboembolism and certain neoplasms.[50] Furthermore, effectiveness rates of hormonal contraception decrease with obesity. Women seeking reversible contraception following bariatric surgery should be recommended barrier methods or intrauterine contraceptive devices instead of hormonal contraception.

SUMMARY

When a person has been medically qualified for bariatric surgery for at least one year, an individualized weight management plan should include strategic nutrition, tight medical management, and a surgical intervention. More data are needed on treatment interventions for adolescents. The increasing array of surgeries makes selecting the most appropriate procedure very important and the patient can benefit from primary care provider guidance. Both former obesity and surgical treatment of obesity require lifelong medical considerations where nutrients and dietary modifications can be effective adjunctive treatment.

REFERENCES

1. Sjostrom, L. et al., Lifestyle, diabetes, and cardiovascular risk factors 10 years after bariatric surgery, *N. Engl. J. Med.*, 351, 2683–2693, 2004.
2. McTigue, K.M. et al., Screening and interventions for obesity in adults: summary of the evidence for the U.S. preventive services task force, *Ann. Intern. Med.*, 139, 933–949, 2003.
3. Badman, M.K. and Flier, J.S., The gut and energy balance: visceral allies in the obesity wars, *Science*, 307, 1909–1914, 2005.
4. Park, M.I. and Camilleri, M., Gastric motor and sensory functions in obesity, *Obes. Res.*, 13, 491–500, 2005.
5. Al-Momen, A. and El-Mogy, I., Intragastric balloon for obesity: a retrospective evaluation of tolerance and efficacy, *Obes. Surg.*, 15, 101–105, 2005.
6. Shikora, S.A., Implantable gastric stimulation for the treatment of severe obesity, *Obes. Surg.*, 14, 545–548, 2004.
7. Cigaina, V., Long-term follow-up of gastric stimulation for obesity: the Mestre 8-year experience, *Obes. Surg.*, 14 (Suppl. 1), S14–S22, 2004.
8. Xu, X., Zhu, H., and Chen, J.D., Pyloric electrical stimulation reduces food intake by inhibiting gastric motility in dogs, *Gastroenterology*, 128, 43–50, 2005.
9. Cigaina, V. and Hirschberg, A.L., Gastric pacing for morbid obesity: plasma levels of gastrointestinal peptides and leptin, *Obes. Res.*, 11, 1456–1462, 2003.
10. Thorne, A. et al., A pilot study of long-term effects of a novel obesity treatment: omentectomy in connection with adjustable gastric banding, *Int. J. Obes. Relat. Metab. Disord.*, 26, 193–199, 2002.
11. National Institutes of Health, Gastrointestinal surgery for severe obesity, *Consens Statement*, 9, 1–20, 1991.
12. Solga, S. et al., Dietary composition and nonalcoholic fatty liver disease, *Dig. Dis. Sci.*, 49, 1578–1583, 2004.
13. Sachan, D.S., Rhew, T.H., and Ruark, R.A., Ameliorating effects of carnitine and its precursors on alcohol-induced fatty liver, *Am. J. Clin. Nutr.*, 39, 738–744, 1984.
14. Sugerman, H.J., Effects of increased intra-abdominal pressure in severe obesity, *Surg. Clin. North Am.*, 81, vi, 1063–1075, 2001.
15. Sugerman, H.J. et al., Gastric surgery for pseudotumor cerebri associated with severe obesity, *Ann. Surg.*, 229, 634–640, discussion 640–642, 1999.

16. Stern, L. et al., The effects of low-carbohydrate versus conventional weight loss diets in severely obese adults: one-year follow-up of a randomized trial, *Ann. Intern. Med.*, 140, 778–785, 2004.

17. Digiesi, V. et al., L-Carnitine adjuvant therapy in essential hypertension, *Clin. Ter.*, 144, 391–395, 1994.

18. Buchwald, H. et al., Bariatric surgery: a systematic review and meta-analysis, *J. Am. Med. Assoc.*, 292, 1724–1737, 2004.

19. Boger, R.H. and Ron, E.S. L-Arginine improves vascular function by overcoming deleterious effects of ADMA, a novel cardiovascular risk factor, *Altern. Med. Rev.*, 10, 14–23, 2005.

20. Midaoui, A.E. et al., Lipoic acid prevents hypertension, hyperglycemia, and the increase in heart mitochondrial superoxide production, *Am. J. Hypertens.*, 16, 173–179, 2003.

21. Fernandez, A.Z., Jr. et al., Multivariate analysis of risk factors for death following gastric bypass for treatment of morbid obesity, *Ann. Surg.*, 239, 698–702, discussion 702–703, 2004.

22. Alaud-din, A. et al., Assessment of cardiac function in patients who were morbidly obese, *Surgery*, 108, 809–818, discussion 818–820, 1990.

23. Gurlek, A. et al., The effects of L-carnitine treatment on left ventricular function and erythrocyte superoxide dismutase activity in patients with ischemic cardiomyopathy, *Eur. J. Heart Fail.*, 2, 189–193, 2000.

24. Rizos, I., Three-year survival of patients with heart failure caused by dilated cardiomyopathy and L-carnitine administration, *Am. Heart J.*, 139, S120–S123, 2000.

25. Woodard, C.B., Pregnancy following bariatric surgery, *J. Perinat. Neonatal Nurs.*, 18, 329–340, 2004.

26. Borcea, V. et al., alpha-Lipoic acid decreases oxidative stress even in diabetic patients with poor glycemic control and albuminuria, *Free Radic. Biol. Med.*, 26, 1495–1500, 1999.

27. Dixon, J.B. and O'Brien, P.E., Neck circumference a good predictor of raised insulin and free androgen index in obese premenopausal women: changes with weight loss. *Clin. Endocrinol. (Oxf.)*, 57, 769–778, 2002.

28. Thaisetthawatkul, P. et al., A controlled study of peripheral neuropathy after bariatric surgery, *Neurology*, 63, 1462–1470, 2004.

29. Tankova, T., Koev, D., and Dakovska, L., Alpha-lipoic acid in the treatment of autonomic diabetic neuropathy (controlled, randomized, open-label study), *Rom. J. Intern. Med.*, 42 , 457–464, 2004.

30. Fujioka, K., Follow-up of nutritional and metabolic problems after bariatric surgery, *Diabetes Care*, 28, 481–484, 2005.

31. Marcason, W., What are the dietary guidelines following bariatric surgery? *J. Am. Diet Assoc.*, 104, 487–488, 2004.

32. Visser, M. et al., Elevated C-reactive protein levels in overweight and obese adults, *J. Am Med. Assoc.*, 282, 2131–2135, 1999.

33. Gahtan, V. et al., Body composition and source of weight loss after bariatric surgery, *Obes. Surg.*, 7, 184–188, 1997.

34. Riedt, C.S. et al., Overweight postmenopausal women lose bone with moderate weight reduction and 1 g/day calcium intake, *J Bone Miner. Res.*, 20, 455–63, 2005.

35. Backhed, F. et al., Host-bacterial mutualism in the human intestine, *Science*, 307, 1915–1920, 2005.

36. Zemel, M.B., Calcium and dairy modulation of obesity risk, *Obes. Res.*, 13, 192–193, 2005.

37. Zemel, M.B. et al., Dairy augmentation of total and central fat loss in obese subjects, *Int. J. Obes. Relat. Metab. Disord.*, 29, 391–397, 2005.

38. Alvarez-Leite, J.I., Nutrient deficiencies secondary to bariatric surgery, *Curr. Opin. Clin. Nutr. Metab. Care*, 7, 569–575, 2004.

39. Grange, D.K. and Finlay, J.L., Nutritional vitamin B12 deficiency in a breastfed infant following maternal gastric bypass, *Pediatr. Hematol. Oncol.*, 11, 311–318, 1994.

40. Sjostrom, C.D. et al., Reduction in incidence of diabetes, hypertension and lipid disturbances after intentional weight loss induced by bariatric surgery: the SOS intervention study, *Obes. Res.*, 7, 477–484, 1999.

41. Bralley, J.A. and Lord, R.S., *Laboratory Evaluations in Molecular Medicine*, The Institute for Advances in Molecular Medicine, Norcross, GA, 2001, p. 365.

42. Xu, H. et al., Chronic inflammation in fat plays a crucial role in the development of obesity-related insulin resistance, *J. Clin. Invest.*, 112, 1821–1830, 2003.

43. Saltzman, E. et al., Criteria for patient selection and multidisciplinary evaluation and treatment of the weight loss surgery patient, *Obes. Res.*, 13, 234–243, 2005.

44. Willett, W.C. and Leibel, R.L., Dietary fat is not a major determinant of body fat, *Am. J. Med.*, 113 (Suppl. 9B), 47S–59S, 2002.

45. Gifford, K.D., Dietary fats, eating guides, and public policy: history, critique, and recommendations, *Am. J. Med.*, 113 (Suppl. 9B), 89S–106S, 2002.

46. Wutzke, K.D. and Lorenz, H., The effect of L-carnitine on fat oxidation, protein turnover, and body composition in slightly overweight subjects, *Metabolism*, 53, 1002–1006, 2004.

47. Shankar, S.S. et al., L-Carnitine may attenuate free fatty acid-induced endothelial dysfunction, *Ann. N. Y. Acad. Sci.*, 1033, 189–197, 2004.

48. Eck, L.H. et al., Differences in macronutrient selections in users and nonusers of an oral contraceptive, *Am. J. Clin. Nutr.*, 65, 419–424, 1997.

49. Physicians' Desk Reference, 2005.

50. Burkman, R., Schlesselman, J.J., and Zieman, M., Safety concerns and health benefits associated with oral contraception, *Am. J. Obstet. Gynecol.*, 190 (Suppl. 4), S5–S22, 2004.

17 Malnutrition: Applying the Physiology of Food Restriction to Clinical Practice

Altoon S. Dweck, M.D., M.P.H.

CONTENTS

PHYSIOLOGY OF FOOD RESTRICTION

Starvation is the result of a serious or total lack of nutrients needed for the maintenance of life.[1] The physiology of starvation is the same whether the cause is anorexia nervosa, cancer, hunger strike, famine, severe gastrointestinal disease, or being a refugee. In order to combat malnutrition, the body breaks down its own fat stores and eventually its own tissue. This destructive process affects both the structure and function of the body and causes a variety of symptoms. The body adapts to starvation in an attempt to survive with a complex series of metabolic alterations to decrease metabolic rate, maintain glucose homeostasis, conserve body nitrogen, and increase the use of adipose tissue triglycerides to meet energy needs.

The body prioritizes utilization of energy differently in the fed state compared to the fasting or starvation states. In the normal fed state, the body utilizes energy first to meet the need for immediate metabolism. Once those requirements are met, energy is used to expand liver and muscle glycogen reserves and to replace muscle protein. Finally, as the last priority, the body converts excess energy into triglyceride and stores the calories in adipose tissue.[2] In the normal anabolic state, the glycogen turnover rate is high at approximately 50% per day, the protein replacement rate is low at less than 2% of body stores, and fat stores replacement rate is even lower at 0.3% per day.[3]

Conversely, in starvation, the priorities are reversed. The body shifts from an anabolic state to a catabolic state and lipolysis replaces gluconeogenesis (see Figure 17.1). The body undergoes many changes to catabolize adipose tissue and muscle to make ketones and free fatty acids available as an energy source so that ketone bodies and free fatty acids can be used to replace glucose as the major energy source. Catabolism of fat and muscle results in a loss of lean muscle mass, water and minerals, and intracellular loss of electrolytes.

The initial response to starvation involves breaking down glycogen and protein to provide glucose as the major energy fuel. At the metabolic level, a decrease in plasma insulin, a rise in plasma catecholamines, and an increase in lipolytic sensitivity to catecholamines occurs and stimulates mobilization of fatty acids from adipose tissue. As insulin decreases and glucagon increases, gluconeogenesis accelerates with a rapid conversion of glycogen stores into glucose.

During the early stage of starvation, protein stores are utilized as energy, with ketoacids serving as the major muscle and brain fuel. Muscle mass decreases in a linear fashion with the severity and duration of fasting. This loss of protein tissue slows metabolism, thereby decreasing energy requirements. With continued starvation, the body relies more on adipose tissue which decreases at a slower rate resulting most likely because of the high energy density of fat. After 2 to 3 days of fasting, adipose tissue provides more than 90% of the daily energy requirements, saving the ketoacids for the brain.[3] The proportion of energy mobilized from protein is dependent upon the percentage of body fat. People with high body

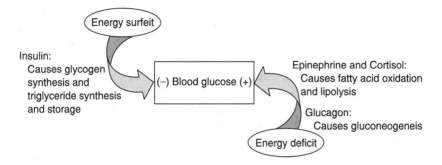

FIGURE 17.1 Metabolic regulation of blood sugar during the fed and food-restricted states.

fat stores exhibit a blunted increase in lipolysis and mobilize less energy from protein to conserve muscle protein.[4]

The switch to using ketone bodies as fuel for the brain is controlled by the concentration of ketone bodies in the blood rather than a direct hormonal effect on the brain. Cahill and Owens demonstrated that the human brain can derive energy from storage fat allowing starving, normal-weight individuals to survive for up to 2–2.5 months and obese individuals to survive up to a year.[5] During the initial phases of starvation, the body utilizes fat stored as adipose tissue to obtain energy. As starvation progresses, the body resorts to using fat contained in the visceral organs. Because visceral fat is involved in essential functions, organ failure is associated with later stages of starvation.

The body adapts to undernourishment by decreasing the basal metabolic rate (BMR) as much as 20 to 25% in order to conserve energy for survival.[6] The exact mechanisms involved in downregulating the BMR have yet to be elucidated but the process is thought to be multifactorial and may be caused by the decrease in thyroid hormone secretion as well as the loss of lean body mass. This is evidenced by the fact that the amount of weight and fat-free mass lost during starvation influences the degree of BMR reduction.[2,7] Data from patients with anorexia nervosa show that the decrease in the resting energy expenditure (REE) is proportional to the loss of lean body mass. A relative reduction in oxygen consumption and energy expenditure are additional adaptations to the low energy state of undernourishment.

CLINICAL FINDINGS ASSOCIATED WITH FOOD RESTRICTION

Physical exam reflects the physiology described earlier. On vital sign assessment, hypotension, bradycardia, and hypothermia are often seen in patients with extremely low weight.[8] Malnourished patients tend to have body temperatures below normal. Data from World War II and from patients with anorexia nervosa document temperatures below 33°C and even as low as 27°C in those exposed to severe cold.[8,9]

Anthropometric measurements such as weight and triceps skin-fold may be below normal. However, if the malnutrition has been chronic allowing the body to adapt, specific measures such as albumin, transferrin, and muscle mass may be within normal limits. Also note that obesity may mask food deprivation.

Malnutrition may cause depletion of skin, protein, and collagen, causing the skin to become dry, thin and wrinkled. Scalp hair becomes thin, sparse and easy to pull out. In women with anorexia nervosa, Savvas et al. documented thin skin with reduced collagen content that bruises easily.[6,9] These changes are similar to the changes that occur in postmenopausal women and are thought to be due to a common etiology of estrogen deficiency, as estrogen seems to have a direct effect on collagen metabolism.[6] Skin conditions can be exacerbated by micronutrient deficiency, particularly vitamin C.

Even though many malnourished patients are intravascularly volume depleted due to inadequate water and sodium intake, edema is often noted and usually manifested in the lower extremities. Total body water is usually greater in malnourished individuals and may be increased by as much as 20 to 25% with total body water levels reaching 89% of body weight in some cases.[10] The water accumulation and swelling are mostly due to dysfunction of the enzyme Na–K-ATPase, hypoalbuminemia, and a fall in plasma osmotic pressure.[10]

Often there is a reduction in muscle mass causing weakness. Both the loss of muscle mass and impaired metabolism decrease muscle function. A metabolic myopathy, resulting in impaired muscle function, has been documented in patients with severe malnutrition. Decreased sodium pump activity results in an increase in intracellular sodium and a decrease in intracellular potassium. This affects myocyte electrical potential and contributes to fatigue.

Additionally, the heart, lungs, ovaries, and testes, and their functions can be affected. However, the integrity of the brain is preserved at the expense of all other organs, and tissues and the brain and spinal cord lose very little weight and protein content. Even in Keys et al.'s experiment on starvation, the neurological changes were minimal with a diminution of the response of the tendon reflexes being the most common finding.[11] Cardiac muscle mass decreases and there is fragmentation of the myofibrils. Bradycardia, even as low as 40 beats per minute, and decreased stroke volume can cause a decrease in cardiac output and low blood pressure.[3] EKG changes may include decreased amplitude of all deflections (P wave, QRS, complex, T wave) and marked right axis shift of the QRS axis and T axis.[11] There is a decrease in vital capacity, tidal volume, minute ventilation, and diminished respiratory muscle function. This could lead to air trapping and lung hyperinflation, thereby causing a deterioration in respiratory defense mechanisms.

A malnutrition–infection synergy has been described since malnutrition is thought to suppress critical immune functions rendering patients immuno-compromised. Malnourished patients often have a loss of resistance to infection along with poor wound healing. In addition, there is atrophy of all lymphoid tissues, including the thymus, tonsils, and lymph nodes.

Malnutrition results in growth retardation in children, which is generally classified as wasting, stunting, and underweight. These anthropometric parameters place children at increased risk of having diarrhea and acute respiratory infections.[12]

Because of the decreased ability to digest and absorb food, patients may experience chronic diarrhea. Starvation causes structural and functional disturbances of the intestinal tract, pancreas and liver that limit the gastrointestinal tract's ability to digest and absorb food. The changes include mucosal atrophy with disappearance of the villous structure, reduced synthesis of mucosal and pancreatic digestive enzyme, decreased gastric and biliary secretions, and reduced total mass and protein content of the intestinal mucosa and pancreas. Most of these adverse effects disappear within 1 to 2 weeks of refeeding.

There are many laboratory parameters which are altered during food restriction. Anemia may be the first sign of malnutrition in adults, resulting from suppression of red blood cell production.

A number of endocrine abnormalities, including anovulation, elevated growth hormone, elevated cortisol levels, and low thyroxine levels, have been documented in starvation. These changes result from upregulation in the hypothalamic–pituitary–adrenal axis; however, the reason this occurs is unknown.[13] With weight recovery, all of these endocrine abnormalities resolve.

Anovulation has been documented in patients undernourished due to war, famine, and anorexia nervosa. Anovulation is a screening tool for anorexia among female athletes. At low body weight, circulating levels of luteinizing hormone (LH) are depressed, probably due to inadequate stimulation of the pituitary gonadotrophins. While the exact mechanism of anovulation is unknown, a threshold level of approximately 80% of standard body weight (the average weight of individuals of the same age, sex, and height) is thought to be necessary for normal release of gonadotropin-releasing hormone.[8,14]

Elevated levels of growth hormone (GH) and plasma cortisol are frequently described in malnourished patients. Data from patients with anorexia nervosa reveal hypercortisolism with elevated corticotrophin-releasing hormone (CRH) and blunted ACTH responses to CRH, as well as increased GH levels.[13] The elevation of GH is probably an adaptation to undernourishment since GH helps to mobilize fat tissue to combat hypoglycemia.[14]

Patients in starvation frequently exhibit a sick euthyroid syndrome with low thyroxine levels and a decreased conversion of thyroxine to triiodothyronine. Because thyroid hormone is catabolic, a decrease in thyroid hormone production may be a compensatory mechanism and probably contributes to the hypothermia mentioned previously.[14]

Adipocytes secrete leptin, a protein that is involved in body weight regulation. In lab animals, leptin induces satiety and decreases with fasting prior to weight loss. In patients with anorexia nervosa, low serum leptin levels have been found. With weight recovery, the leptin levels increase but still remain below normal.[15] Herpertz et al. showed a time-delayed relationship between letpin and insulin with insulin peaks preceding leptin increases following food ingestion. This study also demonstrated that leptin levels correlated with body mass index (BMI) supporting the idea that leptin functions as a signal generated by the increasing fat mass.[13] Further research is needed to define the exact role of leptin in weight regulation, whether starvation can actually trigger leptin resistance and leptin's function in signaling other hormonal systems.

There is significant variability in mortality as a direct result of severe malnutrition, ranging from 5 to 10% in refugee camp conditions and from 20 to 40% in hospitals.[16] That variability might exist because of the significant number of comorbidities that result from malnutrition. The duration of survival during starvation depends on the amount of available body fuels and lean body mass. The time until death is determined primarily by the size of fat stores and the time to reach the 3% level of essential fat. In humans, typical fat stores are 10 to 15 kg, or approximately 27% of body weight which should be enough to sustain life for 60 to 70 days. Some propose that lethal levels of body weight loss (40% of body weight), protein depletion (30 to 50% of body protein), fat depletion (70 to 95% of body fat stores) or BMI of 13 for men and 11 for women and perhaps even as low as 10 under conditions of specialized hospital care.[17] The mechanisms responsible for death due to starvation are not well understood. The literature demonstrates that women have a lower mortality risk from severe starvation. This is attributed to women usually having a higher initial level of body fat with subsequent reduced loss of protein and lean body mass during fasting. In addition, women usually have lower body mass and less lean body mass to maintain than men.

CLINICAL APPLICATIONS

Assess for Malnutrition

Malnutrition occurs in diverse clinical settings, and tends to be more prevalent than generally recognized. The increasing prevalence of obesity adds to the difficulty of diagnosing malnutrition. A tool known as the subjective global assessment (SGA) was developed to screen surgical patients for malnutrition and is now being used more broadly.[18] The SGA measures physical exam features outlined in the preceding text, with emphasis on weight loss and muscle wasting. A recent American study applied SGA to patients with colorectal cancer, finding that 52% had some degree of malnutrition. The degree of malnutrition was able to predict survival.[19] SGA has also been shown to predict cost impact in surgical patients.[20]

TREAT ELECTROLYTE AND NUTRITIONAL IMBALANCES

The incidence of electrolyte disturbances is not known. One complicating factor is that the clinical features can be subtle and unless the electrolyte deficit is severe, it may not be clinically manifested. Furthermore, the plasma concentrations do not necessarily reflect total body stores. Even so, plasma electrolytes should be monitored before and during refeeding specifically for sodium, potassium, phosphate, and magnesium as well as glucose. In addition, urinary electrolytes should be monitored, a urine sodium concentration of less than 10 mmol/l may be a sign of saline depletion, and urine magnesium, phosphate, and potassium can help to indicate body losses of these electrolytes. Before initiating refeeding, electrolyte disorders should be corrected.

Vitamin deficiencies should also be corrected prior to refeeding. While folate has not been shown to prevent the refeeding syndrome, some clinicians recommend giving various doses of thiamine in order to prevent thiamine deficiency.[21]

Zinc may be a novel nutritional intervention during malnutrition, especially anorexia nervosa. The connection between zinc deficiency and anorexia nervosa is discussed in detail because it is a simple intervention that is under-recognized. Zinc deficiency and anorexia have a number of symptoms in common including weight loss, decreased appetite, sexual dysfunction, and amenorrhea. Hence similar features such as poor growth/weight loss, skin abnormalities (acrodermatitis enteropathica), and amenorrhea are seen in patients with both conditions.[22]

There are differences between zinc deficiency and anorexia nervosa. The pathonomonic features of anorexia nervosa including distorted body image, fear of fat, excessive exercising, self-induced vomiting, and laxative abuse are not present in zinc deficiency. Conversely, signs and symptoms of zinc deficiency, such as depression, skin lesions, and impaired taste, are not usually present in patients with anorexia nervosa. Zinc deficiency can be a complication of anorexia nervosa, triggered by increased urinary losses of zinc from stress and decreased intake from starvation.

Open trials with zinc supplementation have been shown to improve weight gain in anorexia nervosa patients.[23] One study done by Katz et al. showed that patients given zinc supplementation had a significant decrease in the level of depression, greater weight gain, and an increase in height. This study suggests individuals with anorexia nervosa may be at risk for zinc deficiency and may respond favorably after zinc supplementation.[24,25] Another study by Birmingham et al. found that the rate of increase of BMI in the zinc supplementated group was double that of the placebo group.[26] Hence, the literature indicates that zinc supplementation increases the rate of recovery of anorexia nervosa patients by enhancing weight gain and decreasing their levels of depression and anxiety.

Furthermore, evidence from animal studies show that zinc promotes bone formation *in vitro* and bone growth and mineralization in newborn rats.[27] Zinc is thought to play a critical role in protein synthesis. Cavan et al. reported in zinc deficiency a shift towards fat tissue deposition in place of muscle.[28]

Based on studies with lab animals, when zinc deficient rats were given a choice between carbohydrate, fat and protein, carbohydrate intake fell significantly. Therefore zinc not only regulates food intake but also appears to regulate nutrient selection.[29] The exact role of zinc in food intake and the connection between zinc and anorexia have yet to be defined. A recent theory involves neuropeptide Y (NPY) in zinc-regulated feeding mechanisms. NPY regulates a variety of physiologic functions and is known to be a powerful regulator of feeding behavior. It appears to act as a stimulator of food intake when administered centrally, is increased in the hypothalamus by food restriction, and specifically stimulates carbohydrate intake. Previous hypotheses, which have not borne out, implicated disruption of NPY synthesis, processing or receptor function in zinc deficiency.[29] But a recent study by Huntington et al. revealed that zinc deficiency appears to prevent the release of NPY from the paraventricular nucleus of the hypothalamus.[30] The exact mechanism and role of zinc needs to be elucidated, but zinc supplementation may play a role in treating malnourished patients.

Clinicians should be aware of the associated conditions of zinc deficiency and anorexia nervosa. Although the causal link has not been fully established, treatment may be warranted. Prior to initiating zinc supplementation, clinicians may wish to quantify a patients' mineral status using the provoked urine specimen detailed in Jaffe's chapter on xenobiotics.

TAKE STEPS TO PREVENT REFEEDING SYNDROME

Malnutrition should be identified because it places persons at risk for life-threatening refeeding syndrome. Refeeding syndrome is broadly defined as the complications associated with the initiation of feeding in malnourished individuals. Adverse cardiovascular effects account for the majority of the morbidity and mortality associated with the syndrome. Other complications include fluid and electrolyte shifts, especially phosphorous, potassium, magnesium, and associated musculoskeletal, hematological, cardiopulmonary, and neurological complications.

The syndrome was discovered at the end of World War II as relief teams began noting similar events among malnourished survivors of concentration camps and prisoners of war. With the initiation of refeeding, many apparently "healthy" malnourished survivors suddenly developed cardiovascular and neurological symptoms; some died abruptly of cardiac failure.[31,32] Keys' Minnesota Experiment (1944 to 1946) confirmed these findings. During 6 months of starvation, the subjects exhibited no cardiovascular symptoms. With refeeding, however, Keys et al. documented diminished cardiovascular reserve, and some subjects suffered cardiac failure.[11] More recently, the introduction of enteral nutrition has rekindled interest in the syndrome. It has been documented in patients undergoing refeeding orally, enterally, parenterally, and in a patient with anorexia nervosa who was overeating at home.[33]

With prolonged inadequate calorie intake, catabolism of fat and muscle leads to a loss of lean muscle mass, water, and minerals resulting in a depletion of

TABLE 17.1
Patients at risk for refeeding syndrome

Classic kwashiorkor
Classic marasmus
Patient unfed in 7 to 10 days with evidence of stress and depletion
Prolonged fasting — hunger strikes
Prolonged vomiting and diarrhea
Massive weight loss in obese patients — after duodenal-switch operations
Chronic alcoholism
Prolonged intravenous fluid repletion
Anorexia nervosa
Cancer chemotherapy
Malnourished elderly
Postoperative patients
Homelessness

minerals such as phosphorous, potassium, and magnesium. Upon refeeding, there is a sudden shift from fat to carbohydrate metabolism and glucose again becomes the major energy source, stimulating the release of insulin. The body shifts from catabolism to anabolism and immediately begins to rebuild lost tissues. Both carbohydrate repletion and insulin release lead to transcellular shifts of glucose, phosphorous, potassium, and magnesium. The combination of depletion of total body minerals during catabolic starvation and increased cellular demands for minerals during anabolic refeeding can result in hypophosphatemia, hypomagnesemia, and hypokalemia.

Starvation causes complex metabolic aberrations making therapeutic replenishment difficult and puts one at risk for refeeding syndrome. It is unclear why every patient who is refed does not develop refeeding syndrome; however those suffering from chronic starvation, especially if there has been more than 10% weight loss over a couple of months, are at higher risk. Since the syndrome is often under-recognized, a key factor in diagnosing refeeding syndrome is for clinicians to recognize the signs and symptoms and have a high index of suspicion in high-risk patients, listed in Table 17.1. Any patient with a history of poor oral intake for even a few days should be suspected of having refeeding syndrome if they develop symptoms of confusion, weakness, dyspnea, tachycardia, paresthesias, or lab evidence of hypophosphatemia, hypomagnesemia, hypokalemia, or hyperglycemia.[31]

Monitor Laboratory Tests

The following are laboratory "red flags" for refeeding syndrome.

Abnormal Fluid Balance

Refeeding with carbohydrates results in insulin secretion, which can reduce water and sodium excretion. This coupled with concurrent increased sodium intake may lead to an expansion of the extracellular-fluid compartment and weight gain, predisposing patients to fluid overload. Hence, refeeding with carbohydrate loads may result in a misleading weight gain which is just a reflection of extracellular fluid retention.[34] In contrast, refeeding with protein or fat can result in continued weight loss and urinary sodium excretion leading to a negative sodium balance. High protein feeding can also result in hypernatremia associated with hypertonic dehydration, azotemia, and metabolic acidosis. Fluid intolerance can result in cardiac failure, dehydration, fluid overload, hypotension, prerenal failure, or sudden death.[21]

Altered Glucose Metabolism

Glucose refeeding can suppress gluconeogenesis which is an important adaptive mechanism during starvation. Once gluconeogenesis has been suppressed, ingesting more glucose, in the form of carbohydrates, can result in hyperglycemia and potentially evoke a variety of adverse effects including hyperosmolar nonketotic coma, ketoacidosis, metabolic acidsosis, osmotic diuresis, and dehydration. In addition, glucose can be converted to fat through lipogenesis potentially evoking hypertriglyceridemia, fatty liver, and a higher respiratory quotient resulting in increased carbon dioxide production, hypercapnia, and respiratory failure. Therefore, it is critical that fat intake does not exceed the maximum lipid-elimination capacity, which is about 3.8 g of lipid per kilogram of body weight per day.[35]

Vitamin B1 (Thiamine) Deficiency

Based on the current research, it is unclear whether thiamine deficiency is a contributing factor in the refeeding syndrome.[21] Carbohydrate refeeding may cause increased cellular thiamine utilization because it is a cofactor for various enzymatic activities, including carbohydrate metabolism. While thiamine deficiency is usually associated with chronic alcohol abuse, its most severe manifestation, Wernicke's encephalopathy, can develop in anyone with a poor nutritional state. Provision of thiamine with refeeding may prevent or reduce symptoms of post-refeeding thiamine deficiency.

Hypophosphatemia

With refeeding, carbohydrate becomes the body's major energy source, stimulating insulin release, and enhancing the uptake of phosphate necessary for protein synthesis and glycogen formation. The combination of total body phosphorous depletion and an increased intracellular uptake of phosphorous due to refeeding leads to severe extracellular hypophosphatemia. The clinical manifestations of hypophosphatemia include cardiac, hematologic, neurologic, respiratory, and musculoskeletal effects. Cardiovascular effects include cardiomyopathy and arrhythmias, specifically intermittent ventricular tachycardia and myocardial depression. Two possible mechanisms have been postulated: reduced phosphorous leads to depleted ATP levels depressing myocardial sarcomere contractility, or low phosphorous directly causes acute myocardial damage.[21,36] Hematologic effects include a decrease in red cell 2,3-DPG causing impaired oxygen release from hemoglobin to the peripheral tissues. In addition, hemolysis, red blood cell dysfunction, and depressed leukocyte function have been described.[34] Neurological manifestations can range from change in mental status to seizures, and include weakness, confusion, coma, paraesthesia, and convulsions. Respiratory consequences include acute respiratory failure due to respiratory muscle fatigue and respiratory depression. There are reports of failure to wean patients from mechanical ventilators due to impaired diaphragmatic contractility thought to be due to a reduction in ATP. Musculoskeletal consequences include rhabdomyolysis, usually manifesting as impaired skeletal-muscle function, weakness and myopathy. During rhabdomyolysis, serum phosphate levels may actually normalize from phosphate released from muscle breakdown. Furthermore, hypophosphatemia can lead to both osteopenia and osteomalacia because phosphorous depletion directly affects osteoclastic resorption of bone.[36] With long-term hypophosphatemia there is increased bone resorption to correct the low serum phosphate, which can result in ostomalacia. This is particularly important in malnourished patients who are already at risk for bone disease.

Monitoring phosphate in malnourished patients during refeeding can be challenging since serum phosphate levels may be misleading and do not necessarily reflect total body stores. For example, with starvation, total body phosphorus stores are depleted yet serum phosphate levels are often maintained by transcellular shifts of phosphate, via increased bone mobilization of PO_4 and an adjustment in renal excretion of phosphate.

Hypomagnesemia

Magnesium is an essential metal that acts as a cofactor for many enzymes. It is found mainly in bone and muscle and is essential for lean tissue anabolism, with 0.5 mEq of magnesium retained for every gram of nitrogen.[6] Like potassium, magnesium is more concentrated inside cells. Plasma levels only indicate extracellular volume, which are not always indicative of total body levels. Carbohydrate refeeding restores depleted magnesium levels within the cells, triggering a drop in plasma magnesium which can have serious clinical consequences. Additional factors may also exist with chronic alcoholics and patients on diuretics at higher risk for hypomagnesemia. While most cases of hypomagnesemia due to refeeding are clinically insignificant, severe hypomagnesemia (plasma concentration less than 0.5 mmol/l) can result in cardiac arrhythmias. There have also been reports of abdominal discomfort, anorexia, nausea, depression, irritability, and neuromuscular features such as tremor, paresthesia, tetany, hyperreflexia, seizures, irritability, confusion, weakness, and ataxia.[21]

Hypokalemia

Potassium is primarily an intracellular cation found primarily in lean tissue; the loss of lean tissue during starvation reduces total body potassium. Hypokalemia during refeeding results from potassium's use in glycogen synthesis, hyperinsulinemia and increased lean tissue anabolism.[6] Hence, hypokalemia may develop during refeeding if inadequate potassium is supplied to meet the new anabolic requirements. Hypokalemia, defined as a plasma potassium concentration less than 3.0 mmol/l, can result in cardiac arrhythmias, convulsions, lethargy, muscle weakness, confusion, coma, rhadbomyolysis, and respiratory depression.

Hypocalcemia

Hypocalcemia may develop secondary to malabsorption, causing true loss of calcium, or it can be secondary to magnesium deficiency. Therefore magnesium should be checked and corrected if necessary. Hypocalcemia can cause tetany and convulsions.

Hepatic Steatosis

With overfeeding, especially of carbohydrates via TPN, there can be an accumulation of hepatic fat. While the exact mechanism for hepatic steatosis is not known, it seems that the fat accumulation in the liver is derived from exogenous lipid or from a redistribution of fat from adipose tissue.[37] Elevated transaminases associated with tender hepatomegaly may result from fatty infiltration of the liver.

ESTABLISH GUIDELINES

There are presently no accepted evidence-based guidelines for the management of refeeding syndrome. The following are considerations.

- Oral or enteral tube feedings are preferred over parenteral feeding because there are fewer serious complications and it allows for enhanced gastrointestinal tract recovery.

- Feedings should be given in small amounts at frequent intervals to prevent overwhelming the body's limited capacity for nutrient processing and to prevent hypoglycemia, which can occur during brief nonfeeding intervals.
- Many nutrients, particularly nitrogen, phosphorus, potassium, magnesium, and sodium are needed to restore lean body mass. Inadequate intake of one nutrient may impair retention of others during refeeding.
- Refeeding should begin with less than full restoration of fluid and calorie needs. Changes in body weight provide a useful guide for evaluating the efficacy of fluid administration. Weight gain greater than 0.25 kg/d, or 1.5 kg/wk, probably represents fluid accumulation.
- Begin calorie repletion at approximately 15 to 20 kcal/kg/d or an average of 1,000 kcal/d. Using the Harris–Benedict equation, one can predict basal energy expenditure (BEE) and start feeding at 100 to 120% of the BEE or resting energy expenditure (REE).[6] Klein et al. recommend initiating feeding at 50% or less of the patient's energy goal and advancing gradually as some patients may require 72 h or more to reach and tolerate the goal for feeding.[37]
- The usual protein requirement is 1.2 to 1.5 g/kg or about 0.17 g of nitrogen/kg /d. Others advocate estimating the previous intake of calories and begin by providing at least that amount plus replenishing protein stores at 1.2 to 1.5 g/kg of protein based on the ideal body weight.[21]
- Liberal amounts of phosphorus, potassium, and magnesium should be given to patients who have normal renal function tests results.
- Daily monitoring of volume status and electrolyte values should include body weight, fluid intake, urine output, phosphorous, potassium, magnesium, and glucose. These values are critical during early refeeding (the first 3 to 7 days), so that nutritional therapy can be appropriately adjusted when necessary.

TREAT RELATED MUSCULOSKELETAL CONDITIONS

The Malnutrition–Obesity Connection

During weight recovery, regardless of the cause of the initial weight loss (malnutrition, famine, or anorexia nervosa) body fat recovers at a rate that is disproportionately greater than that of lean tissue.[38,39] Keys et al. referred to this phenomenon as "post-starvation" obesity and attributes it to overeating after a period of starvation.[11] Weight recovery data from adults with anorexia nervosa show a significant increase in trunk fat with the development of truncal obesity. Increased cortisol levels may lead to a more central fat distribution which might account for this phenomenon. Dulloo et al. showed that the human body's energy balance system that modulates the pattern of lean and fat tissue mobilization during weight loss also operates during weight recovery to modulate the pattern of lean and fat tissue deposition. Moreover, the initial percent body fat is the most important predictor for the pattern of lean and fat tissue deposition in weight recovery. This may partially explain why there is so much human variability in the pattern of lean and fat deposition during weight recovery.[39]

Loss of Lean Tissue

Skeletal and cardiac muscle dysfunction can occur within the first week of refeeding and may manifest itself as weakness, myalgia, rhabdomyolysis, or diaphragmatic weakness. The etiology of the muscle dysfunction is probably from the depletion of myocyte ATP and may be from CPK dysfunction as well. Muscle weakness may also result from altered neuromuscular function due to hypokalemia and hypomagnesemia. Cardiac muscle is also compromised. There is a reduced total heart volume, end diastolic volume, and left ventricular mass. This can lead to impaired cardiac output.[21]

Changes in muscle morphology and muscle energy metabolism following malnutrition have been studied. Muscle dysfunction has been documented in patients with anorexia nervosa, with proximal muscle weakness complaints.[40] Franssen et al. reviewed studies on the effects of anorexia nervosa on skeletal muscle fiber and reports the primary pathology is muscle fiber atrophy, particularly type II fibers. However, a muscle fiber type redistribution does not seem to occur as the relative proportions of the different fiber types (types I, IIA, and IIB) seem to within normal limits. With regard to muscle energy metabolism, decreased activity of enzymes involved in glycolytic and mitochondrial pathways have been reported in muscle biopsies from anorexic patients. Other findings associated with the myopathy include abnormal accumulation of glycogen within muscle fibers, diminished lactate response to exercise and reduced serum carnosinase activity.[41]

Life-long Osteoporosis Risk

Malnutrition during adolescence prevents acquisition of peak bone mass, as discussed by Lamb and Nadelson. Anorexic patients with an average duration of illness of 5.8 years were found to have an annual fraction rate seven times higher than healthy women of the same age.[42] Mineral loss is estimated to occur at a rate of approximately 3% per year of disease.[14] Bone loss occurs very early after the onset of amenorrhea, which may be as short as 6 months of illness.[43] The important predictors of low bone mineral density include the duration of amenorrhea, years of physiologic estrogen exposure after weight gain, lean body mass, and duration of emaciation below a BMI of 15 kg/m^2.[44,45] Anderson et al. found that men with anorexia nervosa are more deficient in BMD than women with anorexia nervosa.[46]

Disagreement exists as to whether full recovery of bone is possible. There are studies showing recovery with weight restoration and others showing only partial improvement.[42,44,47,48] Studies analyzing the long-term effects of anorexia nervosa on bone mineral density found that even after physical recovery, bone density may remain below the normal range for age.[45] Moreover, there is a difference between trabecular and cortical bone. Cortical bone mineral density, which if recovery is possible, will proceed very slowly.[49–51]

Hypogonadism is probably a major factor in the osteopenia of anorexia nervosa. Studies have shown that a longer duration of amenorrhea correlates with more severe osteopenia.[52] However, patients with anorexia nervosa have a more profound bone loss than amenorrheic athletes without anorexia nervosa.[53] Based on the association between bone loss and hypogonadism, hormone replacement therapy (HRT) may seem to be helpful and 78% of doctors treating patients with anorexia nervosa prescribe some form of HRT to prevent or reverse osteoporosis.[54] However, to date there is very little evidence of HRT as an effective therapy to prevent or reverse bone loss in patients with anorexia nervosa.

Calcium supplementation at 1500 mg daily did not preserve bone density in anorectic patients in one study.[55] A prospective study of calcium supplementation in patients with anorexia nervosa showed that calcium did not reverse bone loss.[56] Therefore, a more comprehensive bone nutrient regiment is recommended (Chapters 25 to 27).

The role of physical activity in anorexia is complex. While physical activity is necessary for bone mineral acquisition and maintenance, it has both a protective and harmful effect on bone density in patients with anorexia nervosa. Therefore, physical activity must be monitored to ensure that it is done moderately because excess can result in further weight loss and prevention of menses and may be detrimental to bone density.

MALNUTRITION CAN AFFECT THE NEXT GENERATION

Malnourished women experience miscarriages at a rate of 30 vs. 16% according to a case control study.[57] There does not seem to be a difference in the rate of miscarriage or mean birth weight between women who are anorexic during pregnancy and those who are recently recovered.[58] There are more premature births and cesarean deliveries among malnourished women and mean gestational weight for live births is significantly lower. For more information on maternal nutrition of offspring, refer to Chapter 3 and a recent workshop compilation.[59]

Editor's Note

Our definition of malnutrition tends to be insufficiently broad. As a result, several conditions are underdiagnosed: Osteoporosis decades after adolescent food restriction, sarcopenia in the elderly, obesity from maternal malnutrition while *in utero*, refeeding syndrome, anorexia nervosa, binge eating disorder, and nutrient deficiencies in immigrants.

REFERENCES

1. Starvation. Dr Joseph F Smith Medical Library at http://www.chclibrary.org/micromed/00066230.html (accessed September 2004).
2. Cahill, G.F., Starvation in man, *Clin. Endocrinol. Metab.*, 5, 397–415, 1976.
3. Klein, S., Protein-energy malnutrition, in *Goldman: Cecil Textbook of Medicine*, 21st ed., W.B. Saunders Company, Philadelpha, PA, 2000, pp. 1312–1318.
4. Melchior, J.C., From malnutrition to refeeding during anorexia nervosa, *Curr. Opin. Clin. Nutr. Metab. Care*, 1, 481–485, 1998.
5. Cahill, G.F., Survival in starvation, *Am. J. Clin. Nutr.*, 68, 1–2, 1998.
6. Savvas, M., Treasure, J., Studd, J., Fogelman, I., Moniz, C., and Brincat, M., The effect of anorexia nervosa on skin thickness, skin collagen and bone density, *Br. J. Obstet. Gynaecol.*, 96, 1392–1394, 1989.
7. Apovian, C.M., McMahon, M.M., and Bistrian, B.R., Guidelines for refeeding the marasmic patient, *Crit. Care Med.*, 18, 1030, 1990.
8. Becker, A.E., Grinspoon, A.K., Klibanski, A., and Herzog, D., Eating disorders, *N. Engl. J. Med.*, 340, 1092–1098, 1999.
9. Burger, G.C.E., Drummond, J.C., and Sandstead, H.R., Eds., *Malnutrition and Starvation in Western Netherlands: September 1944- July 1945, Part I*, General State Printing Office, The Hague, 1948, p. 87.
10. Goulet, O., Nutritional support in malnourished paediatric patients, *Baillieres Clin. Gastroenterol.*, 12, 843–876, 1998.
11. Keys, A., Brozek, J., Henschel, A., Mickelsen, O., and Taylor, H.L., *The Biology of Human Starvation, Vol. 1*, University of Minnesota Press, Minneapolis, 1950, p. 712.
12. Nandy, S., et al., Poverty, child undernutrition and morbidity: new evidence from India, *Bull. World Health Organ.*, 83, 210–216, 2005.
13. Herpertz, A., Albers, N., Wagner, R., Pelz, B., Kopp, W., Mann, K., Blum, W.F., Senf, W., and Hebebrand, J., Longitudinal changes of circadian leptin, insulin and cortisol plasma levels and their correlation during refeeding in patients with anorexia nervosa, *Eur. J. Endocrinol.*, 142, 373–379, 2000.
14. Herzog, W., Deter, H.-C., and Vandereycken, W., Eds., *The Course of Eating Disorders: Long Term Follow Up Studies of Anorexia and Bulimia Nervosa*, Springer-Verlag, Berlin, 1992, p. 261.
15. Palacio, A.C., Perez-Bravo, F., Santos, J.L., Schlesinger, L., and Monckeberg, F., Leptin levels and IgF binding proteins in malnourished children: effect of weight gain, *Nutrition*, 18, 17–19, 2002.

16. Golden, M.H., The development of concepts of malnutrition, *J. Nutr.*, 132, 2117S–2122S, 2002.
17. *Auerbach Wilderness Medicine*, 4th ed., Mosby, 2001.
18. Ottery, F.D., Patient-generated subjective global assessment of nutritional status, *Nutr. Oncol.*, 2, 8–9, 1996.
19. Gupta, D., et al., Prognostic significance of Subjective Global Assessment (SGA) in advanced colorectal cancer, *Eur. J. Clin. Nutr.*, 59, 35–40, 2005.
20. Raga, R., et al., Malnutrition screening in hospitalized patients and its implication on reimbursement, *Intern. Med. J.*, 34, 176–181, 2004.
21. Solomon, S.M. and Kirby, D.F., The refeeding syndrome: a review, *JPEN J. Parenter. Enteral Nutr.*, 14, 90–97, 1990.
22. Quirk, C.M., et al., Acrodermatitis enteropathica associated with anorexia nervosa, *J. Am. Med. Assoc.*, 288, 2655–2656, 2002.
23. Bakan, R., The role of zinc in anorexia nervosa: etiology and treatment. *Med. Hypotheses*, 5, 731–736, 1979.
24. Bailey, D.A., A six year longitudinal study of the relationship of physical activity to bone mineral accrual in growing children: the University of Saskatchewan Bone Mineral Accrual Study, *J. Bone Miner. Res.*, 14, 1672–1679, 1999.
25. Katz, R.L., Keen, C.L., Litt, I.F., Hurley, L.S., Kellams-Harrison, K.M., and Glader, L.J., Zinc deficiency in anorexia nervosa, *J. Adolesc. Health Care*, 8, 400–406, 1987.
26. Birmingham, C.L., Goldner, E.M., and Bakan, R., Controlled trial of zinc supplementation in anorexia nervosa, *Int. J. Eat. Disord.*, 15, 251–255, 1994.
27. Doherty, C.P., Crofton, P.M., Sarkar, M.A., Shakur, M.S., Wade, J.C., Kelnar, C., Elmlinger, M.W., Ranke, M.B., and Cutting, W.A., Malnutrition, zinc supplementation and catch-up growth: changes in insulin-like growth factor I, its binding proteins, bone formation and collagen turnover, *Clin. Endocrinol.*, 57, 391–399, 2002.
28. Cavan, K.R., Gibson, R.S., Grazioso, C.F., Isalgue, A.M., Ruz, M., and Solomons, N.W., Growth and body composition of periurban Guatemalan children in relation to zinc status: a cross-sectional study, *Am. J. Clin. Nutr.*, 57, 334–343, 1993.
29. Levenson, C.W., Zinc regulation of food intake: new insights on the role of neuropeptide Y, *Nutr. Rev.*, 61, 247–249, 2003.
30. Huntington, C.E., Shay, N.F., Grouzmann, E., Arseneau, L.M., and Beverly, J.L., Zinc status affects neurotransmitter activity in the paraventricular nucleus of rats, *J. Nutr.*, 132, 270–275, 2002.
31. Marinella, M.A., Refeeding syndrome: implications for the inpatient rehabilitation unit, *Am. J. Phys. Med. Rehabil.*, 83, 65–68, 2004.
32. Beumont, P.J.V. and Large, M., Hypophosphatemia, delirium and cardiac arrhythmia in anorexia nervosa, *Med. J. Aust.*, 155, 519–522, 1991.
33. Fisher, M., Simpson, E., and Schneider, M., Hypophospatemia secondary to oral refeeding in anorexia nervosa, *Int. J. Eat. Disord.*, 28, 181–187, 2000.
34. Marinella, M.A., The refeeding syndrome and hypophospatemia, *Nutr. Rev.*, 61, 320–323, 2003.
35. Crook, M.A., Hally, V., and Panteli, J.V., The importance of the refeeding syndrome, *Nutrition*, 17, 632–637, 2001.
36. Subramanian, R. and Khardori, R., Severe hypophosphatemia. Pathophysiologic implications, clinical presentations, and treatment, *Medicine (Baltimore)*, 79, 1–8, 2000.

37. Klein, C.J., Stanek, G.S., and Wiles, C.E., Overfeeding macronutrients to critically ill adults: metabolic complications, *J. Am. Diet. Assoc.*, 98(7): 795–806, 1998.

38. Faintuch, J., Soriano, F.G., Ladeira, J.P., Janiszewski, M., Velasco, I.T., and Gama-Rodrigues, J.J., Refeeding procedure after 43 days of total fasting, *Nutrition*, 17, 100–104, 2001.

39. Dulloo, A.G., Jacquet, J., and Girardier, L., Autoregulation of body composition during weight recovery in human: the Minnesota Experiment revisited, *Int. J. Obes. Relat. Metab. Disord.*, 20, 393–405, 1996.

40. Franssen, F.M., Wouters, E.F., and Schols, A.M., The contribution of starvation, deconditioning and ageing to observed alterations in peripheral skeletal muscle in chronic organ diseases, *Clin. Nutr.*, 21, 1–14, 2002.

41. McLoughlin, D.M., Wassif, W.S., Morton, J., Spargo, E., Peters, T.J., and Russell, G.F., Metabolic abnormalities associated with skeletal myopathy in severe anorexia nervosa, *Nutrition*, 16, 192–196, 2000.

42. Zipfel, S., Seibel, M.J., Lowe, B., Beumont, P.J., Kasperk, C., and Herzog, W., Osteoporosis in eating disorders: a follow-up study of patients with anorexia and bulimia nervosa, *J. Clin. Endocrinol. Metab.*, 86, 5227–5233, 2001.

43. Bachrach, L.K., Guido, D., Katzman, D.K., Litt, I.F., and Marcus, R., Decreased bone density in adolescent girls with anorexia nervosa, *Pediatrics*, 86, 440–447, 1990.

44. Mehler, P.S., Osteoporosis in anorexia nervosa: prevention and treatment, *Int. J. Eat. Disord.*, 33, 113–126, 2003.

45. Bruni, V., Dei, M., Vicini, I., Beninato, L., and Magnani, L., Estrogen replacement therapy in the management of osteopenia related to eating disorders, *Ann. N Y Acad. Sci.*, 900, 416–421, 2000.

46. Anderson, A.E., Watson, T., and Schlechte, J., Osteoporosis and osteopenia in men with eating disorders, *Lancet*, 355, 1967–1968, 2000.

47. Hartman, D., Crisp, A., Rooney, B., Rackow, C., Atkinson, R., and Patel, S., Bone density of women who have recovered from anorexia nervosa, *Int. J. Eat. Disord.*, 28, 107–112, 2000.

48. Klibanski, A., Biller, B.M., Schoenfeld, D.A., Herzog, D.B., and Saxe, V.C., The effects of estrogen administration on trabecular bone loss in young women with anorexia nervosa, *J. Clin. Endocrinol. Metab.*, 80, 898–904, 1995.

49. Herzog, W., Minne, H., Deter, C., Leidig, G., Schellberg, D., Wuster, C., Gronwald, R., Sarembe, E., Kroger, F., Bergmann, G., et al., Outcome of bone mineral density in anorexia patients 11.7 years after first admission, *J. Bone Miner. Res.*, 8, 597–605, 1993.

50. Bachrach, L.K., Katzman, D., Litt, I., Guido, D., and Marcus, R., Recovery from osteopenia in adolescent girls with anorexia nervosa, *J. Clin. Endocrinol. Metab.*, 72, 602–606, 1991.

51. Rigotti, N.A., Neer, R.M., Ridgeway, L., Skates, S.J., Herzog, D.B., and Nussbaum, S.R., The clinical course of osteoporosis in anorexia nervosa, *J. Am. Med. Assoc.*, 265, 1133–1138, 1991.

52. Biller, B.M., Saxe, V., Herzog, D.B., Rosenthal, D.I., Holzman, S., and Klibanski, A., Mechanism of osteoperosis in adult and adolescent women with anorexia nervosa, *J. Clin. Endocrinol. Metab.*, 68, 548–554, 1989.

53. Grinspoon, S., Gulick, T., Askari, H., and Landt, M., Serum leptin levels in women with anorexia nervosa, *J. Clin. Endocrinol. Metab.*, 81, 3861–3863, 1996.

54. Robinson, E., Bachrach, L.K., and Katzman, D.K., Use of hormone replacement therapy to reduce the risk of osteopenia in adolescent girls with anorexia nervosa, *J. Adolesc. Health*, 26, 343–348, 2000.
55. Rock, C.L., Nutritional and medical assessment and management of eating disorders, *Nutr. Clin. Care*, 2, 332–343, 1999.
56. Treasure, J. and Serpell, L., Osteoporosis in young people, *Psychiatr. Clin. North Am.*, 24, 359–370, 2001.
57. Bulik, C.M., Sullivan, P.F., Fear, J.L., Pickering, A., Dawn, A., and McCullin, M., Fertility and reproduction in women with anorexia nervosa: a controlled study. *J. Clin. Psychiatry*, 60, 130–135, 1999.
58. Finfgeld, D.L., Anorexia nervosa: analysis of long term outcomes and clinical implications, *Arch Psychiatr. Nurs.*, 16, 176–186, 2002.
59. Hornstra, G., Uauy, R., and Yang, X., Eds., *The Impact of Maternal Nutrition on the Offspring*, Karger, Farmington, CN, 2005.

Section IV

Muscle Tissue

18 Muscle Atrophy During Aging

Kevin R. Short, Ph.D.

CONTENTS

INTRODUCTION

Skeletal muscle is vitally important for posture, balance, and locomotion and acts as a major metabolic organ. Loss of muscle mass and function with age puts older people at risk for falls, obesity, diabetes, and dependent living. Muscle loss may be a marker of aging itself. This chapter considers the mechanisms, consequences, and treatments for age-related decline in skeletal muscle size and function, also referred to as sarcopenia.

DEFINITION AND PREVALENCE OF SARCOPENIA

Sarcopenia is most commonly defined as the loss of muscle mass and strength. Sarcopenia can be quantified in several ways, some of which are described in

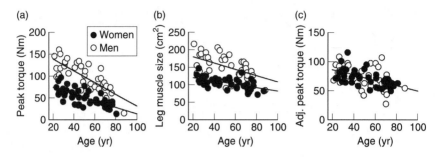

FIGURE 18.1 Decline in leg muscle strength and size with age in healthy men and women: (a) knee extensor isokinetic peak torque measure at 180°/s; (b) cross-sectional area of the thigh muscles measured by computed tomography. Significant differences in muscle size and strength are present between men and women but the changes with age are similar. (c) The decline in knee extensor torque with age persists even after adjustment for muscle cross-sectional area. This demonstrates that muscle quality is reduced with aging. (Adapted from Short, K.R., Vittone, J.L., Bigelow, M.L., Proctor, D.N., Coenen-Schimke, J., Rys, P., and Nair, K.S., *J. Appl. Physiol.*, 2005, in press. With permission.).

Chapter 1. Size and peak contractile strength of leg and arm muscles decline with age in healthy men and women.[1-9] In a group of healthy, nonexercise trained, men and women, cross-sectional area of the thigh muscles declined 5% per decade while peak knee extensor strength declined 10% per decade.[10] The best predictor of muscle strength is muscle size, measured as cross-sectional area, even though correction for muscle size does not fully eliminate the decline in strength (Figure 18.1).

In general, muscle quality, defined as muscle strength per unit muscle mass or area, declines with age.[1,7,8] In our studies, gender did not influence the age-related decline in muscle size and strength. The decline appeared to be linear throughout the adult lifespan. In other studies, muscle strength and size did not decline significantly before the age of 40 to 50 years.[2,3,5,9] The variability in study results may be because of differences in diet, physical activity, or health status of study participants. Each of these potential variables is discussed in this chapter.

Simply measuring height and weight is not an adequate screen for sarcopenia. Measurements of body composition described in Chapter 1 can provide a more accurate assessment. The loss of muscle mass with age is often masked by a corresponding gain in body fat so that body mass is a poor predictor of sarcopenia.[11-14] Much of the increase in adiposity is in the abdominal area. The loss of leg muscle mass and increase in abdominal fat with age is demonstrated in Figure 18.2. The shift in body composition is the major contributing factor for the age-related decline in insulin sensitivity because skeletal muscle is the major site of insulin-stimulated glucose uptake and abdominal fat is closely related to insulin action.[13,15,16] There are smaller increases in inter- and intramuscular fat in limb muscles with aging that also contribute to the decline in muscle quality and insulin sensitivity.[17,18] A recent prospective study of 26 elderly African-American

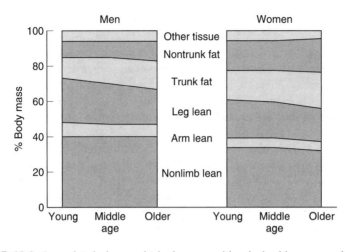

FIGURE 18.2 Age-related changes in body composition in healthy men and women. Body composition was measured in 100 men and 135 women using dual x-ray absorptiometry in subjects combined from two recent studies.[26,36] Subjects were grouped as young (18 to 33 years), middle aged (35 to 57 years), or older (60 to 89 years). Subjects with body mass index between 19 and 32 kg/m^2 were used for this analysis. The most notable change with age in both sexes was a decline in leg lean mass and an increase in trunk fat. Nontrunk fat also increased significantly with age.

women used magnetic resonance imaging over a 2-year study period. These women, who were 75 years old at baseline, showed significant decline in limb muscle mass and increase in intramuscular and visceral fat.[18] These data suggest that the frequent coexistence of obesity and muscle loss in older people can lead to underdiagnosis of sarcopenia.[19]

Among the first studies to measure sarcopenia prevalence was a survey of 883 elderly residents of New Mexico.[6] Appendicular muscle mass was estimated from limb anthropometry and cross-validated in a subset of the group. Sarcopenia was defined as having skeletal muscle mass equal to or less than two standard deviations (SD) below the mean. Based on this criterion, prevalence of sarcopenia among persons under 70 was 15% for men and 23% for women. For people over 80 years of age the prevalence was 43 to 60%, consistent with other estimates of prevalence.[20–22] Sarcopenia was associated with increased risk of physical disability and history of injury, including problems with gait or balance, use of a cane or walker, and history of falls and bone fractures.

CLINICAL SIGNIFICANCE OF SARCOPENIA

Reduced muscle mass and strength increase the risk of disability.[6,21,22] Rantanen showed that in a group of 1000 community-dwelling women over the age of

65 years, reduced muscle strength was closely related to the ability to perform a variety of activities of daily living.[23] Muscle dysfunction resulted in lower capacity to perform physical activities, which could exacerbate muscle loss.[23] An 8-year prospective study of 451 men and women classified participants as obese and sarcopenic at baseline.[19] The 30% of participants who were both obese and sarcopenic were two to three times more likely to experience disability compared with those with healthy body composition, obesity without sarcopenia, and sarcopenia without obesity.

Sarcopenia compounds morbidity and mortality among people who already have compromised health status. In a study of 660 elderly patients followed for 1 year after hospital discharge, mortality risk was greatest for those patients with low body weight at baseline, which in this case was defined as body mass index (BMI) <20 kg/m^2.[24] There is also evidence that older people with low body weight and low intake of protein and energy are more likely to have poor wound healing and development of pressure sores during hospitalization.[25]

Peak aerobic exercise capacity declines with age and this is due in part to reduced muscle mitochondrial function.[26–28] The decline in peak aerobic capacity is approximately 8% per decade in healthy, non-exercise trained people, even after correcting for muscle or total body lean mass. The decline in aerobic capacity also occurs in well-trained individuals.[29,30] Mitochondrial dysfunction may contribute to reduced glucose tolerance and increased insulin resistance in older people and people with type 2 diabetes.[31–33] The lower capacity of mitochondrial oxidation is hypothesized to result in greater fuel storage as intramuscular lipids, which in turn interfere with normal insulin-mediated glucose metabolism.[31,33,35]

Editor's Note

Loss of muscle tissue is often offset by an increase in fat, which can mask age-related muscle loss. Fat has on average only one third the metabolic rate of muscle so the loss of muscle contributes to an age-related decline in resting metabolic rate, as well as declining overall musculoskeletal health. When loss of muscle size and strength is detected early, nutritional interventions can be effective.

POTENTIAL MECHANISMS OF SARCOPENIA

The major component of skeletal muscle, after water, is protein. The balance between protein synthesis and protein breakdown therefore determines the mass of muscle and other tissues. Protein turnover is an essential process through which each cell can regulate size and function (Chapter 6). The rate of whole body protein turnover declines with age at approximately 5% per decade, even after adjustment for the age-related decline in fat-free mass.[36] Potential mechanisms of protein loss are a topic of current study.

Whole body protein turnover measurements average the contribution from all of the body protein pools. Because the size and metabolic rate of these pools change with age, protein turnover measurements can be difficult to interpret. Skeletal muscle is the largest single protein pool in the body, comprising approximately 45 to 50% of body mass and 80% of lean mass in young people, but because of its slow rate of protein turnover muscle accounts for only 30% of the whole body protein turnover rate at rest.[37,38] In older people, muscle may account for only 35% of body mass and 40% of lean tissue mass; nonmuscle organs therefore contribute more to the rate of whole body protein turnover. Turnover rates during steady-state conditions vary widely among different tissues, e.g., 1 to 2% per day in muscle and skin, 5 to 7% per day in heart, 18 to 21% per day in liver, and up to 31 to 48% per day in the gut.[39–41]

Skeletal muscle is a reservoir of amino acids that can be used to supply other body tissues. Following an overnight fast, the balance of amino acids in leg muscles is negative, meaning that amino acid release into the circulation exceeds the rate of uptake.[42,43] With continued fasting up to 3 days, the rate of amino acid release from muscles is further increased.[44] In contrast, amino acid balance in the splanchnic tissues remains positive between meals,[45,46] presumably so that the liver can continue to produce essential proteins such as albumin and clotting factors. Thus, it seems that muscle plays a critical role in providing amino acids to the liver between meals. Following a meal amino acid uptake rapidly increases in muscle and splanchnic tissues.[43] On the basis of tissue mass, however, the total amino acid uptake into skeletal muscles is much greater than other organs.

A decline in muscle protein synthesis and an increase in breakdown could both contribute to muscle loss. Several studies have reported that in human leg muscles the fractional synthesis rate of total mixed muscle proteins, myofibrillar (contractile) proteins, and mitochondrial proteins is reduced with age.[36,37,44–47] Work from our group demonstrated that with age there was a decline in synthesis rates of mitochondrial proteins and myosin heavy chain, which is the major contractile protein. There was no decline in synthesis of sarcoplasmic proteins, which are soluble cellular proteins.[37] This distinction highlights the fact that some muscle proteins are more likely to be affected by the aging process. Not all research groups have found a decline in muscle protein synthesis rate with age. In a comparison between healthy young and old men, Volpi and colleagues[48] reported that there was no significant difference in either leg muscle protein synthesis or breakdown rates. Volpi and colleagues[49] elected not to control diet or exercise habits prior to their measurements and participants self-reported to the testing center on the morning of the study, rather than staying overnight. The rationale presented for this approach was that subjects were studied under a more free-living state, although this may have added variability to the measurements. These studies demonstrate that age effects vary among older subjects, suggesting a critical role for diet and exercise.

There are additional reasons to expect that muscle protein synthesis rate declines with age through reductions in transcription of messenger RNA (mRNA) and translation of proteins decline. Additionally, oxidative damage to mitochondrial DNA, proteins, lipids, and other cellular components increases in skeletal muscle and other organs increase.[50–54] Oxidative damage to proteins, lipids, and other cellular components.[50–56] Activity of antioxidant defense enzymes is altered[57] and antioxidant therapies may attenuate age-related degenerative processes.[58–61] Proteins undergo several other forms of post-translational modification, including phosphorylation, nitrosylation, glycation, and methylation, which adversely affect protein function.[50,61]

Another potential mechanism for sarcopenia is loss of motor neurons. Lexell and colleagues[62,63] demonstrated that in human quadriceps muscle, the total number of muscle fibers is reduced with age and that there is preferential atrophy of the type II (fast twitch) fibers. The loss of muscle fibers may be due to a decrease in motor nerves, because other studies have found evidence of fewer motor units, reinnervation changes, and deterioration of motor endplates in older muscles.[64–66] Muscle fibers in older muscles are clustered into larger motor units that are less randomly distributed than in younger muscles, suggesting that reorganization occurs during aging.[65,66] Frail older people often have decreased neurological function as well as sarcopenia, providing support for a causal association.[66,67]

EXERCISE CAN ATTENUATE SARCOPENIA AND ITS EFFECTS

Skeletal muscle is the major site of insulin-mediated glucose uptake, storage, and oxidation and aerobic exercise can further enhance this capacity.[68–71] The most prominent change in muscle in response to aerobic training is stimulation of mitochondrial biogenesis.[72] A classic study by Holloszy[73] was the first to demonstrate that regular treadmill running produced enhancements in mitochondrial function in rodents. Subsequent work in humans has shown that the capacity to improve mitochondrial function in response to exercise remains largely intact in old age.[13,74,75] In a 4-month program of moderate intensity bicycle exercise, improvements in peak aerobic capacity, activity of oxidative enzymes in skeletal muscle, and expression level of mRNA transcripts encoding mitochondrial proteins were increased to a similar extent in younger, middle-age, and older men and women.[13] Older people who regularly perform aerobic exercise also have increased muscle capillary density.[74,75] Collectively, these enhancements can contribute to decreased muscle fatigability in older people.

Aerobic exercise, however, has not been shown to increase muscle mass.[13,76] Recent studies have shown that both young and old experience an increase in muscle protein synthesis following either a single session of treadmill walking[77] or a 4-month program of bicycle training.[13] In view of the fact that this type of activity does not alter muscle mass, the enhanced rate of protein synthesis may be primarily directed at increasing mitochondrial proteins and may improve muscle quality by replacement of damaged proteins. Further work is required to identify the specific proteins that are affected.

Resistance training is required for improvement of muscle size and strength and it is a safe and effective means for older people to achieve strength gains.[78,79] In most cases, the percentage increase in strength and muscle size is similar in healthy older men and women compared to younger people when following a standardized program. Even frail older people can benefit from resistance exercise.[80,81] However, for older people living in supervised care facilities, there may be significant deconditioning, which results in slower strength gain. Orthopedic, posture, or balance issues may need to be overcome, but there is usually some type of activity that can be successfully implemented.

The increase in muscle strength with resistive training typically exceeds the change in muscle size in both younger and older people. In older men, for example, 12 weeks of resistance training increased leg extensor strength 110% but quadriceps cross-sectional area only 9%.[82] The greater increase in strength is accomplished through alterations in motor unit firing, i.e., increased synchronization of agonists and reduced firing of antagonists, in both young and old individuals.[83,84] These studies show that even though there appear to be fewer motor units in old muscles, the existing neural networks remain highly adaptable. The fact that motor unit plasticity is still present in aging muscles, despite several quantitative and qualitative changes, is a positive sign that exercise interventions may help to attenuate the aging process.

Resistance training ranging from 2 weeks to 4 months increases muscle protein synthesis, especially contractile proteins.[44,47,85–88] Less is known about protein breakdown because it is technically more difficult to measure. Exercise is thought to increase protein breakdown as part of an overall increase in turnover;[89] net protein synthesis occurs as evidenced by protein accumulation (Chapter 6).

DIETARY PROTEIN AND AMINO ACIDS PLAY A ROLE IN PREVENTING SARCOPENIA

Total energy and protein intake decline with age.[90,91] There has been ongoing debate about whether dietary protein needs change with age and whether recommendations for older people to increase dietary protein are beneficial and safe. In 1985, the World Health Organization established a recommended daily allowance (RDA) of 0.6 g of high-quality protein per kilogram body weight per day for older people, but this estimate was challenged and the current RDA is 0.8 g/kg/d.[92,93] According to work by Campbell and colleagues,[94–96] protein requirements in the elderly may actually be closer to 0.9 or even 1 g/kg/d. They arrived at these values after performing studies with experimentally controlled diets and monitoring nitrogen balance for up to 14 weeks. The requirement of 0.9 to 1.0 g protein/kg/d to achieve nitrogen balance was determined from four studies lasting 10–20 days.[95] Such short-term studies may not be adequate to achieve a steady state in nitrogen balance when manipulating dietary protein intake.[96] Campbell and colleagues,[94] therefore, performed a 14-week study in which healthy older men and women consumed 0.8 g protein/kg/d. The subjects in that study were able to maintain body weight but they experienced a 2% decline in thigh muscle area and a 20% reduction in urinary nitrogen excretion, which suggests a compensatory mechanism to slow the loss of lean tissue. Thus, in these healthy older people, protein needs appear to exceed the current RDA. In addition to the role of protein in maintaining muscle mass, protein intake is inversely related to the risk for hip fractures in older people, even after controlling for factors such as physical activity, BMI, and calcium and vitamin D status.[97]

However, before recommending that older people consume more protein it is important to consider current dietary intakes and potential risk factors. A survey of 7207 community-dwelling adults in the United States revealed that the total energy intake declines with age but the mean percentage of energy as protein remains approximately 17% in both men and women.[91] Thus, habitual protein intake per unit of body mass tends to decline from 1.10 to 1.15 g protein/kg body mass/day in people 25 to 50 years of age to values of 0.88 g/kg/d in people over 75 years of age. The oldest people were also more likely to consume less than the RDA for protein; from the ages of 25 to 74 years, 20 to 30% of people were below the RDA but this figure rose to 40% of people over 75 years of age. Of note was that protein intake was not associated with morbidity in women, while in men protein intake below the RDA was associated with a small but significant increase in morbidity. In the United States, protein intake of older people is more likely to be inadequate in people living in rural areas and from lower socioeconomic groups.[98] In some populations, however, protein intakes have been shown to be much higher. A national survey of Germans over the age of 65 years revealed a median protein intake of 1.2 g/kg/d[99] with only 14 and 6% of people below 0.8 and 0.6 g/kg/d, respectively. Similar findings were reported in a study of older Spanish people.[100] A smaller study of 54 Japanese men and women, mean age 74 years, revealed that protein intake, mainly from seafood sources, was surprisingly high for both women (1.5 g/kg/d) and men (1.8 g/kg/d).[101]

There is so far no clear evidence that protein requirements adjusted for body mass and energy expenditure are different in younger and older people.[102–104] Older people, however, are at greater risk of acquiring inadequate dietary protein because, as noted above, the ratio of protein energy to total energy intake often remains stable as people decrease energy intake with age and sedentary lifestyle. Thus, while dietary protein intake should remain in the range of 0.8 to 1.0 g/kg/d for most adults, this requires that protein intake must account for an increasing percentage of calories consumed with advancing age.[93,103]

Increasing protein intake beyond 1 g/kg body weight/day has been shown to alter protein turnover in older people, but there is no evidence to date that this results in any beneficial effects on muscle mass or function. In a study by Pannemans, younger and older healthy men and women consumed diets containing either adequate protein (0.8 to 1.0 g/kg/d) or high protein (1.4 to 1.8 g/kg/d) for 3 weeks.[105] With the adequate protein diet both younger and older people were in nitrogen balance but whole body protein turnover rates were reduced in the older group. In comparison, the high protein diet resulted in higher rates of whole body protein turnover in both groups but nitrogen balance was only increased in the young. Measurements of muscle mass or strength were not reported in this study. Other studies are in agreement that increasing daily protein intake results in increased whole body protein turnover, including protein oxidation.[106,107] Once protein balance is achieved, consumption of additional protein is largely used as a fuel source. One group that may benefit from additional protein intake is frail elders. Chevalier and colleagues[108] studied a group of nine older women with diminished muscle mass but who still performed daily living activities with minimal assistance. When these women were switched from a diet containing 0.87 g protein/kg/d to an isoenergetic diet containing 1.23 g protein/kg/d for 12 days they experienced an improvement in nitrogen retention, although there were no changes in whole body protein turnover. Further work is required to determine whether a longer dietary intervention of increased protein consumption could stimulate gains in lean tissue or improve health in frail elderly people.

Measurements of protein metabolism in each of the above studies were performed in the resting state, typically in sedentary individuals. Physical activity and exercise training result in increased energy and protein requirements.[104,109] Millward[104] has proposed that accommodation to regular exercise occurs so that protein utilization becomes more efficient, resulting in slower rise in dietary protein needs with increasing levels of physical activity. For example, when older men performed resistance training for 12 weeks, nitrogen excretion decreased 10 to 15%, thereby lowering dietary requirements.[110] Half of the men in that study were fed a diet containing the RDA of 0.8 g protein/kg/d and the other half consumed twice that amount of protein. There was no apparent benefit on muscle strength or mass from consuming the higher protein intake. In fact, the most notable effect of the higher protein diet was increased protein oxidation. In another study, frail nursing home residents were randomized to a program of resistance exercise with or without a liquid meal supplement or given the meal supplement alone.[80] In both exercise groups there were significant increases in muscle mass and strength but no effect of the meal supplement. Welle and Thornton[111] found that acute consumption of meals containing 0.6, 1.2, or 2.4 g protein/kg body weight did not have a significant effect on rates of myofibrillar protein synthesis in older men and women following resistance exercise training.

An emerging concept of protein nutrition that may be beneficial for protein accretion in older people is manipulating the timing of protein meals. Arnal et al.[112] assigned older women to receive 80% of their daily protein intake at their mid-day meal or distributed over four smaller meals each day for 14 days. The group consuming the larger mid-day meal experienced greater protein retention during this short study. Timing of protein intake following exercise may also be important. It is well established that resistance training has an acute stimulatory effect on muscle protein synthesis and that consuming protein or amino acids can further enhance the protein synthesis response. When older men performing a 12-week resistance training program consumed a liquid meal supplement (10 g protein, 7 g carbohydrate, 3 g fat) immediately after each exercise session they were more likely to demonstrate increased leg muscle mass compared to men who waited 2 h after exercise to consume the supplement.[113] This was a small study though (only six to seven men per group), and muscle hypertrophy responses are known to vary among people so replication is needed. Still this promising finding highlights the value of consuming nutrients after exercise.

The structural composition of meal proteins is also important for regulating digestion rate, meal appearance, and protein retention. Boirie et al.[114] introduced the concept of "slow" and "fast" proteins, such as casein and whey, respectively, which when studied separately can be shown to leave the gut at different rates, in a manner that is analogous to simple (fast) vs. complex (slow) carbohydrates. In young men casein consumption produced a lower but more sustained increase in plasma amino acid levels and higher deposition of amino acids compared to whey protein.[115] However, older men demonstrated higher protein gain with the rapidly digested whey protein. Following meal ingestion the percentage of amino acids that are extracted by the splanchnic bed before appearing in the circulation is increased in older people.[116,117] Thus, consuming larger meals or faster-digesting proteins may be useful for older people to introduce more amino acids into the circulation for deposition in peripheral tissues.

One of the concerns of advocating high-protein diets for older people is the risk on renal function, which is often reduced with age.[118] Older patients with chronic renal insufficiency are often recommended to follow a reduced protein diet to avoid exacerbating their condition. This could be expected to result in deleterious loss of body protein stores but diet and exercise strategies may help ameliorate these events. In a controlled trial in older people with mild renal insufficiency, Bernhard et al.[119] reduced dietary protein intake from 1 to 0.7 g/kg/d over a 3-month period, but kept total energy intake close to 31 kcal/kg/d to maintain energy balance. Body mass was maintained and amino acid oxidation and appearance rate (a measure of protein breakdown) both declined, indicative of protein sparing. The authors proposed that the key to maintaining body protein stores is consuming sufficient energy so that amino acids are efficiently used for protein deposition and not as fuel. In another study, older people with mild renal insufficiency who had already adapted to a low protein diet (0.64 g/kg/d) were randomized to 12 weeks of resistance training or control activity.[120] Those in the exercise group had increased muscle fiber size and strength and maintained body weight compared to controls that lost weight. Careful selection and timing of dietary protein, coupled with exercise, are critical therapy for older people with diminished renal or liver function.

The selective use of amino acid supplements could also be valuable, especially for those with diminished renal or liver function and for persons on calorie restriction. The potential advantage is that the caloric density of an amino acid supplement should be less than either a protein or mixed meal supplement. Several studies have demonstrated that individual amino acids, particularly the branched-chain amino acids (BCAAs: leucine, isoleucine, valine), have stimulatory effects on muscle protein synthesis and inhibit protein breakdown.[38,121] BCAAs have also been shown to activate anabolic signaling pathways in muscle that result in regulated translation of specific gene transcripts.[122,123] Activation of these pathways, however, also results in reduced muscle glucose uptake during insulin stimulation, perhaps as a means to limit the uptake of nutrients.[124,125] Guillet et al.[126] recently showed that the inhibitory effect of hyperaminoacidemia on glucose disposal is blunted in older people compared to young people, but this is probably due to the fact that older people already had reduced insulin action on glucose metabolism at baseline.

There may be a benefit to glucose metabolism from increasing mixed amino acid or protein intake in older patients with poorly controlled diabetes. In a recent randomized, crossover trial, fasting insulin glucose and glycosylated hemoglobin were shown to decrease over a 4-month period when older men and women with diabetes consumed a liquid amino acid mixture twice per day.[130] It is important to point out that total energy intake was the same and protein intake remained at 15% of energy intake in both study phases so the amino acid mixture was a meal replacement, rather than a supplement. A similar reduction in glucose, insulin, and glycosylated hemoglobin was also demonstrated when older patients with untreated type 2 diabetes switched to a higher protein, low-carbohydrate diet for 5 weeks.[131] The benefit of these diets probably derives from the lower carbohydrate intake, which results in lower excursions in plasma glucose concentration following meals. It is also likely, although yet to be proven, that the additional energy from amino acids in these diets is used as an alternate fuel source. The interaction of these higher protein diets with diabetic medications has not yet been tested.

Volpi and colleagues have actively investigated the role of amino acid supplements in older people. They have shown that both oral and intravenous delivery of a 40-g mixture containing all 20 amino acids stimulates amino acid uptake into leg muscle over a 3-h period in older people.[127,128] While intriguing, this has not been a consistent finding.[124,129]

Consuming a supplement containing one or more of the essential amino acids (EAA) may be sufficient to stimulate muscle protein synthesis in the elderly. When older people received an infusion of either 18 g of EAA or 18 g EAA plus 22 g non-EAA, the resulting stimulation in muscle protein synthesis was similar,[132] implying that the EAA were sufficient for the effect and that the non-EAA had no additive effect despite the additional nitrogen intake. In a follow-up study, a 15-g dose of EAA was given orally and found to stimulate muscle protein synthesis rate in both young and older subjects.[133] How long the stimulatory effects of EAA last beyond the 3-h measurement period and whether the time course differs with age or dose has not been determined. Neither has it been determined if adding glucose to the EAA supplement results in the same blunted effect on protein synthesis in older people as occurred with mixed protein intake.[129] It also remains to be shown whether adding an EAA or individual amino acid supplement to normal meals would have a beneficial effect on muscle mass or function when consumed over several weeks or months. Controlled trials are needed given the potential value of amino acid supplementation.

In summary, it has been shown that up to 40% of older people do not consume the RDA of protein and many are probably not consuming adequate calories to maintain energy balance. Therefore, treatment strategy should be to assure that older individuals are regularly consuming between 0.8 and 1.0 g protein/kg body weight/day as this level has been shown to be adequate to maintain nitrogen balance. In some frail elderly people, 1.25 g protein/kg/d may be beneficial. In contrast, people with reduced renal or liver function need to reduce protein intake to 0.6 to 0.8 g/kg/d, but maintaining adequate energy intake and performing resistance training can help these patients preserve lean tissue mass. Recent studies have provided promising results that amino acid supplementation, particularly essential and branched-chain amino acids like leucine, stimulate muscle protein synthesis and might be valuable for older people. Further work is needed to determine if chronic amino acid supplementation has beneficial effects on muscle mass and function.

ADDITIONAL DIETARY SUPPLEMENT STRATEGIES IN TREATING SARCOPENIA

There are numerous dietary nutrients required for musculoskeletal health, many of which are described in detail in other chapters. Since oxidative stress may contribute to muscle loss through mechanisms described earlier, increasing intake of antioxidant nutrients may be of benefit, although largely unstudied. Here we briefly consider three nutrients that have attracted attention for their proposed usefulness in older adults.

Vitamin D has long been known to play an important role in bone metabolism, but recent data suggest that it may also be vital for maintaining muscle size and strength. In a study of 270 older community-dwelling Italian men and women, serum vitamin D levels were positively associated with muscle strength and self-reported physical performance in women, but not in men.[134] The prevalence of hypovitaminosis D (<37.5 nmol/l) was also higher in women (55% of those studied) than in men (35%). This sexual dimorphism was not observed in a larger study of 4100 American men and women aged between 60 and 90 years.[135] Subjects in this study were all living at home and ambulatory. The major finding was that after adjustment for variables such as age, calcium intake, and comorbidities, serum vitamin D levels were positively correlated with walking speed and the ability to perform repeated chair-rises. Functional ability on these tasks did not vary much for people with serum vitamin D above 40 nmol/l, but below this level there was a rapid decline in performance. Furthermore, in a prospective study of 1000 Dutch men and women over the age of 65 years, it was shown that after 3 years of follow-up people with low serum vitamin D concentration at baseline were up to two times more likely to develop a significant decline in grip strength and muscle mass.[136] Not all studies have shown equal promise,[137–140] because the role of vitamin D in muscle metabolism is currently being quantified (Chapter 10). In summary, prevalence of vitamin D insufficiency in older people is higher than generally appreciated and increased intakes could be useful.[141]

L-Carnitine is an essential cofactor for fatty acid transport into mitochondria where fats are oxidized. Carnitine deficiency is associated with decreased fat oxidation and muscle fatigue. A recent study in rats showed that carnitine levels in brain, muscle, and heart were reduced 20% in older animals compared to young.[142] Furthermore, dietary supplementation of carnitine (100 mg/kg/d) increased tissue carnitine concentration in old rats to levels comparable with young animals and had positive effects on plasma lipid profile.[142] Other studies showed that carnitine supplementation for 2 to 3 weeks increased the activity of mitochondrial respiratory enzymes in muscles from old but not young rats, suggesting that baseline carnitine levels were deficient in the older animals.[143,144] There are very little data available on the effects of age on muscle carnitine content in humans. One study showed that people over the age of 65 years who were undergoing surgery for hip fracture were more likely to have low muscle carnitine levels than healthy controls,[145] but it is difficult to determine whether muscle carnitine levels contributed to hip fracture, or decreased as a result of the injury. Another study performed on healthy men found no effect of age in muscle carnitine levels, although the groups compared had average ages of 27 and 49 years. Thus, a reduction in carnitine with advancing age cannot be excluded.[146] There may be a benefit of carnitine supplementation in older people but the available data to date on this topic are also limited. Pistone and colleagues[147] performed a randomized placebo-controlled study in older men and women, 70 to 92 years old, with muscle fatigue during daily activities. The group that received two grams of L-carnitine twice daily for 30 days had decreased body fat mass, increased lean tissue, positive changes in blood lipids, and less fatigue compared to baseline and control subjects taking the placebo. There were no reported side effects in the group that received L-carnitine.

Chromium is a trace mineral that has been shown to regulate insulin action and therefore can affect glucose metabolism and blood lipids. As described by Anderson,[148] when dietary chromium intake is low, diabetes and cardiovascular disease risk rise. Replacement of chromium to optimal levels has been shown to improve glucose tolerance and diabetes and it was proposed that chromium supplementation may stimulate muscle growth. Chromium supplementation is only beneficial if pretreatment levels are suboptimal and if the duration of treatment continues for at least 3 months (Chapter 9).[149–151]

GROWTH HORMONE AND MUSCLE MASS

The involvement of anabolic hormones and growth factors have long been implicated as regulators of sarcopenia because circulating levels of hormones such as growth hormone (GH), insulin-like growth hormone-I (IGF-I), testosterone, and dehydroepiandrosterone (DHEA) have pronounced reductions with age. In this section, the efficacy of hormone replacement for treatment of sarcopenia is considered.

It has been shown in some studies that GH administration in healthy older adults raises IGF-I levels and increases total body lean mass, muscle mass, and strength.[152–154] The effect of GH on muscle protein synthesis has been equivocal with one study showing a large increase in elderly women after a month of use,[153] while in another study there was no effect on muscle protein synthesis after 3 months of use of a slightly higher dose.[152] An important finding has been that the effects of GH on muscle anabolism are smaller when compared to resistance training. Furthermore, when combined with a resistance-training program GH replacement has shown little or no additional effect on gains in muscle size and strength or muscle protein synthesis rate.[87,88,155–158] GH use was discontinued in some subjects due to undesirable side effects and therefore there is currently less enthusiasm for GH replacement in older people compared to10 years ago. Still, there may be some benefit to using GH to reduce abdominal fat in patients with obesity. Franco and colleagues[159] reported that obese women who were treated with 0.67 mg GH/d for 12 months had reductions in abdominal fat and liver fat content, resulting in improved insulin sensitivity. These women also experienced an increase in leg muscle mass.

INSULIN-LIKE GROWTH HORMONE I AND MUSCLE MASS

Out of concern for the side effects associated with GH, there has been interest in administration of IGF-I, which is largely responsible for anabolic actions of GH. The presence of low levels of IGF-I in older women is associated with lower leg muscle strength and reduced walking speed.[160]

Infusion of IGF-I stimulates an acute increase in muscle amino acid uptake in humans.[161,162] The stimulatory effect IGF-I on protein synthesis during systemic infusion appears to be primarily in skeletal muscle compared to other tissues.[163] There are limited data on the effect of IGF-I replacement on skeletal muscle. A study performed in older women tested the effects of three doses given twice-daily for 4 weeks.[153] All three doses raised circulating IGF-I levels but only the two highest doses resulted in increased whole body and muscle protein synthesis. It was not reported if there were any changes in muscle strength or size, but some of the subjects experienced undesirable side effects at the higher doses. This same research team then studied a group of older women who took daily injections of the lower dose (0.015 mg/kg body weight twice daily) for 1 year.[164] Circulating IGF-I levels were increased almost fivefold, which is in the normal range for young women. However, there were no significant changes in lean mass or muscle strength and the authors reported that they ended the study early as a result. These findings suggest that neither GH nor IGF-I replacement may be viable treatment strategies for sarcopenia.

TESTOSTERONE AND MUSCLE MASS

The effects of testosterone replacement have been studied in men. Serum testosterone concentration is associated with lean mass and muscle strength[165] as well as the capacity to improve strength in response to resistance training in middle-aged and older men and women.[166,167] Because of the importance and the controversies regarding androgen replacement in men there are other more comprehensive reviews available with varied opinions on the usefulness of this approach.[168–170] In older men with low baseline testosterone, administration of daily injections to achieve levels comparable to young men has been shown to produce significant increases in muscle strength in trials lasting 1 to 6 months[171–173] and up to 36 months.[174] The effect of testosterone treatment on muscle protein metabolism is increased net protein balance, albeit through different mechanisms in different studies. In older men who received testosterone for 4 wk[171] and in younger hypogonadal men receiving testosterone for 6 months,[175] there were significant increases in muscle protein synthesis rate. In more recent studies lasting 6 months lean body mass and muscle volume were increased in older men receiving weekly injections of testosterone enanthate. No change in muscle protein synthesis rate was reported in those latter studies but muscle anabolism was achieved through decreased rate of protein breakdown.[172,176] These men also had increased IGF-I expression and decreased activity the ubiquitin–proteosome catabolism pathway, which may help explain the reduction in protein breakdown rate.

Studies by Bhasin and colleagues[177,178] have demonstrated that physiological outcomes to testosterone occur in a dose–response manner in both younger and older men. In their studies younger and older men with normal baseline testosterone levels were assigned to receive one of five doses of testosterone enanthate for 20 weeks (25 to 600 mg/week) and endogenous testosterone production was pharmacologically suppressed. The increase in body lean mass and leg muscle strength was positively related to testosterone dose and was similar in young and older men. The authors cautioned, however, that older men were more likely to experience side effects such as increased hematocrit, leg edema, and prostate problems, especially at the higher doses. Therefore, they suggested that the intermediate dose of 125 mg/week might have the best clinical application since this dose was sufficient to produce significant gains in muscle.

OXANDROLONE AND MUSCLE MASS

A related androgen that has shown some promise is the synthetic compound oxandrolone. Oxandrolone is an analog of testosterone that can be taken orally and appears to have greater anabolic and lower androgenic effects compared to testosterone.[179] Five days of oxandrolone (15 mg/d) use in young healthy men results in a significant increase in muscle protein synthesis[180] and the normal stimulation of protein synthesis rate by amino acid infusion is maintained.[181] Schroeder et al.[182,183] reported that administering a dose of 20 mg/d for 12 weeks resulted in proportional increases in muscle strength and size and reduced abdominal fat. When subjects were retested 12 weeks after stopping the oxandrolone use, fat reduction persisted, but gains in muscle strength and mass were lost. This implies that long-term use would be required to maintain benefits.

ESTROGEN AND MUSCLE MASS

Unlike the anabolic effect of testosterone replacement observed in men, estrogen replacement in older women does not appear to have a beneficial effect on muscle mass. Kenny et al.[184] measured limb muscle mass in postmenopausal women aged 59 to 78 years who had been using estrogen for at least 2 years. Women who used estrogen replacement had nearly the same prevalence of sarcopenia (23.8%, defined as 2 SD below the mean of a young reference group) as women who did not use estrogen (22.6%). Instead, the primary predictors of sarcopenia were BMI, muscle strength, and serum testosterone concentration. Other reports suggest that estrogen may provide some anabolic effects on muscle, but if so, the consensus is that this occurs through its conversion to testosterone.[185]

DHEA AND MUSCLE MASS

DHEA, produced primarily by the adrenal gland, is a weak androgenic steroid precursor for estrogen and testosterone and has the highest circulating concentration of any hormone in humans.[186] DHEA levels peak at age 20 years and then decline continuously during the adult lifespan leading to speculation that it may be somehow linked to a variety of age-related changes in body function.[187] Despite the fact that DHEA is a steroid precursor, not available in the human food chain, and is banned from use by international athletes out of concern that it may influence performance, the United States Food and Drug Administration removed restrictions on its commercial sale in 1994 following the passage of the Dietary and Supplement Health and Education Act. Although specific claims are not supposed to be included as a marketing tool for "nutritional" products, DHEA is widely touted as a potential antiaging compound, is widely available in shops, and more than 400,000 internet websites have some mention of DHEA.[187]

Whether DHEA replacement has any beneficial effects is far from clear. Until recently it has been difficult to determine if DHEA has any inherent biologic activity of its own or if it serves only as a precursor for other compounds. A specific DHEA receptor has not yet been identified, although evidence of binding activity and postreceptor signaling events has been shown in muscle and vascular epithelial cells.[188] Such observations have helped keep enthusiasm for the potential benefit of DHEA replacement high. Further interest in DHEA replacement arose from early studies in which rodents were given suprapharmacologic doses, resulting in some positive changes in body composition and modest improvement of longevity in short-lived mouse strains.[186] However, the relevance of DHEA studies in rodents has been sharply questioned because rodent adrenal glands do not produce DHEA and circulating levels are much lower than in humans.[221,222]

To date there is little or no evidence of beneficial effects of DHEA administration on skeletal muscle in humans. When young men performed an 8-week resistance training program, subjects who took a daily 150 mg dose of DHEA had no increase in serum testosterone and muscle strength improvement was not different from subjects given a placebo.[189] One could reason that the benefits of DHEA might be expected to be small in young men because endogenous DHEA levels are already at relatively high levels. However, muscle mass and strength were not increased in most of the clinical trials that have been conducted in older people.[187] One exception was a trial in which 16 men and women, aged 50 to 65 years, received 100 mg DHEA per day for 6 months.[190] In that study, there was a 6% decrease in body fat and a 15% increase in leg muscle strength in men only; in women body composition and muscle strength were unchanged, but women did have a 2% increase in body mass. Although intriguing, these findings need to be replicated in carefully controlled trials with larger numbers of participants followed beyond 6 months.

There may be beneficial effects of DHEA on other body tissues and functions besides muscle. Recently, it has been reported that DHEA administration (50 mg/d) for 6 months can decrease abdominal fat and increase insulin sensitivity in older people.[191] Likewise, DHEA replacement at 50 mg/d for 12 weeks in hypoadrenal women, who have an absence of basal DHEA production, has been shown to improve insulin-mediated glucose uptake.[192] These effects may be because of the action of DHEA on fat cells as it has been shown in cell culture studies that human adipose cells exposed to DHEA show increased glucose uptake via signaling mechanisms that appear to be distinct from insulin.[193]

DHEA replacement may also have a role in restoring the balance between circulating DHEA and cortisol. In some people DHEA levels fall with age more than cortisol, and in older people treated with glucocorticoids for inflammatory conditions the DHEA-to-cortisol ratio can also decrease, creating a potentially catabolic hormonal milieu.[194] When older people were given a high dose of DHEA (200 mg/d) for 4 weeks, both mean and peak 24-h cortisol levels were reduced.[195] When older men with partial androgen deficiency used a smaller dose (25 mg/d) for 1 year, there were increased levels of several hormones, including serum GH, IGF-I, and testosterone, but cortisol levels remained unchanged, therefore creating a large shift in the DHEA-to-cortisol ratio. In this latter study, indices of body composition were not reported but there were improvements in mood, fatigue, and joint pain.[196]

As a final note on hormone replacement, there appear to be some potential benefits in selected patients, especially in those with clearly defined hormone deficiencies. Effects on skeletal muscle mass and function in older people have been mixed, with testosterone showing the most frequent positive effects. However, as recommended in other recent reviews,[168,197] when interpreting existing data one must consider that most of the randomized, controlled trials to date have been performed in relatively healthy people. Positive effects on overall health and function in older men may be small and side effects are dose dependent.[168] Ongoing and future clinical trials will need to carefully monitor long-term safety issues and determine when hormone replacement is most warranted.

SUMMARY AND RECOMMENDATIONS

The prevalence of sarcopenia increases with age and is closely associated with risk for obesity, physical disability, and falls. Identifying at-risk individuals can be done through assessing muscle mass and strength using body composition measurements and clinical exam testing.

Better understanding of the mechanisms that regulate the decline in skeletal muscle size, strength, and oxidative capacity will translate into clinical recommendations to break the "vicious loops" that interconnect sarcopenia with malnutrition, loss of body protein reserves, reduced protein synthesis, neuromuscular impairment, fall and fractures, and immobilization in a type of feed-forward progression.[198]

The most effective means of maintaining or increasing muscle mass and function is through exercise: resistance training for improving size and strength, and aerobic training for improving oxidative metabolic function. Nutrition is necessary both to repair exercising muscles and protect muscle from oxidative damage potentially induced by exercise. While exercise and nutrition both alter the hormonal environment, there may be a role for exogenous hormone treatment as well, to restore age-appropriate physiologic hormone levels.

REFERENCES

1. Lindle, R.S., Metter, E.J., Lynch, N.A., Fleg, J.L., Fozard, J.L., Tobin, J., Roy, T.A., and Hurley, B.F., Age and gender comparisons of muscle strength in 654 women and men aged 20–93 years, *J. Appl. Physiol.*, 83, 1581–1587, 1997.
2. Larsson, L., Grimby, G., and Karlsson, J., Muscle strength and speed of movement in relation to age and muscle morphology, *J. Appl. Physiol.*, 46, 451–456, 1979.
3. Larsson, L., Karlsson, J., Isometric and dynamic endurance as a function of age and skeletal muscle characteristics.,*Acta Physiol. Scand.*, 104, 129–136, 1978.
4. Izquierdo, M., Ibanez, J., Gorostiaga, E., Garrues, M., Zuniga, A., Anton, A., Larrion, J.L., and Hakkinen, K., Maximal strength and power characteristics in isometric and dynamic actions of the upper and lower extremities in middle-aged and older men, *Acta Physiol. Scand.*, 167, 57–68, 1999.
5. Janssen, I., Heymsfield, S.B., Wang, Z., and Ross, R., Skeletal muscle mass and distribution in 468 men and women aged 18–88 years. J Appl Physiol 2000; 89:81–88.
6. Baumgartner, R.N., Koehler, K.M., Gallagher, D., Romero, L., Heymsfield, S.B., Ross, R.R., Garry, P.J., and Lindeman, R.D., Epidemiology of sarcopenia among the elderly in New Mexico, *Am. J. Epidemiol.*, 147, 755–763, 1998.

7. Klitgaard, H., Mantoni, M., Schiaffino, S., Ausoni, S., Gorza, L., Laurent-Winter, C., Schnohr, P., and Saltin, B., Function, morphology and protein expression of ageing skeletal muscle: a cross-sectional study of elderly men with different training backgrounds, *Acta Physiol. Scand.*, 140, 41–54, 1990.

8. Lynch, N.A., Metter, E.J., Lindle, R.S., Fozard, J.L., Tobin, J., Roy, T.A., Fleg, J.L., and Hurley, B.F., Muscle quality. I. Age-associated differences between arm and leg muscle groups, *J. Appl. Physiol.*, 86, 188–194, 1999.

9. Metter, E.J., Conwitt, R., Tobin, J., and Fozard, J.L., Age-associated loss of power and strength in the upper extremities in women and men, *J. Gerontol. A: Biol. Sci. Med. Sci.*, 52, B267–B276, 1997.

10. Short, K.R., Vittone, J.L., Bigelow, M.L., Proctor, D.N., Coenen-Schimke, J., Rys, P., and Nair, K.S., Changes in myosin heavy chain mRNA and protein expression in human skeletal muscle with age and endurance exercise training, *J. Appl. Physiol.*, 2005, in press.

11. Newman, A., Kupelian, V., Visser, M., Simonsick, E., Goodpaster, B., Nevitt, M., Kritchevsky, S., Tylavsky, F., Rubin, S., Harris, T., Investigators HAS, Sarcopenia: alternative definitions and associations with lower extremity function, *J. Am. Geriatr. Soc.*, 51, 1602–1609, 2003.

12. Short, K.R. and Nair, K.S., Mechanisms of sarcopenia of aging, *J. Endocrinol. Invest.*, 22, 95–105, 1999.

13. Short, K.R., Vittone, J.L., Bigelow, M.L., Proctor, D.N., Rizza, R.R., Coenen-Schimke, J.M., and Nair, K.S., Impact of aerobic training on age-related changes in insulin action and muscle oxidative capacity, *Diabetes*, 52, 1888–1896, 2003.

14. Gallagher, D., Ruts, E., Visser, M., Heshka, S., Baumgartner, R.N., Wang, J., Pierson, R.N., Pi-Suyner, F.X., and Heymsfield, S.B., Weight stability masks sarcopenia in elderly men and women, *J. Appl. Physiol.*, 279, E366–E375, 2000.

15. Khort, W.M., Kirwin, J.P., Staten, M.A., Bourey, R.E., King, D.S., and Holloszy, J.O., Insulin resistance in aging is related to abdominal obesity, *Diabetes*, 42, 273–281, 1993.

16. Basu, R., Breda, E., Oberg, A.L., Powell, C.C., Dalla Man, C., Basu, A., Vittone, J.L., Klee, G,G., Arora, P., Jensen, M.D., Toffolo, G., Cobelli, C., and Rizza, R.A., Mechanisms of the age-associated deterioration in glucose tolerance: contribution of alterations in insulin secretion, action, and clearance, *Diabetes*, 52, 1738–1748, 2003.

17. Goodpaster, B.H., Carlson, C.L., Visser, M., Kelley, D.E., Scherzinger, A., Harris, T.B., Stamm, E., and Newman, A.B., Attenuation of skeletal muscle and strength in the elderly: The Health ABC Study, *J. Appl. Physiol.*, 90, 2157–2165, 2001.

18. Song, M., Ruts, E., Kim, J., Janumala, I., Heymsfield, S., and Gallagher, D., Sarcopenia and increased adipose tissue infiltration of muscle in elderly African American women, *Am. J. Clin. Nutr.*, 79, 874–880, 2004.

19. Baumgartner, R.N., Wayne, S.J., Waters, D.L., Janssen, I., Gallagher, D., Morley, J.E., Sarcopenic obesity predicts instrumental activities of daily living disability in the elderly, *Obes. Res.*, 12, 1995–2004, 2004.

20. Iannuzzi-Sucich, M., Prestwood, K., and Kenny, A., Prevalence of sarcopenia and predictors of skeletal muscle mass in healthy, older men and women, *J. Gerontol. A: Biol. Sci. Med. Sci.*, 57, M772–M777, 2002.

21. Janssen, I., Heymsfield, S.B., and Ross, R., Low relative skeletal muscle mass (sarcopenia) in older persons is associated with functional impairment and physical disability, *J. Am. Geriatr. Soc.*, 50, 889–896, 2004.

22. Janssen, I., Baumgartner, R., Ross, R., Rosenberg, I., and Roubenoff, R., Skeletal muscle cutpoints associated with elevated physical disability risk in older men and women, *Am. J. Epidemiol.*, 159, 413–421, 2004.

23. Rantanen, T., Guralnik, J.M., Sakari-Rantala, R., Leveille, S., Simonsick, E.M., Ling, S., and Fried, L.P., Disability, physical activity, and muscle strength in older women: the women's health and aging study, *Arch. Phys. Med. Rehabil.*, 80, 130–135, 1999.

24. Liu, L., Bopp, M.M., Roberson, P.K., and Sullivan, D.H., Undernutrition and risk of mortality in elderly patients within 1 year of hospital discharge, *J. Gerontol. A: Biol. Sci. Med. Sci.*, 57, M741–M746, 2002.

25. Mathus-Vliegen, E.M.H., Old age, malnutrition, and pressure sores: an ill-fated alliance, *J. Gerontol. A: Biol. Sci. Med. Sci.*, 59, 355–360, 2004.

26. Short, K.R., Bigelow, M.L., Kahl, J., Singh, R., Coenen-Schimike, J., Raghavikaimal, S., and Nair, K.S., Decline in skeletal muscle mitochondrial function with aging in humans, *Proc. Natl. Acad. Sci. USA*, 2005, in press.

27. Hepple, R.T., Hagan, J.L., Krause, D.J., and Jackson, C.C., Aerobic power declines with aging in rat skeletal muscles perfused at matched convective O_2 delivery, *J. Appl. Physiol.*, 94, 744–751, 2002.

28. Haseler, L.J., Lin, A.P., and Richardson, R.S., Skeletal muscle oxidative metabolism in sedentary humans: ^{31}P-MRS assessment of O_2 supply and demand limitations, *J. Appl. Physiol.*, 97, 1077–1081, 2004.

29. Trappe, S.W., Costill, D.L., Vukovich, M.D., Jones, J., and Melham, T., Aging among elite distance runners: a 22-year longitudinal study, *J. Appl. Physiol.*, 80, 285–290, 1996.

30. Tanaka, H., DeSouza, C.A., Jones, P.P., Stevenson, E.T., Davy, K.P., and Seals, D.R., Greater rate of decline in maximal aerobic capacity with age in physically active vs. sedentary healthy women, *J. Appl. Physiol.*, 83, 1947–1953, 1997.

31. Petersen, K.F., Befoy, D., Dufour, S., Dziura, J., Ariyan, C., Rothman, D.L., DiPietro, L., Cline, G.W., and Shulman, G.I., Mitochondrial dysfunction in the elderly: possible role in insulin resistance, *Science*, 300, 1140–1142, 2003.

32. Kelley, D.E., He, J., Menshikova, E.V., and Ritov, V.B., Dysfunction of mitochondria in human skeletal muscle in type 2 diabetes, *Diabetes*, 51, 2944–2950, 2002.

33. Petersen, K.F., Dufour, S., Befroy, D., Garcia, R., and Shulman, G.I., Impaired mitochondrial activity in the insulin-resistant offspring of patients with type 2 diabetes, *N. Engl. J. Med.*, 350, 664–671, 2004.

34. Ritov, V.B., Menshikova, E.V., He, J., Ferrell, R.E., Goodpaster, B.H., and Kelley, D.E., Deficiency of subsarcolemmal mitochondria in obesity and type 2 diabetes, *Diabetes*, 54, 8–14, 2005.

35. Kelley, D.E. and Goodpaster, B.H., Skeletal muscle triglyceride: an aspect of regional adiposity and insulin resistance, *Diabetes Care*, 24, 933–941, 2001.

36. Short, K.R., Vittone, J.L., Bigelow, M.L., Proctor, D.N., and Nair, K.S., Age and aerobic exercise training effects on whole body and muscle protein metabolism, *Am. J. Physiol. Endocrinol. Metab.*, 286, E92–E101, 2004.

37. Balagopal, P., Rooyackers, O.E., Adey, D.B., Ades, P.A., and Nair, K.S., Effects of aging on in vivo synthesis of skeletal muscle myosin heavy-chain and sarcoplasmic protein in humans, *Am. J. Physiol. Endocrinol. Metab.*, 273, E790–E800, 1997.

38. Nair, K.S., Halliday, D., and Griggs, R.C., Leucine incorporation into mixed skeletal muscle protein in humans, *Am. J. Physiol. Endocrinol. Metab.*, 254, E208–E213, 1988.

39. Garlick, P.J., McNurlan, M.A., and Caso, G., Critical assessment of methods used to measure protein synthesis in human subjects, *Yale J. Biol. Med.*, 70, 65–76, 1997.

40. Baumann, P.Q., Stirewalt, W.S., O'Rourke, B.D., Howard, D., and Nair, K.S., Precursor pools of protein synthesis: a stable isotope study in a swine model, *Am. J. Physiol. Endocrinol. Metab.*, 267, E203–E209, 1994.

41. Charlton, M., Ahlman, B., and Nair, K.S., The effect of insulin on human small intestinal mucosal protein synthesis, *Gastroenterology*, 118, 299–306, 2000.

42. Meek, S.E., Persson, M., Ford, G.C., and Nair, K.S., Differential regulation of amino acid exchange and protein dynamics across splanchnic and skeletal muscle beds by insulin in healthy human subjects, *Diabetes*, 47, 1824–1835, 1998.

43. Nygren, J. and Nair, K.S., Differential regulation of protein dynamics in splanchnic and skeletal muscle beds by insulin and amino acids in healthy human subjects, *Diabetes*, 52, 1377–1385, 2003.

44. Yarasheski, K.E., Zachwieja, J.J., and Bier, D.M., Acute effects of resistance exercise on muscle protein synthesis rate in young and elderly men and women, *Am. J. Physiol. Endocrinol. Metab.*, 265, E210–E214, 1993.

45. Welle, S., Thornton, C., Jozefowicz, R., Statt, M., Myofibrillar protein synthesis in young and old men, *Am. J. Physiol. Endocrinol. Metab.*, 264, E693–E698, 1993.

46. Welle, S., Thornton, C., Statt, M., and McHenry, B., Postprandial myofibrillar and whole body protein synthesis in young and old human subjects, *Am. J. Physiol. Endocrinol. Metab.*, 267, E599–E604, 1994.

47. Hasten, D.L., Pak-Loduca, J., Obert, K.A., and Yarasheski, K.E., Resistance exercise acutely increases MHC and mixed muscle protein synthesis rates in 78–84 and 23–32 year olds, *Am. J. Physiol. Endocrinol. Metab.*, 278, E620–E626, 2000.

48. Volpi, E., Sheffield-Moore, M., Rasmussen, B., and Wolfe, R.R., Basal muscle amino acid kinetics and protein synthesis in healthy young and older men, *JAMA*, 286, 1206–1212, 2001.

49. Volpi, E., Rasmussen, B., Sheffield-Moore, M., and Wolfe, R.R., Muscle protein synthesis in younger and older men (reply), *JAMA*, 287, 318, 2002.

50. Mecocci, P., Fano, G., Fulle, S., MacGarvey, U., Shinobu, L., Polidori, M.C., Cherubini, A., Vecchiet, J., Senin, U., and Beal, M.F., Age-dependent increases in oxidative damage to DNA, lipids, and proteins in human skeletal muscle, *Free Radic. Biol. Med.*, 26, 303–308, 1999.

51. Pesce, V., Cormio, A., Fracasso, F., Vecchiet, J., Felzani, G., Lezza, A.M.S., Cantatore, P., and Gadaleta, M.N., Age-related mitochondrial genotypic and phenotypic alterations in human skeletal muscle, *Free Radic. Biol. Med.*, 30, 1223–1233, 2001.

52. Michikawa, Y., Mazzucchelli, F., Bresolin, N., Scarlato, G., and Attardi, G., Aging-dependent large accumulation of point mutations in the human mtDNA control region for replication, *Science*, 286, 774–779, 1999.

53. Hamilton, M.L., Van Remmen, H., Drake, J.A., Yang, H., Guo, Z.M., Kewitt, K., Walter, C.A., and Richardson, A., Does oxidative damage to DNA increase with age? *Proc. Natl. Acad. Sci. USA*, 98, 10469–10474, 2001.

54. Wei, Y.-H., Oxidative stress and mitochondrial DNA mutations in human aging, *Proc. Soc. Exp. Biol. Med.*, 217, 53–63, 1998.

55. Grune, T., Shringarpure, R., Sitte, N., and Davies, K., Age-related changes in protein oxidation and proteolysis in mammalian cells, *J. Gerontol. A: Biol. Sci. Med. Sci.*, 56, B459–B467, 2001.

56. Bassett, C.N. and Montine, T.J., Lipoproteins and lipid peroxidation in Alzheimer's disease, *J. Nutr. Health Aging*, 7, 24–29, 2003.
57. Pansarasa, O., Bertorelli, L., Vecchiet, J., Felzani, G., and Marzatico, F., Age-dependent changes of antioxidant activities and markers of free radical damage in human skeletal muscle, *Free Radic. Biol. Med.*, 27, 617–622, 1999.
58. Liu, J., Head, E., Gharib, A.M., Yuan, W., Ingersoll, R.T., Hagen, T.M., Cotman, C.W., and Ames, B.N., Memory loss in old rats is associated with brain mitochondrial decay and RNA/DNA oxidation: partial reversal by feeding acetyl-L-carnitine and/or R-alpha-lipoic acid, *Proc. Natl. Acad. Sci. USA*, 99, 2356–2361, 2002.
59. Hagen, T.M., Liu, J., Lykkesfeldt, J., Wehr, C.M., Ingersoll, R.T., Vinarsky, V., Bartholomew, J.C., and Ames, B.N., Feeding acetyl-L-carnitine and lipoic acid to old rats significantly improves metabolic function while decreasing oxidative stress, *Proc. Natl. Acad. Sci. USA*, 99, 1870–1875, 2002.
60. Sumien, N., Forster, M.J., and Sohal, R.S., Supplementation with vitamin E fails to attenuate oxidative damage in aged mice, *Exp. Gerontol.*, 38, 699–704, 2003.
61. Leeuwenburgh, C., Hansen, P., Shaish, A., Holloszy, J.O., and Heinecke, J.W., Markers of protein oxidation by hydroxyl radical and reactive nitrogen species in tissues of aging rats, *Am. J. Physiol. Regul. Integr. Comp. Physiol.*, 274, R453–R461, 1998.
62. Lexell, J., Taylor, C., and Sjostrom, M., What is the cause of the aging atrophy? Total number, size and proportion of different fibre types studied in whole vastus lateralis muscle from 15- to 83-year old men, *J. Neurol. Sci.*, 84, 275–294, 1988.
63. Lexell, J. and Downham, D., What is the effect of ageing on type 2 muscle fibres? *J. Neurol. Sci.*, 107, 250–251, 1992.
64. Balice-Gordon, R.J., Age-related changes in neuromuscular innervation, *Muscle Nerve*, Suppl. 5, S83–S87, 1997.
65. Ansved, T. and Larsson, L., Quantitative and qualitative morphological properties of the soleus motor nerve and the L5 ventral root in young and old rats. Relation to the number of soleus muscle fibres, *J. Neurol. Sci.*, 96, 269–282, 1990.
66. Doherty, T.J., Invited review: aging and sarcopenia, *J. Appl. Physiol.*, 95, 1717–1727, 2003.
67. Kinney, J.M., Nutritional frailty, sarcopenia and falls in the elderly, *Curr. Opin. Clin. Nutr. Metab. Care.*, 7, 15–20, 2004.
68. Dengel, D.R., Pratley, R.E., Hagberg, J.M., Rogus, E.M., and Goldberg, A.P., Distinct effects of aerobic exercise training and weight loss on glucose homeostasis in obese sedentary men, *J. Appl. Physiol.*, 81, 318–325, 1996.
69. Ryder, J.W., Chibalin, A.V., and Zierath, J.R., Intracellular mechanisms underlying increases in glucose uptake in response to insulin or exercise in skeletal muscle, *Acta Physiol. Scand.*, 171, 249–257, 2001.
70. Zierath, J.R., He, L., Guma, A., Wahlstrom, E., Klip, A., and Wallberg-Henriksson, H., Insulin action on glucose transport and plasma membrane GLUT4 content in skeletal muscle from patients with NIDDM, *Diabetologia*, 39, 1180–1189, 1996.
71. Garvey, W.T., Maianu, L., Zhu, J.H., Brechtel-Hook, G., Wallace, P., and Baron, A.D., Evidence for defects in the trafficking and translocation of GLUT4 glucose transporters in skeletal muscle as a cause of human insulin resistance, *J. Clin. Invest.*, 101, 2377–2386, 1998.
72. Booth, F.W., Molecular and cellular adaptation of muscle in response to exercise: perspectives of various models, *Physiol. Rev.*, 71, 541–585, 1991.

73. Holloszy, J.O., Effects of exercise on mitochondrial oxygen uptake and respiratory enzyme activity in skeletal muscle, *J. Biol. Chem.*, 242, 2278–2282, 1967.

74. Coggan, A.R., Spina, R.J., King, D.S., Rogers, M.A., Brown, M., Nemeth, P.M., and Holloszy, J.O., Skeletal muscle adaptations to endurance training in 60- to 70-year-old men and women, *J. Appl. Physiol.*, 72, 1780–1786, 1992.

75. Proctor, D.N., Sinning, W.E., Walro, J.M., Sieck, G.C., and Lemon, P.W., Oxidative capacity of human muscle fiber types: effects of age and training status, *J. Appl. Physiol.*, 78, 2033–2038, 1995.

76. Hurley, B.F. and Hagberg, J.M., Optimizing health in older persons: aerobic or strength training? *Exer. Sport Sci. Rev.*, 26, 61–90, 1998.

77. Sheffield-Moore, M., Yeckel, C.W., Volpi, E., Wolf, S.E., Morio, B., Chinkes, D.L., Paddon-Jones, D., and Wolfe, R.R., Postexercise protein metabolism in older and younger men following moderate-intensity aerobic exercise, *Am. J. Physiol. Endocrinol. Metab.*, 287, E513–E522, 2004.

78. Hunter, G., McCarthy, J., and Bamman, M., Effects of resistance training on older adults, *Sports Med.*, 34, 329–348, 2004.

79. Macaluso, A. and De Vito, G., Muscle strength, power and adaptations to resistance training in older people, *Eur. J. Appl. Physiol.*, 91, 450–472, 2004.

80. Fiatrone, M.A., O'Neill, E.F., Ryan, N.D., Clements, K.M., Solares, G.R., Nelson, M.E., Roberts, S.B., Kehayias, J.J., Lipsitz, L.A., and Evans, W.J., Exercise training and nutritional supplementation for physical frailty in very elderly people, *N. Engl. J. Med.*, 330, 1769–1775, 1994.

81. Fiatarone, M.A., Marks, E.C., Ryan, N., Meredith, C.N., Lipsitz, L.A., and Evans, W.J., High-intensity strength training in nonagenarians. Effects on skeletal muscle, *JAMA*, 263, 3029–3034, 1990.

82. Frontera, W.R., Meredith, C.N., O'Reilly, K.P., Evans, W.J., Strength conditioning in older men: skeletal muscle hypertrophy and improved function, *J. Appl. Physiol.*, 64, 1038–1044, 1988.

83. Sale, D.G., MacDougall, J.D., Jacobs, I., and Garner, S., Interaction between concurrent strength and endurance training, *J. Appl. Physiol.*, 68, 260–270, 1990.

84. Sipila, S. and Suominen, H., Effects of strength and endurance training on thigh and leg muscle mass and composition in elderly women, *J. Appl. Physiol.*, 78, 334–340, 1995.

85. Welle, S., Thornton, C., and Statt, M., Myofibrillar protein synthesis in young and old human subjects after three months of resistance training, *Am. J. Physiol. Endocrinol. Metab.*, 268, E422–E427, 1995.

86. Yarasheski, K.E., Pak-Loduca, J., Hasten, D.L., Obert, K.A., Brown, M.B., and Sinacore, D.R., Resistance exercise training increases mixed muscle protein synthesis rate in frail women and men = 76 years old, *Am. J. Physiol. Endocrinol. Metab.*, 277, E118–E125, 1999.

87. Yarasheski, K.E., Zachwieja, J.J., Campbell, J.A., and Bier, D.M., Effect of growth hormone and resistance exercise on muscle growth and strength in older men, *Am. J. Physiol. Endocrinol. Metab.*, 268, E268–E276, 1995.

88. Yarasheski, K.E., Campbell, J.A., Smith, K., Rennie, M.J., Holloszy, J.O., and Bier, D.M., Effect of growth hormone and resistance exercise on muscle growth in young men, *Am. J. Physiol. Endocrinol. Metab.*, 262, E261–E267, 1992.

89. Tipton, K.D. and Wolfe, R.R., Exercise-induced changes in protein metabolism, *Acta Physiol. Scand.*, 162, 377–387, 1998.

90. Morley, J., Anorexia, sarcopenia, and aging, *Nutrition*, 17, 660–663, 2001.

91. Kant, A.K. and Schatzkin, A., Relation of age and self-reported chronic medical condition status with dietary nutrient intake in the US population, *J. Am. Coll. Nutr.*, 18, 69–76, 1999.

92. Food and Nutrition Board Institute of Medicine, Protein and amino acids, in *Dietary Reference Intakes for Energy, Carbohydrates, Fiber, Fat, Protein and Amino Acids*, Institute of Medicine, Ed., The National Academies Press, Washington, DC, 2002, pp. 465–608.

93. Beaufrere, B., Castaneda, C., de Groot, L., Kurpad, A., Roberts, S., and Tessari, P., Report of the IDECG working group on energy and macronutrient metabolism and requirements of the elderly, *Eur. J. Clin. Nutr.*, 54, S162–S163, 2000.

94. Campbell, W.W., Trappe, T.A., Wolfe, R.R., and Evans, W.J., The recommended dietary allowance for protein may not be adequate for people to maintain skeletal muscle, *J. Gerontol. A: Biol. Sci. Med. Sci.*, 56, M373–M380, 2001.

95. Campbell, W., Crim, M., Dallal, G., Young, V., and Evans, W., Increased protein requirements in elderly people: new data and retrospective reassessments, *Am. J. Clin. Nutr.*, 60, 501–509, 1994.

96. Morse, M., Haub, M., Evans, W., and Campbell, W., Protein requirement of elderly women: nitrogen balance responses to three levels of protein intake, *J. Gerontol. A: Biol. Sci. Med. Sci.*, 56, M724–M730, 2001.

97. Wengreen, H.J., Munger, R.G., West, N.A., Cutler, D.R., Corcoran, C.D., Zhang, J., and Sassano, N.E., Dietary protein intake and risk of osteoporotic hip fracture in elderly residents of Utah, *J. Bone Miner. Res.*, 19, 537–545, 2004.

98. Lewis, S.M., Mayhugh, M.A., Freni, S.C., Cardoso, S.S., Buffington, C., Jairaj, K., Turturro, A., and Feuers, R.J., Assessment and significance of 24-h energy intake patterns among young and aged non-affluent southern US women, *J. Nutr. Health Aging*, 7, 78–83, 2003.

99. Volkert, D., Kreuel, K., Heseker, H., and Stehle, P., Energy and nutrient intake of young-old, old-old and very-old elderly in Germany, *Eur. J. Clin. Nutr.*, 58, 1190–1200, 2004.

100. Garcia-Arias, M.T., Villarino Rodriguez, A., Garcia-Linares, M.C., Rocandio, A.M., and Garcia-Fernandez, M.C., Daily intake of macronutrients in a group of institu-tionalized elderly people in Leon, Spain, *Nutricion Hospitalaria*, 18, 87090, 2003.

101. Watanabe, R., Hanamori, K., Kadoya, H., Nishimuta, M., and Miyazaki, H., Nutritional intakes in community-dwelling older Japanese adults: high intakes of energy and protein based on high consumption of fish, vegetables and fruits provide sufficient micronutrients, *J. Nutr. Sci. Vitaminol.*, 50, 184–195, 2004.

102. Kurpad, A. and Vaz, M., Protein and amino acid requirements in the elderly, *Eur. J. Clin. Nutr.*, 54 (Suppl. 3), S131–S142, 2000.

103. Millward, D.J., Macronutrient intakes as determinants of dietary protein and amino acid adequacy, *J. Nutr.*, 134, 1588S–1596S, 2004.

104. Millward, D.J., Protein and amino acid requirements of adults: current controver-sies, *Can. J. Appl. Physiol.*, 26, S130–S140, 2001.

105. Pannemans, D.L.E., Halliday, D., Westerterp, K.R., and Kester, A.D.M., Effect of variable protein intake on whole-body protein turnover in young men and women, *Am. J. Clin. Nutr.*, 61, 69–74, 1995.

106. Young, V.R., El-Khoury, A.E., Raguso, C.A., Forslund, A.H., and Hambraeus, L., Rates of urea production and hydrolysis and leucine oxidation change linearly over widely varying protein intakes in healthy adults, *J. Nutr.*, 130, 761–766, 2000.

107. Gibson, N.R., Fereday, A., Cox, M., Halliday, D., Pacy, P.J., and Millward, D.J., Influences of dietary energy and protein on leucine kinetics during feeding in healthy adults, *Am. J. Physiol. Endocrinol. Metab.*, 270, E282–E291, 1996.

108. Chevalier, S., Gougeon, R., Nayar, K., and Morais, J.A., Frailty amplifies the effects of aging on protein metabolism: role of protein intake, *Am. J. Clin. Nutr.*, 78, 422–429, 2003.

109. Tarnopolsky, M.A., Atkinson, S.A., MacDougall, J.D., Chesley, A., Phillips, S., and Schwarcz, H.P., Evaluation of protein requirements for trained strength athletes, *J. Appl. Physiol.*, 73, 1986–1995, 1992.

110. Campbell, W.W., Crim, M.C., Young, V.R., Joseph, L.J., and Evans, W.J., Effects of resistance training and dietary protein intake on protein metabolism in older adults, *Am. J. Physiol. Endocrinol. Metab.*, 268, E1143–E1153, 1995.

111. Welle, S. and Thornton, C.A., High-protein meals do not enhance myofibrillar synthesis after resistance exercise in 62- to 75-year-old men and women, *Am. J. Physiol. Endocrinol. Metab.*, 274, E677–E683, 1998.

112. Arnal, M., Mosoni, L., Boirie, Y., Houlier, M., Morin, L., Verdier, E., Ritz, P., Antoine, J., Prugnaud, J., Beaufrere, B., and Mirand, P., Protein pulse feeding improves protein retention in elderly women, *Am. J. Clin. Nutr.*, 69, 1202–1208, 1999.

113. Esmarck, B., Andersen, J.L., Olsen, S., Richter, E.A., Mizuno, M., and Kjaer, M., Timing of postexercise protein intake is important for muscle hypertrophy with resistance training in elderly humans, *J. Physiol.*, 535, 301–311, 2001.

114. Boirie, Y., Dangin, M., Gachon, P., Vasson, M.-P., Maubois, J.-L., and Beaufrere, B., Slow and fast dietary proteins differently modulate postprandial protein accretion, *Proc. Natl. Acad. Sci. USA*, 94, 14930–14935, 1997.

115. Dangin, M., Guillet, C., Garcia-Rodenas, C., Gachon, P., Bouteloup-Demange, C., Reiffers-Magnani, K., Fauquant, J., Ballevre, O., and Beaufrere, B., The rate of protein digestion affects protein gain differently during aging in humans, *J. Physiol.*, 549, 635–644, 2003.

116. Boirie, Y., Gachon, P., and Beaufrere, B., Splanchnic and whole-body leucine kinetics in young and elderly men, *Am. J. Clin. Nutr.*, 65, 489–495, 1997.

117. Volpi, E., Mittendorfer, B., Wolf, S.E., and Wolfe, R.R., Oral amino acids stimulate muscle protein anabolism in the elderly despite higher first-pass splanchnic extraction, *Am. J. Physiol. Endocrinol. Metab.*, 277, E513–E520, 1999.

118. Fliser, D., Zeier, M., Nowack, R., and Ritz, E., Renal functional reserve in healthy elderly subjects, *J. Am. Soc. Nephrol.*, 3, 1371–1377, 1993.

119. Bernhard, J., Beaufrere, B., Laville, M., and Fouque, D., Adaptive response to a low-protein diet in predialysis chronic renal failure patients, *J. Am. Soc. Nephrol.*, 12, 1249–1254, 2001.

120. Castaneda, C., Gordon, P.L., Uhlin, K.L., Levey, A.S., Kehayias, J.J., Dwyer, J.T., Fielding, R.A., Roubenoff, R., and M.F. S., Resistance training to counteract the catabolism of a low-protein diet in patients with chronic renal insufficiency. A randomized, controlled trial, *Ann. Intern. Med.*, 135, 975–976, 2001.

121. Nair, K.S. and Short, K.R., Hormonal and signaling role of amino acids, *J. Nutr.*, 2005, in press.

122. Kimball, S.R. and Jefferson, L.S., Amino acids as regulators of gene expression, *Nutr. Metab.*, 1, 2004; http://www.nutritionandmetabolism.com/content/1/1/3 (last accessed January 24, 2004).

123. Kimball, S.R. and Jefferson, L.S., Molecular mechanisms through which amino acids mediate signaling through the mammalian target of rapamycin, *Curr. Opin. Clin. Nutr. Metab. Care*, 7, 39–44, 2004.

124. Nair, K.S., Matthews, D.E., Welle, S.L., and Braiman, T., Effect of leucine on amino acid and glucose metabolism in humans, *Metabolism*, 41, 643–648, 1992.

125. Patti, M.-E., Brambilla, E., Luzi, L., Landaker, E.J., and Ronald Kahn, C., Bidirectional modulation of insulin action by amino acids, *J. Clin. Invest.*, 101, 1519–1529, 1998.

126. Guillet, C., Zangarelli, A., Gachon, P., Morio, B., Giraudet, C., Rousset, P., and Boirie, Y., Whole body protein breakdown is less inhibited by insulin, but still responsive to amino acid, in nondiabetic elderly subjects, *J. Clin. Endocrinol. Metab.*, 89, 6017–6024, 2004.

127. Volpi, E., Ferrando, A.A., Yeckel, C.W., Tipton, K.D., and Wolfe, R.R., Exogenous amino acids stimulate net muscle protein synthesis in the elderly, *J. Clin. Invest.*, 101, 2000–2007, 1998.

128. Rasmussen, B., Wolfe, R., and Volpi, E., Oral and intravenously administered amino acids produce similar effects on muscle protein synthesis in the elderly, *J. Nutr. Health Aging*, 6, 358–362, 2002.

129. Volpi, E., Mittendorfer, B., Rasmussen, B.B., and Wolfe, R.R., The response of muscle protein anabolism to combined hyperaminoacidemia and glucose-induced hyperinsulinemia is impaired in the elderly, *J. Clin. Endocrinol. Metab.*, 85, 4481–4490, 2000.

130. Solerte, S.B., Gazzaruso, C., Schifino, N., Locatelli, E., Destro, T., Ceresini, G., Ferrari, E., and Fioravanti, M., Metabolic effects of orally administered amino acid mixture in elderly subjects with poorly controlled type 2 diabetes mellitus, *Am. J. Cardiol.*, 93, 23A–29A, 2004.

131. Gannon, M.C. and Nuttall, F.Q., Effect of a high-protein, low-carbohydrate diet on blood glucose control in people with type 2 diabetes, *Diabetes*, 53, 2375–2382, 2004.

132. Volpi, E., Kobayashi, H., Sheffield-Moore, M., Mittendorfer, B., and Wolfe, R., Essential amino acids are primarily responsible for the amino acid stimulation of muscle protein anabolism in healthy elderly adults, *Am. J. Clin. Nutr.*, 78, 250–258, 2003.

133. Paddon-Jones, D., Sheffield-Moore, M., Zhang, X., Volpi, E., Wolf, S., Aarsland, A., Ferrando, A., and Wolfe, R., Amino acid ingestion improves muscle protein synthesis in the young and elderly, *Am. J. Physiol. Endocrinol. Metab.*, 286, E321–E328, 2004.

134. Zamboni, M., Zoico, E., Tosoni, P., Zivelonghi, A., Bortolani, A., Maggi, S., Di Francesco, V., and Bosello, O., Relation between vitamin D, physical performance, and disability in elderly persons, *J. Gerontol. A: Biol. Sci. Med. Sci.*, 57, M7–M11, 2002.

135. Bischoff-Ferrari, H.A., Dietrich, T., E.J. O, F.B. H, Zhang, Y., Karlson, E.W., and Dawson-Hughes, B., Higher 25-hydroxyvitamin D concentrations are associated with better lower-extremity function in both active and inactive persons aged = 60 y, *Am. J. Clin. Nutr.*, 80, 752–758, 2004.

136. Visser, M., Deeg, D.J., Lips, P., Low vitamin D and high parathyroid hormone levels as determinants of loss of muscle strength and muscle mass (sarcopenia): the Longitudinal Aging Study Amsterdam, *J. Clin. Endocrinol. Metab.*, 88, 5766–5772, 2003.

137. Pfeifer, M., Begerow, B., Minne, H.W., Abrams, C., Nachtigall, D., and Hansen, C., Effects of a short-term vitamin D and calcium supplementation on body sway and secondary hyperparathyroidism in elderly women, *J. Bone Miner. Res.*, 15, 11113–11118, 2000.

138. Bischoff, H.A., Stahelin, H.B., Dick, W., Akos, R., Knecht, M., Salis, C., Nebiker, M., Theiler, R., Pfeifer, M., Begerow, B., Lew, R.A., and Conzelmann, M., Effects of vitamin D and calcium supplementation on falls: a randomized controlled trial, *J. Bone Miner. Res.*, 18, 343–351, 2003.

139. Grady, D., Halloran, B., Cummings, S., Leveille, S., Wells, L., Black, D., and Byl, N., 1,25-Dihydroxyvitamin D3 and muscle strength in the elderly: a randomized controlled trial, *J. Clin. Endocrinol. Metab.*, 73, 1111–1117, 1991.

140. Kenny, A.M., Biskup, B., Robbins, B., Marcella, G., and Burleson, J.A., Effects of vitamin D supplementation on strength, physical function, and health perception in older, community-dwelling men, *J. Am. Geriatr. Soc.*, 51, 1762–1767, 2003.

141. Hanley, D.A. and Davison, K.S., Vitamin D insufficiency in North America, *J. Nutr.*, 135, 332–337, 2005.

142. Tanaka, Y., Sasaki, R., Fukui, F., Waki, H., Kawabata, T., Okazaki, M., Hasegawa, K., S. A., Acetyl-L-carnitine supplementation restores decreased tissue carnitine levels and impaired lipid metabolism in aged rats, *J. Lipid Res.*, 45, 729–735, 2004.

143. Kumaran, S., Subathra, M., Balu, M., and Panneerselvam, C., Age-associated decreased activities of mitochondrial electron transport chain complexes in heart and skeletal muscle: role of L-carnitine, *Chem. Biol. Interact.*, 148, 11–18, 2004.

144. Iossa, S., Mollica, M.P., Lionetti, L., Crescenzo, R., Botta, M., Barletta, A., G. L., Acetyl-L-carnitine supplementation differently influences nutrient partitioning, serum leptin concentration and skeletal muscle mitochondrial respiration in young and old rats, *J. Nutr.*, 132, 636–642, 2002.

145. Gonzalez-Crespo, M.R., Arenas, J., Gomez-Reino, J.J., Campos, Y., Borstein, B., Martin, M.A., Cabello, A., Garcia-Rayo, R., and Ricoy, J.R., Muscle dysfunction in elderly individuals with hip fracture, *J. Rheumatol.*, 26, 2229–2232, 1999.

146. Starling, R.D., Costill, D.L., and Fink, W.J., Relationships between muscle carnitine, age and oxidative status, *Eur. J. Appl. Physiol.*, 71, 143–146, 1995.

147. Pistone, G., Marino, A., Leotta, C., Dell'Arte, S., Finocchiaro, G., and Malaguarnera, M., Levocarnitine administration in elderly subjects with rapid muscle fatigue: effect on body composition, lipid profile and fatigue, *Drugs Aging*, 20, 761–767, 2003.

148. Anderson, R.A., Chromium in the prevention and control of diabetes, *Diabetes Metab.*, 26, 22–27, 2000.

149. Lukaski, H.C., Bolonchuk, W.W., Siders, W.A., and Milne, D.B., Chromium supplementation and resistance training: effects on body composition, strength, and trace element status of men, *Am. J. Clin. Nutr.*, 63, 954–965, 1996.

150. Hallmark, M.A., Reynolds, T.H., DeSouza, C.A., Dotson, C.O., Anderson, R.A., and Rogers, M.A., Effects of chromium and resistive training on muscle strength and body composition, *Med. Sci. Sports Exer.*, 28, 139–144, 1996.

151. Campbell, W.W., Joseph, L.J., Davey, S.L., Cyr-Campbell, D., Anderson, R.A., and Evans, W.J., Effects of resistance training and chromium picolinate on body composition and skeletal muscle in older men, *J. Appl. Physiol.*, 86, 29–39, 1999.

152. Welle, S., Thornton, C., Statt, M., and McHenry, B., Growth hormone increases muscle mass and strength but does not rejuvenate myofibrillar protein synthesis

in healthy subjects over 60 years old, *J. Clin. Endocrinol. Metab.*, 81, 3239–3243, 1996.

153. Butterfield, G.E., Thompson, J., Rennie, M.J., Marcus, R., Hintz, R.L., and Hoffman, A.R., Effect of rhGH and rhIGF-I treatment on protein utilization in elderly men, *Am. J. Physiol. Endocrinol. Metab.*, 272, E94, 1997.

154. Rudman, D., Feller, A.G., Nagraj, H.S., Gergans, G.A., Lalitha, P.Y., Goldberg, A.F., Schlenker, R.A., and Cohn, L., Effects of human growth hormone in men over 60 years old, *New Engl. J. Med.*, 323, 1–6, 1990.

155. Taffe, D.R., Pruitt, L., Reim, J., Hintz, R.L., Butterfield, G., Hoffman, A.R., and Marcus, R., Effect of recombinant human growth hormone on the muscle strength response to resistive exercise in elderly men, *J. Clin. Endocrinol. Metab.*, 79, 1361–1366, 1994.

156. Taffe, D.R., Jin, I.H., Vu, T.H., Hoffman, A.R., and Marcus, R., Lack of effect of recombinant human growth hormone (GH) on muscle morphology and GH-insulin-like growth factor expression in resistance trained elderly men, *J. Clin. Endocrinol. Metab.*, 81, 421–425, 1996.

157. Hennessey, J.V., Chromiak, J.A., DellaVentura, S., Reinert, S.E., Puhl, J., Kiel, D.P., Rosen, C.J., Vandenburgh, H., and MacLean, D.B., Growth hormone administration and exercise effects on muscle fiber type and diameter in moderately frail older people, *J. Am. Geriatr. Soc.*, 49, 852–858, 2001.

158. Yarasheski, K.E., Zachwieja, J.J., Angelopoulos, T.J., and Bier, D.M., Short-term growth hormone treatment does not increase muscle protein synthesis in experienced weight lifters, *J. Appl. Physiol.*, 74, 3073–3076, 1993.

159. Franco, C., Brandberg, J., Lonn, L., Andersson, B., Bengtsson, B.A., and Johannsson, G., Growth hormone treatment reduces abdominal visceral fat in post-menopausal women with abdominal obesity: a 12-month placebo-controlled trial, *J. Clin. Endocrinol. Metab.*, 90, 1466–1474, 2005.

160. Cappola, A.R., Bandeen-Roche, K., Wand, G.S., Volpato, S., and Fried, L.P., Association of IGF-I levels with muscle strength and mobility in older women, *J. Clin. Endocrinol. Metab.*, 86, 4139–4146, 2001.

161. Russel-Jones, D.L., Umpleby, A.M., Hennessy, T.R., Bowes, S.B., Shojaee-Moradie, F., Hopkins, K.D., Jackson, N.C., Kelly, J.M., Jones, R.H., and Sonksen, P.H., Use of a leucine clamp to demonstrate that IGF-I activity stimulates protein synthesis in normal humans, *Am. J. Physiol.*, 267, E591–E598, 1994.

162. Fryburg, D.A., Jahn, L.A., Hill, S.A., Oliveras, D.M., and Barrett, E.J., Insulin and insulin-like growth factor-I enhance human skeletal muscle protein anabolism during hyperaminoacidemia by different mechanisms, *J. Clin. Invest.*, 96, 1722–1729, 1995.

163. Bark, T.H., McNurlan, M.A., Lang, C.H., and Garlick, P.J., Increased protein synthesis after acute IGF-I or insulin infusion is localized to muscle in mice, *Am. J. Physiol. Endocrinol. Metab.*, 275, E118–E123, 1998.

164. Friedlander, A.L., Butterfield, G.E., Moynihan, S., Grillo, J., Pollack, M., Holloway, L., Friedman, L., Yesavage, J., Matthias, D., Lee, S., Marcus, R., and Hoffman, A.R., One year of insulin-like growth factor I treatment does not affect bone density, body composition, or psychological measures in postmenopausal women, *J. Clin. Endocrinol. Metab.*, 86, 1496–1503, 2001.

165. Bhasin, S., Testosterone supplementation for aging-associated sarcopenia, *J. Gerontol. A: Biol. Sci. Med. Sci.*, 58, 1002–1008, 2003.

166. Hakkinen, K. and Pakarinen, A., Serum hormones and strength development during strength training in middle-aged and elderly males and females, *Acta Physiol. Scand.*, 150, 21–219, 1994.

167. Hakkinen, K., Pakarinen, A., Kraemer, W., Newton, R., and Alen, M., Basal concentrations and acute responses of serum hormones and strength development during heavy resistance training in middle-aged and elderly men and women, *J. Gerontol. A: Biol. Sci. Med. Sci.*, 55, B95–B105, 2000.

168. Liu, P.Y., Swerdloff, R.S., and Veldhuis, J.D., The rationale, efficacy and safety of androgen therapy in older men: future research and current practice recommendations, *J. Clin. Endocrinol. Metab.*, 89, 4789–4796, 2004.

169. Mudali, S. and Dobs, A., Effects of testosterone on body composition of the aging male, *Mech. Ageing Dev.*, 125, 297–304, 2004.

170. Herbst, K.L. and Bhasin, S., Testosterone action on skeletal muscle, *Curr. Opin. Clin. Nutr. Metab. Care*, 7, 271–277, 2004.

171. Urban, R.J., Bodenburg, Y.H., Gilkison, C., Foxworth, J., Coggan, A.R., Wolfe, R.R., and Ferrando, A., Testosterone administration to elderly men increases skeletal muscle strength and protein synthesis, *Am. J. Physiol. Endocrinol. Metab.*, 269, E820–E826, 1995.

172. Ferrando, A.A., Sheffield-Moore, M., Yeckel, C.W., Gilkison, C., Jiang, J., Achacosa, A., Lieberman, S.A., Tipton, K., Wolfe, R.R., and Urban, R.J., Testosterone administration to older men improves muscle function: molecular and physiological mechanisms, *Am. J. Physiol. Endocrinol. Metab.*, 282, E601–E607, 2002.

173. Tenover, J.S., Effects of testosterone supplementation in the aging male, *J. Clin. Endocrinol. Metab.*, 75, 1092–1098, 1992.

174. Snyder, P.J., Peachey, H., Hannoush, P., Berlin, J.A., Loh, L., Lenrow, D.A, Holmes, J.H., Dlewati, A., Santanna, J., Rosen, C.J., and Strom, B.L., Effect of testosterone treatment on body composition and muscle strength in men over 65 years of age, *J. Clin. Endocrinol. Metab.*, 84, 2647–2653, 1999.

175. Brodsky, I.G., Balagopal, P., and Nair, K.S., Effects of testosterone replacement on muscle mass and muscle protein synthesis in hypogonadal men: a clinical research center study, *J. Clin. Endocrinol. Metab.*, 81, 3469–3475, 1996.

176. Ferrando, A., Sheffield-Moore, M., Paddon-Jones, D., Wolfe, R., and Urban, R., Differential anabolic effects of testosterone and amino acid feeding in older men, *J. Clin. Endocrinol. Metab.*, 88, 2003.

177. Bhasin, S., Woodhouse, L., Casaburi, R., Singh, A.B., Bhasin, D., Berman, N., Chen, X., Yarasheski, K.E., Magliano, L., Dzekov, C., Dzekov, J., Bross, R., Phillips, J., Sinha-Hikim, I., Shen, R., and Storer, T.W., Testosterone dose–response relationships in healthy young men, *Am. J. Physiol. Endocrinol. Metab.*, 281, E1172–E1181, 2001.

178. Bhasin, S., Woodhouse, L., Casaburi, R., Singh, A.B., Mac, R.P., Lee, M., Yarasheski, K.E., Sinha-Hikim, I., Dzekov, C., Dzekov, J., Magliano, L., and Storer, T.W., Older men are as responsive as young men to the anabolic effects of graded doses of testosterone on the skeletal muscle, *J. Clin. Endocrinol. Metab.*, 90, 678–688, 2005.

179. Orr, R. and Fiatarone Singh, M., The anabolic androgenic steroid oxandrolone in the treatment of wasting and catabolic disorders: review of efficacy and safety, *Drugs*, 64, 725–750, 2004.

180. Sheffield-Moore, M., Urban, R.J., Wolf, S.E., Jiang, J., Catlin, D.H., Herndon, D.N., Wolfe, R.R., and Ferrando, A.A., Short-term oxandrolone administration stimulates net muscle protein synthesis in young men, *J. Clin. Endocrinol. Metab.*, 84, 2705–2711, 1999.

181. Sheffield-Moore, M., Wolfe, R.R., Gore, D.C., Wolf, S.E., Ferrer, D.M., and Ferrando, A.A., Combined effects of hyperaminoacidemia and oxandrolone on skeletal muscle protein synthesis, *Am. J. Physiol. Endocrinol. Metab.*, 278, E273–E279, 1999.

182. Schroeder, E.T., Terk, M., and Sattler, F.R., Androgen therapy improves muscle mass and strength but not muscle quality: results from two studies, *Am. J. Physiol. Endocrinol. Metab.*, 285, E16–E24, 2003.

183. Schroeder, E.T., Zheng, L., Ong, M.D., Martinez, C., Flores, C., Stewart, Y., Azen, C., and Sattler, F.R., Effects of androgen therapy on adipose tissue and metabolism in older men, *J. Clin. Endocrinol. Metab.*, 89, 4863–4872, 2004.

184. Kenny, A., Dawson, L., Kleppinger, A., Iannuzzi-Sucich, M., and Judge, J., Prevalence of sarcopenia and predictors of skeletal muscle mass in nonobese women who are long-term users of estrogen-replacement therapy, *J. Gerontol. A: Biol. Sci. Med. Sci.*, 58, M436–M440, 2003.

185. Roubenoff, R. and Hughes, V.A., Sarcopenia: current concepts, *J. Gerontol. A: Biol. Sci. Med. Sci.*, 55, M716–M724, 2000.

186. Buvat, J., Androgen therapy with dehydroepiandrosterone, *World J. Urol.*, 21, 346–355, 2003.

187. Dhatariya, K. and Nair, K., Dehydroepiandrosterone: is there a role for replacement? *Mayo Clin. Proc.*, 78, 1257–1273, 2003.

188. Liu, D. and Dillon, J.S., Dehydroepiandrosterone activates endothelial cell nitric-oxide synthase by a specific plasma membrane receptor, *J. Biol. Chem.*, 24, 21379–21388, 2002.

189. Brown, G.A., Vukovich, M.D., Sharp, R., Reifenrath, T.A., Parsons, K.A., and King, D.S., Effect of oral DHEA on serum testosterone and adaptations to resistance training in young men, *J. Appl. Physiol.*, 87, 2274–2283, 1999.

190. Morales, A.J., Haubrich, R.H., Hwang, J.Y., Asakura, H., and Yen, S.S., The effect of six months treatment with a 100 mg daily dose of dehydroepiandrosterone (DHEA) on circulating sex steroids, body composition and muscle strength in age-advanced men and women, *Clin. Endocrinol.*, 49, 421–432, 1998.

191. Villareal, D.T. and Holloszy, J.O., Effect of DHEA on abdominal fat and insulin action in elderly women and men: a randomized controlled trial, *JAMA*, 292, 2243–2248, 2004.

192. Dhatariya, K., Bigelow, M.L., and Nair, K.S., Effect of dehydroepiandrosterone replacement on insulin sensitivity and lipids in hypoadrenal women, *Diabetes*, 54, 765–769, 2005.

193. Perrini, S., Natalicchio, A., Laviola, L., Belsanti, G., Montrone, C., Cignarelli, A., Minielli, V., Grano, M., De Pergola, G., Giorgino, R., and Giorgino, F., Dehydroepiandrosterone stimulates glucose uptake in human and murine adipocytes by inducing GLUT1 and GLUT4 translocation to the plasma membrane, *Diabetes*, 53, 41–52, 2004.

194. Valenti, G., Adrenopause: an imbalance between dehydroepiandrosterone (DHEA) and cortisol secretion, *J. Endocrinol. Invest.*, 25, 29–35, 2002.

195. Kroboth, P., Amico, J., Stone, R., Folan, M., Frye, R., Kroboth, F., Bigos, K., Fabian, T., Linares, A., Pollock, B., and Hakala, C., Influence of DHEA administration on 24-hour cortisol concentrations, *J. Clin. Psychopharmacol.*, 23, 96–99, 2003.
196. Genazzani, A.R., Inglese, S., Lombardi, I., Pieri, M., Bernardi, F., Genazzani, A.D., Rovati, L., Luisi, M., Long-term low-dose dehydroepiandrosterone replacement therapy in aging males with partial androgen deficiency, *Aging Male*, 7, 133–143, 2004.
197. Arlt, W., Dehydroepiandrosterone and ageing, *Best Pract. Res. Clin. Endocrinol. Metab.*, 18, 363–380, 2004.
198. Muhlberg, W. and Sieber, C., Sarcopenia and frailty in geriatric patients: implications for training and prevention, *Z. Gerontol. Geriatr.*, 37, 2–8, 2004.

19 Muscle Strain

*Ingrid Kohlstadt, M.D., M.P.H.,
Eric Schweitzer, D.P.T., M.T.C.,
Karen Mutter, D.O., and
Lawrence B. Godwin, M.Ac., L.Ac.*

CONTENTS

INTRODUCTION

Muscle strain is the stretching or tearing of muscle fibers, usually at the musculo-tendinous junction. Strain occurs when biomechanical forces are in excess of what the muscle–tendon unit can bear. Sometimes strain of the muscle-tendon is the direct result of biomechanical loading of extreme or repetitive forces. At other times the muscle-tendon unit is weak, unable to withstand even small forces. Injuries to the rotator cuff, for example, occur in baseball pitchers following extreme forces, and in the elderly with sarcopenia and degenerating tissues, forces so minor the patient is not able to recall when it happened. Irrespective of person and force, strain launches a body response of pain, swelling, tissue damage, and inflammatory cascade.

Molecular methods show that many techniques reduce the inflammation and tissue-damage of muscle strain. These include surgery, medications, physical therapy, osteopathic manipulation therapy, chiropractic, acupuncture, and nutrition.

337

Combining techniques provides additional and sometimes synergistic benefit in reducing pain, tissue damage, and inflammation. Combining techniques to improve healing is particularly relevant to muscle strain, since strain occurs frequently[1] and often during fitness pursuits. Muscle strains can take a long time to heal and are a major reason for occupational time-loss.[2]

BIOMECHANICS

A strain of the tissue ensues with the muscle fibers being stretched beyond the physiologic limit resulting in muscle fiber destruction.[3] Disruptions that interrupt the alignment of the myofilaments interfere with the tension-gathering ability of these contractile elements.[4] The muscle–tendon unit then gives way at its weakest point, often the musculotendinous junction.[1,2] Figure 19.1 depicts the stress–strain curve for a muscle–tendon tissue. The range at which the stress and the tissue length are linear is the elastic range. If the stress to the tissue is released within the elastic range, the stretched tissue will return to prestretch length without any permanent deformation. Beyond the elastic range is the plastic range of the stress–strain curve, which is not linear, because tissue has an ability to elongate under stress and the capacity to realign the collagen fibrous networks within these tissues.[5] If stress is maintained into the plastic range, the tissue permanently deforms and returns to a new resting length. If the load is maintained beyond the plastic range, tissue strain occurs and soon after tissue failure will ensue.

Stress applied to tissues can occur as a single episode or cumulatively as in repetitive strain and overuse injuries. A single episode causing acute injury is the most common type of strain injury seen in athletics. A common mechanism

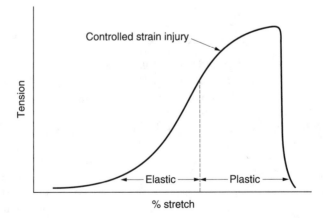

FIGURE 19.1 Stress–strain curve. Mechanical failure occurs when the applied load exceeds the tissue's physiological range of motion.

of this type of strain injury occurs when the entire muscle–tendon system must dissipate the stored energy forces within a muscle when decelerating a body segment. If deceleration forces exceed the capabilities of the muscle, injury to any part of the system, including the muscle or tendon, can occur.[6] Strains most commonly occur in biarthrodial muscles, those which cross two joints and produce and control motion at both joints. The most common biarthrodial muscles strained are the hamstrings, quadriceps, and the gastrocnemius muscles.[7]

When repeated or sustained force is applied in either the elastic or plastic range of the stress–strain curve, it can damage the muscle tendon unit. Tendons that commonly suffer repetitive injury are the rotator cuff, achilles and patellar tendons, extensor carpi radialis brevis, adductor longus, long head of the biceps muscle, tibialis posterior, and flexor hallucis longus.[7] Overuse injuries occur most frequently with sustained postures and eccentric muscle contractions. Eccentric contraction is a type of dynamic muscle loading where muscle tension develops while the muscle is lengthening. The increase in strain injuries with eccentric loading may be due to the significantly greater force produced by eccentric contractions as compared to concentric or isometric contractions.[6,8] Because of maximal muscle force being generated during eccentric work, damage to the contractile components of the muscle fibers decrease force generation capability and the perception of soreness often results.[6] Overuse injury involves histopathological changes in eccentric muscles, including engorgement of muscle cells, increased fibroblastic activity, production of collagen and ground substance, and infiltration of inflammatory cells.[9]

TISSUE RESPONSE TO BIOMECHANICAL FORCES

Tissue injured by biomechanical forces becomes inflamed. Clinically, the presence of inflammation is noted by swelling, erythema, increased temperature, pain and reduced function. At the cellular level, macrophages migrate to the site of injury to remove necrotic debris, thereby preparing the zone of injury for tissue restoration. Inflammation consists of tissue edema, fibrin exudation, infiltration of the inflammatory cells such as neutrophils, monocytes, and macrophages, production of fibronectin, capillary wall thickening, and capillary occlusions.[10] Muscle precursors called satellite cells are activated to redevelop normal muscle structure.[11] Activation of macrophages by phagocytosis results in the synthesis of several important proinflammatory cytokines[2]. Cytokines increase vascular permeability, attract additional mononuclear cells to the injury site, lead to lymphocyte proliferation and differentiation, and stimulate additional release of proinflammatory cytokines. Neutrophils release free radicals as part of the host defense, also leading to ischemia-related tissue injury.[9] Complex coordinated vascular, cellular, and chemical events control the inflammation process, which finally results in tissue regeneration and repair, or in the less optimal scenario, chronic degenerative tissue and scar formation.[10]

Editor's Note

Patients recover more quickly from muscle strain when medicine, nutrition, and structural health techniques are used together. Quick recovery enables patients to resume physical activity quickly and more safely, return to work sooner, reduce the risk of injury recurrence, and minimize the need for pain medications.

PHYSICAL THERAPY

Physical therapy treatments for muscle strain are phase dependent. Physical therapy classifies rehabilitation of muscle strain as follows: acute, subacute, advanced strengthening, and return-to-function.[8,25]

ACUTE PHASE

Management in the acute phase, which lasts up to 4 days, focuses on curtailing cell death by minimizing the amount of acute inflammatory exudates. Certain modalities have been advocated for use during the acute phase of healing for their ability to minimize active inflammation.

The application of ice in the treatment of acute injury was first mentioned by Hippocrates around 400 B.C. and has been widely used ever since. As tissue temperature decreases, cutaneous receptors are stimulated exciting the sympathetic adrenergic fibers to constrict local arterioles and venules. Vasoconstriction leads to decreased rate of metabolism, production of metabolites, and decreased oxygen requirements, thereby limiting the extent of the injury to uninjured tissues.[7] Bleakley et al. performed a systematic review of randomized controlled trials of cryotherapy treatment for acute soft tissue injury.[12] Few studies in his review assessed the effectiveness of ice on closed soft tissue injury and no studies discussed the optimal mode of delivery or duration of treatment.

Merrick reviewed multiple studies demonstrating that high-voltage pulsed electrical stimulation limits edema in animal models. Theories on electrical stimulation's anti-inflammatory effects stem from the concept that the electrical current combats the vasodilation of the capillaries during the initial influx of acute inflammatory exudates.[13] It has also been proposed that electrical stimulation may improve the pumping action of the muscles which, in turn, improves venous return.[13,14] Pulsed ultrasound is also a common treatment for acute muscle strain. Pulsed ultrasound uses acoustic energy beyond audible range emitted in such a fashion to minimize thermal effects of the ultrasonic energy. Theoretically, pulse ultrasound can stimulate soft tissue repair early after an injury when, due to active inflammation, a thermal effect is not desired.[13] Soft tissue repair occurs with ultrasound via increased cell membrane and vascular permeability, increased extensibility of connective tissue, enhanced absorption of interstitial fluid, stimulation of tissue regeneration, and release of histamine from the mast cells by degranulation, which is particularly helpful in the first 72 h postinjury.[5,14] Low-power laser therapy, or "cold" laser, has gained popularity as an early intervention treatment with muscle injury.[15] "Cold" lasers, named such because thermal effects are considered minimal, have a maximum output of less than 50 mW and are commonly used in the treatment of soft tissue injuries. Cold lasers of varying intensity may reduce pain and muscle spasm, increase mitochondrial activity, elevate blood cortisol levels, decrease edema, and improve collagen formation.[16] All of these effects may increase the rate of tissue healing. An immediate analgesic effect may be noted in the treatment of acute conditions. Beckerman et al. performed a criteria-based meta-analysis of randomized controlled trials of the efficacy of laser therapy and reported the efficacy of laser therapy for musculoskeletal disorders seems, on average, to be larger than the efficacy of a placebo treatment. More specifically, for myofascial pain among other conditions, laser therapy seems to have a substantial specific therapeutic effect.[15]

SUBACUTE PHASE

The subacute phase of connective tissue healing begins as inflammation decreases, fibrous clot resolution begins, and repair of the injured site is initiated. The hallmark of this healing stage is the synthesis and deposition of new collagen fibers. Initially, the collagen fibers are small and randomly aligned, and gradually larger bundles of fibers in more parallel alignment are formed.[5] Growth of capillary beds into the injured area takes place, improving transportation of nutrients for development of new collagen tissue. Fibroblastic activity, collagen formation and granulation all strengthen the damaged tissue enough for controlled stress to be initiated. At first the connective tissue produced is thin, fragile, unorganized, and easily injured if overstressed.[8,13] Yet, if insufficient force is applied, the newly formed fibers can stay in a randomized fashion, increasing the chance of scar formation. The development of scar formation and localized fibrosis may be a factor in the propensity for reoccurrence of previous strain injury.[17]

Treatment in the subacute phase focuses on facilitating the synthesis and deposition of collagen in a nonrandomized fashion and preventing development of adhesions within the connective tissue. As the subacute phase progresses, treatment focuses on increasing the length of the muscle, increasing surrounding joint mobility, increasing the overall strength of the connective tissue and ultimately preparing the tissue for more complex activities associated with the advanced strengthening and return to function phases.[13]

Modalities considered beneficial during subacute muscle strain healing usually increase tissue temperature. Raising tissue temperature increases arteriolar dilation, decrease blood viscosity, and increase permeability of capillary membranes. Clinically, tissue heating decreases pain and increases extensibility of the muscle tendon unit, thereby increasing tolerance to muscle stretching, joint manipulation and therapeutic exercise.

Thermal agents can be divided into superficial and deep heating modalities. Superficial heat modalities, including hot packs, paraffin, fluidotherapy, and infrared radiation, are widely used in the treatment of soft tissue injury both for pain reduction and tissue healing qualities. Clinically, superficial heat is commonly used to relieve pain, subdue muscle spasm and prepare the tissues for further treatment such as manual physical therapy (i.e., joint or soft tissue manipulation, manual muscle stretching) or therapeutic exercise. Deeper heating modalities include continuous ultrasound and diathermy. Therapeutic ultrasound is administered as a continuous sound wave, which produces kinetic and thermal energy. Ultrasound enhances chemical reactions, increases membrane permeability, deforms the molecular structure of loosely bonded substances, and increases the extensibility of tendons.[18] Diathermy is a deep heating modality which uses shortwave electromagnetic energy to increase tissue temperature. Diathermy's advantage over ultrasound is that it can be used to treat a large surface area such as a hamstring. Hecox et al. reported several studies showing increased stretch following muscle heating by use of shortwave diathermy.[14]

Soft tissue manipulation is a useful intervention for a muscle strain in the subacute phase of healing. Soft tissue manipulation is defined as the forceful passive movement of the musculofascial elements through its restrictive directions. Soft tissue manipulation during this phase of muscle healing relieves pain, releases muscle spasm or tension, stretches abnormal fibrous tissue, releases fascial adhesions, increases blood flow, and restores structural harmony and balance.[19] Muscle energy techniques and proprioceptive neuromuscular facilitation are two such examples. Mechanical tension and manual compression of the muscle enhances tissue remodeling, stimulates collagen synthesis, increases tissue strength, and helps to align the repair cells and collagen fibers. Lack of tension leaves the repair tissue cells and matrix disoriented. Biomechanical testing shows accelerated recovery of tissue strength in mobilized muscles.[2] This is important when one considers that, despite an average muscle strain appearing to be resolved after 2 to 3 weeks of physical therapy, recent evidence shows that there is still ongoing muscle regeneration in the presence of mature scar tissue formation.[20] Scar tissue at the musculotendinous junction may be responsible for the increased risk of reinjury during the early postinjury period and it has been proposed that treatment should aim to minimize the scar tissue formation.[21]

Another manual treatment that may be implemented during the subacute phase is joint manipulation. Whereas soft tissue manipulation addresses adhesions in the musculofascial tissue, all intensities of joint manipulation (grades I–V) can be used to stimulate joint nutrient circulation and release joint adhesions secondary to disuse of the tissues since onset of injury. Grades I and II manipulation move the joint through the beginning of the range of motion not aiming to deform the joint capsule but rather to stimulate nutrient flow through the available range of motion. Grades III–V manipulation move the joint to the end range of motion and beyond the end range with intention to stretch the joint capsule and cause increased joint range of motion. There is some evidence all grades of joint manipulation also result in firing of sensory receptors and release of endorphins which may cause local skeletal muscle tissue relaxation providing pain relief and increased freedom of movement. Joint manipulation also allows water and other nutrient delivery to a joint unable to travel through its full range of motion secondary to a local strained muscle.[22]

ADVANCED STRENGTHENING PHASE

During the advanced strengthening phase intensity, the strengthening exercises can increase and strength imbalances can be prevented. Strength imbalances can be precipitated by injuries and are associated with reinjury. For example, preseason hamstring weakness has been identified as a risk factor for hamstring muscle strains in soccer players.[23] Strength imbalance was also found to be a risk factor to lower extremity injuries in female collegiate athletes.[24] Strength training involves adaptations in all fiber types and improves firing of motor neurons for more synchronous muscle activation, described in the return-to-function phase. The maximum percentage of an injured muscle's fibers that can be firing at the same time ranges from 60 to 90%. The percentage correlates with the degree of strength training the muscle has undergone.[2] During the subacute phase, newly formed connective tissue is fragile. This is demonstrated by Nikolaou et al. who report a 50% decrease in contractile ability following a controlled strain injury in animals.[17] Another factor to consider when applying therapeutic exercise to a healing muscle strain is the statistically significant decrease in the percent length increase to rupture (79%) and peak load (63%) sustained by the muscle when compared to a healthy control.[1]

RETURN-TO-FUNCTION PHASE

The principle behind the return-to-function phase is regaining agility, coordination, and proprioception. Kinetic chain strengthening entails viewing muscles as a complete system requiring coordinated action to produce precise movement. For athletes, abrupt movements such as hopping, jumping, and bounding, known collectively as plyometrics, use the kinetic chain to further strengthen the healing tissue while preparing it for demands associated with the patient's goals.[25] For example, a basketball player healing from a gastrocnemius muscle strain may begin performing jump shots as an exercise in this phase. The return-to-function phase also uses the kinetic chain concept to strengthen nonathletes. For example, a construction worker who sustained a strain to his or her rotator cuff may begin to lift objects as an exercise in this phase. Muscles at the center of the body provide a stable base of support and generate force. Energy is transmitted to more peripheral muscles successively. Retraining the afferent pathways is critical for shortening of the time lag of muscular reaction to counteract the excessive strain on the passive structures and guard against future injury.[26]

TABLE 19.1
Summary of physical therapy treatments of muscle strain

Phase	Time postinjury	Modalities and techniques	Treatment goals
Acute	1 to 4 days	Cryotherapy, electrical stimulation, ultrasound, laser therapy	Decrease inflammation through vasoconstriction, decreasing permeability of the capillaries, stimulation of release of histamine from the mast cells
Subacute	4 to 21 days	Superficial heat modalities, laser therapy, electrical stimulation, ultrasound, diathermy, soft tissue and joint manipulation, muscle energy, and proprioceptive neuromuscular facilitation	Increases rate of tissue healing; increase strength and length of newly formed tissue; initiate muscle balance and coordination
Advanced strengthening and return-to-function	22 to 360 days	Therapeutic exercise, proprioceptive exercise, plyometrics	Increase strength/energy generating capabilities of individual muscle and entire kinetic chain; regain agility, coordination and proprioception; activity-based strengthening

Table 19.1 summarizes the physical therapist's approach to injury of the muscle–tendon unit. Once the recovered muscle has full range of motion, full strength, and can participate as an active member of the kinetic chain, the patient can gradually resume full participation in his or her desired activities. It should be noted that when a patient appears to have met the criteria for full participation, basic science studies show us that healing is much slower than our clinical findings would indicate and the patient must be educated they are temporarily at increased risk for reinjury.[20]

OSTEOPATHIC APPROACH

Osteopathy emphasizes that the condition of the musculoskeletal system is fundamental to the health of the whole being. Osteopathy also focuses on the body's self-healing capacity. The training curriculum for doctors of osteopathic medicine (D.O.) is similar to that of doctors of medicine. Additionally, D.O. training includes osteopathic manipulation therapy (OMT). OMT is a hands-on method to treat musculotendinous strain and to assist in restoring balance to the musculoskeletal system. This therapy, like chiropractic, involves manipulation of the entire body including all joints and soft tissue. Osteopathy asserts that the neuromuscular system is functionally and inextricably linked with all body systems via neural and humoral pathways.[28]

Osteopaths view acute and chronic musculotendinous strain as an imbalance of the neuromusculoskeletal system and refer to this injury as somatic dysfunction. The presence of normal passive motion in one direction of one plane of motion and resistance in the other is presumptive evidence of somatic dysfunction.[27] In addition, there may be changes in tissue texture and temperature, diminished range of motion, and asymmetry of the affected region. Acute ankle sprain is an example of a common musculotendinous injury where OMT has been shown to be beneficial. In a recent study, patients with acute ankle injuries were randomized to OMT or no OMT. Those receiving OMT demonstrated clinically significant improvement in edema and pain. On follow-up, patients in the OMT group had significant improvement in ankle range of motion over the control group.[29]

Osteopathic techniques may be classified as direct or indirect. This classification refers to a restrictive barrier which can be defined simply as a zone of restricted movement.[30] Direct techniques engage the restrictive barrier by positioning the patient's somatic dysfunction in the direction of the restrictive barrier. Indirect techniques involve positioning away from the restrictive barrier. Indirect techniques are gentle and effective for acute strain or injury because the tissues are being moved in the direction of freedom, and release of restriction is by inherent forces, not those imposed by the physician. Examples of direct techniques include soft tissue, articulation, myofascial, muscle energy, and thrust techniques. Examples of indirect techniques are counterstrain or positional release, Sutherland ligamentous release, and unwinding. Direct and indirect techniques may be used in combination.

The cascade of inflammation that occurs in musculoskeletal injury is necessary for tissue repair. However, neurogenic inflammation occurs when nerve endings at the site of trauma release neuropeptides to the spinal cord and local tissue, thereby perpetuating a cycle of inflammation. Neurogenic inflammation at this stage is a homoeostatic mechanism gone awry.[31] "A noxious stimulus, such as a muscle strain, triggers the release of a neuropeptide, substance P (SP), from the peripheral terminal of the primary afferent nociceptor (PAN). SP triggers the release of histamine from the surrounding mast cells, prostaglandins from the capillary endothelial cells, and the formation of bradykinin from the plasma protein preprobradykinin. White blood cells migrate to the tissue and release proinflammatory cytokines. Many of these substances are capable of triggering increased activity of the PAN and further secretion of neuropeptides. Thus a feed forward situation is established, leading to edema in the local tissue with sensitization of the PAN."[32] PAN activity contributes to hyperalgesia and lowered threshold for pain at the injured site. Nociceptive information processed by spinal neurons is relayed upstream to the brainstem and thalamus en route to the cerebral cortex. The arousal system of the brainstem is activated through the reticular activating system. This in turn initiates a strong systemic sympathetic nervous system response along with the hypothalamic–pituitary–adrenal axis causing release of catecholamines and adrenal cortical steroid hormones. Norepinephrine and cortisol in turn modify the release of various cytokines by the immune system. The cytokines can interact at the spinal cord level to alter pain thresholds and in the brain to alter the function of this neuroendocrine-immune network. This feedback loop between the site of somatic dysfunction and the central nervous system is the basis for spinal facilitation.

Spinal facilitation is a state of over-excitation of the spinal cord central motor neurons. It occurs at the level in the spinal column corresponding to the region of somatic dysfunction. It is measurable by electromyography.[33] Spinal facilitation perpetuates neurogenic inflammation at the injured site and may delay healing. OMT can interrupt the cycle of spinal facilitation and promote healing.

Reflex sympathetic dystrophy, also known as complex regional pain syndrome (CRPS) is a clinical example of how muscle strain can precipitate neurogenic inflammation with resultant spinal facilitation. CRPS is characterized by pain, exaggerated response to minimal stimulus, and autonomic dysfunction resulting in excessive sweating, swelling, and temperature differences at the injured site.[34] OMT can be applied to the affected spinal segments to interrupt spinal facilitation and neurogenic inflammation triggered by the initial extremity muscle injury. A case study published in the *Journal of Orthopedic Sports Physical Therapy* demonstrated immediate improvement in a patient with CRPS after vertebral manipulation. The patient experienced improvement in hand temperature and sweating, reduction in pain, and increase in shoulder range of motion.[35]

In summary, the goals of osteopathic intervention are to alleviate pain by correcting bony alignment and soft tissue strain, to improve circulation to and from the injured site including lymphatic, venous, arterial, and neural pathways, and to restore optimal physiologic functioning of the entire patient.

ACUPUNCTURE

Acupuncture is performed in the context of a larger total body treatment. Most Western trained traditional Chinese medicine acupuncturists are not trained to undertake rigorous physical examination of their patients, assuming most issues are internal imbalances of the organs.[36] Japanese acupuncturists focus on palpation as the main diagnostic tool. Japanese-style acupuncture can be applied to various muscle strains.

The acupuncturist is taught to diagnose by listening, seeing, hearing, and feeling. Acupuncturists examine the 20 muscles involved in shoulder movement and carefully map myofascial constriction, with particular attention to tender points. This, in combination with the patient's history of the incident, provides information about the progress of dysfunction, that is, the predictable cascade of injury weakened muscles requiring associated muscle systems to act in movement which cause them to weaken and incur trauma.[37,38] Tender points have many different presentations from feeling like twisted fibers of macaroni to grains of sand under the skin. The size of the tender points can vary from very fine grains to knots; associated inflammation can reduce their definition.

Needling sensitive points was first described in the fifth century by Sun Si-Miao, who referred to them as *Ah-Shi* points.[38] The Chinese texts describe the *Shi* point as any point where the patient expresses discomfort upon the application of pressure. The Japanese use the idea of *kori* points to describe areas of myofascial constriction that can be felt by the practitioner although they may or may not cause discomfort. The Japanese consider *kori* a blockage to lymphatic drainage, nervous conduction, venous and arterial circulation. Travell and Simons called tender points trigger points (TrPs) and defined them as points of hyperirritable tissue, that when compressed may be tender or refer pain and tenderness, autonomic phenomena, and disturbance of proprioception.[39,40] Seem describes how unblocking the *qi* by dispersing the *Shi* point with acupuncture produces the same response as myofascial release.[36]

Four ways that TrPs generate nociceptor activity are: (1) trauma (the subjection of a muscle to high intensity stimulation, either direct injury or repeated overloading); (2) anxiety or chronic stress (the holding of a group of muscles persistently contracted due to sympathetic nerve over activity); (3) radicular compression (the result of spinal nerve root entrapment and seen in cervical and lumbar disk prolapse); and (4) muscle wasting.[41]

When TrPs become active, they release calcitonin from the nociceptor sensory afferents. This in turn causes excessive release of acetylcholine from dysfunctional motor endplates causing marked contraction and contraction knots as identified by Simons and Stolov in 1976. The pain developing from active TrPs is the result of activation and sensitization of Group IV nociceptors. Nociceptors are activated and sensitized by either a high intensity noxious stimulus of a Group IV sensory afferent resulting in the propagation of potentials, or the release of SP and calcitonin which has a vasodilatory effect, causing edema and algesic vasoneuroactive substances such as bradykinin, serotonin, potassium ions, and histamine to be liberated. Bradykinin may also be responsible for sensitizing nociceptors and lowering of their threshold to high intensity and low intensity innocuous stimuli. Bradykinin also affects the release of prostaglandins which have a strong sensitizing effect on nociceptors. It is the sensitization of the nociceptors that makes TrPs sensitive to direct pressure.[41]

In 1972, during a goodwill mission by President Nixon to China, the President's personal physician, Walter Tkach, observed and later reported on the use of acupuncture analgesia. Scientists have worked diligently to understand the mechanisms of superficial dry needling (SDN) in producing analgesia. The study of acupuncture analgesia lends itself to scientific observation and has provided the opportunity to unravel some of the body's responses to SDN. Much more can be learned and, importantly, acupuncture analgesia is just a small part of a much larger Asian medical tradition.

Studies have correlated electro-acupuncture (EA), low frequency/high intensity, with the release of endogenous opioid peptide (EOP) in the cerebrospinal fluid and pain relief. EA stimulation results in the release of met- and leu-enkephalin and dynorphins at three sites; the dorsal horn, the midbrain, and the hypothalamus/pituitary complex. In the dorsal horn, EA applied to A and Types II and III muscle sensory afferents causes EOP release and the blocking of any information generated by C and unmyelinated Type IV muscle sensory afferents. In the midbrain, an enkephalin release activates the serotoninergic-mediated pain inhibitory system. And in the hypothalamus/pituitary complex, EA causes a release of adrenocorticotrophic (ACTH) hormone.[41]

The needling of TrPs results in release of spinal segmental endorphins. This explains why needling LI-4, found in the first interosseous muscle, provides analgesia for facial pain and not the abdomen. Needling specific acupuncture points provides highly correlated results, for example, Types II and III fibers provide total-body effect as EOPs are released from the midbrain and pituitary. In the ACTH-directed release of cortisol, acupuncture generates an anti-inflammatory effect on tissues, as well as a bronchodilator effect.[42] Research continues to provide insight into thousands of years of observations documenting the response to and use of acupuncture techniques.

A recent application of this ancient tradition is using electric stimulation on *kori* points. Electrical measurement shows that acupuncture points have electrical resistance lower than the surrounding skin. Points are real and they are not necessarily features of the body's nervous system.[38] Science has yet to identify the existence of meridians, which may be described as an early myofascial map.[36] In 1982, Macdonald described how 85% of his patients with chronic musculoskeletal pain and no knowledge of meridian systems were able to draw precise tracts of specific meridians.[41]

Complex myofascial patterns of constriction are common in neck and shoulder injury. Travel and Simons suggest the practitioner first correlate subjective experiences of shoulder pain and discomfort reported by the patient with the TrPs causing the pain. Palpation of the TrPs prior to therapy will often allow the patient to validate the existence of the referral pattern prior to therapy. While TrPs may appear in patterns of multiple muscles, single muscle patterns of the extensor carpi radialis brevis are common. TrP referal to the epicondyle results in tennis elbow. If the TrPs refer to the attachment point on the third carpal, it can send pain to the back of the wrist and hand, a feeling of tightness, burning on the extensor side of the forearm, and if the shortened muscle traps the radial nerve it may cause numbness and tingling in the hand, common in computer users. A painful shoulder is generally the result of soft tissue damage in the area of the glenohumeral joint or primary TrPs in related muscles groups. Soft tissue disorders of the glenohumeral joint may have been diagnosed by a medical doctor as rotator cuff tendonitis, subacromial bursitis, bicipital tendonitis, and capsulitis. Acupuncturists describe chronic shoulder pain as a combination of primary TrP activation and secondary activation from chronic pain, guarding, lack of movement, faulty posture occurring in the neck, shoulder girdle, upper arm, and anterior and posterior axillary folds. The longer arm and shoulder movement is restricted the higher the likelihood of capsulitis (frozen shoulder). A middle-aged woman developed capsulitis following an injury to her left shoulder. She received two cortisone shots and 10 weeks of physical therapy. With persistent pain, guarding, decreased shoulder range of motion, and disturbed sleep she consulted an acupuncturist. TrPs were mapped in the muscles of the rotator cuff and neck. Six acupuncture treatments focusing on TrPs were provided including electro-stimulation over an 8 week period, which resulted in full recovery of range of motion and no residual pain.[43]

In summary, acupuncture promotes pain relief and relaxation in single muscles as well as entire areas. Sympathetic hyperactivity responds to stimulation–relaxation of smooth muscle in associated areas, supporting muscle health generally by relieving vasospasm and lymph constriction.[36]

NUTRITION

Nutrition plays a role in preventing tissue breakdown and inflammation, thereby reducing pain and preserving strength. Strategic nutrition can also strengthen the muscle-tendon unit and improve biomechanics. For nutrient delivery, muscle strain resembles a traffic jam. Egress of lactic acid, inflammatory debris, and exuded extracellular fluid is impaired. Transport of oxygen, electrolytes, glucose, protein, and antioxidants into the injured region is similarly impaired. The previously described approaches to structural health improve nutrient import and toxin export of strained muscles. Nutrition interventions are generally whole body interventions, equipping the body to triage nutrients to the site of injury.

Muscle strain can occur during physical activity, a time when the body is depleting glycogen stores, protein stores, and water. Glycogen is the major fuel of muscle activity. The body replenishes glycogen stores most quickly in the 2 h following muscle damage, provided that dietary carbohydrate is available. Skeletal muscle breakdown from muscle strain can be intensified by inadequate dietary protein. One amino acid, l-creatine, has been found to be beneficial in reducing cell damage and inflammation after long distance exercise.[44] Hydration promotes muscle recovery, and sodium increases water absorption and intake into the cells. Since sweat reduces sodium, sometimes salt replacement is needed (Chapter 8). Carbohydrate enhances water absorption, especially when glycogen is depleted (Chapter 5).

Muscle strain is associated with oxidative stress and therefore increased antioxidant demand. The body has a reserve of diverse antioxidants as described in Chapter 7. Dietary supplementation with antioxidants can be beneficial if antioxidant stores are depleted. Whey protein has the amino acids needed to synthesize the peptide glutathione, an aqueous-phase antioxidant of high potency. Therefore, whey protein may provide essential amino acids for both muscle protein synthesis and glutathione synthesis. One particular antioxidant, vitamin C, is also needed for muscle formation.[45] Extreme deficiency in vitamin C led to a medial head tear of the gastrocnemius in a 22-year-old man.[46] Repleting vitamin C improves clinical response to healing musculoskeletal strain.[46,47] Fruits and vegetables are good dietary sources of vitamin C and other antioxidants, and they are also alkalinizing. Since muscle strain is a state of regional metabolic acidosis, in theory, dietary and nutritional supplement selections which are alkalinizing could be advantageous to healing. Patients can test for both vitamin C and pH with urine dipstick tests described in Chapter 25.

Omega-3 essential fats, such as those found in fish oil, are incorporated into the cell membrane where they modulate the inflammatory cascade. The Western diet is associated with low total omega-3 intake, low intake of omega-3 with respect to omega-6 and consumption of *trans* fats. Restoring omega-3 concentrations, the balance between omega-3 and omega-6 fats and the absence of *trans* fats improves recovery from muscle strain.

Using the aforementioned knowledge of antioxidants and essential fats, researchers at the University of Florida developed a dietary supplement containing mixed tocopherols (various forms of the antioxidant vitamin E), flavonoids (plant-derived antioxidants) and DHA (an omega-3 essential fat). The supplement was given to the test group during a 14 day experimental protocol, which induced an acute phase injury via eccentric arm curl exercise. Both groups experienced injury as evidenced by increases in CK, LDH, pain and decreased range of motion 3 days after the exercise. At day 10, the placebo group had significantly greater increases in IL-6 and C reactive protein (CRP), biochemical markers of systemic inflammation, than the treatment group.[48]

Minerals influence the body's ability to recover from muscle strain. Sodium is required for adequate hydration. Chromium is needed for muscle cells to replenish glucose after exercise, as described in Chapter 11. Suboptimal zinc impairs tissue healing; zinc purportedly serves as a cofactor for over 300 enzymes including carbonic anhydrase which removes carbon dioxide from cells and lactate dehydrogenase, which converts lactate to pyruvate.[49] Iron deficiency reduces oxygenation of tissue because of associated anemia. Insufficient magnesium is prevalent and impairs tissue healing. Dietary intake of magnesium among women athletes is estimated at 65% of the current RDA of 280 mg/d,[49] suggesting that suboptimal magnesium is common. Supplementation is associated with reduction in muscle spasm, reduction in serum lactate, and increase in muscle strength.[49,50]

Muscle strain can bring an underlying acquired or inherited myopathy to clinical attention. Statin-induced myopathy as well as the more common myalgias may be ameliorated by coenzyme Q supplementation.[51] Inherited metabolic myopathies have been considered degenerative. However, enzyme therapy using recombinant DNA techniques and other medical advances extend the possibility that in the near future early diagnosis, medical treatment and dietary intervention can prevent degeneration.[52] Optimizing vitamin B12 in persons with inadequate absorption and dietary intake may also improve recovery from muscle strain, presumably by correcting early changes in erythropoesis, energy metabolism and the kinetic chain.

Nutrition can also decrease biomechanical forces on a muscle tendon unit. Examples are hydration and weight reduction for muscle strain of the lower back. Hydration can restore the vertebral disks' ability to absorb biomechanical forces (Chapter 8). Weight reduction improves function,[53] while obesity increases risk of low back pain[54] and makes acute muscle strain more likely to become chronic.[55]

SUMMARY

Common muscle strains occur when the tissue's strength is overcome by biomechanical forces. The molecular process of inflammation ensues. Various structural interventions work synergistically with nutrition to reduce inflammation, strengthen tissue, and reduce biomechanical forces on the muscle–tendon unit.

REFERENCES

1. Taylor, D.C., Dalton, J.D., Seaber, A., and Garrett, W., Experimental muscle strain inury: early functional and structural deficits and the increased risk of reinjury, *Am. J. Sports Med.*, 21, 11; 190–194, 1993.
2. Buckwalter, J.A., Einhorn, T.A., and Simon, S.R., *Orthopaedic Basic Science*, 2nd ed., American Academy of Orthopaedic Surgeons, 2000, p. 63, 588, 700, 702.
3. Sahrmann, S.A., *Diagnosis and Treatment of Movement Impairment Syndromes*, Mosby, St. Louis, 2002.
4. Lieber, R.L., Woodburn, T.M., and Friden, J., Muscle damage induced by eccentric contractions of 25% strain, *J. Appl. Physiol.*, 70, 2498–2507, 1991.
5. Lundon, K., *Orthopedic Rehabilitation Science*, Butterworth Heinmann, New York, 2003.
6. LaStayo, P.C., Woolf, J.M., Lewek, M.D., et al., Eccentric muscle contractions: their contribution to injury, prevention, rehabilitation, and sport, *J. Orthop. Sports Phys. Ther.*, 33, 557–571, 2003.
7. Brukner, P. and Khan, K., *Clinical Sports Medicine*, 2nd ed., McGraw-Hill Company, New York, 2002.
8. Kisner, C. and Colby, L., *Therapeutic Exercise: Foundations and Techniques*, 3rd ed., F.A. Davis Co, Philadelphia, PA, 1996.
9. Toumi, H. and Best, T.M., The inflammatory response: friend or enemy for muscle injury? *Br. J. Sports Med.*, 37, 284–286, 2003.
10. Kannus, P., Parkkari, J., Jarvinen, T.L.N., Jarvinen, T.A.H., and Jarvinen, M., Basic science and clinical studies coincide: active treatment approach is needed after a sports injury, *Scand. J. Med. Sci. Sports*, 13, 150–154, 2003.
11. Bedair, H.S., Ho, A.M., Fu, F.H., and Huard, J., Skeletal muscle regeneration: an update and recent findings, *Curr. Opin. Orthop.*, 15, 360–363, 2004.
12. Bleakley, C., McDonough, S., and MacAuley, D., The use of ice in the treatment of acute soft tissue injury: a systematic review of randomized controlled trials, *Am. J. Sports Med.*, 32, 251–261, 2004.

13. Merrick, M.A., Therapeutic modalities as an adjunct to rehabilitation, in *Physical Rehabilitation of the Injured Athlete*, 3rd ed., Andrews, J.R., Harrelson, G.L., and Wilk, K.E., Eds., Saunders, Philadelphia, PA, 2004.

14. Hecox, B., Mehreteab, T.A., and Weisberg, J., *Physical Agents*, Appleton & Lange, Norwalk, CT, 1994.

15. Beckerman, H., et al., The efficacy of laser therapy for musculoskeletal and skin disorders: a criteria-based meta-analysis of randomized clinical trials, *Phys. Ther.*, 72, 483–491, 1992.

16. Stergiolas, A., Low-level laser therapy treatment can reduce edema in second degree ankle sprains, *J. Clin. Laser Med. Surg.*, 22, 125–128, 2004.

17. Nikolaou, P., MacDonald, B., Glisson, R., Seaber, A., and Garrett, W., Biomechanical and histological evaluation of muscle after controlled strain injury, *Am. J. Sports Med.*, 15, 9–13, 1987.

18. Kahn, J., *Principles and Practice of Electrotherapy*, 3rd ed., Churchill Livingstone, New York, 1994.

19. Grodin, A.J. and Cantu, R.I., *Myofascial Manipulation Course Manual*, University of St. Augustine Press, St. Augustine, FL, 1999.

20. Orchard, J. and Best, T., The management of muscle strain injuries: an early return versus the risk of reoccurrence, *Clin. J. Sport Med.*, 12, 3–5, 2002.

21. Best, T.M., Shehadeh, S.E., Leverson, G., Michel, J.T., Corr, D.T., and Aeschlimann, D., Analysis of changes in mRNA levels of myoblast- and fibroblast-derived gene products in healing skeletal muscle using quantitative reverse transcription polymerase chain reaction, *J. Orthop. Res.*, 19, 565–572, 2001.

22. Paris, S.V. and Loubert, P.V., *Foundations of Clinical Orthopaedics*, Institute Press, St. Augustine, FL, 1999.

23. Orchard, J., Marsden, J., Lord, S., and Garlick, D., Preseason hamstring muscle weakness associated with hamstring muscle injury in Australian footballers, *Am. J. Sports Med.*, 25, 81–85, 1997.

24. Knapik, J.J., Bauman, C.L., Jones, B.H., Harris, J.McA, and Vaughan, L., Preseason strength and flexibility imbalances associated with athletic injuries in female collegiate athletes, *Am. J. Sports Med.*, 19, 76–81, 1991.

25. Dale, R.B., Harrelson, G.L., and Leaver-Dunn, D., Principles of rehabilitation, in *Physical Rehabilitation of the Injured Athlete*, 3rd ed., Andrews, J.R., Harrelson, G.L., and Wilk, K.E., Eds., Philadelphia, PA, Saunders, 2004.

26. Voight, M.L., Hoogenboom, B., Blackburn, T.A., and Cook, G., Functional training and advanced rehabilitation, in *Physical Rehabilitation of the Injured Athlete*, 3rd ed., Andrews, J.R., Harrelson, G.L., and Wilk, K.E., Eds., Saunders, Philadelphia, PA, 2004.

27. Kappler, R.E. and Kuchera, W.A., Diagnosis and plan for manual treatment: a prescription, in *Foundations for Osteopathic Medicine*, Ward, R.C., Ed., Lippincott Williams & Wilkins, Philadelphia, PA, 2003, 574–579.

28. Seffinger, M.A., Development of osteopathic philosophy, in *Foundations for Osteopathic Medicine*, Ward, R.C., Ed., Lippincott Williams & Wilkins, Baltimore, MD, 1997, pp. 3–7.

29. Eisenhart, A.W., Gaeta, T.J., and Yens, D.P., Osteopathic manipulative treatment in the emergency department for patients with acute ankle injuries, *J. Am. Osteopath. Assoc.*, 103, 417–421, 2003.

30. Kimberly, P.E., Formulating a prescription for osteopathic manipulative treatment, in *The Principles of Palpatory Diagnosis and Manipulative Technique*, Beal, M.C., Ed., 1979, pp. 146–152.

31. Willard, F.H., Nociception, the neuroendocrine immune system, and osteopathic medicine, in *Foundations for Osteopathic Medicine*, Ward, R.C., Exec. Ed., Lippincott Williams & Wilkins, Philadelphia, PA, 2003, pp. 137–154.

32. Willard, F.H., Neuroendocrine-immune network, nociceptive stress, and the general adaptive response. in *Physiotherapy in Mental Health: A Practical Approach*, Everett, T., Dennis, M., and Ricketts, E., Eds., Butterworth-Heinemann, Oxford, UK, 1995, pp. 102–126.

33. Denslow, J.S. and Hassett, C.C., Central excitatory state associated with postural abnormalities, *J. Neurophysiol.*, 5, 393–402, 1942.

34. Engstrom, J. and Martin, J., Disorders of the autonomic nervous system, in *Harrison's Principles of Internal Medicine*, 14th ed., Fauci, A.S., et al., Ed., McGraw-Hill, New York, 1998, pp. 2375–2376.

35. Menck, J.Y., Requejo, S.M., and Kulig, K., Thoracic spine dysfunction in upper extremity complex regional pain syndrome Type I, *J. Orthop. Sports Phys. Ther.*, 30, 401–409, 2000.

36. Seem, M., *A New American Acupuncture, Acupuncture Osteopathy (The Myofacial Release of the Bodymind's Holding Patterns)*, 1st ed., 7th printing, Blue Poppy Press, Boulder, CO, 1999, pp. 16–17, 148.

37. Bonica, J.J. and Sola, A.E., Other painful disorders of the upper limb, in *The Management of Pain*, 2nd ed., Bonica, J.J., Loeser, Chapman, C.R., et al., Eds., Lea & Febiger, Philadelphia, PA, 1990.

38. Birch, S.J. and Felt, R.L., *Understanding Acupuncture*, Churchill Livingstone, New York, 1999, p. 46, 154, 170.

39. Travell, J.G. and Simons, D.G., *Myofascial Pain and Dysfunction: The Trigger Point Manual*, vol. 1, Williams & Wilkins, Baltimore, MD, 1983, p. 4.

40. Davies, C., *The Trigger Point Workbook, Your Self-Treatment Guide for Pain Relief*, New Harbinger Publications, Inc., Oakland, 2001.

41. Baldry, P.E., *Acupuncture, Trigger Points and Musculoskeletal Pain*, 3rd ed., Elsevier Churchill Livingstone, Philadelphia, PA, 2005, pp. 76–77, 82–83, 117.

42. Worsley, J.R., *Traditional Chinese Acupuncture, Meridians and Points*, Element Books, Inc., Boston, MA, Reprinted 1988, p. 296.

43. Godwin, L., Acupuncture in capsulitis management: a clinical case, Personal communication.

44. Santos, R.V., Bassit, R.A., Caperuto, E.C., and Costa Rosa, L.F., The effect of creatine supplementation upon inflammatory and muscle soreness markers after a 30 km race, *Life Sci.*, 75, 1917–1924, 2004.

45. Boyle, P.E. and Irving, J.T., Skeletal muscle changes in scurvy with a note on the mechanism of the attachment of myofibrils to tendon, *Science*, 114, 572–573, 1951.

46. Keenan, A., Mitts, K.G., and Kurtz, C.A., Scurvy presenting as a medial head tear of the gastrocnemius, *Orthopedics*, 25, 689–691, 2002.

47. Kearns, S.R., Daly, A.F., Sheehan, K., Murray, P., Kelly, C., and Bouchier-Hayes, D., Oral vitamin C reduces the injury to skeletal muscle caused by compartment syndrome, *J. Bone Joint Surg. Br.*, 86, 906–911, 2004.

48. Phillips, T., Childs, A.C., Dreon, D.M., Phinney, S., and Leeuwenburgh, C., A dietary supplement attenuates IL-6 and CRP after eccentric exercise in untrained males, *Med. Sci. Sports Exerc.*, 35, 2032–2037, 2003.

49. Lukaski, H.C., Vitamin and mineral status: effects on physical performance, Nutrition, 20, 632–644, 2004.

50. Brilla, L.R. and Haley, T.F., Effect of magnesium supplementation on strength training in humans, *J. Am. Coll. Nutr.*, 11, 326–329, 1992.

51. Rosenson, R.S., Current overview of statin-induced myopathy, *Am. J. Med.*, 116, 408–416, 2004.

52. Kishnani, P.S. and Howell, R.R., Pompe disease in infants and children, *J. Pediatr.*, 114 (Suppl. 1), S35–S43, 2004.

53. Melissas, J., Kontakis, G., Volakakis, E., et al., The effect of surgical weight reduction on functional status in morbidly obese patients with low back pain, *Obes. Surg.*, 15 (3): 378–81, 2005.

54. Andersen, R.E., Crespo, C.J., Bartless, S.J., et al., Relationship between body weight and significant knee, hip and back pain in older Americans, *Obes. Res.*, 11, 1159–1162, 2003.

55. Fransen, M., Woodward, M., Norton, R., et al., Risk factors associated with the transition from acute to chronic occupational back pain, *Spine*, 27, 92–98, 2002.

20 Muscle Hypertrophy

Stephen E. Alway, Ph.D.

CONTENTS

MUSCLE GROWTH

INTRODUCTION

Skeletal muscle hypertrophy can develop in response to overload or resistance training exercise. Muscle hypertrophy occurs as a result of an increase in proteins, leading to elevations in muscle cross-sectional area, length, or muscle mass. Advances in cellular and molecular research over the past two decades have provided a basis for understanding some of the mechanisms that contribute to these responses leading to muscle hypertrophy.

MUSCLE HYPERTROPHY RESULTS FROM INCREASED PROTEIN ACCUMULATION

If muscle hypertrophy is to occur, there must be a net increase in protein accumulation. This can occur through an increase in protein synthesis, a decrease in protein degradation, or both. It is clear that exercise and various types of overload have a profound effect on muscle protein metabolism. If the stimulus is sufficient, net protein synthesis will increase, resulting in muscle hypertrophy. Recent improvements in the methods used to study muscle hypertrophy including the use of isotopic tracers and muscle biopsies to identify muscle protein synthesis and the use of magnetic resonance imaging or computerized tomographic scanning to carefully document changes in muscle cross-sectional area or muscle volume have advanced our understanding of mechanisms leading to muscle hypertrophy.

EXERCISE AS A STIMULUS FOR MUSCLE GROWTH

Acute resistance exercise stimulates increased protein synthesis,[1] but aging may increase the need for available amino acids to induce muscle growth.[2] The summation of acute responses of protein synthesis to exercise or overload results in chronic increases in net protein accumulation or muscle hypertrophy.[3] Long-term adaptations to resistance exercise might result in protein synthesis rates not significantly different from those of untrained muscles as a plateauing effect.[4] It is possible that increasing the intensity of the training or improving the amino acids or other nutrients required for protein synthesis could improve muscle hypertrophy[5] once this plateau has been reached. However, in a study by Chesley et al.,[6] muscle protein was not increased in spite of an intensive training stimulus, and this suggests that nutritional or other elements are at least as important as the training stimulus for inducing muscle hypertrophy.

MUSCLE HYPERTROPHY REQUIRES ADDING NEW NUCLEI

Because myonuclei are postmitotic,[7] satellite cells, which are also called muscle precursor cells (MPCs), provide the only important source for adding new nuclei to initiate muscle regeneration, muscle hypertrophy, and postnatal muscle growth in muscles of both young and aged humans.[7] MPCs are critical for muscle growth because muscle hypertrophy is markedly reduced or eliminated completely after irradiation to prevent MPC activation.[8] An example of activated MPCs is shown in Figure 20.1. Growth of adult skeletal muscle requires activation and differentiation of MPCs and increased protein synthesis and accumulation of proteins.

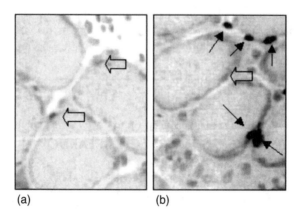

(a)   (b)

FIGURE 20.1 Satellite cells, also called muscle precursor cells, proliferate to add new nuclei during muscle hypertrophy. a. Control muscle has myonuclei that are not capable of proliferating. Myonuclei examples are shown with open arrows. b. Satellite cells or MPCs are activated and proliferate in loaded muscles. Closed arrows show examples of activated satellite cells that have a marker incorporated for DNA synthesis. The open arrow shows an example of a nonproliferating myonucleus.

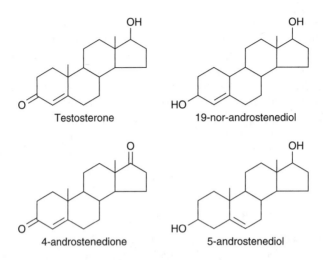

FIGURE 20.2 Chemical structures of anabolic hormones.

A proposed model of how MPC activation may lead to greater muscle hypertrophy after anabolic steroid treatement is presented in Figure 20.2.

Editor's Note

Exogenous anabolic steroids, which excede physiologic levels, cause nutrients to be used for muscle growth instead of other, perhaps more crucial, functions. Laboratory and clinical data provide a rationale for treating anabolic steroid-induced nutrient imbalances.

THE STIMULUS FOR MUSCLE GROWTH MAY ALSO INCREASE MUSCLE BREAKDOWN

ACUTE EXERCISE MAY INCREASE MUSCLE PROTEIN BREAKDOWN

The net effects of muscle growth in response to an exercise or overload stimulus depend upon an elevation in protein synthesis and any changes in net protein degradation. Studies conducted over the past two decades have shown divergent results. Indirect evaluations of muscle protein breakdown via urea and 3-methylhistididine excretion suggested that protein degradation increases,[9] decreases,[10] or remains unchanged.[11] More recent methods have examined muscle degradation using isotopic enrichment of the intracellular protein pool and have shown increases in muscle protein degradation after resistance training,[1] although not as much as the increase in protein synthesis. The availability of required nutrients may be a determining factor.

THE STIMULUS FOR MUSCLE GROWTH CAN EXCEED THE BODY'S ABILITY TO ADEQUATELY NOURISH THE MUSCLE

The stimulus for muscle growth (e.g., resistance exercise) includes increases in both muscle protein synthesis and degradation. For a net increase in protein accumulation, the cellular conditions must favor increasing protein synthesis more than protein degradation. This requires a much greater metabolic demand than if only protein synthesis was increased with resistance training. Although the stimulus for hypertrophy is important, dietary composition may be a critical factor regulating the degree of muscle hypertrophy[12] because inadequate nutrients will not position the muscle's environmental milieu to favor net protein synthesis and accumulation.

WHAT LIMITS MUSCLE HYPERTROPHY?

We can learn some clues from what limits hypertrophy by studying aging muscles. Both young adults and aged humans can achieve some degree of muscle hypertrophy as long as muscles are exposed to resistance exercise or overload of adequate intensity and duration.[13] Aging appears to reduce the relative change in muscle mass to loading.[14] Assuming that the stimulus is adequate and the intensity is sufficient to fully activate the mechanical and molecular signaling pathways, the limitations to muscle hypertrophy may occur at several levels. First, the inability to fully recruit adequate MPCs will limit hypertrophy. Secondly, inadequate hormonal environments for activation and differentiation of MPCs will limit hypertrophy. Finally, increases in apoptosis (programmed cell death) that remove activated MPCs will limit or reduce the potential for hypertrophy. Thus, anything that limits activation, proliferation, and differentiation of MPCs will limit muscle hypertrophy.

1. *A low activation of MPCs will limit hypertrophy.* Without sufficient new nuclei, muscle specific gene transcription will be limited, and this will result in less total protein synthesis and muscle hypertrophy even in the face of adequate muscle stimulus for growth.[15]

2. *Apoptosis in response to overload may limit hypertrophy.* MPC proliferation is a critical event that provides additional nuclei, enabling muscle to increase its mass. However, even if MPCs are activated normally during repetitive loading, but they either do not differentiate or do not survive to participate in increased protein synthesis, then muscle hypertrophy cannot occur. One possibility that could explain

the lower differentiation (largely lower survival) of activated MPCs in aging muscles is the result of the elevation of apoptosis protein levels in muscles from aged animals. We have recently shown that the most recently activated MPCs during loading are also the most susceptible to apoptosis.[16] On the basis of these data, we hypothesize that satellite cell activation is lower in muscle of old animals and that apoptosis is higher in these cells, activated during repetitive loading, so fewer MPCs survive and contribute to muscle hypertrophy. Apoptosis might also limit hypertrophy in young athletes, especially in conditions of overtraining.

3. *Inadequate or inappropriate hormonal milieu will limit hypertrophy.* Skeletal muscle tissue constitutes ~40 to 45% of total body weight in humans and is among the body's most metabolically active tissues. The muscle's hormonal environment (i.e., milieu) has a major impact upon protein synthesis and therefore on muscle growth and hypertrophy. Human skeletal muscle undergoes protein turnover even under nonexercised conditions, and protein metabolism increases during hypertrophy. Hormones such as testosterone, growth hormone (GH), insulin, insulin-like growth factor-I (IGF-I), and glucocorticoids are important regulators of muscle remodeling including determining whether muscle growth or atrophy will occur. Furthermore, skeletal muscles act as a reserve for free amino acids, which provide precursors for glucose via gluconeogenesis during caloric restriction, but clearly such conditions are not favorable for muscle hypertrophy.

Some of the hormonal responses occurring in muscle hypertrophy are difficult to characterize *in vivo* because one hormone or metabolite can interact with other hormones or metabolites. A complete review of the endocrine effects on muscle protein turnover is beyond the scope of this chapter; however, the responses of major hormones that affect protein synthesis and degradation will be summarized here. The effects of testosterone and exogenous testosterone will be examined in detail.

- *Insulin.* Shortly after the discovery of insulin, it was found that exogenous insulin reduced muscle wasting, which is often associated with diabetes. Anecdotal and case study evidence also indicates that insulin therapy improves muscle hypertrophy in athletes (especially those who have diabetes). Nevertheless, the literature has conflicting data evaluating the efficacy of insulin on *in vivo* protein synthesis. Part of the confusion may be the manner in which insulin is studied. For example, infusion of insulin to the venous systems causes a significant reduction in blood amino acid levels. This reduces the available amino acids that can be provided to a muscle for protein synthesis. Thus, when amino acid levels are not increased along with insulin, there is no increase in protein synthesis,[17,18] but if amino acids are elevated during insulin therapy, protein synthesis can be increased[19] even in atrophic muscle.[20] Insulin has also been shown to reduce protein catabolism, thereby improving net protein accumulation and muscle mass in healthy subjects.[21]

- *Growth hormone and insulin-like growth factor-I.* It is thought that the anabolic properties of growth hormone (GH) largely stem from its actions through insulin-like growth factor-I (IGF-I), which is produced in the liver in response to GH. However, both GH and IGF-I have been shown to increase muscle protein synthesis in resting and inactive muscles[22,23] and in atrophic muscles[24] or after resistance exercise,[25] but this may be dependent upon adequate nutrition.[26,27] Nevertheless, other studies have failed to find any increase in muscle protein synthesis by IGF-I or GH in resting or exercised muscles.[28]

It is now understood that tissues other than the liver express IGF-I and that there are local as well as systemic forms of IGF-I that have different functions. Two alternatively spliced variants of IGF-I have been identified so far, and these are both expressed in skeletal muscle. One splice variant is expressed in response to physical activity, which has now been called 'mechano-growth factor' (MGF).[29] The other is similar to the systemic or liver type (IGF-IEa) and is important because it supplies the mature IGF-I required for upregulating protein synthesis in skeletal muscle and other tissues. MGF differs from systemic IGF-IEa in that it has a different peptide sequence, which is responsible for replenishing the MPCs in skeletal muscle. The ability to produce MGF declines with age,[29] and this occurs concomitantly with the decline in circulating GH levels. GH treatment upregulates the level of IGF-I gene expression in older people, and when combined with resistance exercise, more is spliced toward MGF and hence should improve the ability of muscle to respond to physical activity.[29,30]

- *Cortisol.* High levels of cortisol can reduce muscle mass during inactivity or injury and can limit the extent of muscle hypertrophy even given an adequate stimulus for muscle growth.[4,31] The time of day when exercise is done may also affect the level to which cortisol is expressed, with greater levels found during evening exercise sessions.[32] Presumably, reduced cortisol levels should reduce protein catabolism and improve protein accumulation, and this can at least be partially accomplished by providing higher levels of amino acids and other nutrients.[33]
- *Testosterone.* Exogenous testosterone and testosterone derivatives have received considerable political and press attention and have been the focus of numerous studies. Most studies examining androgens and testosterone has been aimed at hypogonadal men,[34] in persons having muscle-wasting diseases,[35] or aging-associated (sarcopenia) muscle loss.[36] Compounds such as nandrolone decanoate have been used to improve tendons and rotator cuff tendon healing.[37] However, there have been long debates in the scientific literature regarding whether

testosterone and related compounds improve muscle protein synthesis and muscle hypertrophy and whether any anecdotal changes in muscle mass and performance are caused by placebo effects or water retention by subjects. However, Bhasin and colleagues[38] have shown quite clearly that testosterone injections improve muscle mass in nonexercised subjects as compared with placebo injections. The increase in muscle mass occurs from an increase in protein synthesis[39] and may also be in part because of a decrease in protein degradation.[33]

PHYSIOLOGIC EFFECTS OF EXOGENOUS TESTOSTERONE AND NUTRIENTS AIMED AT STIMULATING ENDOGENOUS TESTOSTERONE PRODUCTION

EFFECTS OF EXOGENOUS TESTOSTERONE

Testosterone is a 19-carbon steroid with a 4,5 double bond and a keto-group at position 3 and a hydroxyl group at position 17 of its sterane ring (see Figure 20.3). Androgenic–anabolic steroid testosterone derivatives are synthetically derived versions of testosterone. Early attempts to generate anabolic steroids produced synthetic androgens that retained both androgenic and anabolic properties. The androgenic functions include developing male secondary sexual characteristics including lowering of the tone of the voice, male pattern hair growth, and hair loss. Anabolic effects include increasing muscle mass and strength. The most important anabolic function of testosterone and synthetic derivatives of this hormone is to increase protein synthesis and inhibit protein breakdown.[40]

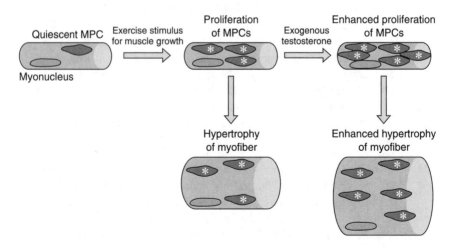

FIGURE 20.3 Proposed model of enhanced satellite cell or muscle precursor cell activation leading to improved muscle hypertrophy with exogenous testosterone.

Testosterone or anabolic steroids administered orally or by intramuscular injection are rapidly metabolized, so they cannot exert any significant effects on the human body. However, pharmacological manipulations of testosterone have been developed to reduce this problem. Three major modifications have been made. These include alkylation at the 17-α position with an ethyl or methyl group, esterification at the 17-β position, and alterations of testosterone's ring structure (see Figure 20.3).

Alkylation is important for creating oral active compounds that slow degradation by the liver. Esterification of testosterone and nortestosterone at the 17-β position slows metabolism and prolongs the effects of the compounds. Injectable oil soluble compounds can remain in the body (and detectable) for several months. Finally, alterations of the testosterone ring structure have been made for both oral and parenteral agents, which increase the activity of these compounds.[40]

MEDICAL USE OF EXOGENOUS TESTOSTERONE

Medical use of anabolic steroids has been prescribed to counteract testicular dysfunction (i.e., low testosterone levels) and improve the hypothalamus–pituitary–gonadal axis (i.e., male hypogonadism). Androgen and anabolic steroid therapy is primarily used in hypogonadal men to improve or maintain muscle strength and function.[41] Anabolic steroids have also been used to improve nitrogen balance to favor muscular anabolism in several muscle wasting conditions[42] including sarcopenia, which is the age-associated loss of muscle mass,[42] and some forms of anemia,[43] hereditary angioneurotic edema,[44] and osteoporosis.[45] Anabolic steroid use is also beneficial for improving respiratory muscle mass and strength in individuals who have tetraplegia and ventilatory insufficiency.[46]

Small amounts of anabolic steroids improve nitrogen balance after trauma and in patients after abdominal surgery and after burn injury,[47] and this should reduce muscle loss in these patients. In addition, patients with chronic obstructive pulmonary disease and HIV have been shown to have improved lean body mass after treatment with anabolic steroids; however, the effect of the improvement also appears to be related to the nutritional status of the patients.[48] Exogenous testosterone and anabolic steroids have been used to treat muscular dystrophies for many years because they improve muscle mass and reduce muscular dysfunction in muscular dystrophy.[49] However, the number of clinical trials has not been extensive, and the degree to which anabolic steroid treatment can improve various wasting diseases has not been widely studied in humans.

TESTOSTERONE THERAPY IN WOMEN

Like men, women have a loss in muscle mass and strength with age.[50] Likewise, there is a decrease in circulating blood levels of testosterone with increasing age

TABLE 20.1
Examples of anabolic androgenic steroids used by athletes

Clostebol	Dianabol
Drostanolone	Ethylestrenol
Fluoxymesterone	Metandren
Mesterolone	Methenolone
Norethandrolone	Nortestosterone
Oxandrolone	Oxymesterone
Oxymetholone	Stanozolol
Stenbolone	Testosterone
Tetrahydrogestrinone	Turinabol

in women, with ~50% of the decrease occurring by the age of 40.[51,52] Although levels of serum estradiol and 25-hydroxy vitamin D have a higher correlation with muscle mass than serum testosterone levels in women over 65 years of age,[52] there have been an insufficient number of studies to fully evaluate the effects of testosterone therapy combined with resistance exercise on muscle mass and strength in postmenopausal women.

TESTOSTERONE THERAPY AND ANABOLIC STEROIDS TO IMPROVE MUSCLE HYPERTROPHY

It is well known that exogenous testosterone in the form of androgenic–anabolic steroids increases the rate of muscle protein synthesis, promotes muscle growth, and reduces fat deposition.[39] Examples of anabolic–androgenic steroids available to athletes are given in Table 20.1.

Several studies have shown that muscle mass increases more than does strength, although both increase with testosterone therapy in men.[53,54] Although muscle hypertrophy occurs with anabolic steroid treatment, the gains are markedly greater when resistance training (to provide a growth stimulus) is combined with anabolic steroid therapy.[38] Women who use anabolic steroids in conjunction with resistance training have increases in both type I (slow twitch) and type II (fast twitch) fiber cross-sectional area,[55] whereas men who use exogenous testosterone and anabolic steroids while resistance training appear to induce preferential type II fiber hypertrophy.[13] The improvement in muscle mass after anabolic steroid treatment appears to be attributable to increased lean tissue rather than hydration.[56] Androgen receptors are preferentially expressed on mature muscle cells and myonuclei[57] and MPCs.[58] A model whereby exogenous testosterone increases satellite cell proliferation to support enhanced muscle hypertrophy is shown in Figure 20.2.

ANABOLIC PROHORMONES — THEIR MISUSE AMONG ATHLETES AND NUTRITIONAL PRODUCT MANUFACTURERS

INTRODUCTION

The prohormone, androstenedione first became available for public consumption over-the-counter in 1996. It is frequently marketed with nutrition products. Subsequently, several other prohormones including androstenediol, norandrostene-dione, and norandrostenediol became available to the public. The manufactures of these compounds claim that peripheral enzymatic conversion of prohormones to testosterone or nortestosterone (via ingestion of androstenedione and androstene-diol or 19-nor-androstenedione and 19-nor-androstenediol, respectively) leads to anabolic or ergogenic effects including improvements in muscle strength and mass. It has also been suggested that prohormones might help to offset the age-associated reduction in endogenous testosterone, DHEA, and sexual interest.[59]

The effects of oral 4-androstenedione administrations have received the most investigation in humans. Although androstenedione is structurally a "steroid," the anabolic effects of this steroid have not been clearly shown in healthy humans. Structurally similar prohormones such as 19-nor-4-androstenedione, 19-nor-4-androstenediol, 4-androstenediol, 5-androstenedione, and 5-androstenediol are also available to the public. There are subtle differences between the structures of prohormones and testosterone. For example, 19-norsteroids contain one less carbon atom in their sterane ring structure than testosterone. 4-androstenedione contains keto groups at positions 3 and 17, instead of one keto and one hydroxyl group, whereas 4-androstenediol contains two hydroxyl groups at these positions. 5-androstenedione and 5-androstenediol have a 5,6 double bond instead of the 4,5 double bond like testosterone (Figure 20.2).

The ubiquitous enzyme 17 regulates the synthesis of testosterone from the -dione, and synthesis of testosterone from -diol prohormones is regulated by 3-β-hydroxysteroid dehydrogenase. The isozymes in this enzyme family have specific metabolic activities and substrate specificity, which makes it likely that prohormone consumption could affect the synthesis of androgenic steroids other than testosterone such as dehydroepiandrosterone, estradiol, or luteinizing hormone either directly or via indirect pathways. In women, the activation of androgens appears to occur in the abdominal visceral and omental adipose tissue,[60] which suggests that adiposity may influence metabolic inactivation of testosterone or prohormone-induced testosterone.

ANDROSTENEDIONE AND DEHYDROEPIANDROSTERONE

Androstenedione (4-androstenedione) is the immediate precursor of testosterone. Androstenedione is produced by the testes and by the adrenal glands from dehydroepiandrosterone (DHEA).[61] Androstenedione supplementation has been speculated to increase plasma testosterone levels and improve muscle hypertrophy.[62] Thus, it is not surprising that androstenedione supplements have become popular for improving performance in athletes. Androstenedione is marketed to increase blood testosterone levels, with the idea that this will directly improve muscle strength and mass. Manufacturer-suggested daily doses for oral use of this prohormone range from 100 to 1200 mg/d. It is also available as patches, percutaneous gels, and sublingual sprays.[63] So far, clinical applications of androstenedione have not been reported.

Although androstenedione has been studied previously in rodents,[64] its use was first described in 1962 as a case study in two women, who were given 100 mg of oral androstenedione.[65] This study reported that the oral androstenedione increased plasma testosterone by fourfold to sevenfold in these two subjects, with peak testosterone levels found within 60 min of ingestion of the prohormone. In spite of these large changes in plasma testosterone, plasma levels of androstenedione that had been undetectable before supplementation only had very small increases 60 to 90 min after androstenedione ingestion.[65] DHEA given at a similar dose was shown to have similar effects with ~4-fold increases in plasma testosterone within 90 min of ingestion. These data suggest that oral supplementation with androstenedione or DHEA improves blood levels of testosterone in women.[65]

Blaquier and coworkers[66,67] reported that 4-androstenediol (androstenediol) exhibited ~2.8-fold greater conversion to testosterone than did 4-androstenedione. This introduces the possibility that 4-androstenediol might provide greater anabolic/androgenic results than 4-androstenedione. This higher efficacy may be because androstenedione is converted to androstenediol before becoming testosterone.[67] It is therefore unclear why most research and earlier marketing focused on androstenedione instead of androstenediol in spite of the greater likelihood for androstenediol to elevate testosterone.

EFFECTS OF ANDROSTENEDIONE ON BLOOD HORMONAL LEVELS AND MUSCLE HYPERTROPHY

The extent by which elevated blood levels of prohormones increase muscle growth is unclear from current studies. A critical review of key studies allows clinicians to decide if the information can be generalized to their patients and if additional nutritional recommendations are needed to increase effectiveness.

King et al.[62] studied 30 untrained normotestoterogenic men who performed 8 weeks of whole-body resistance training. Acute androstenedione (100 mg) had no effect on total testosterone, free testosterone, luteinizing hormone (LH), or follicle stimulating hormone (FSH) but increased serum androstenedione concentrations by 175 to 350%. Serum estradiol concentrations were higher after 2, 5, and 8 weeks of resistance training compared with the androstenedione group. Total testosterone was unaffected by androstenedione ingestion, but the free testosterone concentration was significantly higher at 0 and 8 weeks of the study. Despite the elevated blood levels, androstenedione did not appear to alter body composition, fat free mass, cross-sectional areas of type I and type II fibers from the vastus lateralis, and muscle strength relative to placebo consumption in the trained subjects. The generalizability of the study to competitive athletes may be limited because the men in this study had body fat in excess of 20%. Adipose is likely to minimize the effectiveness because adiposity increases conversion of androstenedione to estrogens because of peripheral aromatization in adipose tissue.[68]

Wallace et al.[69] studied the effects 12 weeks of supplementation with 50 mg two times daily of either androstenedione or DHEA in a group of middle-aged men. No significant improvements in testosterone levels, lean body mass, or strength were observed in either supplement group compared with the placebo group. This lack of effect was the result of the low dose provided to the subjects. The dose is comparable with that used in the treatment of elderly subjects before surgery to preserve muscle and bone. It is not surprising that the positive results of muscle preservation before stress in frail elderly men and women is not generalizable to muscle enhancement in middle-aged men.

Ballantyne et al.[70] examined oral androstenedione supplementation in male subjects over a 24 h period and then gave the subjects 200 mg of oral androstenedione (in two divided doses). Venous blood samples were obtained every 3 h over the following 12 h and then 24 h after ingestion of the final capsule. Heavy resistance training increased serum testosterone, and androstenedione supplementation increased serum androstenedione by ~200% and luteinizing hormone by ~100%, without concomitant increases in serum testosterone, free testosterone, or estradiol. Because most androstenedione is converted first to estrone in blood, bone, skeletal muscle, and adipose tissue rather than to estradiol, it is possible that estrone rather than estradiol levels would have been a more sensitive measure of the effect of androstenedione on serum estrogens.[71] However, exercise in the androstenedione group significantly elevated plasma estradiol by approximately 83% for 90 min. On the basis of the lack of change in testosterone levels, these data suggest that androstenedione may not improve testosterone release or synthesis and therefore may not provide male athletes a marked anabolic improvement above that provided by heavy resistance exercise.[70]

Leder et al.[71] found that healthy men aged 20 to 40 years given 300 mg of oral androstenedione had serum testosterone concentrations increased by 34%; however, baseline testosterone levels, obtained 24 h after androstenedione administration, did not change.[71] Serum estradiol significantly increased by 42 and 128% in subjects consuming 100 and 300 mg/d of androstenedione, respectively. These data suggest that oral androstenedione, when given in dosages of 300 mg/d, increases serum testosterone and estradiol concentrations in some healthy men, but the effects are variable between subjects.[71]

Recent studies by Brown and colleagues[72,73] have evaluated the effectiveness of a nutritional supplement containing androstenedione and herbs that were designed to enhance serum testosterone concentrations and prevent the formation of dehydrotestosterone and estrogens. Healthy 30 to 59 year old men consumed a combination of 300 mg androstenedione, 150 mg dehydroepiandrosterone,

540 mg saw palmetto, 300 mg indole-3-carbinol, 625 mg chrysin, and 750 mg tribulus terrestris per day or a placebo for 28 days. Whereas the ingestion of androstenedione combined with herbal products increased serum-free testosterone concentrations in older men, these herbal products did not prevent the conversion of ingested androstenedione to estradiol and dehydrotestosterone in the short duration of this study.

Broeder and colleagues[74] studied the effects of oral androstenedione and androstenediol supplementation during 12 weeks of intense resistance training in the so called Andro Study. Fifty healthy men (age 35 to 65 years) were randomly assigned to a placebo, androstenedione (200 mg/d taken in two divided doses), or androstenediol (200 mg/d taken in two divided doses) group. Each subject participated 3 days per week in a heavy resistance training program that included an average of three sets of nine exercises (i.e., a total of 81 sets per week) using 60 to 95% of their pre-training 1 repetition maximum. Total and free testosterone levels increased in the androstenedione group over 1 to 2 months but returned to basal concentrations by the third month of the study. Compared with week 0, concentrations of estrone, estradiol, and DHEA-sulfate increased significantly in the androstenedione and androstenediol groups at week 12. Neither androstenedione nor androstenediol supplementation improved the resistance training improvements in muscle strength compared with the placebo group and may have a negative impact on blood lipids and cholesterol.[75] However, the conclusion regarding the impact on muscle mass should be viewed carefully because the subjects were probably hypocaloric because the average energy intake was only ~120 kJ/kg/d or 29 kcal/kg/d, whereas current nutrition recommendations for individuals undergoing intense exercise training suggest that these subjects needed ~3 kJ/kg/d or 13 kcal/kg/d more than they received in this study.[76] Thus, the training program in this study[74] may have been too strenuous or the nutritional intake inadequate, considering that it failed to positively alter improve muscle mass even in the placebo group. This underscores the importance of maintaining adequate or superior nutrition during exercise training such as resistance training and that supplementation per se may be inadequate to invoke changes in muscle mass even given adequate muscle stimulus to hypertrophy and having a muscle milieu that includes potential anabolic compounds.

GENDER DIFFERENCES WITH ANDROSTENEDIONE

Horton and Tait[77] examined the interconversions of androstenedione and testosterone in women. These researchers showed that with intravenous administration of androstenedione and testosterone, ~60% of plasma testosterone is derived from androstenedione, whereas less than 3% of the plasma androstenedione is derived from testosterone. Therefore, the conversion of androstenedione to testosterone contributes largely to the circulating testosterone concentrations in women. In contrast, in men only ~0.3% of plasma testosterone is derived from androstenedione, whereas ~37% of plasma androstenedione is derived from plasma testosterone.

Therefore, men appear to be capable of preferentially converting testosterone into androstenedione, and the contribution of androstenedione to blood testosterone levels is likely to be minimal. From further investigation of gender differences in hormone metabolism, Horton and Tait concluded that men can convert testosterone to androstenedione more easily than women, but women appear to convert androstenedione to testosterone more readily than men. These data provide a rationale for using androstenedione for increasing androgen levels and reducing sarcopenia and osteoporosis in postmenopausal women and hypogonadal men.[78]

PHYSICAL EXAM AND LABORATORY SCREENING — FALSE POSITIVES AND FALSE NEGATIVES

CLINICAL AND LABORATORY CHARACTERISTICS OF EXOGENOUS TESTOSTERONE USE

Exogenous steroid use alters clinical and laboratory findings. Much of the information relating to clinical and laboratory effects of exogenous testosterone is obtained from case reports, which even include fatalities.[79] The long-term clinical health effects are dependent upon the type of exogenous testosterone compound, dose, frequency of use, and age of the athlete. Assessment of health consequences and evaluation of the physical examination are complicated in that some athletes combine one or two anabolic steroids or other hormones and several prohormones or just take prohormones. Some athletes use the compounds in tandem for long periods of time, and some use them more periodically.[80] Comprehensive scientific studies are complicated by the ethical implications of giving volunteers the supramaximal doses typically used by athletes. The final problem is that some of the compounds obtained by athletes are obtained on the "black market," and the quality, amount, and composition of the compounds cannot be known.[81]

There are several physical attributes that might together provide some evidence of exogenous testosterone use, but these must be followed up with more objective data before drawing conclusions on use or misuse. Many of the clinical and laboratory characteristics are summarized in Table 20.2.

Sexual and Physical Characteristics

1. *Gynecomastia.* Gynecomastia in male athletes is a common problem and easily recognized in a physical examination. In addition to the pain that usually accompanies gynecomastia, this creates a cosmetic physical problem, especially for bodybuilders, who are judged by the quality of their physiques, and may require corrective surgery.[82] Development of gynecomastia is the result of converting the large amounts of exogenous testosterone to estrogens.[83] Athletes have been reported to use tamoxifen to prevent gynecomastia, and recent findings suggest that this is an effective treatment.[84]

TABLE 20.2
Examples of physical and clinical effects reported for anabolic–androgenic steroid use

Endocrine changes
    Hypothalamic–pituitary dysfunction
    Altered sexual interest
    Altered glucose tolerance
    Hyperinsulinism

Sexual and physical characteristics in men
    Acne
    Gynecomastia
    Lower sperm production
    Lower endogenous testosterone production
    Infertility
    Increased male pattern baldness
    Prostate hypertrophy
    Testicular atrophy
    Voiding alterations

Sexual and physical characteristics in women
    Acne
    Clitoral hypertrophy
    Deepening of the voice
    Male pattern baldness
    Increased facial and body hair
    Infertility
    Menstrual irregularities

Behavioral changes
    Aggressiveness
    Depression
    Irritability
    Irregular "mood" changes

Immune function
    Decreased immunoglobulins
    Depressed immune responses

Cardiovascular changes
    Potential for elevated systolic or diastolic blood pressure
    Altered blood lipid profile
    Increased levels of C-reactive proteins
    Increased hematocrit and red blood cells
    Decreased high-density lipoprotein
    Increased low-density lipoprotein
    Decreased fibrinolytic inhibition
    Increased triglycerides
    Left ventricular hypertrophy

TABLE 20.2
Continued

Adolescent growth
    Premature epiphyseal closure

Hepatic function
    Altered liver structure
    Hepatocellular adenomas
    Hematocellular hyperplasia
    Cholestatic jaundice
    Peliosis hepatis
    Altered liver enzymes

2. *Acne.* Obvious indicators upon physical examination include acne around the shoulders, upper and middle back, and face of male and female athletes.[85] The acne will clear upon termination of use of exogenous testosterone.[86] Clearly though, acne by itself is not sufficient for diagnosis and must be considered in combination with other clinical tests.

3. *General characteristics in women.* In women, some irreversible physiological changes associated with anabolic steroid use include male pattern baldness, virilization, and deepening of the voice.[87] There may also be menstrual irregularities.[88] However, such changes could also result from androgen-producing ovarian and adrenal neoplasms, and this possibility should be explored by the practitioner.[87]

4. *Sexual characteristics and reproductive system.* Plenty of anecdotal cases have been cited by the lay media; however, what role anabolic steroids and exogenous testosterone might have in the etiology of various diseases in humans or animals is still not known. Testosterone and steroid use in clinical trials and in controlled laboratory studies has been reported to correlate with a number of deleterious changes in risk factors for infertility. In males, anabolic steroid use could result in lower levels of endogenous testosterone, gonadotrophic hormones, sex hormone-binding globulin levels, sperm motility, sperm count, altered sperm structure, and testicular atrophy.[89] However, termination of anabolic steroid use results in a normalization of sperm production and testes function. Menstrual abnormalities, shrinkage of the breasts, and increased sex drive will usually return to normal after steroid termination in women.[86] However, in women, there are some irreversible physiological changes associated with anabolic steroid use[90] including male pattern baldness, deepening of the voice, increased body hair, and clitoris hypertrophy.[91]

Prostate abnormalities have been reported in humans including an increase in prostatic volume, reduction in urine flow rate, and marked changes in voiding patterns.[75] In contrast, 100 mg of androstenedione does not alter serum levels of prostate-specific antigen,[72] suggesting no overall change in prostate function with this prohormone.

Behavioral Changes

It is reasonable to expect that some of the behavioral signs and symptoms accompanying anabolic steroid use are likely overlooked by healthcare professionals, so it is not possible to determine the number or extent of steroid-related behavioral complications.[79] Female athletes have been reported to display increased aggressiveness when using anabolic steroids.[88] A positive correlation has been established between endogenous testosterone levels and aggressive behavior in males, but some people are much more sensitive to changes in mood and others are much more resistant to steroid-induced changes in mood and behavior.[92] Moderate and low doses of exogenous testosterone have failed to produce changes in male aggressiveness, general outlook or mood, and sexual behavior of subjects.[93] However, the high levels of steroids often used by athletes have been reported to induce psychotic and sometimes violent syndromes and, importantly, psychological dependence on the steroids.[94] This psychological dependence explains the severe withdrawal symptoms.[95] Nevertheless, other reports have not supported a close relationship between steroid use and changes in personality or aggression.[96] Although supraphysiological levels of exogenous testosterone have been found to increase both the subjective and objective assessments of aggression, the interpretation of these data are complicated by the fact that several steroid users in this study had personality disorder profiles including Cluster B personality disorder traits for antisocial, borderline, personality disorder; histrionic personality disorder.[94] Thus it is likely that some athletes, if predisposed as a result of some preexisting personality disorder, may have increased aggression and behavioral changes, but others not prone to personality disorders may not be observed clinically to have any changes in behavior or aggression. It has been estimated that ~300,000 athletes use anabolic steroids yearly in the United States;[97] however, only a small percentage of steroid users experience psychological dependence requiring clinical treatment. Thus, the psychological dependence may be overestimated, or most people using anabolic steroids have not developed symptoms of a significant nature that require interventions.

Immune Function

Other potential areas of concerns studied in animals and humans include reduced T-cell and immune function,[91] which has the potential for the athlete to suffer upper respiratory infections or other more complicated problems.

Cardiovascular Risks

Exogenous steroid use has been linked to increased coronary artery disease, cardiomyopathy, and cerebrovascular accidents.[56,98]

1. *Lipoproteins.* Use of exogenous testosterone compounds has been thought to increase cardiovascular risk factors.[99] The most important are changes in lipoproteins, increased levels of triglycerides, and elevated concentrations of several blood clotting factors. Estimates of anabolic steroid-induced changes in blood lipids include a marked decrease in high-density lipoprotein-2 (HDL-2) levels by ~52% and severe decreases in high-density lipoprotein-b (HDL-b) levels by ~78% along with increases in low-density lipoprotein levels (LDLs) by ~36%.[100,101] However, this observation is not universal and may depend on the steroid used because nandrolone has been reported to show no changes in HDL cholesterol (HDL-C), low-density lipoprotein cholesterol (LDL-C), total cholesterol, triglycerides, the total cholesterol to HDL-C ratio, or the LDL-C/HDL-C ratio from 100 mg/wk of nandrolone in men or women.[102] Nevertheless, athletes frequently use much higher levels of nandrolone and combine this with other steroids, and the effects of the higher doses or combinations of several anabolic steroids and prohormones may alter the lipid profiles in these athletes. The changes in blood lipid profiles provide a negative stimulus that would promote cardiovascular disease. Blood lipids and lipoprotein changes favor an increased atherogenic lipid profile that persists after termination of steroid use.[103] As with the findings of King and colleagues,[62] serum concentrations of HDL-C decreased 10% during the first week of androstenedione supplementation and remained depressed thereafter. However, serum concentrations of total testosterone did not change. These data and others[74,75] support data from earlier studies that indicate an increase in serum estrogen and a decrease in HDL-C in response to oral androstenedione.

2. *Blood profiles and lipids.* Urhausen et al.[104] studied 32 male bodybuilders and powerlifters, comparing the blood profiles of current users with those who had terminated anabolic steroid use ~1 year before the study began. The previous users had taken ~720 mg/wk of combined anabolic–androgenic steroids for 26 weeks per year over ~9 years. The athletes who currently used anabolic–androgenic steroids at the time of the study took ~1030 mg/wk of combined steroids for 33 weeks per year for an average of ~8 years. Blood tests showed that erythrocyte and platelet counts in the former steroid users were normal, but in current steroid users, all hematological cell types were increased. Liver alanine aminotransferase levels were increased in some but not all of the former steroid users. The blood cholesterol

and endogenous testosterone levels of the former steroid users were normal. In general, these data show that lipid blood levels return to normal after cessation of exogenous testosterone use.

3. *C-reactive proteins.* A recent observation is that anabolic steroids can elevate C-reactive protein concentrations without any relationship to changes in cardiac troponin T. The higher C-reactive protein concentrations may indicate a greater predisposition to developing peripheral arterial disease.[105]

4. *Cardiomyopathy.* The types and extent of clinical changes vary among different types and doses of anabolic steroids and among individuals. The clinical changes appear to be reversible within several months after cessation of anabolic steroid use.[89,104] However, increased left ventricular mass and dilated cardiomyopathy are not reversible upon cessation of anabolic steroid use.[106] Furthermore, several case reports on athletes have linked anabolic steroid use to nonfatal myocardial infarction, atrial fibrillation, and stroke.[98]

Blood and Thrombogenic Characteristics

Testosterone can potentially alter thromogenic activity by increasing thromboxane A^2 receptor activity and platelet aggregability.[107] However, there is no direct evidence that exogenous testosterone or its anabolic steroid compounds are thrombogenic in humans.[108] On the contrary, the reductions of fibrinolytic inhibition and lipoprotein A in men and women who use anabolic steroids[109,110] are considered favorable effects of androgens with regard to the risk of cardiovascular disease. Anabolic steroid use increases whole-body hematocrit and red blood cell volume, and as a result, anabolic steroids have been used to treat patients with renal failure.[111]

Blood Pressure

The literature concerning potential changes in blood pressure during anabolic steroid use is mixed. Some studies have found no change in blood pressure in healthy athletes,[89,112] whereas others have found an increase in systolic or diastolic blood pressure.[91,113] Thus, although it is not clear that anabolic steroids will increase resting blood pressure levels, androgenic compounds may affect the blood pressure more than anabolic substances do, but the exact mechanism of this is unknown.[114,115]

Hepatic Function

Liver structure and function are changed by steroid use.[116] These include peliosis hepatitis, hepatocellular hyperplasia, hepatocellular adenomas, and cholestatic jaundice.[91,117] It has also been shown that high levels of anabolic steroids may lead to hepatocellular carcinomas.[118,119] Liver changes are associated with use of oral 17-α-alkylated anabolic steroids.[91] An interesting case study reported on a

26 year old jaundiced bodybuilder, whose steroid regimen over 5 weeks before hospitalization was 500 mg testosterone injected intramuscularly injection twice weekly and daily consumptions of 40 mg of oral stanazol and 30 mg of methylandrostenediol.[120] This bodybuilder had high aminotransferase and alanine aminotransferase levels but normal bilirubin levels. However, he was found to have hepatocellular necrosis, based upon pathological analysis of his liver biopsy. Clinical signs and laboratory findings for this bodybuilder improved substantially 12 weeks after he discontinued these testosterone derivatives.[120] This type of damage is, however, unusual, and it is in contrast to other case reports, which primarily report a cholestatic-type liver damage with steroid use.[121] Other reports suggest widespread liver changes even with anabolic steroids thought to have low levels of toxicity. For example, acute stanozolol treatment (5 mg/kg/d) was shown to significantly decrease the levels of cytochrome P450 (Cyt. P450) and cytochrome b5 (Cytb5) during the first 48 hr of treatment in rats, whereas subsequently, at 72 and 96 h, the levels of these enzymes significantly increased. In contrast to the acute treatment, both P450 and Cytb5 enzymes decreased with 60 to 90 days of chronic treatment.[122]

Nevertheless, most reports of anabolic steroid-induced hepatotoxicity in humans are primarily based on elevated levels of aminotransferase, aspartate aminotransferase, and creatine kinase levels, but this may not be sufficient assessment of liver function because athletes using steroids do not have changes in hepatic dysfunction, at least based on gamma-glutamyltranspeptidase levels.[123] In general, the data show that blood levels of liver enzymes return to normal,[104] and other data show that liver tumors regress and there is a return to normal liver function after termination of anabolic steroid use.[89]

Endocrine Modifications

1. *Hypothalamic–pituitary dysfunction.* A case report from van Breda et al.[124] described a competitive bodybuilder who initially presented with gynecomastia and widespread acne. However, the physical examination and subsequent laboratory tests showed that this athlete had a hypothalamic–pituitary dysfunction, which was thought to have persisted for several months even after termination of the anabolic steroid use.[124] This is a rather severe problem, and these investigators suggest that to regain normal hypothalamic–pituitary function in athletes with similar conditions, supraphysiological doses of 200 μg LH-releasing hormone (LH-RH) should be considered when the physiological challenge test with LH-RH (50 μg) fails to show an acceptable response and a return toward normal.[124]

2. *Glucose metabolism.* Hyperinsulinimia and reduced glucose tolerance have also been noted in athletes using various steroids.[89] For example, powerlifters who ingested anabolic steroids had a lower glucose tolerance compared with a control group who did not take steroids, in spite of having significantly higher postglucose serum

insulin concentrations.[125] These results suggest that athletes who use anabolic steroids may have diminished glucose tolerance, which is linked to insulin resistance.

Growth in Adolescents

Several reports suggest premature stunting of growth in adolescent anabolic steroid users, presumably by premature closing of the epiphyseal endplates,[126,127] but this has not been carefully and systematically studied.

DRUG TESTING — FALSE POSITIVES AND FALSE NEGATIVES

The use of androstenedione and DHEA is banned by most sports governing bodies including the International Olympic Committee (IOC).[128,129] The prohormones androstenediol and androstenedione are on the "banned list." The USAA limit for the testosterone-to-epitestosterone (T/E) ratio is 4.0 (as compared to the IOC limit of 6.0). The limit for the 19-norandrosterone urine level is greater than 2 ng/ml and the epitestosterone level is above 200 ng/ml. These more stringent standards increase the likelihood of false positive results, but they also reduce the likelihood of having athletes test negative but actually taking a banned hormone or prohormone for competition or training.

Drug testing for some prohormones has been difficult, but newer methods are improving the detection of these compounds in athletes.[130] The other complication of using prohormones is that some preparations have been found to contain anabolic hormones such as testosterone or 19-nortestosterone, without this information available on the manufacturer's label.[131,132] A study funded by the IOC of 634 nonhormonal supplements found that ~15% contained prohormones that were not listed on the label.[133] These findings were found subsequently by another study.[134]

For more than 20 years, urine analysis of the T/E ratio has been used to provide an indirect marker of testosterone or anabolic steroid use in athletes.[135] The body produces endogenous epitestosterone, the 17-α epimer of testosterone, but it has little anabolic activity. The IOC has set a T/E ratio limit of 6 for competitions.[136]

FALSE NEGATIVE TESTS

Urine analysis is prone to misdiagnosis because some athletes have T/E ratios below 6.0 in spite of using anabolic steroids. Athletes have used epitestosterone to effectively reduce the T/E ratio and therefore become negative for drug use. Because epitestosterone is believed to be a urine-manipulating agent, the IOC has banned it. The epitestosterone that is marketed for normalizing manipulation is synthesized from soybean, which has a low carbon-13 content.[137] These manufactured commercial compounds appear to have lower levels of carbon-13 than endogenously synthesized steroids, and higher levels of carbon-12.[138] Athletes using anabolic steroids and epitestosterone would be expected to have urinary steroids with higher levels of carbon-12 than those athletes who are not taking these compounds. Not surprisingly, recent improvements in drug testing have focused on analysis of the ratio of carbon-13 to carbon-12, using a gas chromatography–combustion–isotope ratio mass spectrometry method (GC/MS).[138] This method is not influenced by athlete ethnicity[139] and does appear to be sensitive and reliable.[138] Although the carbon-13 to carbon-12 ratio appears to be reliable and valid,[138] it is a new method and therefore should be thoroughly tested to minimize the chances of false positives before being used in international competitions.

Four men took up to 150 mg of DHEA for up to 4 days, and urine samples were analyzed using gas chromatography-mass spectrometry (GC-MS) on day 3. Only one of the four subjects had an increase in the T/E ratio above 6.0.[140] However, the doses of DHEA were also lower than suggested by supplement manufacturers, and it is not known if the T/E ratio would exceed the IOC standards to therefore reach a "positive" detection if much higher levels of DHEA are consumed by athletes.

FALSE POSITIVES

On 6 September 1994 a female Olympic 400 m athlete was suspended by the British Athletic Federation Limited for testing positive for testosterone in her urine. Although she was initially suspended, she was reinstated on the basis of the argument that urinary microbes produced testosterone and caused her false positive urine tests for testosterone. The basis of the argument was that unlike prokaryotes (e.g., *Escherichia coli*), many eukaryotic microorganisms can synthesize steroids and steroid substrates including testosterone.[141] Investigation of urine samples of 134 women showed that when normal urine was inoculated with 10,000 or 100,000 CFU/ml of *Candida albicans*, a microbe that is typically found in vaginal flora, the testosterone levels in the urine rose significantly although the absolute increases were small. Although it is potentially possible that a false positive drug evaluation could be made if testosterone alone were examined, this is unlikely because there was a small increase in the absolute concentration of testosterone and a corresponding small increase in the T/E ratios, which are maintained well below 6. The increase in urinary testosterone appears to be caused by conversion of urinary androstenedione rather than by synthesis of testosterone per se. This leaves open the possibility that false positives could arise at least in women with some type of urinary microbe infection.

De la Torre and co-workers[142] investigated the increases in urine testosterone after contamination with 15 different organisms (bacteria, fungi, and molds). In the future, improved handling of urine samples such as freeze-drying will reduce the potential for contamination[143] and false positives. In addition, false positives will be likely reduced by evaluating the isotope ratio of carbon-13 to carbon-12 of urinary steroids to determine whether the testosterone is of exogenous or endogenous origin.[138] An additional reduction in false positives might occur if we compare the testosterone liberated by glucuronidase hydrolysis or that in the free steroid fraction with the total testosterone as a routine test.

Some nutritional supplements have also been found to contain anabolic or androgenic steroids and banned prohormones, which result in positive drug tests, even though the athletes have not knowingly consumed the drugs.[133,144] Athletes can fail a drug test up to 120 h after consuming food supplements,[131] so this could also be viewed as a "false" positive test[145] although it is really a true positive by the IOC regulations. Nandrolone is indirectly detected by identification of its two main metabolites, 19-norandrosterone (19-NA) and 19-noretiocholanolone (19-NE), in the urine. The IOC has set a limit for these metabolites of 2 ng/ml in men and 5 ng/ml in women[146] because endogenous production is known to occur in humans, especially pregnant women.[147]

Athletes who have tested positive for nandrolone have contested positive drug tests on a variety of grounds, including the fact that physical effort alone can produce increased levels of nandrolone.[145] However, Schmitt et al. showed that exhaustive exercise in trained athletes does not significantly increase endogenous nandrolone production and produces nandrolone metabolites in urine levels that are far below the IOC threshold of 2 ng/ml urine in males.[148] However, it is possible to obtain a false positive for drug screen for urinary 19-norandrosterone in a woman athlete who is pregnant.[147]

The potential for false positive drug tests can also arise from testing for specific markers that are naturally occurring in the body. In the case of DHEA or other banned prohormone supplements, urine markers are commonly measured using gas chromatography-mass spectrometry (GC-MS) in methods such as gas chromatography–combustion–isotope ratio mass spectrometry (GC-C-IRMS). A urinary product of DHEA administration is detectable in samples from subjects given multiple doses of DHEA, and was identified in GC-MS experiments to be 3α,5-cyclo-5α-androstan-6β-ol-17-one (3α,5-cyclo). This metabolite occurs naturally, found in urine samples collected from elite athletes; yet, concentrations are markedly elevated after both single and multiple DHEA administrations.[130] Coupling screening of GC-MS and GC-C-IRMS may become the standard method of detecting androstenedione, testosterone, and dehydrotestosterone use, but it is still possible that some false positives may arise.

Van Thuyne and Delbeke[134] report that GC-MS identified dehydrotestosterone in food supplements even though its presence was not listed on the manufacturer's label. However, follow-up studies with GC-MS were unable to confirm its presence in the food supplement. This emphasizes the point that athletes might indeed test positive for prohormone use in some tests but not in others.

Designer Drugs and Getting Around Drug Tests

Some substances are currently undetectable. Tests have been developed for the known drugs, but resourceful entrepreneurs have manufactured new "designer" drugs, and without a "footprint" they cannot be detected using routine methods. The so-called tetrahydrogestrinone designer steroid (THG) was only discovered because a syringe reported to contain an "undetectable steroid" was sent to the U.S. Anti-Doping Agency (USADA) by a track coach. The syringe contents were analyzed using liquid chromatograph and mass spectrometry. The compound resembled somewhat the structures of gestrinone, used to treat endometriosis, and trenbolone, an agriculture anabolic steroid used primarily in cattle and by some athletes because it is believed to be minimally affected by aromatase or 5α-reductase. The investigators synthesized the new drug as a combination of gestrinone and trenbolone and made a new compound called THG. THG was given to an animal, and the urine tested positive for THG, and this was the same signature as the original compound in the syringe sent to the USADA.[149]

CONCLUSION

Although some studies suggest that prohormones may change testosterone blood levels, there is currently no compelling evidence that clearly demonstrates that prohormones are effective in enhancing muscle mass or strength even when combined with heavy resistance training. These prohormones may result in negative health consequences and may also in some cases test positive in routine drug tests.[144] Despite the negative studies, recreational use of anabolic steroids is increasing among fitness club members and other amateur athletes.

Clinical changes resulting from exogenous testosterone administration include increased circulating estrogen changes in blood lipids, which increases the risk factors associated with cardiovascular disease, altered liver function, and cardiac hypertrophy. All except the cardiomyopathic changes appear to be reversible once steroid use is discontinued. As with anabolic steroids, supplementation of prohormones including oral androstenedione elevates circulating estrogens and is associated with small but statistically significant decreases in HDL-C. It is not yet known if the small transient negative changes in blood lipids (i.e., 3 to 6 mg/dl reductions in HDL-C) induced by androstenedione will have a major impact on the risk for cardiovascular disease. Although estrogen may have cardio-protective effects,[150] it is important to determine inflammatory and atherothrombotic indices (e.g., homocysteine and C-reactive protein) that determine the health impact of prohormones on athletes. A future area of study is applying nutrient interventions to treating side effects of anabolic steroid misuse, some which may be lifelong.

REFERENCES

1. Pitkanen, H.T., Nykanen, T., Knuutinen, J., Lahti, K., Keinanen, O., Alen, M., Komi, P.V., and Mero, A.A., Free amino acid pool and muscle protein balance after resistance exercise, *Med. Sci. Sports Exerc.,* 35, 784–792, 2003.

2. Sheffield-Moore, M., Paddon-Jones, D., Sanford, A.P., Rosenblatt, J.I., Matlock, A.G., Cree, M.G., and Wolfe, R.R., Mixed muscle and hepatic-derived plasma protein metabolism is differentially regulated in older and younger men following resistance exercise, *Am. J. Physiol. Endocrinol. Metab.*, 288: E922–E929, 2005.

3. Alway, S.E., MacDougall, J.D., and Sale, D.G., Contractile adaptations in the human triceps surae after isometric exercise, *J. Appl. Physiol.*, 66, 2725–2732, 1989.

4. Phillips, S.M., Tipton, K.D., Ferrando, A.A., and Wolfe, R.R., Resistance training reduces the acute exercise-induced increase in muscle protein turnover, *Am. J. Physiol.*, 276, E118–E124, 1999.

5. Yarasheski, K.E., Exercise, aging, and muscle protein metabolism, *J. Gerontol. A Biol. Sci. Med. Sci.*, 58, M918–M922, 2003.

6. Chesley, A., MacDougall, J.D., Tarnopolsky, M.A., Atkinson, S.A., and Smith, K., Changes in human muscle protein synthesis after resistance exercise, *J. Appl. Physiol.*, 73, 1383–1388, 1992.

7. Schultz, E., and McCormick, K.M., Skeletal muscle satellite cells, *Rev. Physiol. Biochem. Pharmacol.*, 123, 213–257, 1994.

8. Hawke, T.J., and Garry, D.J., Myogenic satellite cells: physiology to molecular biology, *J. Appl. Physiol.*, 91, 534–551, 2001.

9. Mashiko, T., Umeda, T., Nakaji, S., and Sugawara, K., Effects of exercise on the physical condition of college rugby players during summer training camp, *Br. J. Sports Med.*, 38, 186–190, 2004.

10. Reichsman, F., Scordilis, S.P., Clarkson, P.M., and Evans, W.J., Muscle protein changes following eccentric exercise in humans, *Eur. J. Appl. Physiol. Occup. Physiol.*, 62, 245–250, 1991.

11. Carraro, F., Stuart, C.A., Hartl, W.H., Rosenblatt, J., and Wolfe, R.R., Effect of exercise and recovery on muscle protein synthesis in human subjects, *Am. J. Physiol.*, 259, E470–E476, 1990.

12. Thyfault, J.P., Carper, M.J., Richmond, S.R., Hulver, M.W., and Potteiger, J.A., Effects of liquid carbohydrate ingestion on markers of anabolism following high-intensity resistance exercise, *J. Strength Cond. Res.*, 18, 174–179, 2004.

13. Alway, S.E., Grumbt, W.H., Gonyea, W.J., and Stray-Gundersen, J., Contrasts in muscle and myofibers of elite male and female bodybuilders, *J. Appl. Physiol.*, 67, 24–31, 1989.

14. Alway, S.E., Coggan, A.R., Sproul, M.S., Abduljalil, A.M., and Robitaille, P.M., Muscle torque in young and older untrained and endurance-trained men, *J. Gerontol. A Biol. Sci. Med. Sci.*, 51, B195–B201, 1996.

15. Lowe, D.A., and Alway, S.E., Stretch-induced myogenin, MyoD, and MRF4 expression and acute hypertrophy in quail slow-tonic muscle are not dependent upon satellite cell proliferation, *Cell Tissue Res.*, 296, 531–539, 1999.

16. Siu, P.M., and Alway, S.E., Id2 and p53 participate in apoptosis during unloading-induced muscle atrophy, *Am. J. Physiol. Cell Physiol.*, 288: C1058–C1073, 2005.

17. Solerte, S.B., Gazzaruso, C., Schifino, N., Locatelli, E., Destro, T., Ceresini, G., Ferrari, E., and Fioravanti, M., Metabolic effects of orally administered amino acid mixture in elderly subjects with poorly controlled type 2 diabetes mellitus, *Am. J. Cardiol.*, 93, 23A–29A, 2004.

18. Prod'homme, M., Rieu, I., Balage, M., Dardevet, D., and Grizard, J., Insulin and amino acids both strongly participate to the regulation of protein metabolism, *Curr. Opin. Clin. Nutr. Metab. Care*, 7, 71–77, 2004.

19. Prod'homme, M., Balage, M., Debras, E., Farges, M.C., Kimball, S., Jefferson, L., and Grizard, J., Differential effects of insulin and dietary amino acids on muscle protein synthesis in adult and old rats, *J. Physiol.*, 563: 235–248, 2005.

20. Tischler, M.E., Satarug, S., Aannestad, A., Munoz, K.A., and Henriksen, E.J., Insulin attenuates atrophy of unweighted soleus muscle by amplified inhibition of protein degradation, *Metabolism*, 46, 673–679, 1997.

21. Nygren, J., and Nair, K.S., Differential regulation of protein dynamics in splanchnic and skeletal muscle beds by insulin and amino acids in healthy human subjects, *Diabetes*, 52, 1377–1385, 2003.

22. Fryburg, D.A., and Barrett, E.J., Growth hormone acutely stimulates skeletal muscle but not whole-body protein synthesis in humans, *Metabolism*, 42, 1223–1227, 1993.

23. Mauras, N., Rini, A., Welch, S., Sager, B., and Murphy, S.P., Synergistic effects of testosterone and growth hormone on protein metabolism and body composition in prepubertal boys, *Metabolism*, 52, 964–969, 2003.

24. Lang, C.H., Frost, R.A., Svanberg, E., and Vary, T.C., IGF-I/IGFBP-3 ameliorates alterations in protein synthesis, eIF4E availability, and myostatin in alcohol-fed rats, *Am. J. Physiol. Endocrinol. Metab.*, 286, E916–E926, 2004.

25. Farrell, P.A., Fedele, M.J., Hernandez, J., Fluckey, J.D., Miller, J.L., III, Lang, C.H., Vary, T.C., Kimball, S.R., and Jefferson, L.S., Hypertrophy of skeletal muscle in diabetic rats in response to chronic resistance exercise, *J. Appl. Physiol.*, 87, 1075–1082, 1999.

26. Bush, J.A., Kimball, S.R., O'Connor, P.M., Suryawan, A., Orellana, R.A., Nguyen, H.V., Jefferson, L.S., and Davis, T.A., Translational control of protein synthesis in muscle and liver of growth hormone-treated pigs, *Endocrinology*, 144, 1273–1283, 2003.

27. Davis, T.A., Fiorotto, M.L., Burrin, D.G., Vann, R.C., Reeds, P.J., Nguyen, H.V., Beckett, P.R., and Bush, J.A., Acute IGF-I infusion stimulates protein synthesis in skeletal muscle and other tissues of neonatal pigs, *Am. J. Physiol. Endocrinol. Metab.*, 283, E638–E647, 2002.

28. Welle, S., Bhatt, K., Shah, B., and Thornton, C., Insulin-like growth factor-1 and myostatin mRNA expression in muscle: comparison between 62–77 and 21–31 yr old men, *Exp. Gerontol.*, 37, 833–839, 2002.

29. Goldspink, G., Age-related muscle loss and progressive dysfunction in mechanosensitive growth factor signaling, *Ann. N. Y. Acad. Sci.*, 1019, 294–298, 2004.

30. Goldspink, G., and Harridge, S.D., Growth factors and muscle ageing, *Exp. Gerontol.*, 39, 1433–1438, 2004.

31. Brillon, D.J., Zheng, B., Campbell, R.G., and Matthews, D.E., Effect of cortisol on energy expenditure and amino acid metabolism in humans, *Am. J. Physiol.*, 268, E501–E513, 1995.

32. Bird, S.P., and Tarpenning, K.M., Influence of circadian time structure on acute hormonal responses to a single bout of heavy-resistance exercise in weight-trained men, *Chronobiol. Int.*, 21, 131–146, 2004.

33. Paddon-Jones, D., Sheffield-Moore, M., Urban, R.J., Aarsland, A., Wolfe, R.R., and Ferrando, A.A., The catabolic effects of prolonged inactivity and acute hypercortisolemia are offset by dietary supplementation, *J. Clin. Endocrinol. Metab.*, 90: 1453–1459, 2005.

34. Asthana, S., Bhasin, S., Butler, R.N., Fillit, H., Finkelstein, J., Harman, S.M., Holstein, L., Korenman, S.G., Matsumoto, A.M., Morley, J.E., Tsitouras, P., and

Urban, R., Masculine vitality: pros and cons of testosterone in treating the andropause, *J. Gerontol. A Biol. Sci. Med. Sci.,* 59, 461–465, 2004.

35. Choi, H., Gray, P., Storer, T., Calof, O., Woodhouse, L., Singh, A., Padero, C., Mac, R., Sinha-Hikim, I., Shen, R., Dzekov, J., Dzekov, C., Kushnir, M., Rockwood, A., Meikle, A., Lee, M., Hays, R., and Bhasin, S., Effects of testosterone replacement in human immunodeficiency virus-infected women with weight loss, *J. Clin. Endocrinol. Metab.,* 90: 1531–1541, 2005.

36. Schroeder, E.T., Singh, A., Bhasin, S., Storer, T.W., Azen, C., Davidson, T., Martinez, C., Sinha-Hikim, I., Jaque, S.V., Terk, M., and Sattler, F.R., Effects of an oral androgen on muscle and metabolism in older, community-dwelling men, *Am. J. Physiol. Endocrinol. Metab.,* 284, E120–E128, 2003.

37. Triantafillopoulos, I.K., Banes, A.J., Bowman, K.F., Jr., Maloney, M., Garrett, W.E., Jr., and Karas, S.G., Nandrolone decanoate and load increase remodeling and strength in human supraspinatus bioartificial tendons, *Am. J. Sports Med.,* 32, 934–943, 2004.

38. Bhasin, S., Storer, T.W., Berman, N., Callegari, C., Clevenger, B., Phillips, J., Bunnell, T.J., Tricker, R., Shirazi, A., and Casaburi, R., The effects of supraphysiologic doses of testosterone on muscle size and strength in normal men, *N. Engl. J. Med.,* 335, 1–7, 1996.

39. Herbst, K.L., and Bhasin, S., Testosterone action on skeletal muscle, *Curr. Opin. Clin. Nutr. Metab. Care,* 7, 271–277, 2004.

40. Wilson, J.D., Leihy, M.W., Shaw, G., and Renfree, M.B., Androgen physiology: unsolved problems at the millennium, *Mol. Cell. Endocrinol.,* 198, 1–5, 2002.

41. Tenover, J.S., Declining testicular function in aging men, *Int. J. Impot. Res.* 15 (Suppl. 4), S3–S8, 2003.

42. Wolfe, R.R., Regulation of skeletal muscle protein metabolism in catabolic states, *Curr. Opin. Clin. Nutr. Metab. Care,* 8, 61–65, 2005.

43. Umeda, K., Adachi, S., Watanabe, K., Kimura, N., Lin, Y., and Nakahata, T., Successful hematopoietic stem cell transplantation for aplastic anemia following living-related liver transplantation, *Bone Marrow Transplant.,* 30, 531–534, 2002.

44. Helfman, T., and Falanga, V., Stanozolol as a novel therapeutic agent in dermatology, *J. Am. Acad. Dermatol.,* 33, 254–258, 1995.

45. Seeman, E., and Eisman, J.A., Treatment of osteoporosis: why, whom, when and how to treat. The single most important consideration is the individual's absolute risk of fracture, *Med. J. Austr.,* 180, 298–303, 2004.

46. Spungen, A.M., Grimm, D.R., Strakhan, M., Pizzolato, P.M., and Bauman, W.A., Treatment with an anabolic agent is associated with improvement in respiratory function in persons with tetraplegia: a pilot study, *Mt. Sinai J. Med.,* 66, 201–205, 1999.

47. Creutzberg, E.C., and Schols, A.M., Anabolic steroids, *Curr. Opin. Clin. Nutr. Metab. Care,* 2, 243–253, 1999.

48. Creutzberg, E.C., Wouters, E.F., Mostert, R., Pluymers, R.J., and Schols, A.M., A role for anabolic steroids in the rehabilitation of patients with COPD? A double-blind, placebo-controlled, randomized trial, *Chest,* 124, 1733–1742, 2003.

49. Welle, S., Jozefowicz, R., Forbes, G., and Griggs, R.C., Effect of testosterone on metabolic rate and body composition in normal men and men with muscular dystrophy, *J. Clin. Endocrinol. Metab.,* 74, 332–335, 1992.

50. Newman, A.B., Kupelian, V., Visser, M., Simonsick, E., Goodpaster, B., Nevitt, M., Kritchevsky, S.B., Tylavsky, F.A., Rubin, S.M., and Harris, T.B., Sarcopenia: alternative

definitions and associations with lower extremity function, *J. Am. Geriatr. Soc.,* 51, 1602–1609, 2003.

51. Goldstat, R., Briganti, E., Tran, J., Wolfe, R., and Davis, S.R., Transdermal testosterone therapy improves well-being, mood, and sexual function in premenopausal women, *Menopause,* 10, 390–398, 2003.

52. Iannuzzi-Sucich, M., Prestwood, K.M., and Kenny, A.M., Prevalence of sarcopenia and predictors of skeletal muscle mass in healthy, older men and women, *J. Gerontol. A Biol. Sci. Med. Sci.,* 57, M772–M777, 2002.

53. Snyder, P.J., Effects of age on testicular function and consequences of testosterone treatment, *J. Clin. Endocrinol. Metab.,* 86, 2369–2372, 2001.

54. Wittert, G.A., Chapman, I.M., Haren, M.T., Mackintosh, S., Coates, P., and Morley, J.E., Oral testosterone supplementation increases muscle and decreases fat mass in healthy elderly males with low-normal gonadal status, *J. Gerontol. A Biol. Sci. Med. Sci.,* 58, 618–625, 2003.

55. Alway, S.E., Characteristics of the elbow flexors in women bodybuilders using anabolic steroids, *J. Strength Cond. Res.,* 8, 161–169, 1994.

56. Hartgens, F., and Kuipers, H., Effects of androgenic–anabolic steroids in athletes, *Sports Med.,* 34, 513–554, 2004.

57. Monks, D.A., O'Bryant, E.L., and Jordan, C.L., Androgen receptor immunoreactivity in skeletal muscle: enrichment at the neuromuscular junction, *J. Comp. Neurol.,* 473, 59–72, 2004.

58. Sinha-Hikim, I., Taylor, W.E., Gonzalez-Cadavid, N.F., Zheng, W., and Bhasin, S., Androgen receptor in human skeletal muscle and cultured muscle satellite cells: up-regulation by androgen treatment, *J. Clin. Endocrinol. Metab.,* 89, 5245–5255, 2004.

59. Bribiescas, R.G., Age-related differences in serum gonadotropin (FSH and LH), salivary testosterone, and 17-beta estradiol levels among Ache Amerindian males of Paraguay, *Am. J. Phys. Anthropol.,* 2004.

60. Blouin, K., Richard, C., Belanger, C., Dupont, P., Daris, M., Laberge, P., Luu-The, V., and Tchernof, A., Local androgen inactivation in abdominal visceral adipose tissue, *J. Clin. Endocrinol. Metab.,* 88, 5944–5950, 2003.

61. Labrie, F., Adrenal androgens and intracrinology, *Semin. Reprod. Med.,* 22, 299–309, 2004.

62. King, D.S., Sharp, R.L., Vukovich, M.D., Brown, G.A., Reifenrath, T.A., Uhl, N.L., and Parsons, K.A., Effect of oral androstenedione on serum testosterone and adaptations to resistance training in young men: a randomized controlled trial, *JAMA,* 281, 2020–2028, 1999.

63. Bahrke, M.S., and Yesalis, C.E., Abuse of anabolic androgenic steroids and related substances in sport and exercise, *Curr. Opin. Pharmacol.,* 4, 614–620, 2004.

64. Roy, S., Mahesh, V.B., and Greenblatt, R.B., Effect of dehydroepiandrosterone and delta4-androstenedione on the reproductive organs of female rats: production of cystic changes in the ovary, *Nature,* 196, 42–43, 1962.

65. Mahesh, V.B., and Greenblatt, R.B., Isolation of dehydroepiandrosterone and 17alpha-hydroxy-delta5-pregnenolone from the polycystic ovaries of the Stein–Leventhal syndrome, *J. Clin. Endocrinol. Metab.,* 22, 441–448, 1962.

66. Blaquier, J., Forchielli, E., and Dorfman, R.I., In vitro metabolism of androgens in whole human blood, *Acta Endocrinol. (Copenhagen),* 55, 697–704, 1967.

67. Blaquier, J., Dorfman, R.I., and Forchielli, E., Formation of epitestosterone by human blood and adrenal tissue, *Acta Endocrinol. (Copenhagen),* 54, 208–214, 1967.

68. Longcope, C., Dehydroepiandrosterone metabolism, *J. Endocrinol.*, 150 (Suppl.), S125–S127, 1996.

69. Wallace, M.B., Lim, J., Cutler, A., and Bucci, L., Effects of dehydroepiandrosterone vs androstenedione supplementation in men, *Med. Sci. Sports Exerc.*, 31, 1788–1792, 1999.

70. Ballantyne, C.S., Phillips, S.M., MacDonald, J.R., Tarnopolsky, M.A., and MacDougall, J.D., The acute effects of androstenedione supplementation in healthy young males, *Can. J. Appl. Physiol.*, 25, 68–78, 2000.

71. Leder, B.Z., Longcope, C., Catlin, D.H., Ahrens, B., Schoenfeld, D.A., and Finkelstein, J.S., Oral androstenedione administration and serum testosterone concentrations in young men, *JAMA*, 283, 779–782, 2000.

72. Brown, G.A., Vukovich, M.D., Martini, E.R., Kohut, M.L., Franke, W.D., Jackson, D.A., and King, D.S., Effects of androstenedione-herbal supplementation on serum sex hormone concentrations in 30- to 59-year-old men, *Int. J. Vitam. Nutr. Res.*, 71, 293–301, 2001.

73. Brown, G.A., Vukovich, M.D., Martini, E.R., Kohut, M.L., Franke, W.D., Jackson, D.A., and King, D.S., Endocrine and lipid responses to chronic androstenediol-herbal supplementation in 30 to 58 year old men, *J. Am. Coll. Nutr.*, 20, 520–528, 2001.

74. Broeder, C.E., Quindry, J., Brittingham, K., Panton, L., Thomson, J., Appakondu, S., Breuel, K., Byrd, R., Douglas, J., Earnest, C., Mitchell, C., Olson, M., Roy, T., and Yarlagadda, C., The Andro Project: physiological and hormonal influences of androstenedione supplementation in men 35 to 65 years old participating in a high-intensity resistance training program, *Arch. Intern. Med.*, 160, 3093–3104, 2000.

75. Broeder, C.E., Oral andro-related prohormone supplementation: do the potential risks outweigh the benefits? *Can. J. Appl. Physiol.*, 28, 102–116, 2003.

76. Williams, M.H., *Nutrition for Health, Fitness and Sport*, 6th ed., McGraw-Hill, 2002.

77. Horton, R., and Tait, J.F., Androstenedione production and interconversion rates measured in peripheral blood and studies on the possible site of its conversion to testosterone, *J. Clin. Invest.*, 45, 301–313, 1966.

78. Morley, J.E., Anorexia, sarcopenia, and aging, *Nutrition*, 17, 660–663, 2001.

79. Thiblin, I., and Petersson, A., Pharmacoepidemiology of anabolic androgenic steroids: a review, *Fundam. Clin. Pharmacol.*, 19, 27–44, 2005.

80. Gallaway, S., *The Steroid Bible*, BI Press, Sacramento, 1997.

81. Parssinen, M., and Seppala, T., Steroid use and long-term health risks in former athletes, *Sports Med.*, 32, 83–94, 2002.

82. Babigian, A., and Silverman, R.T., Management of gynecomastia due to use of anabolic steroids in bodybuilders, *Plast. Reconstr. Surg.*, 107, 240–242, 2001.

83. Calzada, L., Torres-Calleja, J., Martinez, J.M., and Pedron, N., Measurement of androgen and estrogen receptors in breast tissue from subjects with anabolic steroid-dependent gynecomastia, *Life Sci.*, 69, 1465–1469, 2001.

84. Saltzstein, D., Sieber, P., Morris, T., and Gallo, J., Prevention and management of bicalutamide-induced gynecomastia and breast pain: randomized endocrinologic and clinical studies with tamoxifen and anastrozole, *Prostate Cancer Prostatic Dis.*, 8: 75–83, 2005.

85. Marks, R., Acne and its management beyond the age of 35 years, *Am. J. Clin. Dermatol.*, 5, 459–462, 2004.

86. Triemstra, J.L., and Wood, R.I., Testosterone self-administration in female hamsters, *Behav. Brain Res.*, 154, 221–229, 2004.

87. Derman, R.J., Effects of sex steroids on women's health: implications for practitioners, *Am. J. Med.,* 98, 137S–143S, 1995.
88. Malarkey, W.B., Strauss, R.H., Leizman, D.J., Liggett, M., and Demers, L.M., Endocrine effects in female weight lifters who self-administer testosterone and anabolic steroids, *Am. J. Obstet. Gynecol.,* 165, 1385–1390, 1991.
89. Friedl, K.E., Effect of anabolic steroids on physcial health, in *Anabolic Steroids in Sport and Exercise*, 2nd ed., Yesalis, C.E., Ed., Champaign, 2000, pp. 175–225.
90. Elliot, D.L., and Goldberg, L., Women and anabolic steroids, in *Anabolic Steroids in Sport and Exercise*, Yesalis, C.E., Ed., Human Kinetics, Champaign, 2000, pp. 225–246.
91. Feller, A.A., Mylonakis, E., and Rich, J.D., Medical complications of anabolic steroids, *Med. Health R. I.,* 85, 338–340, 2002.
92. Bahrke, M.S., Yesalis, C.E., III, and Wright, J.E., Psychological and behavioural effects of endogenous testosterone levels and anabolic–androgenic steroids among males. A review, *Sports Med.,* 10, 303–337, 1990.
93. Haren, M.T., Wittert, G.A., Chapman, I.M., Coates, P., and Morley, J.E., Effect of oral testosterone undecanoate on visuospatial cognition, mood and quality of life in elderly men with low-normal gonadal status, *Maturitas,* 50, 124–133, 2005.
94. Perry, P.J., Kutscher, E.C., Lund, B.C., Yates, W.R., Holman, T.L., and Demers, L., Measures of aggression and mood changes in male weightlifters with and without androgenic anabolic steroid use, *J. Forensic Sci.,* 48, 646–651, 2003.
95. Bahrke, M.S., Psychological effects of endogenous testosterone and anabolic–androgenic steroids, in *Anabolic Steroids in Sport and Exercise*, Yesalis, C.E., Ed., Human Kinetics, Champaign, 2000, pp. 247–278.
96. Yates, W.R., Perry, P.J., MacIndoe, J., Holman, T., and Ellingrod, V., Psychosexual effects of three doses of testosterone cycling in normal men, *Biol. Psychiatry,* 45, 254–260, 1999.
97. Kenney, J., Extent and nature of illicit trafficking in anabolic steroids. Report of the International Conference on the Abuse of Trafficking of Anabolic Steroids, United States Drug Enforcement Administration Conference Report, 34–35, 1994, Washington, DC.
98. Payne, J.R., Kotwinski, P.J., and Montgomery, H.E., Cardiac effects of anabolic steroids, *Heart,* 90, 473–475, 2004.
99. Wright, J.E., Anabolic steroids and athletics, *Exerc. Sport Sci. Rev.,* 8, 149–202, 1980.
100. Glazer, G., Atherogenic effects of anabolic steroids on serum lipid levels. A literature review, *Arch. Intern. Med.,* 151, 1925–1933, 1991.
101. Palatini, P., Giada, F., Garavelli, G., Sinisi, F., Mario, L., Michieletto, M., and Baldo-Enzi, G., Cardiovascular effects of anabolic steroids in weight-trained subjects, *J. Clin. Pharmacol.,* 36, 1132–1140, 1996.
102. Glazer, G., and Suchman, A.L., Lack of demonstrated effect of nandrolone on serum lipids, *Metabolism,* 43, 204–210, 1994.
103. Hartgens, F., Rietjens, G., Keizer, H.A., Kuipers, H., and Wolffenbuttel, B.H., Effects of androgenic–anabolic steroids on apolipoproteins and lipoprotein (a), *Br. J. Sports Med.,* 38, 253–259, 2004.
104. Urhausen, A., Torsten, A., and Wilfried, K., Reversibility of the effects on blood cells, lipids, liver function and hormones in former anabolic–androgenic steroid abusers, *J. Steroid Biochem. Mol. Biol.,* 84, 369–375, 2003.

105. Grace, F.M., and Davies, B., Raised concentrations of C reactive protein in anabolic steroid using bodybuilders, *Br. J. Sports Med.,* 38, 97–98, 2004.

106. Urhausen, A., Albers, T., and Kindermann, W., Are the cardiac effects of anabolic steroid abuse in strength athletes reversible? *Heart,* 90, 496–501, 2004.

107. Shapiro, J., Christiana, J., and Frishman, W.H., Testosterone and other anabolic steroids as cardiovascular drugs, *Am. J. Ther.,* 6, 167–174, 1999.

108. Ansell, J.E., Tiarks, C., and Fairchild, V.K., Coagulation abnormalities associated with the use of anabolic steroids, *Am. Heart J.,* 125, 367–371, 1993.

109. Winkler, U.H., Effects of androgens on haemostasis, *Maturitas,* 24, 147–155, 1996.

110. Crook, D., Sidhu, M., Seed, M., O'Donnell, M., and Stevenson, J.C., Lipoprotein Lp(a) levels are reduced by danazol, an anabolic steroid, *Atherosclerosis,* 92, 41–47, 1992.

111. Johnson, C.A., Use of androgens in patients with renal failure, *Semin. Dial.,* 13, 36–39, 2000.

112. LeGros, T., McConnell, D., Murry, T., Edavettal, M., Racey-Burns, L.A., Shepherd, R.E., and Burns, A.H., The effects of 17 alpha-methyltestosterone on myocardial function in vitro, *Med. Sci. Sports Exerc.,* 32, 897–903, 2000.

113. Grace, F., Sculthorpe, N., Baker, J., and Davies, B., Blood pressure and rate pressure product response in males using high-dose anabolic androgenic steroids (AAS), *J. Sci. Med. Sport,* 6, 307–312, 2003.

114. Riebe, D., Fernhall, B., and Thompson, P.D., The blood pressure response to exercise in anabolic steroid users, *Med. Sci. Sports Exerc.,* 24, 633–637, 1992.

115. Kuipers, H., Wijnen, J.A., Hartgens, F., and Willems, S.M., Influence of anabolic steroids on body composition, blood pressure, lipid profile and liver functions in body builders, *Int. J. Sports Med.,* 12, 413–418, 1991.

116. Gragera, R., Saborido, A., Molano, F., Jimenez, L., Muniz, E., and Megias, A., Ultrastructural changes induced by anabolic steroids in liver of trained rats, *Histol. Histopathol.,* 8, 449–455, 1993.

117. Ishak, K.G., Hepatic lesions caused by anabolic and contraceptive steroids, *Semin. Liver Dis.,* 1, 116–128, 1981.

118. Mottram, D.R., and George, A.J., Anabolic steroids, *Baillieres Best Pract. Res. Clin. Endocrinol. Metab.,* 14, 55–69, 2000.

119. Dourakis, S.P., and Tolis, G., Sex hormonal preparations and the liver, *Eur. J. Contracept. Reprod. Health Care,* 3, 7–16, 1998.

120. Stimac, D., Milic, S., Dintinjana, R.D., Kovac, D., and Ristic, S., Androgenic/anabolic steroid-induced toxic hepatitis, *J. Clin. Gastroenterol.,* 35, 350–352, 2002.

121. Simon, D.M., Krause, R., and Galambos, J.T., Peliosis hepatis in a patient with marasmus, *Gastroenterology,* 95, 805–809, 1988.

122. Boada, L.D., Zumbado, M., Torres, S., Lopez, A., Diaz-Chico, B.N., Cabrera, J.J., and Luzardo, O.P., Evaluation of acute and chronic hepatotoxic effects exerted by anabolic–androgenic steroid stanozolol in adult male rats, *Arch. Toxicol.,* 73, 465–472, 1999.

123. Dickerman, R.D., Pertusi, R.M., Zachariah, N.Y., Dufour, D.R., and McConathy, W.J., Anabolic steroid-induced hepatotoxicity: is it overstated? *Clin. J. Sport Med.,* 9, 34–39, 1999.

124. van Breda, E., Keizer, H.A., Kuipers, H., and Wolffenbuttel, B.H., Androgenic anabolic steroid use and severe hypothalamic–pituitary dysfunction: a case study, *Int. J. Sports Med.,* 24, 195–196, 2003.

125. Cohen, J.C., and Hickman, R., Insulin resistance and diminished glucose tolerance in powerlifters ingesting anabolic steroids, *J. Clin. Endocrinol. Metab.,* 64, 960–963, 1987.

126. Rogol, A.D., Sex steroid and growth hormone supplementation to enhance performance in adolescent athletes, *Curr. Opin. Pediatr.,* 12, 382–387, 2000.

127. Houchin, L.D., and Rogol, A.D., Androgen replacement in children with constitutional delay of puberty: the case for aggressive therapy, *Baillieres Clin. Endocrinol. Metab.,* 12, 427–440, 1998.

128. Mottram, D.R., Banned drugs in sport. Does the International Olympic Committee (IOC) list need updating? *Sports Med.,* 27, 1–10, 1999.

129. Chester, N., Reilly, T., and Mottram, D.R., Over-the-counter drug use amongst athletes and non-athletes, *J. Sports Med. Phys. Fitness,* 43, 111–118, 2003.

130. Cawley, A.T., Hine, E.R., Trout, G.J., George, A.V., and Kazlauskas, R., Searching for new markers of endogenous steroid administration in athletes: "looking outside the metabolic box", *Forensic Sci. Int.,* 143, 103–114, 2004.

131. Delbeke, F.T., Van Eenoo, P., Van Thuyne, W., and Desmet, N., Prohormones and sport, *J. Steroid Biochem. Mol. Biol.,* 83, 245–251, 2002.

132. Parr, M.K., Geyer, H., Reinhart, U., and Schanzer, W., Analytical strategies for the detection of non-labelled anabolic androgenic steroids in nutritional supplements, *Food Addit. Contam.,* 21, 632–640, 2004.

133. International Olympic Committee, Analysis of non-hormonal nutritional supplements for anabolic–androgenic steroids, *http://multimedia olympic org/pdf/en_report_324 pdf* 83, 245–251, 2002.

134. Van Thuyne, W., and Delbeke, F.T., Validation of a GC-MS screening method for anabolizing agents in solid nutritional supplements, *Biomed. Chromatogr.,* 18, 155–159, 2004.

135. Schanzer, W., Metabolism of anabolic androgenic steroids, *Clin. Chem.,* 42, 1001–1020, 1996.

136. Catlin, D.H., Cowan, D.A., de la Torre, R., Donike, M., Fraisse, D., Oftebro, H., Hatton, C.K., Starcevic, B., Becchi, M., de la Torre, X., Norli, H., Geyer, H., and Walker, C.J., Urinary testosterone (T) to epitestosterone (E) ratios by GC/MS. I. Initial comparison of uncorrected T/E in six international laboratories, *J. Mass Spectrom.,* 31, 397–402, 1996.

137. Catlin, D.H., Hatton, C.K., and Starcevic, S.H., Issues in detecting abuse of xenobiotic anabolic steroids and testosterone by analysis of athletes' urine, *Clin. Chem.,* 43, 1280–1288, 1997.

138. Aguilera, R., Hatton, C.K., and Catlin, D.H., Detection of epitestosterone doping by isotope ratio mass spectrometry, *Clin. Chem.,* 48, 629–636, 2002.

139. Aguilera, R., Chapman, T.E., Starcevic, B., Hatton, C.K., and Catlin, D.H., Performance characteristics of a carbon isotope ratio method for detecting doping with testosterone based on urine diols: controls and athletes with elevated testosterone/epitestosterone ratios, *Clin. Chem.,* 47, 292–300, 2001.

140. Bowers, L.D., Oral dehydroepiandrosterone supplementation can increase the testosterone/epitestosterone ratio, *Clin. Chem.,* 45, 295–297, 1999.

141. Rizner, T.L., and Zakelj-Mavric, M., Characterization of fungal 17beta-hydroxysteroid dehydrogenases, *Comp. Biochem. Physiol. B Biochem. Mol. Biol.,* 127, 53–63, 2000.

142. de la Torre, R., de la Torre, X., Alia, C., Segura, J., Baro, T., and Torres-Rodriguez, J.M., Changes in androgenic steroid profile due to urine contamination by

microorganisms: a prospective study in the context of doping control, *Anal. Biochem.,* 289, 116–123, 2001.

143. Jimenez, C., Ventura, R., Williams, J., Segura, J., and de la Torre, R., Reference materials for analytical toxicology including doping control: freeze-dried urine samples, *Analyst,* 129, 449–455, 2004.

144. Maughan, R.J., King, D.S., and Lea, T., Dietary supplements, *J. Sports Sci.,* 22, 95–113, 2004.

145. Kohler, R.M., and Lambert, M.I., Urine nandrolone metabolites: false positive doping test? *Br. J. Sports Med.,* 36, 325–329, 2002.

146. Gambelunghe, C., Sommavilla, M., and Rossi, R., Testing for nandrolone metabolites in urine samples of professional athletes and sedentary subjects by GC/MS/MS analysis, *Biomed. Chromatogr.* 16, 508–512, 2002.

147. Van Eenoo, P., Delbeke, F.T., de Jong, F.H., and De Backer, P., Endogenous origin of norandrosterone in female urine: indirect evidence for the production of 19-norsteroids as by-products in the conversion from androgen to estrogen, *J. Steroid Biochem. Mol. Biol.,* 78, 351–357, 2001.

148. Schmitt, N., Flament, M.M., Goubault, C., Legros, P., Grenier-Loustalot, M.F., and Denjean, A., Nandrolone excretion is not increased by exhaustive exercise in trained athletes, *Med. Sci. Sports Exerc.,* 34, 1436–1439, 2002.

149. Ritter, S., Washington, C., and Washington, E.N., Designer steroid rocks sports world, *Chem. Eng. News,* 81, 83–94, 2003.

150. Gross, M.L., Ritz, E., Korsch, M., Adamczak, M., Weckbach, M., Mall, G., Berger, I., Hansen, A., and Amann, K., Effects of estrogens on cardiovascular structure in uninephrectomized SHRsp rats, *Kidney Int.,* 67, 849–857, 2005.

Section V

Soft Tissue

21 Osteoarthritis

Laurie Mischley, N.D. and
David Musnick, M.D.

CONTENTS

DEFINITION

Osteoarthritis (OA) is characterized by progressive degeneration of articular cartilage with resultant joint space narrowing, cysts, and osteophyte formation. OA occurs and progresses when regeneration cannot keep pace with the rate of cartilage loss. Joint deterioration occurs when the biomaterial properties of the articular cartilage are inadequate or the load on the joint is excessive.[1,2] Joint vulnerability can stem from injury, malalignment, muscle weakness, genetic and ethnic predisposition, aging, and nutritional factors. Additional insult on the total joint load can come from the extra weight burden associated with obesity and certain physical activities (i.e., high-impact sports). Nutritional interventions and in particular certain joint support supplements can play a key role in the management of patients with OA.

Pain, stiffness, and loss of function are the most common complaints among individuals with OA, causing it to be the leading cause of physical disability in industrialized societies.[3] Despite the high frequency of disability associated with the disease, OA pain may not correlate with the amount of structural damage within the joint. Several studies have demonstrated joints that show similar amounts of loss on x-ray exhibiting considerable variation in function and pain.[4,5]

Age is the single risk factor most strongly correlated with OA and some studies suggest that more than 80% of individuals over the age of 75 years are affected.[6,7] Age-related tissue changes are believed to be because of a decrease in the repair mechanisms of chondrocytes. With age, chondrocytes are unable to maintain synthetic activity, exhibit decreased responsiveness to anabolic growth factors, synthesize smaller and less uniform proteoglycans and fewer functional link proteins.[7] Given the vulnerability of aging joints and the lack of correlation between symptoms and loss of cartilage, it is advisable to ensure proper joint mechanics and nutrition in all elderly individuals.

Excessive impact loading, such as jobs that require heavy lifting and repetitive, high-impact sports, are strongly associated with joint injury and increase risk of developing OA.[8] It has been theorized that excessive loads may cause microfractures of adjacent bone and subsequent callus formation, resulting in bone that is less effective as a shock absorber and predisposing articular cartilage to excessive impact loading and, eventually, degeneration.[7] More overtly, the increased risk of OA associated with injuries such as ligament tears and meniscal injuries, which are more frequent in athletes, has long been appreciated.[8]

Greater body mass index (BMI) in both women and men has been associated with an increase in risk of OA. Obesity significantly increases the risk of knee symptoms and radiographic osteophytes. Obesity likely contributes to OA by increasing the forces at weight-bearing joints, changing posture, gait, and the physical activity level, any or all of which may further contribute to altered joint biomechanics.[9]

PATHOPHYSIOLOGY

OA is characterized initially by irregularities of the articular cartilage surface, a thickening of subchondral bone, and the formation of marginal osteophytes. Eventually, changes include cartilage softening, ulceration, and focal disintegration within the joint with the most striking changes usually seen in load-bearing areas of the articular cartilage.

Chondrocytes comprise the entire cellular matrix of the joint capsule whereas the substrate of the extracellular matrix consists of collagen and polysaccharides known as glucosaminoglycans (GAGs). Substantial GAGs in the extracellular matrix include hyaluronic acid, chondroitin-4-sulfate, chondrotin-6-sulfate, dermatan sulfate, and keratan sulfate. The primary roles of the extracellular matrix include shock absorption, maintaining viscosity, and the nourishment of the chondrocytes. The primary role of the chondrocytes is the ongoing synthesis of matrix components. In short, the health of the joint is dependent on the function and quality of the chondrocyte and the extracellular matrix.

Early in the course of the disease there is evidence of enhanced chondrocyte replication, suggestive of attempts at repair. In spite of accelerated metabolism within the chondrocyte, the synthesis of matrix substrates is insufficient and results in a decreased concentration of sulfur-containing proteoglycans within the extracellular space. The failure of chondrocytes to compensate for the proteoglycan loss results in a net loss of major matrix contents, including chondrocytes.[10]

The loss of proteoglycan density causes an influx of water into the matrix. The influx of water weakens the chemical bonds within the matrix, decreasing the matrix viscosity as well as its capacity to absorb shock and nourish the chondrocytes. The hypertrophy and subsequent death of the chondrocytes causes hyaline cartilage to degenerate and the matrix begins to calcify.[11,12] The progressive depletion of sulfated proteoglycans from the extracellular matrix of articular cartilage, one of the earliest manifestations of OA, is thought to be because of enhanced activity of the lysosomal enzymes arylsulfatases A and B.[13]

Interleukin-1 (IL-1) is the prototypical inflammatory cytokine implicated in signaling the degradation of cartilage matrix in OA. IL-1 stimulates and upregulates the production of proteinases that cleave proteoglycan. Intra-articular injection of IL-1 induces proteoglycan loss and an IL-1 receptor antagonist slows progression of cartilage loss in animal models of OA.[14] Given the role of IL-1 in promoting cartilage degradation, IL-1 inhibition is a logical treatment target in OA.

In addition to the production of proteinases, IL-1 triggers an entire cascade of proinflammatory and catabolic cytokines including tumor necrosis factor-α (TNF-α), IL-6, IL-8, and PGE2, which act synergistically with IL-1 to perpetuate the proinflammatory cascade.[14] TNF-α induces cartilage degeneration by both sustaining cytokine production and increasing expression of collagenases and proteinases.[15] In response to IL-1, chondrocytes secrete neutral metalloproteinases (MMP) and active oxygen species that are directly implicated in the destruction of cartilage matrix. Moreover, this cytokine is a potent inhibitor of proteoglycan and collagen synthesis.[16]

Editor's Note

When sufficiently available, nutrients provide 24/7 coverage for cartilage repair. The modern diet is low in these primarily sulfur-containing nutrients, and as a result minor trauma is more likely to damage cartilage. Adjusting the diet and incorporating supplemental nutrients is particularly relevant given the prevalence of OA and the side effects of current long-term medical management. Repletion of nutrients generally benefits the entire body, not just the arthritic joint.

TREATMENT GOALS

The primary treatment targets for OA include the reduction of pain and inflammation, restoration of good mechanics, halting degeneration, and encouraging regeneration of cartilage. Nutritional therapies provide the substrate for cartilage regeneration and have demonstrated efficacy in controlling pain and inflammation.

PAIN CONTROL

Pain is the primary complaint among sufferers of OA and, as far as the patient is concerned, the success of any treatment is often measured by its ability to reduce pain. It has long been known that cortisone and hydrocortisone inhibit cartilage growth and matrix formation[11] and for this reason steroids are typically avoided. Conventional pharmacological treatment of OA consists primarily of nonsteroidal anti-inflammatory drugs (NSAIDs) and analgesics.

While NSAIDs are effective in the reduction of pain, the long-term use of NSAIDs is not recommended in OA[17] because of the tremendous side-effect profile of these agents. Each year, as many as 7600 deaths and 76,000 hospitalizations in the United States, 2000 deaths in the United Kingdom, and 365 deaths and 3900 hospitalizations in Canada may be attributable to NSAIDs.[10] Epidemiological data suggest NSAIDs are currently overused in OA management based on the prevalence of the disease and the disproportionate volume of side effects noted. In addition to the inherent side effects of NSAIDs, there is evidence, both in animals with experimental OA and in humans, that administration of NSAIDs may actually accelerate joint destruction[18–21] but this is still debated in the literature.[22] Because of the high incidence of side effects from NSAIDs, clinicians are advised to avoid NSAIDs when possible and use on a short-term basis when necessary.

Several nutritional supplements have been shown to be as effective as NSAIDs in reducing pain and improving functional limitation in patients with OA without adverse effects common to NSAIDs. A 2004 study demonstrated *S*-adenosyl methionine (SAMe) (1200 mg/d) was as effective as a commonly prescribed COX-2 inhibitor, but with a slower onset of action and a lower incidence of side effects.[23] Other nutritional supplements that have shown to alleviate pain in OA are discussed in detail later in this chapter.

BIOMECHANICS

OA occurs more commonly in a number of areas of the body: the C5–7 areas of the cervical spine, the L4–S1 areas of the lumbar spine, the knees, hips, and the

IP and DIP joints of the hands. The hips and knees are weight-bearing joints and excessive or abnormal loads can contribute to the development and progress of OA. Dysfunctional mechanics at a joint can create excessive shearing and abnormal forces on articular cartilage contributing to the progression of Degenerative Joint Disease (DJD). Dysfunctional mechanics can result from alignment dysfunction at the foot, gait dysfunction, overuse in exercise and sports, and poor posture. A patient who has OA of the lower extremity or spine needs a good gait and biomechanics evaluation to evaluate problems with ligament laxity, foot biomechanics, muscle strength, muscle tightness, and joint restriction.

Exercise recommendations (aerobic options, strength and balance exercise) should be given to patients with OA. The clinician should help the patient to choose exercise options that are less likely to cause progression of osteoarthritic changes. Patients with moderately severe OA of the ankle, knee, hip, or low back should limit high-impact aerobic activities such as running and jumping activities.

WEIGHT MANAGEMENT

In patients who are obese and have OA of the ankle, knee, hips, or lumbar spine weight reduction should be targeted as a clinical goal to decrease the abnormal and excessive forces in the ankles, knees, and hips in individuals with an elevated BMI. Obesity can alter the biomechanics of gait and cause abnormal forces especially in the lower extremity.

REDUCE INFLAMMATION

Inflammatory mediators are integral in the pathogenesis of OA. Human OA cartilage expresses modulators of inflammation (COX-2, 5-LOX, FLAP, IL-1α, TNFα)[24] that normal human cartilage does not. Inhibition of inflammatory mediators curbs disease progression and has long been a target for treatment. The past decade has elucidated the mechanism by which several nutritional supplements reduce inflammation. Table 21.1 summarizes the mechanism by which avocado/soybean unsaponifiable residues, omega-3 fatty acids, SAMe, and glucosamine interfere with the inflammatory cascade.

REGENERATE CARTILAGE

Whereas analgesics most effectively address patient concerns in the short term, the regeneration of cartilage must be an emphasis of treatment to avoid disease progression. Substantial evidence, *in vitro* and *in vivo*, attests to the ability of nutritional agents to enhance proteoglycan synthesis, increase the strength of the collagen network, decrease proteinases that degrade collagen and proteoglycans (aggrecanase), and decrease IL-1 and subsequent proinflammatory cytokines that further perpetuate cartilage degradation.

TABLE 21.1

Nutrient	Mechanism of action	Reference
Analgesic		
Avocado/soybean unsaponifiable residues	Analgesic	Lequesne, Maheu et al. (2002)
Chondroitin sulfate	Analgesic	Morreale, Manopulo et al. (1996)
Glucosamine sulfate	Analgesic	Matheson and Perry (2003), Bruyere, Pavelka et al. (2004)
SAMe	Analgesic	Najm, Reinsch et al. (2004)
Modulate inflammation		
Avocado/soybean unsaponifiable residues	Modulate inflammation by suppressing IL-1, PGE-2, IL-6, IL-8	Hauselmann (2001)
Omega-3 fatty acids	Modulate inflammation by suppressing IL-1, TNF-α, PGE-2, 5-LOX, FLAP, COX-2	Curtis (2000)
SAMe	Modulate inflammation by suppressing IL-1, TNF-α	Gloystein, Gillespie et al. (2003)
Glucoasamine	Modulate inflammation by suppressing PGE-2	Nakamura, Shibakawa et al. (2004)
Cartilage regeneration		
Chondroitin sulfate	Increase proteoglycan synthesis	Reginster (2003)
Glucosamine sulfate	Increase proteoglycan synthesis, increase chondrocyte matrix gene expression	Matheson and Perry (2003), Poustie, Carran et al. (2004)
SAMe	Increase proteoglycan synthesis	Gloystein, Gillespie et al. (2003), Bottiglieri (2002)
Vitamin C	Increase proteoglycan synthesis	Schwartz and Adamy (1977)
Avocado/soybean unsaponifiable residues	Increase collagen synthesis, stimulate TGF-β1, stimulate plasminogen activator inhibitor-1 expression	Boumediene, Felisaz et al. (1999), Hauselmann (2001)
Vitamin C	Increase collagen synthesis, stabilization of the mature collagen fibril	Spanheimer, Bird et al. (1986), Peterkofsky (1991)
Decrease degradation		
Glucosamine sulfate	Decrease collagen degradation	Christgau, Henrotin et al. (2004)
n – 3 PUFA	Decreases degradation by inhibiting ADAMTS-4, MMP-3, MMP-13, aggrecanase	Curtis (2000)
Vitamin C	Decrease degradation by inhibiting aggrecanase	Schwartz and Adamy (1977)
Avocado/soybean unsaponifiable residues	Decrease degradation by inhibiting metalloproteinase activity and collagenase synthesis	Henrotin, Labasse et al. (1998), Ernst (2003), Hauselmann (2001)

NUTRITIONAL SUBSTRATES FOR CARTILAGE REPAIR AND REGENERATION

The study of nutrition is especially pertinent in OA, where the pathophysiology is, by definition, an inability to maintain the growth and replacement of damaged components of the joint. Nourishment of the joint is complicated in that cartilage is neither vascularized (except for the outer third of the meniscus cartilage of the knees) nor supplied with nerves or lymphatic vessels. Chondrocytes receive their nourishment from synovial fluid. The use of nutritional supplements to support joints with osteoarthritic changes makes sense primarily if there is cartilage surface remaining as opposed to bone on bone anatomy. Providing substrate for cartilage regeneration has its basis in biochemistry and numerous scientific studies. Most of the studies have been done regarding OA of the knee.

Sulfur is an essential component of the GAGs (i.e. chondroitin sulfate, keratan sulfate) and an essential element for joint health. Sulfur is important in the biochemistry of the cartilage in that it has the potential to bind several molecules of water, which allows the joint to remain appropriately hydrated. It is recommended that patients have adequate amounts of dietary sulfur. Patients should be encouraged to eat the following high-sulfur foods daily: broccoli, cabbage, eggs, garlic, milk, kale, mustard greens, onions, shallots, soy milk, and watercress. Sulfur may also be obtained from supplements including glucosamine sulfate, chondroitin sulfate, alpha-lipoic acid, and methylsulfonylmethane (MSM).

GLUCOSAMINE

N-Acetyl-D-glucosamine is a naturally occurring amino sugar found in all human tissues. It functions as a building block in the synthesis of structural substrates such as glycoproteins, glycolipids, GAGs, hyaluronate, and proteoglycans and is required to manufacture joint lubricants and protective agents such as mucin and mucous secretions.[25]

Although glucosamine is not generally found in the human diet, it is easily obtained from the exoskeletons of shrimp, crabs, and lobsters for use in medical applications. As a supplement glucosamine is available alone or in combination as glucosamine sulfate, glucosamine hydrochloride, and N-acetyl glucosamine. Thus far, the majority clinical research demonstrating efficacy in OA has been conducted with the sulfate form and is thus the recommended form at this time.

When administered orally, the absorption rate for glucosamine sulfate in the human gastrointestinal tract is approximately 87%.[26] In recent years, topical cream containing glucosamine and chondroitin sulfate has shown efficacy in relieving pain in OA of the knee.[27]

In 2004, a hallmark publication was the first to demonstrate that a pharmacological intervention for OA, glucosamine sulfate, had the ability to modify the course of the disease.[28] Prior to this study, OA was understood to be a progressively worsening condition and the therapies only palliative. The vast majority of published clinical research demonstrates that glucosamine is effective for decreasing pain, improving range of motion, and reducing joint space narrowing in patients with OA. The mechanism of action is purported to be the increased availability of substrate for proteoglycan synthesis.[25,28]

While studies of glucosamine and OA are largely positive, there are a few negative studies that raise several interesting questions about whether or not glucosamine may be more effective OA subtypes. In a 2004 study, Christgau et al.[29] explored using specific markers of collagen turnover to help classify patients at baseline. Using these markers, they were able to demonstrate that those patients who initially had high cartilage turnover were particularly responsive to glucosamine therapy. Glucosamine seems to be effective for treating OA of all joints, but the knee has been the most widely studied.

The one constant found in all studies reported in the medical literature is that glucosamine appears to be remarkably safe and well tolerated at 1500 to –2000 mg/d given orally in divided doses. Side effects are significantly less common with glucosamine than either NSAIDs or placebo.[30] Recent studies have addressed concerns that glucosamine, a sugar, can have adverse effects on levels of plasma glucose and insulin but further research has found these concerns to be unfounded.[31–33]

Glucosamine is often derived from shellfish and several authors have expressed concern that the supplement may cause allergic reactions in people who are sensitive to shellfish. Glucosamine is derived from the exoskeletons of shellfish but antibodies in individuals allergic to shellfish are targeted at antigens in the meat, not the shell. Thus far, there have been no documented reports of allergic reactions to glucosamine among shellfish-sensitive patients, but it is prudent to recommend the synthetically derived form of the supplement be used in this population.[34] Most studies have concluded that patients taking glucosamine do not seem to notice much effect for at least 6 weeks.

Chondroitin Sulfate

Chondroitin sulfate, a mucopolysaccharide, is a proteoglycan component that functions in the maintenance of cartilage elasticity, strength, and mass. In humans, chondroitin sulfate is manufactured from glucosamine sulfate derivatives. Chondroitin sulfate, like glucosamine, is not present in significant amounts in the human diet. It is extracted from either bovine or marine sources for use in medical applications.

The medical literature contains numerous positive studies pertaining to the use of chondroitin as a therapy for OA. It has been shown to alleviate pain, decrease NSAID use, improve joint mobility, and stabilize the loss of interarticular space with varying degrees of efficacy in patients with OA.[35–37] Results of chondroitin supplementation typically take 8 to 12 weeks to become apparent, but in most studies the effect persisted for several months, even after discontinuing the medication. The typical study doses ranged from 800 to 1200 mg/d given orally. Some research suggests that the combined use of glucosamine and chondroitin sulfate demonstrates synergistic activity on the maintenance of cartilage and inhibition of its degradation based on demonstrated abilities to aid in the protection of cartilage in different ways.[38]

An important controversy in the medical literature as it pertains to the efficacy of chondroitin is whether or not clinically significant amounts are available to the body via oral dosing given the large size of the molecule. During the past few years, several studies have demonstrated the oral absorption of chondroitin sulfate but absorption estimates across the gut mucosa range from 10 to 70%.[39,40]

Other than mild gastrointestinal distress, the incidence of adverse effects with chondroitin sulfate is extremely low. Chondroitin is typically extracted from bovine trachea and concern has been expressed about the potential risk of contamination by animals infected with bovine spongiform encephalopathy (BSE, mad cow disease). There are currently no documented cases of such contamination and risk of transmission is thought to be low.

S-ADENOSYL METHIONINE (SAMe)

SAMe is present in all organisms and is synthesized endogenously from methionine and adenosine triphosphate. It is a methyl donor to numerous acceptor molecules and plays an essential role in many biochemical reactions involving enzymatic transmethylation. SAMe has been shown to inhibit the synthesis and the activity of IL-1 and TNF-α at multiple locations in its signal transduction pathways and has demonstrated the ability to upregulate the proteoglycan synthesis and proliferation rate of chondrocytes by 50 to 60%, thereby promoting cartilage formation and repair.[38,41]

SAMe is an alternative to NSAIDs for treatment of joint inflammation and pain caused by trauma and disease states such as OA. It is a proven therapy for OA and has a low side-effect profile. The Arthritis Foundation concludes there is sufficient information to support the pain relief claims made for SAMe.[8] The consensus among several published reviews is that SAMe appears to be of equivalent effectiveness to NSAIDs in reducing pain and improving functional limitations, with fewer side effects. One study suggested SAMe has a slower onset of action than NSAIDs with equivalent results at 4 weeks.[42]

Dosage ranges from 200 to 1600 mg have been used for joint support. B12 and folate aid the body in using SAMe, and it may be useful to supplement with these nutrients as well.[38] Supplementation with 400 mg for 7 days significantly increased SAMe concentrations in synovial fluid by three- to fourfold compared with pretreatment values.[43]

HYALURONIC ACID

Hyaluronic acid is the main component of the extracellular matrix within the joint. It is a hydrophilic polysaccharide varying in length from 250 to 25,000 disaccharide units. The large size of this molecule and the water it holds give the matrix solution remarkable viscosity, tensile strength, and shock-absorption properties.

Intra-articular hyaluronans (viscosupplementation) are used to treat pain and mechanical dysfunction associated with OA of the knee because the oral form is not well absorbed. Many controlled clinical studies have demonstrated their efficacy and a low side-effect profile for this indication and application.[44–47] Intra-articular injections of the knee are indicated if the patient has very little cartilage surface and wishes to avoid surgery. Intra-articular injections are carried out once per week for 3 to 5 weeks (depending on the viscosupplementation liquid used). An improvement in pain levels and in function appears to have clinical benefit for 6 to 9 months. The treatment may be repeated but there do not appear to be cumulative effects. Side effects are minimal. It is important to note the oral cartilage support supplements do not appear to have much effect in joints with little surface or meniscus cartilage remaining.

OMEGA-3 FATTY ACIDS

Osteoarthritic cartilage expresses markers of inflammation that contribute to the dysregulation of chondrocyte function and the progressive degradation of the cartilage matrix. *In vitro*, when human OA cartilage explants are exposed to omega-3 polyunsaturated fatty acids, the molecular modulators of inflammation are inhibited. Curtis et al.[24] cultured human OA articular cartilage with various fatty acids and concluded the omega-3 fatty acids, but not other fats, have the capacity to improve late-stage OA chondrocyte function. They found culture for 24 h with omega-3 fatty acids resulted in a decrease loss of GAGs, reduced collagenase cleavage of type II collagen, a dose-dependent reduction in aggrecanases, and all studied modulators of inflammation (COX-2, 5-LOX, FLAP, IL-1α) and joint destruction (ADAMTS-4, MMP-3, MMP-13) were abrogated or reduced.

The concentration and distribution of fatty acids in the diet has long been known to exert influence over the inflammatory cascade (see Chapter 9). While no large-scale clinical studies have yet been done on the influence of omega-3 fatty acids on the symptoms or progression of OA, several clinical studies have demonstrated dietary supplementation with omega-3 fatty acids reduces the inflammatory symptoms of rheumatoid arthritis. When treating patients with omega-3 fatty acids it is reasonable to use fish oil products consisting of EPA and DHA (and primarily of EPA). It is reasonable to choose products that have been tested for purity and that are extremely low in contaminants (PCPs, heavy metals). It is reasonable to use approximately 2 to 4 g of fish oil per day. Side effects are minimal but caution should be used if a patient is on a medication such as Coumadin because of the platelet effects of fish oil. A patented extraction of New Zealand green-lipped mussel powder derived from Perna canaliculus, Lypronol, has been shown to provide significant pain relief and improvement in joint function in 80% of subjects after 8 weeks of treatment without adverse effect. The therapeutic value of Lypronol has been attributed, in part, to its high concentration of omega-3 fatty acids.[50]

Vitamin C (Ascorbic Acid)

Ascorbic acid plays a role in the synthesis of joint components and encourages cartilage synthesis *in vitro*; epidemiologic data suggest dietary intake of ascorbic acid is associated with a reduction of OA progression.

Vitamin C is necessary for the synthesis of collagen and GAGs within the joint capsule. In collagen synthesis, ascorbic acid is a cofactor for enzymes essential for stabilization of the mature collagen fibril.[51,52] The role of vitamin C as a carrier of sulfate groups also makes it a requirement for GAG synthesis.[13]

In vitro, addition of ascorbic acid to OA cultures results in a decreased level of the proteinases responsible for the degradation of proteoglycan. Vitamin C has been shown to significantly increase the biosynthesis of proteoglycan in both normal and osteoarthritic tissues, suggesting it may be helpful in joint repair.[13]

In the Framingham Osteoarthritis Cohort Study, a moderate intake of vitamin C (120 to 200 mg/d) was associated with a threefold lower risk of OA progression. The association was strong and highly significant and was consistent between sexes and among individuals with different severities of OA. The higher vitamin C intake also reduced the likelihood of development of knee pain.[53]

Avocado/Soybean Unsaponifiable Residues (ASU)

ASU is a manufactured product, distributed in France as Piascledine, consisting of one third avocado oil and two thirds soybean unsaponifiables.[54] The unsaponifiable portion of avocado and soybean lipids make up less than 1% of the total lipid content and, thus, sufficient quantities of the ASU are not available from dietary consumption of soy and avocado. Clinical trials suggest that ASU is an effective symptomatic treatment of OA with doses as low as 300 mg ASU per day. Outcome measures have included a reduction in NSAIDs and analgesic intake, a reduction in pain, and an increase in function.[55] Based on both *in vitro* and *in vivo* research, the apparent mechanism of effect of ASU is via the attenuation of inflammatory mediators and the stimulation of anabolic processes within the cartilage.[16,56,57] No serious side effects were reported in any of the published studies.

Niacinamide (Vitamin B3)

Niacin, or vitamin B3, occurs in two forms, nicotinic acid (usually referred to as niacin) and nicotinamide (typically referred to as niacinamide). While both forms have many functions in the body and are crucial to cellular energy production as precursors of NAD and NADP, their therapeutic uses differ considerably.

Niacinamide has been in use as a therapy for OA since the 1940s based on preliminary work by Kaufman.[58–60] In-office clinical research, reported by Kaufman on 455 patients receiving 1500 to 4000 mg/d niacinamide compared against untreated age-matched controls suggested an increase in joint range index and subsequent reduction in pain in 4 to 8 weeks. Recently, investigators have examined efficacy and potential mechanism of action of niacinamide in OA more closely. Jonas et al.[61] demonstrated in a 12-week randomized double-blind placebo-controlled trial ($N = 72$) that patients who took niacinamide (3000 mg daily) experienced an improvement in the global impact of their OA, increased joint flexibility, reduced inflammation, and decrease use of anti-inflammatory medication, compared to controls.

While the mechanism of action of niacinamide in OA has yet to be fully elucidated, current theories suggest that niacinamide acts on chondrocytes to decrease cytokine-mediated inhibition of aggrecan and type II collagen synthesis. In addition, reduction in either production or effect of IL-1 on chondrocytes has been suggested as a plausible mechanism.[41]

Adverse affects have not been widely reported with pharmaceutical-grade niacinamide;[62] however, nausea, heartburn, flatulence, and diarrhea have been reported. Elevated liver enzymes have been reported with the administration of niacinamide[63] and for this reason it is advisable to insure niacinamide supplement quality and evaluate baseline liver function tests prior to, and periodically after, niacinamide administration. While large-scale safety, efficacy, and dosing studies are clearly lacking for the general recommendation of niacinamide treatment for OA, preliminary research suggests the nutrient has therapeutic value and warrants further investigation.

ADDITIONAL NUTRIENTS

Other vitamins and minerals, such as vitamin E, manganese, boron, and vitamin D, likely play an essential role in synthesis and function of the joint. At this time, their role in preventing or treating OA has not been adequately investigated and will, therefore, not be addressed in this chapter. MSM has been commonly used for joint support but the studies do not support its efficacy.

DURATION AND SELECTION OF JOINT SUPPORT SUPPLEMENTATION

The duration of supplementation depends on the pathology that the clinician is treating. For acutely injured joints with articular or meniscus cartilage, supplementation immediately upon diagnosis and continued treatment for approximately 12 weeks is recommended. An x-ray of the joint 6 months after the original injury can evaluate if OA changes have occurred.

A reasonable clinical approach is to start a patient on glucosamine sulfate at the 1500 to 2000 mg/d dose for a minimum of 8 weeks. The clinician can consider adding chondroitin sulfate at the 1200 mg dose to see if there is an added benefit in symptoms and function after 8 to 12 weeks. SAMe can be considered if there is no benefit with the above or as an additional nutrition. Patients can also be educated on how hydration (Chapter 8), healthy dietary fat (Chapter 4), and optimal vitamin C (Chapter 25) enhance cartilage repair.

There is a rational for the use of joint support nutrients after traumatic injury that involves meniscus or articular cartilage. This may involve moderate to severe sprains or contusions to a joint. This would include motor vehicle injuries to the facets of the neck, thoracic and lumbar spine, contusions to the patella, ankle, knee meniscus, and other extremity sprains. There are presently no long-term studies documenting the prevention of OA with joint support nutrients after traumatic injury but the rational of nutritionally supporting the healing and bio-chemical substrates of cartilage healing are very sound. Glucosamine sulfate may be started at the time of the diagnosis and continued for a minimum of 8 weeks and preferably for 12 weeks. There is a definite preventative indication here with low chance of side effects. In addition to traumatic injuries there appears to be good clinical response to the use of glucosamine sulfate in problems involving the articular cartilage of the patella in both patellofemoral tracking syndrome and chondromalacia. The clinician can recommend starting joint support nutrients 6 to 8 weeks before an individual begins a season of high use of the knee in sports.

SUMMARY

A nutritional approach to OA is theoretically justified and has been overwhelmingly validated in laboratory and clinical trails. Whereas conventional therapeutics may offer the most effective short-term pain relief in OA, long-term pain relief and regeneration of the joint is better accomplished with nutritional therapies with surprisingly few side effects.

REFERENCES

1. Felson, D.T., and Schurman, D.J., Risk factors for osteoarthritis: understanding joint vulnerability, *Clin. Orthop.*, 427 (Suppl.), S16–S21, 2004.
2. Brandt, K.D., Osteoarthritis, in *Harrison's Principles of Internal Medicine*, Fauci, A.S. et al., Eds., McGraw-Hill, New York, pp. 1935–1941.
3. Herndon, J.H., Davidson, S.M., and Apazidis, A., Recent socioeconomic trends in orthopaedic practice, *J. Bone Joint Surg. Am.*, 83A, 1097–1105, 2001.
4. Hannan, M.T., Felson, D.T., and Pincus, T., Analysis of the discordance between radiographic changes and knee pain in osteoarthritis of the knee, *J. Rheumatol.*, 27, 1513–1517, 2000.
5. Barker, K. et al., Association between radiographic joint space narrowing, function, pain and muscle power in severe osteoarthritis of the knee, *Clin. Rehabil.*, 18, 793–800, 2004.
6. Badley, E.M., The effect of osteoarthritis on disability and health care use in Canada, *J. Rheumatol. Suppl.*, 43, 19–22, 1995.
7. Di Cesare, P. and Abramson, S., Pathogenesis of osteoarthritis, in *Harris: Kelly's Textbook of Rheumatology*, Harris, E.J. et al., Eds., Elsevier, Amsterdam, 2005, pp. 1493–1537.

8. Conaghan, P.G., Update on osteoarthritis part 1: current concepts and the relation to exercise, *Br. J. Sports Med.*, 36, 330–333, 2002.

9. Jadelis, K. et al., Strength, balance, and the modifying effects of obesity and knee pain: results from the Observational Arthritis Study in Seniors (OASIS), *J. Am. Geriatr. Soc.*, 49, 884–891, 2001.

10. Hungin, A.P. and Kean, W.F., Nonsteroidal anti-inflammatory drugs: overused or underused in osteoarthritis? *Am. J. Med.*, 110, 8S–11S, 2001.

11. Gartner, L. and Hiatt, J., Cartilage and bone, in *Color Textbook of Histology*, W.B. Saunders Company, Philadelphia, 1997, p. 112.

12. Lorenzo, P., Bayliss, M.T., and Heinegard, D., Altered patterns and synthesis of extracellular matrix macromolecules in early osteoarthritis, *Matrix Biol.*, 23, 381–391, 2004.

13. Schwartz, E.R. and Adamy, L., Effect of ascorbic acid on arylsulfatase activities and sulfated proteoglycan metabolism in chondrocyte cultures, *J. Clin. Invest.*, 60, 96–106, 1977.

14. Goldring, S.R., Goldring, M.B., and Buckwalter, J., The role of cytokines in cartilage matrix degeneration in osteoarthritis, *Clin. Orthop.*, 427 (Suppl.), S27–S36, 2004.

15. Dozin, B. et al., Response of young, aged and osteoarthritic human articular chondrocytes to inflammatory cytokines: molecular and cellular aspects, *Matrix Biol.*, 21, 449–459, 2002.

16. Henrotin, Y.E. et al., Effects of three avocado/soybean unsaponifiable mixtures on metalloproteinases, cytokines and prostaglandin E2 production by human articular chondrocytes, *Clin. Rheumatol.*, 17, 31–39, 1998.

17. Bjordal, J.M. et al., Non-steroidal anti-inflammatory drugs, including cyclo-oxygenase-2 inhibitors, in osteoarthritic knee pain: meta-analysis of randomised placebo controlled trials, *Br. Med. J.*, 329, 1317, 2004.

18. Brandt, K.D., Effects of nonsteroidal anti-inflammatory drugs on chondrocyte metabolism in vitro and in vivo, *Am. J. Med.*, 83, 29–34, 1987.

19. Brandt, K.D., Nonsteroidal antiinflammatory drugs and articular cartilage, *J. Rheumatol.*, 14, 132–133, 1987.

20. Brandt, K.D. and Slowman-Kovacs, S., Nonsteroidal antiinflammatory drugs in treatment of osteoarthritis, *Clin. Orthop.*, 213, 84–91, 1986.

21. Rashad, S. et al., Effect of non-steroidal anti-inflammatory drugs on the course of osteoarthritis, *Lancet*, 2, 519–522, 1989.

22. El Hajjaji, H. et al., Celecoxib has a positive effect on the overall metabolism of hyaluronan and proteoglycans in human osteoarthritic cartilage, *J. Rheumatol.*, 30, 2444–2451, 2003.

23. Soeken, K.L. et al., Safety and efficacy of S-adenosylmethionine (SAMe) for osteoarthritis, *J. Fam. Pract.*, 51, 425–430, 2002.

24. Curtis, C.L. et al., Pathologic indicators of degradation and inflammation in human osteoarthritic cartilage are abrogated by exposure to n-3 fatty acids, *Arthritis Rheum.*, 46, 1544–1553, 2002.

25. Matheson, A.J. and Perry, C.M., Glucosamine: a review of its use in the management of osteoarthritis, *Drugs Aging*, 20, 1041–1060, 2003.

26. Setnikar, I. et al., Pharmacokinetics of glucosamine in man, *Arzneimittelforschung*, 43, 1109–1113, 1993.

27. Cohen, M. et al., A randomized, double blind, placebo controlled trial of a topical cream containing glucosamine sulfate, chondroitin sulfate, and camphor for osteoarthritis of the knee, *J. Rheumatol.*, 30, 523–528, 2003.

28. Bruyere, O. et al., Glucosamine sulfate reduces osteoarthritis progression in postmenopausal women with knee osteoarthritis: evidence from two 3-year studies, *Menopause*, 11, 138–143, 2004.

29. Christgau, S. et al., Osteoarthritic patients with high cartilage turnover show increased responsiveness to the cartilage protecting effects of glucosamine sulphate, *Clin. Exp. Rheumatol.*, 22, 36–42, 2004.

30. Anderson, J.W., Nicolosi, R.J., and Borzelleca, J.F., Glucosamine effects in humans: a review of effects on glucose metabolism, side effects, safety considerations and efficacy, *Food Chem. Toxicol.*, 43, 187–201, 2005.

31. Scroggie, D.A., Albright, A., and Harris, M.D., The effect of glucosamine-chondroitin supplementation on glycosylated hemoglobin levels in patients with type 2 diabetes mellitus: a placebo-controlled, double-blinded, randomized clinical trial, *Arch. Intern. Med.*, 163, 1587–1590, 2003.

32. Tannis, A.J., Barban, J., and Conquer, J.A., Effect of glucosamine supplementation on fasting and non-fasting plasma glucose and serum insulin concentrations in healthy individuals, *Osteoarthritis Cartilage*, 12, 506–511, 2004.

33. Virkamaki, A. et al., Activation of the hexosamine pathway by glucosamine in vivo induces insulin resistance in multiple insulin sensitive tissues, *Endocrinology*, 138, 2501–2507, 1997.

34. Gray, H.C., Hutcheson, P.S., and Slavin, R.G., Is glucosamine safe in patients with seafood allergy? *J. Allergy Clin. Immunol.*, 114, 459–460, 2004.

35. Morreale, P. et al., Comparison of the antiinflammatory efficacy of chondroitin sulfate and diclofenac sodium in patients with knee osteoarthritis, *J. Rheumatol.*, 23, 1385–1391, 1996.

36. Rovetta, G. et al., Chondroitin sulfate in erosive osteoarthritis of the hands, *Int. J. Tissue React.*, 24, 29–32, 2002.

37. Reginster, J.Y. et al., Naturocetic (glucosamine and chondroitin sulfate) compounds as structure-modifying drugs in the treatment of osteoarthritis, *Curr. Opin. Rheumatol.*, 15, 651–655, 2003.

38. Gloystein, D.M., Gillespie, M.J., and Schenck, R.C.J., The effects of medications in sports injuries, in *DeLee: DeLee and Drez's Orthopaedic Sports Medicine*, 2nd edn, DeLee, J.C., and Drez, D.J., Eds., Elsevier, Philadelphia, 2003, pp. 129–134.

39. Barthe, L. et al., In vitro intestinal degradation and absorption of chondroitin sulfate, a glycosaminoglycan drug, *Arzneimittelforschung*, 54, 286–292, 2004.

40. Conte, A. et al., Biochemical and pharmacokinetic aspects of oral treatment with chondroitin sulfate, *Arzneimittelforschung*, 45, 918–925, 1995.

41. McCarty, M.F., and Russell, A.L., Niacinamide therapy for osteoarthritis — does it inhibit nitric oxide synthase induction by interleukin 1 in chondrocytes? *Med Hypotheses*, 53, 350–360, 1999.

42. Najm, W.I. et al., *S*-Adenosyl methionine (SAMe) versus celecoxib for the treatment of osteoarthritis symptoms: a double-blind cross-over trial [ISRCTN36233495], *BMC Musculoskelet. Disord.*, 5, 6, 2004.

43. Bottiglieri, T., *S*-Adenosyl-L-methionine (SAMe): from the bench to the bedside — molecular basis of a pleiotrophic molecule, *Am. J. Clin. Nutr.*, 76, 1151S–1157S, 2002.

44. Kelly, M.A., Kurzweil, P.R., and Moskowitz, R.W., Intra-articular hyaluronans in knee osteoarthritis: rationale and practical considerations, *Am. J. Orthop.*, 33 (2 Suppl.), 15–22, 2004.

45. Aggarwal, A. and Sempowski, I.P., Hyaluronic acid injections for knee osteoarthritis. Systematic review of the literature, *Can. Fam. Physician*, 50, 249–256, 2004.

46. Kelly, M.A. et al., Osteoarthritis and beyond: a consensus on the past, present, and future of hyaluronans in orthopedics, *Orthopedics*, 26, 1064–1079 (quiz 1080–1081), 2003.

47. Hammesfahr, J.F., Knopf, A.B., and Stitik, T., Safety of intra-articular hyaluronates for pain associated with osteoarthritis of the knee, *Am. J. Orthop.*, 32, 277–283, 2003.

48. Kremer, J.M., Effects of modulation of inflammatory and immune parameters in patients with rheumatic and inflammatory disease receiving dietary supplementation of *n* - 3 and *n* - 6 fatty acids, *Lipids*, 31 (Suppl.), S243–S247, 1996.

49. Ariza-Ariza, R., Mestanza-Peralta, M., and Cardiel, M.H., Omega-3 fatty acids in rheumatoid arthritis: an overview, *Semin. Arthritis Rheum.*, 27, 366–370, 1998.

50. Cho, S.H. et al., Clinical efficacy and safety of Lyprinol, a patented extract from New Zealand green-lipped mussel (*Perna canaliculus*) in patients with osteoarthritis of the hip and knee: a multicenter 2-month clinical trial, *Allerg. Immunol. (Paris)*, 35, 212–216, 2005.

51. Peterkofsky, B., Ascorbate requirement for hydroxylation and secretion of procollagen: relationship to inhibition of collagen synthesis in scurvy, *Am. J. Clin. Nutr.*, 54 (6 Suppl.), 1135S–1140S, 1991.

52. Spanheimer, R.G., Bird, T.A., and Peterkofsky, B., Regulation of collagen synthesis and mRNA levels in articular cartilage of scorbutic guinea pigs, *Arch. Biochem. Biophys.*, 246, 33–41, 1986.

53. McAlindon, T.E. et al., Do antioxidant micronutrients protect against the development and progression of knee osteoarthritis? *Arthritis Rheum.*, 39, 648–656, 1996.

54. Hauselmann, H.J., Nutripharmaceuticals for osteoarthritis, *Best Pract. Res. Clin. Rheumatol.*, 15, 595–607, 2001.

55. Lequesne, M. et al., Structural effect of avocado/soybean unsaponifiables on joint space loss in osteoarthritis of the hip, *Arthritis Rheum.*, 47, 50–58, 2002.

56. Boumediene, K. et al., Avocado/soya unsaponifiables enhance the expression of transforming growth factor beta1 and beta2 in cultured articular chondrocytes, *Arthritis Rheum.*, 42, 148–156, 1999.

57. Ernst, E., Avocado-soybean unsaponifiables (ASU) for osteoarthritis — a systematic review, *Clin. Rheumatol.*, 22, 285–288, 2003.

58. Kaufman, W., *The Common Form of Joint Dysfunction: its Incidence and Treatment*, Ell. Hildreth Co., Brattleboro, VT, 1949.

59. Kaufman, W., The use of vitamin therapy to reverse certain concomitants of aging, *J. Am. Geriatr. Soc.*, 3, 927, 1955.

60. Kaufman, W., Niacinamide: a most neglected vitamin, *J. Int. Acad. Prev. Med.*, Winter, 5–25, 1983.

61. Jonas, W.B., Rapoza, C.P., and Blair, W.F., The effect of niacinamide on osteoarthritis: a pilot study, *Inflamm. Res.*, 45, 330–334, 1996.

62. Lampeter, E.F., Scherbaum, K.A., and W.A., The Deutsche Nicotinamide Intervention Study: an attempt to prevent type 1 diabetes, *Diabetes*, 47, 980–984, 1998.

63. Knip, M. et al., Safety of high-dose nicotinamide: a review, *Diabetologia*, 43, 1337–1345, 2000.

22 Fibromyalgia

Jacob Teitelbaum, M.D.

CONTENTS

OVERVIEW

Chronic fatigue syndrome (CFS) and fibromyalgia syndrome (FMS) are two common names for an overlapping spectrum of disabling syndromes. It is estimated that FMS alone affects 3 to 6 million Americans, causing more disability than rheumatoid arthritis.[1] Myofacial pain syndrome (MPS) affects many millions more. Although we still have much to learn, effective treatment is now available for the large majority of patients with these illnesses.[2,3]

CFS/FMS/MPS represents a syndrome, a spectrum of processes with a common end point. Because the syndromes affect major control systems in the body, there are myriad symptoms that initially do not seem to be related. Recent research has implicated mitochondrial and hypothalamic and dysfunction as common denominators in these syndromes.[4–7] Dysfunction of hormonal, sleep,

407

and autonomic control centers in the hypothalamus and energy production centers can explain the large number of symptoms and why most patients have a similar set of complaints.

To make it easier to explain to patients, we use the model of a circuit breaker in a house:

> If the energy demands on their body are more than it can meet, their body "blows a fuse." The ensuing fatigue forces the person to use less energy, protecting them from harm. On the other hand, although a circuit breaker may protect the circuitry in the home, it does little good if you do not know how to turn it back on or that it even exists.

This analogy actually reflects what occurs. Research in genetic mitochondrial diseases shows not simply myopathic changes, but also marked hypothalamic disruption. Since the hypothalamus controls sleep, hormonal systems, autonomic systems, and temperature regulation, it has higher energy needs for its size than other areas. Because of this, as energy stores are depleted, hypothalamic dysfunction occurs early on, resulting in the disordered sleep, autonomic dysfunction, low body temperatures, and hormonal dysfunctions commonly seen in these syndromes. In addition, inadequacy of energy stores in a muscle results in muscle shortening and pain, which is further accentuated by the loss of deep sleep. Reductions in stages 3 to 4 of deep sleep results in secondary drops in growth hormone and tissue repair. As discussed below, disrupted sleep causes pain. Therefore, restoring adequate energy production by treating opportunistic infections and giving nutritional, hormonal, and sleep support restores function in the hypothalamic "circuit breaker," which in turn allows muscle relaxation and pain relief. Our placebo controlled study showed that when this is done, 91% of patients improve, with an average 90% improvement in quality of life, and the majority of patients no longer qualified as having FMS in 3 months.[3]

DIAGNOSIS

The criteria for diagnosing CFS are readily available elsewhere. What is important is that these criteria were meant to be used for research and therefore have stringent exclusion criteria to create a research cohort. These exclusionary criteria eliminate approximately 80 to 90% of patients who clinically have CFS, and therefore I do not recommend them for clinical use. For example, anyone who was significantly depressed in the past, even 30 years earlier, can technically never develop CFS.

The American College of Rheumatology (ACR) criteria for fibromyalgia are more useful clinically. According to the ACR, a person can be classified as having fibromyalgia if he or she has:

1. A history of widespread pain. The patient must be experiencing pain or achiness, steady or intermittent, for at least 3 months. At times, the pain must have been present
   - on both the right and the left sides of the body
   - both above and below the waist
   - in the midbody, including the neck, midchest, midback, or back of head.
2. Pain on pressing at least 11 of the 18 spots on the body that are known as tender points.

The presence of another clinical disorder, such as arthritis, does not rule out a diagnosis of fibromyalgia.[8]

Although the tender point exam takes a good bit of time to master, it clinically adds little and will likely be eliminated in the future. Relative to the time they take to learn, the 11/18 tender points offer little predictive value to whether the person will respond to the treatment approach described in this chapter. There is a simpler approach that is very effective clinically. If the patient has the paradox of severe fatigue combined with insomnia, they do not have severe primary depression, and these symptoms do not go away with vacation, they are likely to have a CFS-related process. If they also have widespread pain, fibromyalgia is probably present as well. Both respond well to proper treatment as discussed below. Alternatively, clinicians may wish to ask the patient if he or she has the following symptoms:

- Severe fatigue lasting over 4 months.
- Feeling worse the day after exercise. Patients may even describe this as feeling "hit by a truck."
- Diffuse, often migratory, achiness.
- Disordered sleep. Is the patient able to get 7 to 8 h of uninterrupted sleep at night?
- Difficulty with word finding and substitution, poor short-term memory, and poor concentration, often described as brain fog.
- Bowel dysfunction. Many people diagnosed with irritable bowel syndrome (IBS) or spastic colon have CFS/FMS, and their IBS resolves along with the FMS.
- Recurrent infections such as nasal congestion and sinusitis.
- Chemical/medication sensitivities.

In addition to strengthening the diagnosis of FMS, the above questions show the patient that their health care provider understands their illness.

Fibromyalgia may be secondary to other causes. Secondary causes may be suggested by laboratory findings such as an elevated erythrocyte sedimentation rate, alkaline phosphatase, creatine kinase, or thyroid stimulating hormone (TSH). Depression is less likely to be a secondary cause of fibromyalgia and CFS symptoms in patients who express frustration over not having the energy to do things as opposed to lack of interests. Since MPS is in some ways a localized form of FMS, evaluation for structural problems should also be considered.

Current research and clinical experience show that these patients have a mix of disordered sleep, hormonal insufficiencies, low body temperature, and autonomic dysfunction with low blood pressure and neurally mediated hypotension (NMH). The hypothalamus is the major control center for all four of these functions.

Anything that results in inadequate energy production or energy needs greater than the body's production ability can trigger hypothalamic dysfunction. This includes infections, disrupted sleep, pregnancy, hormonal deficiencies, and other physical or situational stresses. Although still controversial, a large body of research also strongly suggests mitochondrial dysfunction as a unifying theory in CFS/FMS.[7] Some viral infections have been shown to suppress both mitochondrial and hypothalamic function. As noted above, in genetic mitochondrial diseases, severe hypothalamic dysfunction is seen. This is possibly because the hypothalamus has high energy needs. The mitochondrial dysfunction, combined with secondary hypothalamic suppression, can cause the poor function seen in many tissues with high energy needs. This includes dysfunction of the immune system aggravated by glutathione deficiency, dysfunction of the liver with medication or chemical sensitivities secondary to decreased ability to detoxify, irritable bowel syndrome from opportunistic infections and autonomic dysfunction, muscle pain and dysfunction of central nervous system neurotransmitter production and alterations in blood flow.

Editor's Note

Chronic fatigue syndrome is generally a diagnosis of exclusion. However, uncertain disease etiology does not preclude evidence-based treatment. Evidence supports symptom management that incorporates strategic nutritional interventions.

TREATMENT

Two studies[2,3] show an average 90% improvement rate when using the "SHIN" protocol. "SHIN" stands for Sleep, Hormonal support, Infections, and Nutritional support. When a patient has fatigue and insomnia coupled with widespread pain, see them as having a body-wide energy crisis. Treating with the SHIN approach will help them. A recent editorial in the *Journal of the American Academy of Pain Management* notes:

> ... this study by Dr. Teitelbaum et al. confirms what years of clinical success have shown — that the treatment approach described in Chapter 4 of The Trigger Point Manual is effective, that subclinical abnormalities are important and that the comprehensive and aggressive metabolic approach to treatment in Teitelbaum's study is highly successful and makes fibromyalgia a very treatable disorder. The study by Dr. Teitelbaum et al. and years of clinical experience makes this approach an excellent and powerfully effective part of the standard of practice for treatment of people who suffer from FMS and MPS — both of which are common and devastating syndromes.[9]

As discussed above, the acronym SHIN outlines FMS treatment.

DISORDERED SLEEP (S)

The basis of CFS/FMS is the sleep disorder.[10] Many patients wake up at night and only sleep solidly for 3 to 5 h. They lose restorative stage 3 to 4 sleep. Using medications that increase deep restorative sleep, so that the patient gets 7 to 9 h of solid sleep without waking or hangover, is critical. Start treatment with natural therapies or with a low dose of sleep medications that do not decrease stage 3 to 4 sleep. The sedation that some patients experience the next day often resolves in 2 to 3 weeks. If it does not, have the patient take the medication earlier in the evening so that it wears off earlier the next day, or switch to shorter-acting agents such as Ambien, Sonata, or Xanax. Continue to adjust the medications each night until the patient is sleeping 8 h a night without a hangover.

Most addictive sleep remedies, except for clonazepam (Klonopin) and alprazolam (Xanax), actually decrease the time that is spent in deep sleep and can worsen fibromyalgia. Therefore, they are not recommended. There are over 20 natural and prescription sleep aids that can be tried safely and effectively in fibromyalgia and CFS.

Medications with which to begin include the following:

- Zolpidem (Ambien), 5 or 10 mg. Use 5 to 20 mg qhs. This medication is a newer agent with fewer side effects than the other medications. It is very helpful for most patients and is my first choice among the sleep medications. Although only to be used for 1 week in routine insomnia, experience shows that extended use is appropriate and safe in CFS/FMS. Patients can take an extra 5 to 10 mg in the middle of the night if they wake.

- Neurontin, 100 to 900 mg hs can help sleep, pain, and restless leg syndrome (RLS) as well.
- Cyclobenzaprine (Flexeril), 10 mg; Klonopin, 5 mg; or carisprodol (Soma), 350 mg. Use 1/2 to 2 tablets qhs. These medications are often very sedating. Use one of these first if myalgias are a major problem.
- Trazodone (Desyrel), 50 mg. Use 1/2 to 6 tablets qhs. Use this medication first if anxiety is a major problem. Warn patients to call immediately if priapism occurs.
- Amitriptyline (Elavil) or Doxepin, 10 mg. Use a 1/2 to 5 tablets qhs. These drugs cause weight gain and can worsen NMH and RLS.
- Herbal preparations containing a mix of valerian root, wild lettuce, Jamaican dogwood, passionflower, hops, and theanine. These six herbs can help muscle pain and libido as well as improve sleep.[11-15]
- Doxylamine (Unisom for Sleep), 25 mg qhs.

For patients with disabling muscle aches or anxiety, respectively, I recommend Klonopin or Xanax. Begin with 0.25 mg qhs and slowly adjust the dose upward as needed as the next-day sedation diminishes.

Some patients will sleep well with 5 mg of Ambien and others will require all of the above combined. Because the malfunctioning hypothalamus controls sleep and the muscle pain also interferes with sleep, it is often necessary and appropriate to use multiple sleep aids. Zanaflex, Gabatril, and many other nonbenzodiazepines can also help sleep. Because of next-day sedation and each medication having its own independent half-life, CFS/FMS patients do better with combining low doses of several medications than with a high dose of one medication.

Although less common, three other sleep disturbances must be considered and, if present, treated. The first is sleep apnea. This should especially be suspected if the patient snores and is overweight or hypertensive. If two of these three conditions are present and the patient does not improve with our treatment, I would consider a sleep apnea study to include assessment for upper airway resistance syndrome. Preapproval from the patient's insurance company is recommended since the test usually costs $1500 to $2000. Some patients prefer to do their own inexpensive screening by videotaping themselves one night during sleep. Sleep apnea is treated with weight loss and nasal C-pap.

A sleep study will also detect RLS, which is also fairly common in fibromyalgia.[16] The patient with RLS may notice that the bedsheets are scattered when he or she awakes and may also report kicking a spouse during sleep. RLS is treated with Ambien, Klonopin, and/or Neurontin, supplemental magnesium, and by keeping ferritin levels over 50.

HORMONAL DYSFUNCTION (H)

Hormonal imbalance is associated with FMS. Sources of imbalance include hypothalamic dysfunction and autoimmune processes such as Hashimoto's thyroiditis. When the hypothalamus is not able to efficiently regulate hormone balance, medical management can do so until hypothalamic function is restored. When focusing on achieving hormonal balance, the standard laboratory testing aimed at identifying a single hormone deficiency is less effective. For example, increased hormone binding to carrier proteins is often present in CFS/FMS. Because of this, total hormone levels are often normal while the active hormone levels are low. This creates a functional deficiency in the patient. Also, most blood tests use two standard deviations to define blood test norms. By definition, only the lowest or highest 2 to 3% of the population is in the treatment range. This does not work well if over 2.5% of the population has a problem. For example, it is estimated that as many as 20% of women over 60 are hypothyroid. Other tests use late signs of deficiency such as anemia for iron or B12 levels to define an abnormal laboratory value.

The goal in FMS management is to restore optimal function while keeping lab results in the normal range for safety. One way to convey the difference between the normal range based on two standard deviations and the optimal range, which the patient would maintain if they did not have FMS, is as follows:

> Pretend your lab test uses two standard deviations to diagnose a "shoe problem." If you accidentally put on someone else's shoes and had on a size 12 when you wore a size 5, the normal range derived from the standard deviation would indicate you had absolutely no problem. You would insist the shoes did not fit although your shoe size would be in the normal range. Similarly, if you lost your shoes, the doctor would pick any shoes out of the "normal range pile" and expect them to fit you.

Thyroid Function

Suboptimal thyroid function is very common and very important. Because thyroid-binding globulin function and conversion of T_4 to T_3 may be altered in CFS/FMS, it is important to check a free T_4. Thyroid hormone replacement is important in all CFS patients whose T_4 blood levels fall below the 50th percentile of normal. Many CFS/FMS patients also have difficulty in converting T_4, which is fairly inactive, to T_3, the active hormone. Additionally, T_3 receptor resistance may be present, requiring higher levels.[17,18]

Synthroid has only inactive T_4, while Armour Thyroid has both inactive T_4 and active T_3. Many clinicians will give an empiric trial of Synthroid, 25 to 250 μm, or Armour Thyroid, 1/2 to 3 grains every morning, adjusted to the dose that feels best to the patient as long as the free T_4 is not above the upper limit of normal. An empiric trial of thyroid-hormone therapy is given in patients who feel poorly if one or more of the following is true:

- The patient has fibromyalgia.
- The patient's oral temperatures are generally less than 98.0°F.
- The patient has symptoms and signs suggestive of hypothyroidism.
- The patient's TSH test result is less than 0.95 or greater than 3.0.
- The patient's T_3 or T_4 is below the 50th percentile of normal.

Physicians generally interpret a low-normal TSH — that is, 0.5 to 0.95 — as a confirmation of euthyroidism. The rules, however, are different with CFS/FMS. In this setting, hypothalamic hypothyroidism is common and the patient's TSH can be low, normal, or high.[19] Also, if subclinical hypothyroidism is missed, the patient's fibromyalgia/MPS simply will not resolve. The inadequacy of thyroid testing is further suggested by studies that show that most patients with suspected thyroid problems have normal blood studies.[20,21] When patients with symptoms of hypothyroidism and normal labs were treated with thyroid (in this study Synthroid at an average dose of 120 μg every day) a large majority improved significantly.[20]

Clinical management may include the following. If the patient does not respond to Synthroid, switch to Armour Thyroid, and vice versa. For every 50 μg of Synthroid, have the patient take 1/2 grain (30 mg) of Armour Thyroid. If the free or total T_3 result is low or low normal, begin with Armour Thyroid, which has both T_3 and T_4, instead of Synthroid, which has only T_4. I usually recommend beginning with Armour Thyroid.

Adjust the thyroid dose clinically to the dose that feels the best to the patient, as long as the free T_4 test does not show hyperthyroidism. Do not use TSH to monitor thyroid replacement. Because of the hypothalamic suppression, it may be low despite inadequate hormonal dosing. Make sure that the patient does not take any iron supplements within 6 h or calcium within 2 h of the morning thyroid dose or the thyroid hormone will not be absorbed. Have the patient take the iron between 2:00 and 6:00 P.M. — on an empty stomach and away from any hormone treatments. Since thyroid supplementation can increase a patient's cortisol metabolism and unmask a case of subclinical adrenal insufficiency, if the patient feels worse on low-dose thyroid replacement, adrenal support may be needed as well.

Adrenal Insufficiency

The hypothalamic–pituitary–adrenal (HPA) axis does not function well in CFS/FMS.[4,22,23] Because early researchers were not aware of physiologic doses of cortisol, they treated with high doses and their patients developed severe complications. Because of this, many hypoadrenal patients are now treated only when they are ready to go into Addisonian crisis. Research and clinical experience shows that this approach misses many hypoadrenal patients.[2,3,24,25]

Significant toxicity not seen with physiologic dosing of hydrocortisone (Cortef) up to 20 mg/d,[24] which is approximately equivalent in potency to 4 to 5 mg of prednisone.

Symptoms of an underactive adrenal include weakness, hypotension, dizziness, sugar craving, and recurrent infections — all of which are common in CFS/FMS. I often evaluate CFS/FMS patients' adrenal function with a Cortrosyn stimulation test. The test must be done between 7:00 and 9:00 A.M. The patient should be fasting and take no caffeine for 24 h before the test. Check a baseline cortisol level and then give ACTH (Cortrosyn) 25 units or 1 unit IM (current data suggests the 1 unit Cortrosyn test is more reliable) and recheck cortisol levels at 30 min and at 1 h. Although a baseline of 6 μg/dl is often considered normal, most healthy people run approximately 16 to 24 μg/dl at 8:00 A.M.

My treatment guidelines are that if the baseline cortisol is less than 16 μg/dl or the cortisol level does not increase by at least 7 μg/dl at 30 min and 11 μg/dl at 1 h, or does not double by 1 h and is less than 35 μg/dl, I treat with a therapeutic trial of 5 to 15 mg Cortef in the morning, 2.5 to 10 mg at lunchtime, and 0 to 2.5 mg at 4:00 P.M. (maximum of 20 mg/d). Most patients find 5 to 7.5 mg each morning plus 2.5 to 5 mg at noon to be optimal (the equivalent of 1.5 to 3 mg prednisone qd). Cortef is more effective than prednisone in CFS/FMS.

After keeping the patient on the initial dose for 2 to 4 weeks, adjust the dose up to a maximum of 20 mg daily or, if no benefit has been evident, taper it off. Adjust the Cortef to the lowest dose that feels the best. Give most of the Cortef in the morning and at lunchtime. I often tell my patients to take the last dose, 2.5 to 5 mg, no later than 4:00 P.M. Otherwise, the Cortef may keep the patient up at night.

After 9 to 18 months, taper the Cortef off over a period of 1 to 4 months. If the other physiologic stresses, such as infections, have been eliminated, the patient's adrenal function may be adequate or normalized. If symptoms recur off the Cortef, continue treatment with the lowest optimal dose.

Improvement is often dramatic and is usually seen within 2 to 4 weeks. The Cortef should be doubled during periods of acute stress and raised even higher during periods of severe stress such as surgery. Consider also giving the patient 1000 mg of calcium and 400 IU of vitamin D daily with the Cortef if the patient is at high risk for osteoporosis.

There are different approaches to treatment and more is not better. High-dose cortisol taken at night will worsen the already disrupted sleep patterns. In a study by McKenzie, patients were administered a very high dose of about 25 to 35 mg daily, which disrupted their sleep ($p \leq .02$).[26] Although they did not treat the disrupted sleep, most patients still felt somewhat better on treatment. A small percentage of the patients had significantly decreased posttreatment Cortrosyn tests without complications. Based on this study, the authors recommend against using Cortef in CFS/FMS.[27] In contrast, our study did not show adrenal suppression using lower Cortef dosing.[3] Dr. Jefferies, with thousands of patient-years' experience in using low-dose Cortef, recommends an empiric trial of 20 mg/d of Cortef for all patients with severe, unexplained fatigue and has found this to be quite safe for long-term use.[24,25] Our research and clinical experience suggest that using Cortef at 20 mg/d or less in CFS and fibromyalgia patients is safe and often very helpful.

Dehydroepiandrosterone

Dehydroepiandrosterone (DHEA) is a major adrenal hormone that has recently been getting a lot of attention.[28] It is stored as DHEA-sulfate (DHEA-S) and levels of the active free DHEA fluctuate markedly throughout the day. Because of this, I recommend checking DHEA-S levels and not DHEA levels.

Many CFS/FMS patients have suboptimal DHEA-S levels, and the benefit of treatment is often dramatic. Most women need 5 to 25 mg/d and most men 25 to 50 mg/d. I keep the DHEA-S level at 150 to 180 μg/dl in women and 350 to 480 μg/dl in men.

Low Estrogen and Testosterone

Although we are trained to diagnose menopause by cessation of periods, hot flashes, and zelevated FSH and LH, these are late findings. Estrogen deficiency often begins many years before, and may coincide with the onset of fibromyalgia.[29] To compound the problem, research done by Sarrel shows that the majority of women who have a hysterectomy, even with the ovaries left in, begin menopause within 6 months to 2 years.[29] Some physicians suspect that this may also occur in woman who have had a tubal ligation, which may also disrupt the ovarian blood supply.

In her book on estrogen and testosterone deficiency, Dr. Elizabeth Vliet gives a well-referenced, in-depth foundation for evaluation and treatment of these problems.[29] To summarize, the initial symptoms of estrogen deficiency are poor sleep, poor libido, brain fog, achiness, PMS, and decreased neurotransmitter function. Dr. Vliet feels that estradiol levels at midcycle should be at least 100 pg/ml. If a woman's CFS/FMS symptoms are worse at ovulation and the 10 days before menses (when estrogen levels are dropping), then a trial of estrogen is warranted. While a birth control pill can be used, side effects of bleeding and fluid retention are common for the first 3 to 4 months. Bioidentical hormones are better tolerated and likely safer. Therefore, natural 17-B-estradiol as Estrace or Climara patches may be preferable. The usual dose of Climara is one 0.05 to 0.1 mg patch a week and the usual dose of Estrace is 1/2 to 2 mg/d, adjusted to what feels best to the patient. I prefer to use Biest, a compounded natural estrogen that combines estriol with estradiol, which is usually dosed at 1.25 to 2.5 mg/d.

Early data on estriol suggest that estriol does not raise the risk of breast cancer and may actually lower it (Jonathan Wright, M.D., personal communication). In addition, it also has immune modulating and other properties that can be beneficial in FMS. In the absence of a hysterectomy, progesterone should be added to prevent uterine cancer. Natural progesterone is available from most pharmacies as Prometrium 100 mg and is better tolerated than Provera. The dose is 100 mg at bedtime (qhs), instead of Provera 2.5 mg, or 200 mg/d for 10 to 14 days a month, instead of Provera 10 mg. If you are prescribing the Bi-Est cream, have the compounding pharmacist make a combination of Bi-Est 2.5 mg plus progesterone 30 to 50 mg, plus testosterone 4 mg, all in 0.2 cm^3 of cream.

Testosterone Deficiency

Testosterone deficiency is important in both men and women. It is important to check a free testosterone level rather than total testosterone, since free testosterone is a better measure of testosterone function. If the age-adjusted free testosterone is in the lowest quartile for age, a trial of treatment is often very helpful. Among my CFS/FMS patients, 70% of men and many women have free testosterone levels in the lowest quartile while their total testosterone levels are normal. A recently completed study found that treating low testosterone in women decreases FMS pain. Be sure the free testosterone normal range is age-adjusted using 10 year age groups, since a normal range that includes both 20- and 80-year-olds is not clinically meaningful.

In women, acne, intense dreams, or darkening of facial hair suggest that testosterone replacement is too high. An elevated testosterone in women can also increase insulin resistance. Symptoms are generally reversible. These side effects can also be caused by low estrogen relative to the testosterone level, and may be avoided in women by supplementing both together. As noted above, this can be done easily by adding 3–5 mg of testosterone to the estrogen cream.

In men, acne suggests the dose is too high. Monitor levels because elevated levels can cause elevated blood counts, liver inflammation, reversibly decreased sperm counts with infertility, and elevated cholesterols with increased risk of heart disease. These are the symptoms seen in athletes given many times the recommended physiologic dose to enhance sports performance. Because of this, in men it is prudent to monitor a CBC, cholesterol, and liver enzymes intermittently. Testosterone supplementation can also cause elevated thyroid hormone levels in those taking thyroid supplements. If the patient is on thyroid supplements, I would recheck thyroid hormone levels after 6 to 12 weeks or sooner if palpitations, anxiety, or hyperactive feelings occur. Despite the concerns about athletes using very high levels of synthetic testosterone, it is important to remember that research shows that raising a low testosterone level in men using natural testosterone actually results in lower cholesterol, decreased angina and depression, and improved diabetes.[30]

IMMUNE DYSFUNCTION AND INFECTIONS (I)

The other name for CFS is CFIDS, which stands for chronic fatigue and immune dysfunction syndrome. CFIDS correctly suggests that immune dysfunction is part of the syndrome. Opportunistic infections present in CFIDS/FMS include chronic upper respiratory infections, sinusitis, bowel infections, and chronic, low-grade prostatitis. These need to be treated.

Chronic sinusitis responds poorly to antibiotics but responds well to antifungals. Conservative measures such as saline nasal rinsing and avoiding refined carbohydrates are more appropriate than chronic antibiotics.[31]

Bowel infections with alterations of normal bacterial flora, fungal overgrowth, and parasitic infections are generally present. Because of the lack of a definitive test for gastrointestinal yeast overgrowth, there is little research published in this area and treatment is controversial. Treatment is empiric, and based on the patient's history. Yeast vaginitis, onchomycosis, sinusitis, or a history of frequent antibiotic use such as tetracycline for acne warrants an empiric therapeutic antifungal trial. Bowel symptoms of gas, bloating, diarrhea, or constipation also warrant an empiric trial of antifungal medication. Many CFIDS/FMS patients who have failed other therapies for spastic colon or sinusitis have responded dramatically to antifungal treatments.

Treatment consists of nystatin, two 500,000 IU tablets po, bid, or tid, begun slowly, for 5 months. The patient's symptoms, especially fibromyalgia pain, may flare initially as the yeast die off. Therefore, begin with one 500,000 unit tablet of nystatin once a day and increase by one tablet every 1 to 3 days, as tolerated, up to two tablets tid. After 4 weeks on the nystatin, add 200 mg of fluconazole (Diflucan) or itraconazole (Sporanox) qd for 6 weeks. I usually use Diflucan. Rare and mild liver enzyme elevations are sometimes seen with Diflucan and Sporanox in this population. Supplementing with alpha lipoic acid may decrease this side effect. If symptoms are only partially relieved or recur after the first 6 weeks on Diflucan or Sporanox, I recommend repeating the 200 mg/d dose for another 6 weeks. If no benefit is derived from the first course, I do not recommend repeating it. Patients should continue nystatin for a total of 5 to 8 months. I recommend patients be on nystatin while they are taking Sporanox or Diflucan to avoid development of resistant organisms. *Lactobacillus acidophilus*, a probiotic, should also be taken at 4 to 8 billion units per day to help restore normal bowel flora.

Parasitic infections, often with nonpathogenic or normally self-limiting organisms, are common. Stool samples should be sent to a lab specializing in Parasitology for O & P and *Clostridium difficile*. One-sixth of our study patients had a positive test for parasites. Laboratory reporting of bacteria varies.[‡] If the patient has parasites, even if nonpathogenic, treat them, as these patients should be considered immune suppressed.

In patients with low-grade fevers or chronic lung congestion, occult infections such as *Chlamydia* and *Mycoplasma incognitus* are being found. Empiric therapy with doxycycline 100 mg bid for 6 months to 2 years, while on nystatin, can be very helpful. Recent research shows that human herpes virus 6 (HHV-6), cytomegalovirus (CMV), and Epstein–Barr virus (EBV) are also sometimes active in CFS/FMS.

[‡] I only do my O&P testing by mail through Great Smokies Diagnostic Labs (800-522-4762) and the Parasitology Center (480-767-5855).

NUTRITIONAL DEFICIENCIES (N)

CFS/FMS patients are often nutritionally deficient. This occurs because of (1) malabsorbtion from bowel infections, (2) increased needs due to the illness, and (3) inadequate diet. B-vitamins, magnesium, ribose, iron, coenzyme Q_{10}, malic acid, and carnitine are essential for mitochondrial function.[7,32] These nutrients are also critical for many other processes. Our recently completed study showed that ~2/3 of the fibromyalgia patients improved significantly after 1 month of ribose.Although blood testing is not reliable or necessary for most nutrients, I do recommend that you check B_{12}, Fe, total iron-binding capacity (TIBC), and ferritin levels.

I begin patients with CFS/FMS on the following nutritional regiment:

1. A quality multivitamin suited for their needs. It should contain at least a 50 mg B Complex, 150 mg of magnesium glycinate, 900 mg of malic acid, 600 mg of vitamin D, 500 mg of vitamin C, 200 mg zinc, 200 µg selenium, 200 µg chromium, and amino acids. A powdered vitamin is generally better tolerated, better absorbed, and less expensive as a single drink can replace over 35 tablets or capsules and 50 nutrients each day. This should be taken long term.

2. If the iron percent saturation is under 22 or the ferritin is under 40 mg/ml, supplement with iron. I recommend Chromagen FA, 1 qd for 4 months. It should be taken on an empty stomach, since food decreases absorption by over 60%. It should not be taken within 6 h of thyroid hormone, since it blocks thyroid absorption. Caution should be taken in supplementing with iron since continuing supplementation beyond the requirement can result in increased body iron stores. Even one dose of iron can be harmful in persons with primary hemochromatosis. Continue treatment until the ferritin level is over 50 and the iron percent saturation is over 22.

3. Chromium at 200 µg daily, which should be contained in the multiple vitamin, is important for maintaining lean muscle mass. Refer to the chapter on this trace mineral. It is mentioned specifically here since chronium helps prevent the drops in blood sugar which often accompany suboptimal adrenal function.

4. If the B_{12} level is under 540 pg/ml, I recommend B_{12} injections, 3000 µm IM three times a week for 15 weeks, then as needed based on the patients clinical response. Recent reports on CFS show absent or near-absent CSF B_{12} levels despite normal serum B_{12} levels.[33] Metabolic evidence of B_{12} deficiency is seen even at levels of 540 pg/ml or more.[34] Severe neuropsychiatric changes are seen from B_{12} deficiency even at levels of 300 pg/ml (a level over 209 is technically normal).[35] As an editorial in *The New England Journal of Medicine*

suggests, the old-time doctors may have been right about giving B_{12} shots.[36] Compounding pharmacies can make B_{12} at 3000 $\mu g/cm^3$ concentrations. I use hydroxycobalmin. The multivitamin should also contain at least 500 μg of B_{12} for ongoing use.

5. Coenzyme Q_{10}, 100 to 200 mg/d because it is a conditionally essential nutrient that improves energy production in patients with CFS/FMS. It is especially critical in patients on Mevacor-family cholesterol treatments (which can actually cause fibromyalgia pain).

6. Potassium-magnesium aspartate. This is very helpful in fatigue states.[7] The dose is 500 mg, 2 bid for 3 months. The magnesium in this supplement is in addition to what is in the multiple vitamin.

7. Treating with acetyl-L-carnitine 500 mg twice daily for 4 months is strongly recommended. Biopsies show CFS patients to be routinely low. This not only causes weakness but also contributes to the average 32 lb weight gain seen in CFS and fibromyalgia.

8. Vitamin D insufficiency is associated with seasonal affective disorder symptoms, deep muscle pain, and compromised immunity. It can exacerbate these symptoms, which are already present in persons with CFS/FMS. Diagnosis of insufficient vitamin D can be delayed by CFS/FMS masking the vitamin deficiency. Supplemental vitamin D_3 of 1000 IU daily is recommended. See the chapter on vitamin D.

9. The patient should avoid sugar, caffeine, and excessive alcohol. The patient should be informed that there may be a 7 to 10 day withdrawal period when coming off the sugar and caffeine.

GENERAL PAIN RELIEF

Although pain will often resolve within 3 months of simply treating SHIN. as discussed above, it is also critical to eliminate pain directly. Many studies show a marked analgesic and anti-inflammatory effect from adequate doses of two herbals, willow bark (containing at least 240 mgd of salicin) and boswellia (900+ mgd), which have been shown to be as or more effective than NSAIDs and COX 2 inhibitors but without the GI or other toxicity.[37–54] These herbals are excellent for arthritic, inflammatory, and other pains as well. Herbs that can be helpful for sleep, including Jamaican dogwood, wild lettuce and hops, can also help muscle pain. Other natural remedies that help pain include 5-HTP, 300 mg at bedtime, high-dose curcumin, and ginger. Neurontin, Ultram, and Skelaxin are also far more effective for fibromyalgia pain than NSAIDs.

AUTONOMIC DYSFUNCTION

This is especially important to treat in patients under 18 years of age. Blood pressure and dizziness, increased thirst, polyuria, cold extremities, and night sweats are a few of the symptoms that reflect autonomic dysfunction in CFS/FMS. A recent study at John Hopkins Hospital showed that a majority of CFS patients had NMH on tilt table testing.[55] This means that CFS/FMS patients can severely drop their blood pressure with standing or minimal exertion. If the patient has a low blood pressure or dizziness or a positive tilt table test, a treatment trial is appropriate. I predominantly use clinical history or the "poor man's tilt table test," which consists of having the patient stand while leaning against the wall for 10 min. If this aggravates symptoms, the test is positive. Treatment consists of markedly increasing salt and water intake. In children, fludrocortisone (Florinef), 1/10 mg tablets, 1 to 2 qd, can be helpful, although it is usually not helpful in adults. Florinef helped only 14% of adult CFS patients in a recent study, vs. 10% of placebo patients. Fluoxetine (Prozac), sertraline (Zoloft), and dextroamphetamine (Dexedrine) are clinically much more effective in treating NMH in CFIDS patients, and I rarely use Florinef in anyone over 18 years old.

PSYCHOLOGICAL WELL-BEING

Many illnesses are associated with various psychological profiles. In CFS/FMS, a common profile is a "mega-type-A" overachiever who, because of childhood low self-esteem, overachieves to get approval. They tend to be perfectionists and have difficulties protecting their boundaries — that is, they say yes to requests when they feel like saying no. Instead of responding to their bodies' signal of fatigue by resting, they redouble their efforts. Taking time to rest, and getting and staying out of abusive work environments is critical. As they start to feel better, they need to be instructed to take it slowly and not to go back to the level of overfunctioning that made them sick in the first place. They especially need to be instructed not to make up for lost time.

REFERENCES

1. Wolfe, F., Ross, K., Anderson, J. et al., The prevalence and characteristics of fibromyalgia in the general population, *Arthritis and Rheumatism*, 38, 19–28, 1995.
2. Teitelbaum, J. and Bird, B., Effective treatment of severe chronic fatigue: a report of a series of 64 patients, *Journal of Musculoskeletal Pain*, 3, 91–110, 1995.
3. Teitelbaum, J.E., Bird, B., and Greenfield, R.M. et al., Effective treatment of CFS and FMS: a randomized, double-blind placebo controlled study, *Journal of Chronic Fatigue Syndrome*, 8, 3–25, 2001 (the full text of the study can be found at www. Vitality101.com).
4. Demitrack, M.A., Dale, K., Straus, S.E. et al., Evidence for impaired activation of the hypothalamic-pituitary-adrenal axis in patients with chronic fatigue syndrome, *Journal of Clinical Endocrinology and Metabolism*, 73, 1223–1234, 1991.
5. Teitelbaum, J., Estrogen and testosterone in CFIDS/FMS, *The From Fatigued To Fantastic Newsletter*, 1, 1–8, Feb. 1997.
6. Behan, P.O., Post-viral fatigue syndrome research, in *The Clinical and Scientific Basis of Myalgic Encephalitis and Chronic Fatigue Syndrome*, Hyde, B., Goldstein, J., and Levine, P., Eds., Nightingale Research Foundation, Ottawa, 1992, p. 238.

7. Teitelbaum, J., Mitochondrial dysfunction [in CFS/FMS], *The From Fatigued to Fantastic Newsletter*, 1, 1–8, 1997.

8. Wolfe, F. et al. The American College of Rheumatology 1990 Criteria for the Classification of Fibromyalgia: Report of the Multicenter Criteria Committee, *Arthritis and Rheumatology*, 33, 160–172, 1990.

9. Blatman, H., Editorial, *Journal of the American Academy of Pain Management*, Apr. 2002.

10. Conference on the Neuroscience and Endocrinology of Fibromyalgia Syndrome, sponsored by the National Institutes of Health, Jul. 16–17, 1996.

11. Fleming, T., Ed., Jamaica dogwood, in *PDR for Herbal Medicines*, Medical Economics Company, Montvale, NJ, 1998, pp. 428–429.

12. Humulus lupus (monograph), *Alternative Medicine Review*, 8, 190–192, 2003.

13. Cronin, J.R., Passionflower — reigniting male libido and other potential uses, *Alternative and Complementary Therapies*, Apr., 89–92, 2003.

14. Dhawan, K., et al., Reversal of morphine tolerance and dependence by passiflora incarnata, *Pharmaceutical Biology*, 40, 576–580, 2002.

15. Hadley, S. et al., Valerian, *American Family Physician*, 67, 1755–1758, 2003.

16. Yunus, M.B. and Aldag, J.C., Restless legs syndrome and leg cramps in fibromyalgia syndrome: a controlled study, *British Medical Journal*, 312, 1339, 1996.

17. Lowe, J.C., Garrison, R.L., Reichman, A.J., Yellin, J., Thompson, M., and Kaufman, D., Effectiveness and safety of T3 therapy for euthyroid fibromyalgia: a double-blind, placebo-controlled response driven crossover study, *Clinical Bulletin of Myofascial Therapy*, 2, 31–58, 1997.

18. Lowe, J.C., Reichman, A.J., and Yellin, J., The process of change during T3 treatment for euthyroid fibromyalgia: a double-blind, placebo-controlled, crossover study, *Clinical Bulletin of Myofascial Therapy*, 2, 91–124, 1997.

19. Faglia, G., Bitensky, L., Pinchera, A. et al., Thyrotropin secretion in patients with central hypothyroidism: evidence for reduced biological activity of immunoreactive thyrotropin, *Journal of Clinical Endocrinology and Metabolism*, 48, 989–998, 1979.

20. Skinner, G.R.B., Holmes, D., Ahmad, A. et al., Clinical response to thyroxine sodium in clinically hypothyroid but biochemically euthyroid patients, *Journal of Nutritional and Environmental Medicine*, 10, 115–125, 2000.

21. Nordyke, R.A., Reppun, T.S., Madanay, L.D. et al., Alternative sequences of thyrotropin and free thyroxine assays for routine thyroid function testing quality and cost, *Archives of Internal Medicine*, 158, 266–272, 1998.

22. Griep, E.N., Boersma, J.N., and de Kloet, E.R., Altered reactivity of the hypothalamic-pituitary axis in the primary fibromyalgia syndrome, *Journal of Rheumatology*, 20, 469–474, 1993.

23. McCain, G.A. and Tilbe, K.S., Diurnal hormone variation in fibromyalgia syndrome and a comparison with rheumatoid arthritis, *Journal of Rheumatology*, 25, 469–474, 1993.

24. Jefferies, W.M., *Safe Uses of Cortisol*, 2nd ed. (monograph), Charles C. Thomas, Springfield, IL, 1996.

25. Jefferies, W.M., Low-dosage glucocorticoid therapy. An appraisal of its safety and mode of action in clinical disorders, including rheumatoid arthritis, *Archives of Internal Medicine*, 119, 265–278, 1967.

26. McKenzie, R., O'Fallon, A., Dale, J. et al., Low-dose hydrocortisone for treatment of chronic fatigue syndrome: a randomized controlled trial, *Journal of the American Medical Association*, 280, 1061–1066, 1998.

27. Teitelbaum, J.E., Bird, B., Weiss, A. et al., Low dose hydrocortisone for chronic fatigue syndrome, *Journal of the American Medical Association*, 281, 1887–1888, 1999.
28. Morales, A.J., Nolan, J.J., Nelson, J.C. et al., Effects of replacement dose of dehydroepiandrosterone in men and women of advancing age, *Journal of Clinical Endocrinology and Metabolism*, 78, 1360–1367, 1994.
29. Lee Vliet, E., *Screaming to Be Heard: Hormone Connections Women Suspect ... and Doctors Ignore*, M. Evans and Company, New York, 1995.
30. Wright, J.V. and Lenard, L., *Maximize Your Vitality and Potency, for Men over 40*, Smart Publications, 1999 (an excellent reference for those who would like to explore the topic further).
31. Ivker, R.S., *Sinus Survival*, Tarcher/Putnam, New York, 2000.
32. Becker, W.M., Reece, J.B., and Poenie, M.F. et al., *The World of the Cell*, 3rd ed., Benjamin Cummings, San Francisco, CA, 1996.
33. Regland, B., Andersson, M., Abrahamsson, L. et al., Increased concentrations of homocysteine in the cerebrospinal fluid in patients with fibromyalgia and chronic fatigue syndrome, *Scandinavian Journal of Rheumatology* 26, 301–307, 1997.
34. Lindenbaum, J., Rosenberg, I.H., Wilson, P.W. et al., Prevalence of cobalamin deficiency in the Framingham elderly population, *American Journal of Clinical Nutrition*, 60, 2–11, 1994.
35. Lindenbaum, J., Healton, E.B., Savage, D.G. et al., Neuropsychiatric disorders caused by cobalamin deficiency in the absence of anemia or macrocytoses, *The New England Journal of Medicine*, 318, 26, 1720–1728, 1988.
36. Beck, W.S., Cobalmin and the nervous system (editorial), *The New England Journal of Medicine*, 318, 26, 1752–1754, 1988.
37. Beck, W.S.; as cited in Chrubasik, S. et al., Treatment of low back pain exacerbations with willow bark extract: a randomized double-blind study, *American Journal of Medicine*, 109, 9–14, 2000.
38. Chrubasik, S., Kunzel, O. et al., Potential economic impact of using a proprietary willow bark extract in outpatient treatment of low back pain: an open non-randomized study, *Phytomedicine*, 8, 241–251, 2001.
39. Marz, R.W. and Kemper, F., Willow bark extract — effects and effectiveness. Status of current knowledge regarding pharmacology, toxicology and clinical aspects, *Wiener medizinische Wochenschrift*, 152, 354–359, 2002 (in German).
40. Schmid, B. et al., Efficacy and tolerability of a standardized willow bark extract in patients with osteoarthritis: randomized placebo-controlled, double blind clinical trial, *Phytotherapy Research*, 15, 344–350, 2001.
41. Highfield, E.S. and Kemper, K.J., *White Willow Monograph*, Longwood Herbal Task Force, http://www.mcp.edu/herbal/willowbark/willow.pdf.
42. Hedner, T. and Everts, B., The early clinical history of salicylates in rheumatology and pain, *Clinical Rheumatology*, 17, 17–25, 1998.
43. Chrubasik, S. and Eisenberg, E., Treatment of rheumatic pain with herbal medicine in Europe, *Pain Digest*, 8, 231–236, 1998.
44. Meier, B., Sticher, O., and Julkunen-Tiitto, R., Pharmaceutical aspects of the use of willows in herbal remedies, *Planta Medica*, 559–560, 1988.
45. Singh, G.B. and Atal, C.K., *Agents and Actions*, 18, 407, 1986.
46. Sharma, M.L. et al., *Agents and Actions*, 24, 161, 1986.
47. Sharma, M.L. et al., *International Journal of Immunopharmacology*, 11, 647, 1989.
48. Kar, A. and Menon, M.K., *Life Sciences*, 8, 1023, 1969.

49. Menon, M.K. and Kar, A., *Planta Medica*, 19, 333, 1971.
50. Sander, O., Herborn, G., and Rau, R. Is H15 (resin extract of *Boswellia serrata*, "incense") a useful supplement to established drug therapy of chronic polyarthritis? Results of a double-blind pilot study, *Zeitschrift fur Rheumatologie*, 57, 11–16, 1998 (in German).
51. Sharma, M.L. et al. *Agents and Actions*, 24, 161, 1988.
52. Etzel, R. *Phytomedicine*, 3, 91–94, 1996.
53. Kimmatkar, N., Thawani, V., Hingorani, L. et al., *Phytomedicine*, 10, 3–7, 2003.
54. Safayhi, H. et al., Inhibition by Boswellic acids of human leukocyte elastase, *Journal of Pharmacological Experimental Theory*, 281, 460–463, 1997.
55. Rowe, P.C., Bou-Holaigah, I., Kan, J.S. et al., Is neurally mediated hypotension an unrecognized cause of chronic fatigue? *The Lancet*, 345, 623–624, 1995.

23 Gout

Tony Helman, M.B., B.S.

CONTENTS

CLINICAL PRESENTATION

Gout is a clinical disorder that results from the deposition of urate crystals (monosodium urate monohydrate) from supersaturated body solution into soft tissue or joints. It is common – affecting more than 2 million people in the United States (e.g. Kramer et al.).[1]

Typically, gout presents with an acute onset of swelling and severe pain from inflammation of tendons and one or more joints, usually the smaller ones such as the big toe. For most patients the first acute episode of gout resolves within a week or several weeks, and a significant proportion of patients never have a relapse thereafter. But in other cases further episodes do occur, and may do so with increasing severity and frequency leading to the development of prominent tophi in connective tissues.[2]

ETIOLOGY

Gout has been recognised as a disease since ancient times, and it was always seen as something linked with nutrition. For example, a medical publication dating from the 16th century expressed the view popular over many centuries that gout is a disease of 'overindulgent lifestyle.' Its author especially commends the avoidance of "inordinate eating and drinking" and "mixing one's wines."[3]

In the context of this long scope of history, the understanding of the central role of urate in gout has been relatively recent. Urate (for the purposes of this chapter is essentially the same thing as uric acid) is produced in the body as a product of the catabolism of purine nucleotides, and therefore is related to the rate of cell death, and the recycling of the constituents of cellular DNA.

Urate crystals are deposited in gout either because of an excess production of uric acid, or because of a decrease in its renal clearance. The latter may, in turn, be due to a variety of conditions, including renal disease, hypertension, chronic lead exposure and treatment with certain drugs such as some diuretics.[4] Niacin is a nutrient that when used as a pharmacological supplement for treatment of hyperlipidemia can also decrease urinary uric acid excretion.[5]

Hyperuricemia is thus a major risk factor for gout. However, it is important to realize that it is entirely possible to have hyperuricemia without gout, and that conversely some patients with acute gout do not have hyperuricemia.[5] Admittedly, most gout patients do, and if absent this is usually only a transient finding during the acute attack, possibly due to the deposition of urate crystals having removed some of the excess urate from the blood.[2,5]

NUTRITIONAL FACTORS

The obvious place to begin in looking at nutritional factors involved in gout is with those which cause elevated levels of uric acid. Note that many non-nutritional factors can cause hyperuricemia, for example, diseases such as cancer (particularly hematological cancer), which increase cellular turnover and thus purine breakdown. Indeed it has been estimated that purine in the diet contributes only around 15% to total blood urate.[5]

URATE FORMATION

Foremost amongst the nutritional factors that increase uric acid levels in the body is consumption of purine-rich foods — see Table 23.1. Purine content is affected by food storage and cooking. Boiling, for example, generally reduces purine content through loss into the cooking water.[6] Moreover, not all purines have equal effects on urate levels — it depends on how much of the uricogenic bases xanthine and hypoxanthine the purines contain.[2]

The traditional notion that gout sufferers should avoid excess protein is an oversimplification, even though the purine-rich foods listed in Table 23.1 are primarily proteins. Observational studies have not found a direct relationship between protein intake and uric acid levels, whilst dairy foods have been shown to have a lowering effect on blood urate level.[7–10] Whether they do so because they replace more purine-rich foods as a source of protein in the diet or via some direct effect of casein and lactalbumin is not clear.[10]

Elements of the diet apart from purine content can also elevate uric acid levels. For example, coffee and fructose can raise urate levels, whilst cherries can

TABLE 23.1
Purine-rich foods

Meat (especially organ meats), seafood
Yeast products, including alcoholic drinks
Legumes (peas and beans)
Oatmeal, wheat bran
Spinach, cauliflower, asparagus, mushrooms
Tea, coffee, cola drinks

lower it.[5,7,11,12] Obesity and a high rate of weight gain are both associated with gout.[13,14] Obesity and hyperuricemia are also part of the metabolic syndrome.

Excess alcohol consumption has been understood to be involved in gout since ancient times and this is not surprising since it both increases production and decreases excretion of urate.[5] Recent observational data reported a dose–response effect on gout incidence, in which alcohol intake increased the risk of gout by a third at intakes of 10 to 15 g/d and by two and a half times at intakes over 50 g/d.[15] Amongst alcoholic beverages, beer has a greater association, probably because it is a source of purines (e.g., from yeast).[15]

ANTIOXIDANTS

The question of whether gout is a pro-oxidant condition in which antioxidant nutrients might have a role is intriguing, because uric acid *in vitro* is actually a powerful antioxidant.[16] There is some evidence that uric acid can combine with nitrous oxide to remove free radicals.[17] One interesting speculation is that elevated urate might not only cause inflammation, but also be produced in response to the pro-oxidant state produced by inflammation. If this were true, it would be one rationale for giving antioxidant nutrients to gout sufferers.

Additionally, a Russian study reported that free-radical concentrations in gout patients were positively correlated with the severity of the disease.[18] A Japanese study found higher levels of oxidized LDL in gout patients, and that these levels were lowered with allopurinol treatment to lower the urate.[19]

However, there is as yet no human clinical trial evidence to support the use of antioxidants in treating gout. Vitamin C supplements are uricosuric, although whether this has any practical impact on gout is doubtful.[20] Whilst a diet with plenty of fruit and vegetables — rich sources of antioxidants — is associated with lower risk of gout, this could also be because such diets result in a person consuming less hyperuricemic foods.[13] Such diets are also alkalinizing.

XANTHINE OXIDASE INHIBITORS

Some nutritional factors are known to inhibit the enzyme xanthine oxidase, which is involved in the conversion of xanthine to urate. Folate is one of these — it is a weak inhibitor of this enzyme, but a very small, human trial of high-dose folate failed to lower urate.[21] Curcumin (an active compound in the spice turmeric) is another dietary element that inhibits xanthine oxidase.[22]

CALCIUM AND VITAMIN D

The relationship of gout to calcium and vitamin D is complex. Hyperuricemic patients can certainly develop calcium stones, a combination known as hyperuricosuric calcium urolithiasis, but whether the patient gets this pattern of gout depends on the pH as much as on the urate or calcium concentrations.[23] In parathyroid disorders calcium and vitamin D certainly impact on uric acid metabolism, and one study has found that patients with gout have lower vitamin D3 levels correlated with higher urate.[24,25] Yet synthesis of this same vitamin has been found in synovial cells from gouty joints.[26] In short, no consistent relationship has been demonstrated between calcium homoeostasis and gout.

Editor's Note

A patient with gout is likely to have more musculoskeletal health conditions than the inflamed joint. Gout is linked to both obesity and the treatment of obesity. Eating less and exercising more may exacerbate gout because muscle breakdown increases purine levels. Gout is also associated with insulin resistance, low vitamin D levels, and inflammation, all of which interfere with muscle synthesis. Evidence is increasing that gout represents a pro-oxidative state with lipid oxidation and higher concentrations of free radicals. Ongoing metabolic research suggests there may be a clinical a role for antioxidants (Chapter 7) and vitamin D (Chapter 10) in gout management.

CLINICAL APPLICATIONS

All this information about nutritional factors is interesting, but what is its practical relevance to clinical disease? In addressing this question, we have to be careful to distinguish between hyperuricemia and gout itself.

Hyperuricemia is involved in disease outcomes unrelated to gout. For example, it is one of a cluster of closely related but independent risk factors that constitute the metabolic syndrome.[27] Since metabolic syndrome is a prelude to diabetes and heart disease, the treatment of hyperuricemia might feasibly make a significant contribution to health outcomes related to this syndrome.[28] There is certainly room for scepticism as to whether gout per se, rather than hyperuricemia, is associated with cardiovascular disease risk.[29,30]

A randomized trial of dairy vs. no dairy intake found significant difference in plasma uric acid level after several weeks, but this was because the urate increased in the non-dairy diet group, rather than decreasing in the dairy group.[9] Some have suggested that it might be useful to follow a higher-protein and lower-carbohydrate, unsaturated fat diet to improve insulin sensitivity, on the grounds that hyperuricemia through the decreased urate clearance mechanism may be related to insulin resistance.[31,32] At present, this remains a hypothesis.

Dietary approaches in gout have focused on secondary prevention, i.e. minimizing the risk of a further attack in someone who has already had one. Most medical textbooks and recommendations on gout include a role for some or all of the following: an increase in fluid intake, moderating the intake of alcohol and purine-rich foods and reducing weight where appropriate.[31] Others no longer recommend routine purine avoidance on the grounds that drug treatments are sufficiently effective.[33] Surprisingly, although it is clear that such approaches can reduce hyperuricemia (e.g., Scott et al.)[34], there is not so much evidence showing that dietary approaches prevent the actual recurrence of gout. It would be reasonable to say that this is more an accepted part of clinical practice than an evidence-based conclusion.

Research may cast better light on the role of free radicals and antioxidants and vitamin D. The present consensus for dietary advice in gout management is increased fluids and moderation in purine-rich food and alcohol intake, along with reduction of any excess weight.

REFERENCES

1. Kramer, H.M. et al., The association between gout and nephrolithiasis: the National Health and Nutrition Examination Survey III, 1988–1994, *Am. J. Kidney. Dis.*, 37–42, 2002.
2. Ball, L.C. et al., Gout: aetiology and nutritional management, in *Encyclopedia of Human Nutrition*, Vol. 2, Sadler, M.J., Strain, J.J., and Caballero, B., Eds., Academic Press, San Diego, CA, 1999.
3. Copeman, W.S. et al., The first medical monograph on the gout, *Med. Hist.*, 13, 288–293, 1969.
4. Slot, O., Hyperuricemia, *Ugeskr. Laeger*, 156, 2396–2401, 1994.
5. Emmerson, B.T., The management of gout, *N. Engl. J. Med.* 334, 445–451, 1996.
6. Colling, M. et al., Effect of cooking on the purine content of foods, *Z. Ernahrungswiss.*, 26, 214–218, 1987.
7. Choi, H.K. et al., Intake of purine-rich foods, protein, and dairy products and relationship to serum levels of uric acid: the Third National Health and Nutrition Examination Survey, *Arthritis Rheum.*, 52, 283–289, 2005.
8. Choi, H.K. et al., Purine-rich foods, dairy and protein intake, and the risk of gout in men, *N. Engl. J. Med.*, 350, 1093–1103, 2004.
9. Ghadirian, P. et al., The influence of dairy products on plasma uric acid in women, *Eur. J. Epidemiol.*, 11, 275–281, 1995.
10. Garrel, D.R. et al., Milk- and soy-protein ingestion: acute effect on serum uric acid concentration, *Am. J. Clin. Nutr.*, 53, 665–669, 1991.
11. Jacob, R.A. et al., Consumption of cherries lowers plasma urate in healthy women, *J. Nutr.*, 133, 1826–1829, 2003.

12. Kiyohara, C. et al., Inverse association between coffee drinking and serum uric acid concentrations in middle-aged Japanese males, *Br. J. Nutr.*, 82, 125–130, 1999.

13. Lyu, L.C. et al., A case-control study of the association of diet and obesity with gout in Taiwan, *Am. J. Clin. Nutr.*, 78, 690–701, 2003.

14. Roubenoff, R. et al., Incidence and risk factors for gout in white men, *J. Am. Med. Assoc.*, 266, 3004–3007, 1991.

15. Choi, H.K. et al., Alcohol intake and risk of incident gout in men: a prospective study, *Lancet*, 363, 1277–1281, 2004.

16. Kirschbaum, B., Renal regulation of plasma total antioxidant capacity, *Med. Hypotheses*, 56, 625–629, 2001.

17. Squadrito, G.L. et al., Reaction of uric acid with peroxynitrite and implications for the mechanism of neuroprotection by uric acid, *Arch. Biochem. Biophys.*, 376, 333–337, 2000.

18. Agureev, A.P. et al., Generation of superoxide anion and lipid peroxidation in serum of gout patients, *Vopr. Med. Khim.*, 38, 29–31, 1992.

19. Tsutsumi, Z. et al., Oxidized low-density lipoprotein autoantibodies in patients with primary gout: effect of urate-lowering therapy, *Clin. Chim. Acta*, 339, 117–122, 2004.

20. Stein, H.B. et al., Ascorbic acid-induced uricosuria. A consequence of megavitamin therapy, *Ann. Intern. Med.*, 84, 385–388, 1976.

21. Boss, G.R. et al., Failure of folic acid (pteroylglutamic acid) to affect hyperuricemia, *J. Lab. Clin. Med.*, 96, 783–789, 1980.

22. Lin, J.K. et al., Inhibitory effect of curcumin on xanthine dehydrogenase/oxidase induced by phorbol-12-myristate-13-acetate in NIH3T3 cells, *Carcinogenesis*, 15, 1717–1721, 1994.

23. Pak, C.Y. et al., Biochemical distinction between hyperuricosuric calcium urolithiasis and gouty diathesis, *Urology*, 60, 789–794, 2002.

24. Yoneda, M. et al., Parathyroid function and uric acid metabolism, *Nippon Naibunpi Gakkai Zasshi*, 59, 1738–1751, 1983.

25. Takahashi, S. et al., Decreased serum concentrations of 1,25(OH)2-vitamin D3 in patients with gout, *Metabolism*, 47, 336–338, 1998.

26. Hayes, M.E. et al., Synthesis of the active metabolite of vitamin D, 1,25(OH)2D3, by synovial fluid macrophages in arthritic diseases, *Ann. Rheum. Dis.*, 48, 723–729, 1989.

27. Vazquez-Mellado, J. et al., Primary prevention in rheumatology: the importance of hyperuricemia, *Best Pract. Res. Clin. Rheumatol.*, 18, 111–124, 2004.

28. Daskalopoulou, S.S. et al., Prevention and treatment of the metabolic syndrome, *Angiology*, 55, 589–612, 2004.

29. Gelber, A.C. et al., Gout and risk for subsequent coronary heart disease. The Meharry–Hopkins Study, *Arch. Intern. Med.*, 157, 1436–1440, 1997.

30. Roubenoff, R., Gout and hyperuricemia, *Rheum. Dis. Clin. North. Am.*, 16, 539–550, 1990.

31. Schlesinger, N. et al., Gout: can management be improved? *Curr. Opin. Rheumatol.*, 13, 240–244, 2001.

32. Marangella, M., Uric acid elimination in the urine. Pathophysiological implications, *Contrib. Nephrol.*, 147, 132–148, 2005.

33. Anon. Gout, section in crystal-induced conditions, in *The Merck Manual of Diagnosis and Therapy*, chap. 55, http://www.merck.com/mrkshared/mmanual/section5/chapter55/55a.jsp (accessed Mar. 9, 2005).

34. Scott, J.T. et al., The effect of weight loss on plasma and urinary uric acid and lipid levels, *Adv. Exp. Med. Biol.*, 76B, 274–277, 1977.

24 Oral Markers of Tissue Health

Helyn Luechauer, D.D.S. and
Kathryn Poleson, D.M.D.

CONTENTS

The 21st century patient expects to be weighed, measured for height, body temperature, and blood pressure, frequently asked for a urine sample, and routinely examined in the eyes, ears, nose, and throat. They expect to be comprehensively evaluated, sometimes even demanding that these health conditions be considered in an overall treatment plan. They want health care professionals to be sensitive to the body's lack of isolated and noncommunicating compartments.[1] The rapid response of oral tissues to metabolic changes provides many clues to deficiency states long before the condition is classified as a disease.

In this day of patient demand for prevention of disease as well as treatment, the physician examining the patient, regardless of the symptoms presented, will discover that performing a cursory, quick check of the oral cavity, is quite beneficial. While examining the tonsils or other structures in the throat area, some physicians may be missing an opportunity to note that the tongue, teeth, palate, and gums offer a wealth of potential disease information that develops in a remarkably short period of time.[2] The wooden tongue depressor and a mouth mirror are the only instruments needed to note normal and abnormal appearances in the lip, tongue, teeth, gingiva, palate, and saliva. Abnormalities are generally considered to be signs of a nutritional deficiency.

THE TONGUE, PALATE, GUMS, AND GINGIVA

The tongue is one of the most prominent responders to metabolic disorders or deficiencies.[3-6] An oversized tongue, thick in a dorsal–ventral direction, with indented or scalloped borders (from slight indentations to almost pedunculated formations) is a well-described sign of an underfunctioning and underdeveloped thyroid gland. Early signs, even in children, are the slight tooth-mark indentations on the lateral margins of the tongue. Because of the thyroid gland's importance in metabolism, these tongue formations are a valuable sign of nutritional dysfunction.

A coated tongue appears in as few as 12 h after a dietary overload or deficiency. Because of its papillary structure, it is an instant incubator for *Candida* and other oral infections. Coatings are usually white, with the exception that "smokers' tongue" coatings range from tan to black. A dry, glistening tongue, atrophied in appearance, may signal lack of saliva from medications taken, a stroke, or senility.[7-9]

In deficiency states, the normally pink palate may be coated overall and be patchy or have ulcerative patches. A posterior palate showing a red color is the initial sign of oral candidiasis.

Red, swollen, boggy gums are the signs of periodontal infection. There is much ongoing research on the possible systemic disease link to periodontal disease, which involves loss of attachment of the gingiva to the tooth, increased pocket depth, and loss of alveolar bone, especially interproximally.[10,11] Ideal gingival architecture is a triangle of gum tissue that extends tightly between the teeth and around the buccal and lingual surfaces of the tooth, is pale salmon pink in color in persons of light skin, and has varying degrees of pigmentation in persons of darker skin color. There is no expressible exudate from the sulcus. Recession apically of the gingiva along the root of the tooth without a change in color or form is not an inflammatory condition and is not yet fully understood. Recession of the gingiva appears to follow bone loss, most apparently in the mandible. Receding gums is the focus of the current study, and an association with osteoporosis appears likely.

Cracks on the corners of the mouth, known as cheilosis, have long been considered a B vitamin deficiency and are now recognized as a primary result of a *Candida* infection superimposed on a B vitamin deficiency.[12,13]

Cold sores are herpetic lesions that recur under conditions of physical stress when there is an underlying imbalance in the ratio of the amino acids arginine and lysine. Supplementation with 1 g of lysine on an empty stomach three times daily has been demonstrated to shorten the course of the disease.[14]

EXAMINING TEETH

Teeth work automatically in mastication with rare sensory output, erupt more or less unobtrusively over a 20 year period when other systems demand much more attention, have no early warning system when attacked, and do not cause pain until the breakdown of the system is far advanced, irreversibly in many instances.

The teeth, by their absence or presence, indicate nutritional (metabolic) changes that are taking or have taken place in the body.[15] There is evidence that a minimum of 12 posterior or 20 overall teeth are necessary to properly masticate a bolus of food. Heart disease correlates with having less than 20 teeth.[16] Missing teeth often indicate an immune system failure and may be markers of radiation therapy outside the oral cavity.[17]

The presence of third molars has also been noted in an atherosclerosis study by the University of North Carolina as having a possible negative impact on periodontal disease in the 52- to 74-year-old participants.[18] Almost universally, the wisdom tooth disrupts the occlusion of the proximal tooth and interferes with mastication.

A single missing tooth causes a malocclusion in the bite, a shifting of the dental arch, and loss of efficiency in chewing. Moreover, the teeth on either side drift out of contact and the matching tooth in the opposite arch continues to erupt into the space of the lost tooth, interrupting occlusion and mastication. Digestion of protein is compromised and dietary intake of whole foods is often reduced because of discomfort.

The absence of enamel on the lingual surfaces of the teeth is a strong indicator that the patient is bulimic or anorexic and purges, leaving a heavy stomach-acid residue on the lingual surface of the teeth, which over time dissolves the enamel and leaves the exposed yellow dentin vulnerable to caries.[19]

Stains on the teeth, intrinsic in many cases, are noticeable on cursory examination but are rarely congenital. Most common in this intrinsic category are discoloration bands in the enamel caused by antibiotics, particularly tetracycline, administered during infancy and early childhood when the enamel is forming within the jawbone, long before the tooth erupts. Other drugs and smoking stain the enamel and support a huge cosmetic remodeling subspecialty in dentistry today.

Untreated caries on the occlusal surfaces of posterior teeth are easily visible and may extend onto the surfaces between the teeth.[20] An acid pH (6.3 or less) fosters bacterial infection and decay. The pH of the saliva can be assayed during examination of the oral cavity.

Calculus (tartar), especially on the inside of the lower front teeth, is a metabolic sign of imbalance in nutrition and seems to accompany or cause bone loss around the teeth involved. Composed primarily of calcium oxalate, calculus may result from an interaction between calcium, magnesium, and vitamin D. Additional research is ongoing.

OBSERVING SALIVA

Sticky, slimy saliva is another oral indicator of an acid pH.[20] Its causes include a sugar diet, lack of saliva from medications, stroke, old age, or the result of radiation or chemotherapy.

Xerostomia, the drying up of saliva flow, has been the topic of several dental conferences in the past decade.[21,22] Of concern to the dental provider are the sequelae, i.e., increased caries, especially at the gum line, loss of gingiva around the teeth and accompanying bone loss, and a dry, glossy, denuded tongue. The oral examiner may see these results of diminished salivary flow even before the patient is aware of the condition. Body secretions, saliva constituents, bony elements, and their possible connection or relationship to oral and systemic diseases are the substance of ongoing research.[23–25]

There are easy-to-use paper strips available, which indicate the pH of the saliva. Placed on the tongue for a few seconds, the strips can be read immediately and are an indication of dietary sugar intake. Salivary pH correlates to total body acid–base balance.[26,27] How acidity damages bone and a method by which to test the body's acidity burden are presented in Chapter 25.

Use of high-carbohydrate sports drinks has been demonstrated to reduce pH and accelerate enamel erosion.[28,29] Sports drinks contain three times the amount of refined carbohydrate needed for electrolyte repletion (Chapter 8).

While most refined carbohydrates promote tooth decay, sugar alcohols actually have a protective effect. Sugar alcohols, such as xylitol and mannitol, are refined and sweet, yet cannot be metabolized by oral bacteria. For this reason sugar alcohols are found in chewing gum and toothpaste. Xylitol has been demonstrated to exert a positive effect on the pH of the oral cavity, by selectively promoting healthful commensal oral flora and preventing the overgrowth of harmful microorganisms.[30] Both maternal and pediatric use of xylitol has been shown to reduce dental caries.[31–33]

VITAMIN C FOR SOFT TISSUE HEALTH

Inflamed gums are an early sign of vitamin C deficiency.[34] Over two centuries ago, Linn of the British Navy classified scurvy from the oral markers he saw in vitamin C-deprived sailors. Also, the principal author of this chapter finds that red, swollen, bleeding gums around the teeth are benefited by oral supplementation with vitamin C well beyond the recommended daily allowance dosage, especially if the inflamed gingiva are coupled with any history or observation of bruising.[34–36] Vitamin C is a precursor for hyaluronic acid, necessary for regeneration and maintenance of bone and cartilage. Consistent with the biochemistry, vitamin C supplementation facilitates the healing of dental procedures involving gingival attachment and regrowth of trabecular and cortical bone.

OSTEOPOROSIS

Periodontal disease is associated with osteoporosis,[11,37–44] insulin resistance, diabetes, and heart disease.[17,45–51] Alveolar bone loss and osteoporosis are two conditions where the dental and the all-body studies overlap;[25,52,53] both diseases are primary factors in the study of nutritional deficiencies and aging.

One dietary link is magnesium deficiency. Aikawa locates 60% of the body stores of magnesium in bone and designates it as a "surface-limited-ion,"[54–58] which helps to explain the rapid disappearance of the skeletal bone and the alveolar ridge in magnesium-deficient states.[4,19,59,60] As discussed in Chapter 9, refining carbohydrates reduces dietary intake of magnesium: 80% loss in refining wheat, 83% loss in polishing rice, 99% loss in extracting sugar from molasses, and 97% loss in producing starch from corn.[54] Carbohydrates "unchaperoned" by magnesium facilitate erosion of the dental enamel.

IATROGENIC HEAVY-METAL EXPOSURE

Heavy-metal toxicity and the possible deleterious effects of silver-amalgam restorations in the teeth is a contentious issue at all levels of prevention and treatment.[54,61] One of the most compelling clinical observations is a black mole-like lesion called an amalgam tattoo. Amalgam tattoos are sometimes seen in the gingiva, the palate, and even in the lip, not far from the site of an amalgam restoration or an extraction (surgical) site.[62] The nidus is a residual piece of metal incorporated accidentally into the soft tissue at the treatment site. The tissue responded by leaching out some of the metallic ions into the surrounding connective tissue and epithelium, causing a black mole-like area. They are considered harmless unless they spread, at which time they are removed. A potential link between amalgam tattoos and whole-body mercury stores has not been investigated.

Mercury toxicity results in many musculoskeletal conditions, as discussed in Chapter 29. Whether mercury amalgams are a significant, iatrogenic source remains unresolved.[63–65] Several European countries no longer use mercury–silver fillings; the American Dental Association continues to state that there is no harmful effect from mercury–silver amalgam to the human body. The outcome is likely to be decided on an entirely different level: patients' desires. Given the choices of dark, unaesthetic, and controversial metal fillings vs. tooth-colored, virtually undetectable restorative materials, the decision is, with rare exception, for more natural-looking, tooth-colored material. The mercury issue may pass into evolutionary extinction.

CONCLUSION

Teeth constitute only a fraction of the structures within the oral cavity that influence and are influenced by the musculoskeletal system of which they are an integral part. The agenda envisioned by Dr. Richard Carmona, Surgeon General of the United States, that begins with health promotion and disease prevention should include the care of the oral cavity.[66,67]

Too often the mouth is the "stepchild" in the maintenance of health, coming into focus only after disease has a firm foothold in the body. Yet the mouth is inextricably linked with health and is vital to the development of the individual. An all-encompassing review of nutrition's relationship to dental health and oral markers is impossible to present in one chapter. The mouth is a factor in musculoskeletal, indeed in total body health care.[68,69] Some additional topics of interest are magnesium deficiency in diabetes,[5,54,70,71] coronary heart disease, stroke, osteoporosis[41] and arthritis,[7] protein synthesis,[72] bone loss,[40,73] tooth loss and ma nutrition,[74] protein metabolism effects on bone mineral density and rate of bone loss,[75] protein and calcium balance,[18] acid–alkaline balance,[26,27] calcium and vitamin D levels,[19,76–78] sugar–fructose effects,[24] and B complex vitamin absorption.[15] The interactions are endless, and many deficiencies first emerge in the mouth.[79,80] In summary, physicians and dentists, working together, can accomplish mutual goals of preventing and, when necessary, treating disease.

Editor's Note

The mouth serves as an early detection system for nutritional deficiencies. Examining the oral cavity can reveal "jaw-droppingly" useful information about less visible portions of the musculoskeletal system.

REFERENCES

1. Weil, A., The significance of integrative medicine for the future of medical education, *Am. J. Med.*, 108, 441–443, 2000.
2. Halstead, C.L., Blozis, G.G., Drinnan, A.J., and Gier, RE, *Physical Evaluation of the Dental Patient*, CV Mosby, St Louis, 1982.
3. Academy of Oriental Heritage, *The Chinese Classics of Tongue Diagnosis*, Academy of Oriental Heritage, Vancouver, BC, 1980 (translated by Lu, H.C.).
4. Barnes, B.O. and Galton, L., *Hypothyroidism: The Unsuspected Illness*, Thos Crowell Co., New York, 1976.
5. Beaven, D.W. and Brooks, S.E., *Color Atlas of the Tongue*, Wolfe Medical Publications, U.K., 1988.
6. Braverman, L.E. and Utiger, R.D., *Werner and Ingabar's The Thyroid*, JB Lippencott, Philadelphia, 1991.
7. Bohmer, T. and Mowe, M., The association between atrophic glossitis and protein-calorie malnutrition in old age, *Age Ageing*, 29, 47–50, 2000.
8. Navazesh, M., Rhodus, N., and Ship, J., Zeroing in on xerostomia, paper presented at American Dental Association 144th Annual Scientific Session, San Francisco, 2003.

9. Walsh, N.P. et al., Saliva parameters as potential indices of hydration status during acute dehydration, *Med. Sci. Sports Exerc.*, 36, 1535–1542, 2001.
10. British Nutrition Foundation 1998, Task force: regarding oral health — diet and other factors, *Am. J. Clin. Nutr.*, 169, 2000.
11. Hamilton, J, The link between periodontal disease and systemic disease: state of the evidence 2005; *CA Dent. J.*, 2005.
12. Odds, F.C., *Candida and Candidosis*, Leicester University Press, Leicester, U.K., 1979, pp. 96–97.
13. Shephard, M.G., Candidiasis — an infectious disease of increasing importance, *N. Z. Dent. J.*, 78, 89–93, 1982.
14. Elter, J.R. et al., Prevalence of coronary heart disease, *J. Periodont.*, 75, 782–790, 2004.
15. Page, D.C., Tooth loss as an independent predictor of abnormal heart findings, *J. Dent. Res.*, 80, 1648–1652, 2001.
16. Page, D.C., *Your Jaws — Your Life, Alternative Medicine*, Smileage Corp., Baltimore, MD., 2003, p. 72.
17. Joshipura, K.C., Douglass, C., and Willett, W.C., Possible explanations for the tooth loss and cardiovascular relationship, *Ann. Periodontol.*, 3, 175–183, 1998.
18. U. NC, Negative impact of third molars on periodontal disease, *J. Oral Maxillofac. Surg.*, 2005.
19. Krall, E.A. et al., Calcium and vitamin D supplements reduce tooth loss in the elderly, *Am. J. Med.*, 111, 452–456, 2001.
20. Steinberg, S., Caries risk and saliva testing, *J. Pract. Hyg.*, 25, 2005.
21. Guggenheimer, J. and More, P., Xerostomia: etiology, recognition, and treatment, *J. Am. Dent. Assoc.*, 134, 61–69, 2003.
22. Lipski, E., *Functional Medicine and Functional Testing in Digestive Wellness*, 3rd ed., McGraw-Hill, New York, 2005, pp. 98–106.
23. Nizel, A.E. and Papas, A.S., *Nutrition in Clinical Dentistry*, 3rd ed., W.B. Saunders, Philadelphia, 1989, pp. 163–164.
24. Page, R.C., The pathobiology of periodontal disease may affect systemic diseases: inversion of a paradigm, *Ann. Periodont.*, 108–120, 1998.
25. Taguchi, A. et al., Relationship between dental panoramic radiographic findings and biochemical markers of bone turnover, *J. Bone Miner. Res.*, 18, 1689–1694, 2003.
26. Brown, S., *Better Bones, Better Body*, 2nd ed., Keats Publishing, Los Angeles, 2000, 294–297.
27. Brown, S. and Jaffe, R., Acid–alkaline balance and its effect on bone health, *Int. J. Integr. Med.*, 2, 7–15, 2000.
28. Hooper, S., West, N.X. et al., A comparison of enamel erosion by a new sports drink compared to two proprietary products: a controlled, crossover study in situ, *J. Dent.*, 32, 541–545, 2004.
29. von Fraunhofer, J.A. and Rogers, M.M., Effects of sports drinks and other beverages on dental enamel, *Gen. Dent.*, 53, 28–31, 2005.
30. Thaweboon, S., Thaweboon, B. et al., The effect of xylitol chewing gum on mutans streptococci in saliva and dental plaque, *Southeast Asian J. Trop. Med. Public Health*, 35, 1024–1027, 2004.
31. Makinen, K.K., Isotupa, K.P. et al., Six-month polyol chewing-gum programme in kindergarten-age children: a feasibility study focusing on mutans streptococci and dental plaque, *Int. Dent. J.*, 55, 81–88, 2005.

32. Thorild, I., Lindau, B. et al., Effect of maternal use of chewing gums containing xylitol, chlorhexidine, or fluoride on mutans streptococci colonization in the mothers' infant children, *Oral Health Prev. Dent.*, 1, 53–57, 2003.

33. Widome, R., What can oral public health learn from Finland? *Am. J. Public Health*, 94, 1842–1843, 2004.

34. Lewin, S., *Vitamin C: Its Molecular Biology and Medical Potential*, Academic Press, New York, 1976.

35. Khaw, K.T., Bingham, S. et al., Relation between plasma ascorbic acid and mortality in men and women in EPIC-Norfolk prospective study: a prospective population study, *Lancet*, 357, 657–663, 2001.

36. Paolini, M., Biagi, F.L. et al., Plasma ascorbic acid in heart disease, *Lancet Lett.*, 358, 71, 2001.

37. Krall, E.A., The periodontal-systemic connection: implications for treatment of patients with osteoporosis and periodontal disease, *Ann. Periodontol.*, 6, 209–213, 2001.

38. Inagaki, K., Kurosu, Y., Kamiya, T., Kondo, F., Yoshinari, F., and Noguchi, T., Low metacarpal bone density, tooth loss, and periodontal disease, *J. Dent. Res.*, 80, 1818–1822, 2001.

39. Mohammed, A.R. and Brunsvold, M., The strength of the association between systemic postmenopausal osteoporosis and periodontal disease, *Int. J. Prosthodont.*, 9, 479–483, 1996.

40. Mohammed, A., Hooper, D., Vermilyea, S., Mariotti, A., and Preshaw, P., An investigation of the relationship between systemic bone density and clinical periodontal status in post-menopausal Asian–American women, *Int. Dent. J.*, 53, 121–125, 2003.

41. Nizel, A.E. and Papas, A.S., *Nutrition in Clinical Dentistry*, 3rd ed., W.B. Saunders, Philadelphia, 1989, pp. 155–159.

42. Phillips, H.B. and Ashley, F.P., The relationship between periodontal disease and a metacarpal bone index, *Br. Dent. J.*, 134, 237–239, 1973.

43. Tezal, M., Wactawski-Wende, J., Grossi, S.G. et al., The relationship between bone mineral density and periodontitis in post-menopausal women, *J. Periodont.*, 71, 1492–1498, 2000.

44. Wactawski-Wende, J., Periodontal disease and osteoporosis: association and mechanisms, *Ann. Periodont.*, 6, 197–208, 2001.

45. Beck, J.D., Pankow, J., Tyroler, H.A., and Offenbacher, S., Dental infections and atherosclerosis, *Am. Heart J.*, 138, S528–S533, 1999.

46. Kinane, D.F., Periodontal disease's contributions to cardiovascular disease: an overview of potential mechanisms, *Ann. Periodont.*, 3, 142–150, 1998.

47. Larkin, M., Link between gum disease and heart disease disputed, *Lancet*, 358, 303, 2001.

48. Hujoel, P., No connection between tooth loss and heart disease, *J. Am. Dent. Assoc.*, 132, 883–889, 2001.

49. Mohammed, A.R., Bauer, R.L. and Yeh, C.K., Spinal bone density and tooth loss in a cohort of postmenopausal women, *Int. J. Prosthodont.*, 10, 381–385, 1997.

50. Haraszthy, V.I., Zambon, J.J. et al., Identification of periodontal pathogens in atheromatcus plaques; *J. Periodontol.*, 71, 1554–1560, 2000.

51. Noack, B. and Genco, R.J., Periodontal infections contribute to elevated systemic C-reactive protein level, *J. Periodontol.*, 72, 1221–1227, 2001.

52. Ward, V.J. and Manson, J.D., Alveolar bone loss in periodontal disease and the metacarpal index, *J. Periodontol.*, 44, 763–769, 1973.

53. Dawson-Hughes, B. and Harris, S.S., Calcium intake influences the association of protein intake with rates of bone loss in elderly men and women, *Am. J. Clin. Nutr.*, 75, 773–779, 2002.

54. Aikawa, J., *Magnesium: Its Biologic Significance*, CRC Press, Boca Raton, FL, 1981, pp. 61 (mercury), 71 (loss of Mg in processing grains), see also 95, 110, 111.

55. Feskanich, D., Willett, W.C., and Colditz, G.A., Calcium, vitamin D, milk consumption, and hip fractures: a prospective study among postmenopausal women, *Am. J. Clin. Nutr.*, 77, 504–511, 2003.

56. Heaney, R.P., Protein and calcium: antagonists or synergists? *Am. J. Clin. Nutr.*, 75, 609–610, 2002.

57. Dawson-Hughes, B., *Oral Health Prev. Dent.*, 1, 2004.

58. Shils, M.E., Olson, J.A. et al., *Modern Nutrition in Health and Disease*, 9th ed., Williams & Wilkins, Baltimore, 1999, p. 182.

59. Gutting, R.D., *Minerals: A Short Course on Description, Use, Functions, Deficiencies*, Tecbook Publications, Topeka, KS, 1978, pp. 11–12.

60. Wallach, S., Magnesium: trace elements, in *Shils*, 9th ed., 1990, p. 172.

61. Siblerud, R.L., Relationship between mercury from dental amalgam and oral cavity health, *Ann. Dent.*, Winter, 6–10, 1990.

62. Callen, J.P., Greer, K.E. et al., *Color Atlas of Dermatology*, W.B. Saunders, Philadelphia, 1993, pp. 376, 386.

63. Effleston, D.W., T-lymphocyte response to dental amalgam, *J. Prosthet. Dent.*, 51, 617–623, 1984.

64. Huggins, H., *It's All in Your Head*: *Diseases Caused by Silver–Mercury Fillings*, 4th ed., Life Sciences Press, Colorado Springs, CO., 1990.

65. Ziff, S., *Silver Dental Fillings — The Toxic Time Bomb*; Aurora Press, New York, pp. 1084, 2002.

66. Carmona, R., Surgeon General of U.S.A., Defining our preventive healthcare agenda, (interview by S. Stephen Coles, editor *e-Jour Med*), 2005.

67. U.S. Department of Health and Human Services, Oral Health in America, A Report of the Surgeon General, Executive Summary National Institute of Dental and Cranofacial Research, National Institutes of Health, 2000.

68. American Dietetic Association, Position paper, Oral health and nutrition, *J. Am. Diet. Assoc.*, 103, 748–765, 2003.

69. Gaby, A.R., Intravenous nutrient therapy: the "Meyers cocktail," *Altern. Med. Rev.*, 7, 389–403, 2002.

70. Brodsky, M. et al., Consensus statement: magnesium supplementation in treatment of diabetes, *Diab. Care*, 19, 593–595, 1996.

71. Dacey, M.J., Hypomagnesemic disorders, *Crit. Care Clin.*, 17, 155–173, 2001.

72. Hu, F.B. and Stampfer, M.J. et al., Dietary protein and risk of ischemic heart disease in women, *Am. J. Clin. Nutr.*, 70, 221–227, 1999.

73. Sebastian, A. et al., Improved mineral balance and skeletal metabolism in postmenopausal women treated with potassium bicarbonate, *N. Engl. J. Med.*, 330, 25, 1776–1781, 1994.

74. Tezal, M., Grossi, S., and Genco, R., Is periodontitis associated with oral neoplasms? *J. Periodontol.*, 76, 406–410, 2005.

75. Rapuri, P.B. et al., Protein intake: effects on bone mineral density and rate of bone loss in elderly women, *Am. J. Clin. Nutr.*, 77, 1517–1525, 2003.

76. Carper, S., *No Milk Today*, Simon & Schuster, New York, 1986.

77. Dawson-Hughes, B. et al., Rates of bone loss in postmenopausal women randomly assigned to one or two dosages of vitamin D, *Am. J. Clin. Nutr.*, 6, 1140–1145, 1995.
78. Holick, M.F., Vitamin D: importance in the prevention of cancers, type I diabetes, heart disease, and osteoporosis, *Am. J. Clin. Nutr.*, 79, 362–371, 2004.
79. Garcia, L.C., Why dental work and infections in the mouth can be the roots of disease, Article #7, Fr. Joseph Mercola's *E-mail to a Friend*, 2004.
80. Harper, L.F., Healthy mouth, healthy body — healthy practice, lecture at CA Dental Association Spring Scientific Session, Anaheim, 2005.

Section VI

Bone

25 Bone Nutrition

Susan E. Brown, Ph.D.

CONTENTS

RETHINKING BONE STRENGTH

The more we consider the issue of bone strength, the more we realize that it is a very complicated phenomenon, which for practical clinical purposes we have tried to make very simple. In the clinical setting bone strength is commonly equated with bone mineral density (BMD). On closer inspection, however, we realize that bone strength encompasses a myriad of considerations beyond BMD.

Although we are yet to understand all the factors influencing bone strength, two major components are clearly bone density and bone quality. While bone density has been well explored, bone quality is an evolving concept. Bone quality includes issues of bone architecture, stiffness, material spatial distribution, turnover, damage accumulation and ability to repair microfractures, mineralization, crystal size and shape, vitality of bone cells, and the structure of bone proteins. A focus on bone quality and overall bone strength leads us to focus on biomechanical determinants and metabolic factors. This chapter discusses the nutritional components of bone strength, information which can be applied to fracture healing, osteoporosis prevention and management, preparation for orthopedic surgery, and for reducing the consequences of immobility.

Editor's Note

In many parts of the world, population rates of fracture are increasing, osteoporosis is occurring in more frequently among perimenopausal women, athletes may have poor bone quality despite high-impact sports, and patients heal at variable rates from the same orthopedic surgery. Inadequate bone nutrition is an underlying cause and is increasingly common across the life span.

BONE RESERVES

Bone plays various important roles beyond providing the body with form, rigidity, and locomotion. Bone serves as an incubator for red blood cells and selected immune cells and provides a protective milieu for the immune system. Bone also serves as a storehouse. The role of bone in calcium storage is well known, daily several hundred milligrams of calcium are taken out of the bone and deposited into the blood to maintain stable serum calcium levels, and ideally the same amount is taken from the blood and deposited into the bone. Without appropriate serum calcium, minute-to-minute survival would be compromised. The importance of adequate serum phosphorus is less well appreciated, as is the role bone plays in phosphorus storage. Phosphorus is required for metabolism by every cell and bone contains a large store of phosphorus comprising nearly 60% of all bone mineral. If the phosphorus levels in the blood entering bone are low, phosphate is extracted from the fluid around the osteoblasts for use in other parts of the body. This creates a local environment of depleted phosphorus, which seriously interferes with osteoblast function, as they too require phosphorus for their metabolism. As a result bone matrix deposition is slowed and osteoblast initiation of mineralization is reduced even more resulting potentially in rickets and osteomalacia.[1]

In addition to the aforementioned functions, bone also serves as an important storage site for minerals and alkalizing compounds. Of equal importance to the storage of mineral in bone is the storage of the anions associated with the mineral (e.g., phosphates and carbonates). It is now clearly documented that bone provides a gigantic reservoir of base, largely in the form of alkaline salts of calcium (phosphates and carbonates), and that these salts are mobilized and released into systemic circulation in response to increased loads of acid. The liberated base mitigates the severity of the attendant systemic acidosis and thus contributes to the maintenance of critical systemic acid–base homeostasis. The liberated calcium and phosphorus, however, are lost in the urine, without compensatory increases in gastrointestinal absorption. Reduction of bone mineral content is an unavoidable consequence of bone's defense of acid–base homeostasis.[2] Bone's role as a storehouse of alkali reserve is a topic of growing scientific interest bearing significant nutritional implications. These implications are detailed in our section on base-forming foods.

The functions of mineral and base storage are more critical than the structural functions of bone, as minute-to-minute survival depends on the availability of these readily exchangeable reserves. As such, the body in its evolutionary adaptive allocation of nutrient resources gives priority to the maintenance of metabolic homeostasis at the expense of the structural integrity of bone.

Each function of bone is tightly woven in to the fabric of human biochemistry. Currently we understand the contributions that many, but not all, nutrients play in bone health development and maintenance. In this chapter we review the major key bone building nutrients, as they are known today. The nutrient categories to be discussed are: (1) protein, (2) minerals, (3) vitamins, (4) essential fatty acids, (5) base-forming foodstuffs, (6) phytoestrogens, and (7) water. While each nutrient is discussed separately, it is important to keep in mind that many are codependent and simultaneously interact with each other, and with genetic and environmental factors. The reader is referred to Table 25.1, "The 19 Key Bone Building Nutrients" for a summary of these nutrients.

PROTEIN

The organic collagen matrix that comprises roughly 50% of bone by volume is formed from protein. Adequate dietary protein is essential for the maintenance of this skeletal protein matrix. Inadequate protein intake, often marked by low serum albumin, is associated with reduced BMD and increased fracture risk amongst the elderly.

TABLE 25.1
The 19 key bone-building nutrients

Nutrient	Adult RDA or AI	Common therapeutic range for bone health*	Dietary considerations
Calcium	800–1200 mg	1000–1500 mg	Typical diet is inadequate, averages 500–600 mg[3,4]
Phosphorus	700 mg	700–1200 mg	Inadequate intake is rare except in elderly and malnourished; excessive intake common with use of processed foods and soft drinks
Magnesium	420 mg men; 320 mg women	400–800 mg	Intake generally inadequate: all ages, sexes, classes, except children less than 5, fail to consume this RDA; 40% of population, 50% of adolescents consume less than 2/3 the RDA[4-7]
Fluoride	4.0 mg men; 3.0 mg women	—	Fluoride overdose has occurred through ingestion of fluoride toothpaste and high fluoride waters[5]
Silica	No values yet set	5–20 mg	Intake is unknown; silica is removed in food processing, current intake is suspected to be low
Zinc	11 mg men; 8 mg women	20–30 mg	Marginal zinc deficiency is common, especially among children (26); average intake was 46–63% the RDA[7]
Manganese	2.3 mg men; 1.8 mg women	10–25 mg	Intakes are generally inadequate, 1.76 mg adolescent girls 2.05 mg women, 2.5 mg males[8]
Copper	900 μg men and women	2–3 mg	75% of diets fail to contain the RDA[7,9]; average intake is below the RDA[5]
Boron	No RDA established	3–4 mg	0.25 mg intake is common[10] to perhaps optimum of 3 mg
Potassium	4700 mg men and women	4700–5000	Adult intake averages 2300 mg for women and 3100 mg for men[11]
Vitamin D	400 IU until age 70; then 600 IU, men and women	800–2000 IU and up as needed	Deficiency is common especially among the elderly, dark skinned and those with little UV sunlight exposure
Vitamin C	90 mg men; 75 mg women	Oral 500 mg; to bowel tolerance as needed	Average daily intake is about 95 mg for women and 107 for men[12]
Vitamin A	2997 IU men; 2,331 IU adult women	5000 IU or less	31% consume less than 70% the RDA[13]; current intake for women is about 2373 μg/d[14]
Vitamin B₆	1.7 mg men; 1.5 mg women	25–50 mg	Studies indicate widespread inadequate vitamin B₆ consumption among all sectors of the population[15]
Folic acid	400 μg men and women	800–1000 mcg	Inadequate intake was common among all age groups, but is improving with food fortification[5]
Vitamin K	120 μg men; 90 μg women	1000 μg	Averages 45–150 μg, which is well below the recommendation AI[16]
Vitamin B₁₂	2.4 mg men and women	100–1000 μg	12% consume less than 70% RDA (119); older people and vegans are especially at risk[5]
Fats	Should comprise 7% of calories minimum, not to exceed 30% of calories	20–30% of total calories is perhaps more ideal	The average American consumes 33% of his or her calories in fat; the consumption of essential acids, however, is frequently inadequate[5]
Protein	0.8 grams per kilo per day men and women; 125 lb person = 45 grams; 175 lb person = 63 grams	1.0 to 1.5 grams per kilo	Intake commonly exceeds 100 grams, but the elderly and women over 50 often have very deficient intakes. Higher protein intakes should be balanced with higher RDA level potassium intakes from food sources (26).

* The common therapeutic dose for bone health may be significantly higher in "special need" cases.

Low protein and low albumin are strongly and independently associated with functional outcome after hip fracture. Higher protein status has been associated with shorter hospital stays, reduced rates of complication and even reduced mortality. Several studies have documented the benefits of using supplemental protein (20 g/d) for hip fracture patients.[17,18] Short-term studies suggest that an abrupt shift to a low-protein diet reduces intestinal calcium absorption to the extent that it causes secondary hyperparathyroidism. Adequate protein is essential for bone growth, maintenance and renewal. While protein consumption of in the United States often exceeds the recommended daily average (RDA), an estimated 30% of all women over the age of 50 consume less than the RDA for protein. Thus, many of those most vulnerable to osteoporosis have inadequate protein intakes. In the Framingham longitudinal study of older men and women, the greatest bone loss over 4 years was observed in those with the lowest animal protein intake.[19] Similarly, the Iowa Women's Health Study reported higher protein intakes to be associated with reduced fracture risk.[20]

In what might initially appear as contrary to the aforementioned studies, excessive animal protein may be deleterious to bone. Some studies suggest that protein intake influences urinary calcium excretion to such an extent that for each 50 g increment of protein consumed an extra 60 mg of urinary calcium is excreted.[21] Thus it follows that uncompensated high protein intake leads to bone loss. Cross-cultural studies suggest that animal protein intake is positively associated with increased hip fracture incidence. Several worldwide surveys document that the countries with highest animal protein intakes are those with highest hip fracture rates.[22,23] In the Study of Osteoporotic Fractures, a high animal protein to vegetable protein ratio was associated with a greater rate of bone loss at the hip and increased hip fracture risk.[24] On the other hand, in a case-controlled study of elderly Utah residents ($n = 2501$), an increase in protein intake was associated with a decreased risk of hip fracture in men and women 50 to 69 years of age but not in those 70 to 89 years of age.[25] The proposed explanation of the relationship between animal protein and hip fracture incidence relates to the fact that animal protein is rich in acid-forming sulfur-containing amino acids. Further, the contemporary cultures consuming a high animal protein diet also tend to under-consume vegetables, fruits, needs, and seeds, food high in base-forming precursors. This combination contributes to chronic low-grade metabolic acidosis and subsequent bone weakening. High dietary protein, if not balanced with high base-forming precursor intake, can have a detrimental impact on bone.

Dietary protein is best considered in the context of the entire diet of each individual, particularity in terms of the balance between acid- and base-forming foodstuffs and overall mineral intake. In order to reconcile what initially seems like contradictory studies on protein intake, consider the human ancestral diet during the Paleolithic Period 100,000 years ago. These early populations developed greater peak bone mass and experienced less age-related bone loss than do age-matched contemporary humans.[26] The diet contained more protein than contemporary diets. These ancestral diets also contained more calcium, potassium, magnesium, and zinc, while low in sodium chloride, sugars, and void of refined carbohydrates.[27] For example, calcium, potassium, and protein intakes were two to three times higher than current intake levels, while sodium intake was seven times lower. These diets were balanced, high protein, high mineral, high phytonutrient, alkalizing diets. For example, Sabastian and colleagues reconstructed the net systemic acid load from 159 ancestral preagricultural diets. Overall, 87% of the 159 prehistoric diets evaluated were estimated to have provided an excess of base, while contemporary Westernized diets provide an excess of acid.[28]

In summary, a low protein, low nutrient diet increases fracture risk and does not favor bone at any life stage. The elderly and underweight frequently exhibit protein intakes below the RDA, which are suboptimal. The adult RDA is currently 0.8 g/kg/d. A high protein diet in association with low intakes of calcium, magnesium, potassium, and other nutrients increases urinary mineral loss and worsens chronic low-grade metabolic acidosis, and is detrimental to bone at all ages. The average American labors under chronic low-grade metabolic acidosis, which is in itself harmful to bone and is exacerbated by excessive protein and inadequate potassium and magnesium intakes. Moderately high protein diets require adequate base-forming foodstuff and nutrients to neutralize net endogenous acid production.[29]

MINERALS

Several minerals are essential for optimal bone health including calcium, phosphorus, magnesium, manganese, zinc, copper, and boron. It is important to keep in mind that these minerals exist in balance with each other. Clinical assessment should evaluate for mineral deficiencies and also screen for toxic minerals. This can be achieved with a D-penicillamine provoked 24-h urine collection as outlined in Chapter 29. Treatment for mineral deficiencies includes increases in dietary consumption of certain foods, as referenced in Table 25.1 and Table 25.2, and the use of multivitamin and mineral supplementation.

CALCIUM

Calcium is the most abundant mineral in the body. This mineral comprises 2% of the adult body weight, with the vast majority found in the hydroxyapatite crystal of bone and teeth. While calcium is clearly an essential nutrient for bone health, the optimum dietary intake of calcium is controversial and appears to depend upon the total diet. For example, authoritative U.S. calcium researcher Robert Heaney suggests that prudent nutritional support for osteoporosis prevention and treatment consists of 1200 to 1600 mg calcium per day together with sufficient vitamin D to maintain serum 25(OH)D levels about 80 nmol/l.[30] In many non-Westernized cultures, however, calcium intakes of 200 to 600 mg are documented to maintain normal bone health and a low incidence of osteoporotic fractures.[31,32] In fact, it has been noted that the countries with the lowest calcium intakes have been found to be those with the lowest fracture rates.[33] Further anthropologist

TABLE 25.2
Clinical considerations for calcium intake

Calcium and other bone building nutrients should be consumed to RDA levels. For RDA levels of the key bone building nutrients see Table 25.1

Calcium therapy will be of greatest benefit to those with the lowest baseline calcium intakes

Calcium doses over 2000–2500 mg/d may pose a risk in relation to the formation of kidney stones, the development of nutrient imbalances and other problems

Supplemental calcium should be used as necessary to meet the RDA and are best taken in divided doses

Magnesium should be supplemented with calcium in a one (Mg) to two (Ca) ratio. Refer to Dr. Buford-Mason's chapter on magnesium

A high-quality vitamin and mineral supplement is recommended to assure adequate levels of, and balance between, other key bone nutrients

Preadolescents through the teens should at least meet, or exceed, the RDA for calcium intakes (RDA = 1300 mg)

Calcium supplements should be taken with food for enhanced absorption as there is a 10–30% greater absorption than if ingested without food

Generally, the preferable forms of calcium supplements are the alkalizing salts of calcium such as calcium citrate, malate, gluconate, acetate, tartrate, fumerate, and carbonate

If protein and calorie intakes are low and suggestive of inadequate phosphorus, calcium in the form of tricalcium phosphate is recommended

High calcium intakes are best taken in balance with other nutrients such as magnesium, phosphorus, iron, and zinc

Iron supplements, if needed, should be taken apart form calcium supplements

Maximum absorption of calcium is obtained when the level of 25(OH) vitamin D is in the top two thirds of the normal range

Stanley Garn measured bone loss over a 50-year period in both North and Central America and failed to find a link between calcium intake and bone loss.[34] Numerous modern population studies make the same observation.

Cross-cultural analysis indicates that there is no one standard ideal calcium intake, neither is a high calcium intake necessary for bone health. As it appears, the adequate calcium intake for any given culture depends on coexisting dietary, lifestyle, and environmental factors. These factors include the balance between, and total intake of other nutrients; consumption of potentially bone-damaging substances like excess salt, protein, alcohol, tobacco, fat, sugar; degree of chronic low-grade metabolic acidosis, use of bone-depleting medications; sunlight exposure; environmental toxins and stress; incidence of sex organ surgeries, degenerative diseases, medications used, etc.

In the United States and other Westernized countries it appears that high calcium intake is needed to maintain positive calcium balance and reduce fracture risk. Calcium authority Robert Heaney.[35] reviewed all published studies on the relationship of calcium and bone health since 1975. Of 52 investigator-controlled calcium intervention studies, all but two showed better bone balance at high intakes, or greater bone gain during growth, or reduced bone loss in the elderly, or reduced fracture risk. Nonetheless, the relationship of current calcium intake and fracture risk is controversial. For example, the large U.S. Study of Osteoporotic Fractures (9704 women 65 years and over followed for 6.6 years) found the current use of calcium supplements was associated with increased risk of hip (RR 1.5) and vertebral (RR 1.4) fractures.[36] The larger U.S. Nurses' Health Study found that among middle aged and older women frequent milk consumption does not provide any substantial protection against hip or forearm fractures. Women consuming greater amounts of calcium from dairy foods had a modestly significant increase in hip fractures while no increase in fractures was observed for the same levels of calcium from nondairy sources.[37]

While calcium is essential to bone, our cultural emphasis on calcium has overshadowed the importance of other key bone-building nutrients of great importance. For example, a large Swedish study (N 65,000 women aged 48 to 80 years) found that when highest quartile of intake was compared to lowest, intakes of iron (OR = 3.3), magnesium (OR = 2.7), and vitamin C (OR = 1.9) were found to be independent risk factors for hip fracture. High calcium intake did not protect against hip fracture.[38] Further, the few intervention trials that have incorporated multi-nutrients have shown positive benefits. For example, a 2-year, placebo controlled trail on 225 postmenopausal women in the United States used three nutrient interventions: (1) calcium alone; (2) zinc, manganese, and copper; and (3) calcium, zinc, manganese, and copper. The only group to experience an improvement in bone mineral density was the group given calcium, zinc, manganese, and copper. Those using the placebo lost on average of 2.23% BMD.[39]

Finally, the important balance among all nutrients, and the fact that high calcium intake is likely to have deleterious effects on the absorption and retention of other minerals, is also often overlooked. For example, calcium and phosphorus maintain an inverse relationship whereby excess in the level of one causes the kidney to excrete the other. Also, calcium competes with iron for absorption and limits calcium absorption. Supplementing with calcium can also increase magnesium losses, and so forth.

The average calcium intake of adult women in the United States is only 60% of the DRI. Further, only 14% of girls and 36% of boys aged 12 to 19 years consume the recommended amount of calcium.[5] See Table 25.2.

PHOSPHOROUS

After calcium, phosphorus is the most abundant mineral in the human body with 85% of the body's phosphorus bound to the skeleton. Phosphorus is required for the appropriate mineralization of bone and depletion of phosphorus leads to impaired bone mineralization and suboptimal osteoblast function.

Recent guidelines have set the RDA for phosphorus well below the recommended adequate intake (AI) for calcium. The average American, however, consumes much more phosphorus than calcium. Dietary phosphorus intake averages 1 to 1.5 g/d and has risen 10 to 15% over the past 20 years, largely because of the increased use of phosphate salts in food additives and cola beverages. Although phosphorous is an essential bone nutrient, there is concern that excess amounts may induce high parathyroid secretion, which suppresses vitamin D production and intestinal calcium absorption, thereby worsening calcium balance. On the other hand, phosphorus also reduces the amount of calcium lost in the urine and thus may offset the adverse effects on calcium absorption. The scientific data on this point is still inconclusive and the effects of high phosphorus intake are likely evident only when combined with a low calcium diet.[40]

The bone health of 10 to 15% of the elderly in the United States is jeopardized by inadequate phosphorus intake. Prolonged dietary phosphorus deficiency and depleted serum levels result in enhanced resorption of minerals from bone. Osteoporosis medications require adequate phosphorus for efficacy. Among the elderly, increased dietary protein intake and supplementation with tricalcium phosphate and vitamin D is associated with decreased fracture risk.[41,42]

MAGNESIUM

Two thirds of the 25 g of magnesium in the human body is found in the skeleton. The average U.S. adult intake of magnesium for males is 323 mg/d and for females is 228 mg/d, these being well below the current RDAs of 420 and 320 mg/d, respectively.[43] Magnesium exists in balance with calcium. In the 1920s, the dietary magnesium/calcium ratio was 1:2, a ratio that has been found to be optimal for retention of each mineral in extensive balance studies in young men and women. As magnesium intake has declined while calcium consumption has increased, the dietary magnesium/calcium ratio is now between 1:3 and 1:4.[44] Information on magnesium's diverse roles in musculoskeletal health is detailed in the chapter by Dr. Burford-Mason. A few small human intervention studies reported that magnesium supplementation (from 250 to 750 mg/d) significantly increased bone density.[45,46]

MANGANESE

Manganese, like zinc and copper, is a trace element that can profoundly affect bone health. Manganese is an important cofactor in the biosynthesis of bone matrix mucopolysacharides.[47] Manganese deficient hens and rats show disproportionate growth of skeleton and under-glycosylation of proteoglycans. Protoglycans are a small but significant component of the mineralized bone matrix, the levels of which appear reduced in manganese deficient animals. Osteoporotic changes in bone can be brought about by manganese deficiency, which appears to increase bone breakdown while decreasing new bone mineralization.[47,48]

Clinical relevance became apparent in the mid-1980s, when researchers trying to understand why the California professional basketball player Bill Walton suffered from joint pain, recurrent bone fractures, and poor fracture healing, discovered that his blood manganese level was undetectable. He was also deficient in copper and zinc, while calcium levels appeared adequate. Supplementation with these trace minerals and calcium restored his bone health.

Greater serum manganese concentrations are associated with decreased bone breakdown and some studies show osteoporotic women to have one quarter the manganese level of nonosteoporotic women.[49] A study of 14 Belgian women with severe osteoporosis, matched by age with nonosteoporotic women, found blood manganese levels in the osteoporotic subjects were one quarter that of the nonosteoporotic subjects. Interestingly, of the 25 variables studied, only manganese was significantly different between osteoporotic and nonosteoporotic women.[50] While there appears to be no mononutrient, manganese-only, human intervention trials, at least three multinutrient human intervention studies have incorporated manganese supplementation.[46,47,51] All three showed an increase in BMD with the multinutrient supplementation.

The current adequate intake for manganese is set at 2.3 mg/d for men and 1.8 mg/d for women. Women consume inadequate amounts of manganese-containing foods such as wheat bran, tea, and spinach, primarily because processed food have less manganese. Absorption of manganese may also be compromised by supplement use, since magnesium, iron, and calcium inhibit manganese uptake.

ZINC

Zinc is present in all organs, tissues, fluids, and secretions of the body. Zinc is primarily an intracellular ion with well over 95% of total-body zinc found within the cells. It is the most abundant intracellular trace element. Of the 1.5 to 2.5 g zinc found in the human body, 57% is located in the skeletal muscle and 29% in the bone. Nearly 90% of the body's zinc is stored in the skeletal muscle and bone. Skeletal muscle and bone likely serve as a zinc reservoir, making the nutrient readily available for the 200 zinc-dependent enzymes.

Zinc functions as a cofactor in over 200 enzymatic reactions, many of these relate to the growth processes. In bone metabolism, zinc is needed for the production of the collagen protein matrix threads upon which the hydroxyapatite crystals are deposited. Zinc deficiency results in impaired DNA synthesis, leading to negative effects on bone formation. Zinc is also needed for the production of enzymes, which degrade and recycle worn-out bits of bone protein. Zinc is required for proper calcium absorption and enhances the biochemical activity of vitamin D. Zinc is essential for bone healing and increased amounts are found at the sites of bone repair.

Osteoporosis has been associated with low zinc levels. In small studies, zinc was found to be 30% lower in osteoporotic women compared to nonosteoporotic women. Bone zinc levels were also 28% lower.[52] Low zinc levels are also found in individuals with advanced jawbone loss. The Rancho Bernardo Study of community dwelling men ages 46 to 92 years reported that dietary zinc intake and plasma concentrations were lower in men with osteoporosis at the hip and spine than in men without osteoporosis at these locations.[53] In another large study

($n = 6576$) of men aged 46 to 68 years, zinc intake in the lowest quintile (10 mg/d) doubled the risk of fractures compared to those in the highest quintile.[54]

Zinc interacts with other nutrients. Large quantities of ingested zinc can interfere with copper bioavailability. Clinical signs of copper deficiency have been documented in individuals taking 150 mg zinc for 2 years. Lower, more typical zinc intake does not affect copper absorption. On the other hand, high copper intakes create a relative zinc deficiency. Supplemental iron inhibits zinc absorption.[55] The Institute of Medicine therefore recommends that all pregnant women receiving more than 60 mg/d of iron also take supplemental zinc. High levels of dietary calcium can impair zinc absorption in animals, and perhaps in humans.[56–58]

While it is held that there is no specific zinc "store" in the body, high dietary zinc increases bone, liver and intestinal zinc levels. Release of zinc from these tissues during depletion may slow the rate of onset of zinc deficiency symptoms. The zinc deficiency induced reduction in cell division and resulting impaired growth may be an adaptive process and represent accommodation to zinc deficit. By reducing growth, including bone protein matrix growth, and by drawing zinc from bone and skeletal muscle, more zinc is made available for critical zinc-dependent metabolic processes.[55] Zinc's important role in maintaining the structure of transcriptional factors and regulating gene expression provides a strong rationale for zinc conservation, and good reason the body might sacrifice bone and muscle zinc in times of deficiency. Just as the body prioritizes the metabolic function of bone over structural functions of bone and gives of is calcium, phosphorus and buffering compound reserves, bone may well also offer trace minerals for systemic use at its own expense. Therefore, marginal zinc nutrient deficiency may adversely impact bone long before manifestation of clinical deficiency.

The current RDA for zinc is 11 mg/d for men and 8 mg/d for women. Zinc inadequacies are common in the United States, particularly among children. While zinc intakes are marginal worldwide, zinc is lost in food processing and depleted by stress and also ejaculated semen. A simple clinical test for zinc adequacy involves the zinc taste test. The perception of the taste of zinc varies according to zinc status. Those with adequate zinc stores note a metallic taste of a zinc solution, while those with inadequate stores of this mineral experience no taste.

COPPER

The adult human body contains only about 50 to 120 mg copper. Approximately one third of body copper stores are in bone, one third in muscle, and one third in liver and brain combined. Insufficient copper leads to anemia, neutropenia, osteoporosis, skeletal abnormalities, and fractures across species. Although severe copper deficiency in humans is rare, a role for copper in the maintenance of human bone health has been determined from observations of osteoporosis in infants recovering from malnutrition, and preterm infants born with inadequate copper reserves. Throughout the lifespan severe copper deficiency is known to cause skeletal abnormalities.

Much of the action of copper in bone health relates to its role as a cofactor in the lysyl oxidase enzyme. This enzyme is copper containing and catalyzes the cross-linking of lysine and hydroxyproline in collagen and elastin. Thus copper aids in the formation of collagen for bone and connective tissue and contributes to the mechanical strength of bone collagen fibrils. Copper also aids in the inhibition of bone resorption through its action as a cofactor for superoxide dismutase. Superoxide dismutase is a copper and zinc containing antioxidant, which neutralizes superoxide radicals produced by osteoclasts during bone resorption.[58]

Copper deficiency results in decreased bone strength in animal studies and inadequate copper levels have been associated with the development of osteoporosis in humans. Copper supplementation (3 mg/d) halted vertebral trabecular bone loss in a placebo-controlled study of middle-aged Irish women (ages 45 to 56 years).[59] Copper, in combination with supplemental calcium, zinc and manganese, increased bone mineral density in two studies of postmenopausal women.[51,60]

High calcium and phosphorus intakes lower copper retention. Additionally, high dose supplementation with zinc and iron can contribute to marginal copper deficiency as might possibly high dose vitamin C and a high fructose intake.[61] The average intake of copper in the United States is below the RDA of 900 μg and it has been suggested that the usual copper intake is marginal and may not support optimum health.

BORON

Boron is a mineral found in substantial amounts in many fruits, vegetables, and beans. Populations with traditional whole food diets may consume up to 10 mg/d as compared with current U.S. intake of 0.50 to 1 mg/d. Animal studies suggest boron enhances bone strength. Early human studies[10] showed 3 mg boron supplementation reduced urine excretion of calcium, magnesium, and phosphorus and increased estrogen and testosterone levels. The mineral-sparing effect of boron appears greatest when intake of magnesium is low. Even though further research is needed to verify and amplify these original observations, increasing boron consumption to at least 3 mg from fruits, vegetables, nuts, beans, and supplements is advisable.

POTASSIUM

The role of potassium in bone health relates to the ability of alkalizing potassium compounds to neutralize metabolic acids. The deleterious impacts of chronic low-grade metabolic acidosis on bone, and the bone-enhancing neutralizing effects of potassium salts, have been documented by several researchers and are discussed in the following section on base-forming foods.

The skeleton serves as an important reservoir of alkaline salts for the maintenance of critical acid-base balance. Less well known is the fact that the initial skeletal response to an acid load involves not bone calcium, but bone carbonate, sodium, and potassium. In the first line of buffering defense protons are taken up into bone and in exchange sodium and potassium are released. Calcium is lost after other bone ions are depleted.[62,63]

Fruits and vegetables provide mineral salts with alkalizing anions useful for neutralizing net endogenous acid production. If these mineral salts are not consumed in adequate amounts, alkalizing bone mineral compounds are drawn upon to help reduce low-grade metabolic acidosis, causing increased bone resorption and enhanced loss of minerals in the urine. Dietary potassium can offset excretion of absorbed calcium to such an extent that calcium authority Dr. Heaney reports that eating one medium baked potato or one large banana can conserve about 60 mg of calcium. Further, recent research by Frassetto and colleagues at the University of California reports the long-term sustained benefits of potassium bicarbonate supplementation. Women receiving potassium bicarbonate supplementation experienced decreased urine calcium loss during the entire three year study period. Those with the highest baseline losses experienced the greatest decreases.[64] Other researchers have found that potassium citrate supplementation attenuated the effects of increased dietary salt on calcium loss.[24]

Vegetables and fruits are high in potassium. Several studies have now found a positive association between fruit and vegetable intake and bone mineral density.[65–67] Urinary potassium as a marker of potassium intake is positively associated with BMD in children.[68,69] In addition to promoting an alkaline environment, a diet high in fruits, vegetables, and legumes provides nutrients such as vitamin C and quercetin, which also promote bone health. Increasing vegetable and fruit intake is the preferred way to increase potassium. The current U.S. adequate intake (AI) for potassium is 4700 mg/d. The average adult daily potassium intake in the United States is below the AI and is reported to average around 2200 mg for women and 3200 mg for men, primarily due to inadequate intake of fruits and vegetables.

VITAMINS

Vitamins A, C, D, K, and folic acid (a B vitamin) are known to be essential for bone health. Vitamin levels can be determined by functional laboratory tests. Vitamin D testing is elaborated by Dr. Holick in his chapter on vitamin D. In addition to laboratory assays, vitamin C can be assessed by the patient with home urine test strips.[*] This chapter describes the vitamins' unique role in bone strength. Most patients' vitamin stores can be optimized with dietary recommendations as outlined in Table 25. 1 and Table 25.2, and simple multivitamin and mineral supplementation.

VITAMIN D

It has long been known that vitamin D is essential for the absorption of calcium and phosphorus and the subsequent development of normal bone health. Low

---

[*] A home urine test kit for vitamin C adequacy is available from the non-profit Osteoporosis Education Project (OEP) at www.betterbones.com in the OEP store section.

vitamin D results in decreased intestinal calcium absorption and lowered serum calcium, which, in turn, triggers increased parathyroid hormone production. Parathyroid hormone stimulates increases in bone resorption and intestinal calcium absorption to normalize serum calcium concentration. A further action of parathyroid hormone is to increase renal clearance of phosphate. By these actions vitamin D deficiency can lead to both osteoporosis and osteomalacia.

The last few years have witnessed an unprecedented expansion of our knowledge about vitamin D and its relation to musculoskeletal and whole body health. In his chapter on vitamin D, Dr. Holick details this exciting new research. Presented here are key findings pertaining to osteoporosis. First, we now know that calcium absorption is optimized by higher than suspected levels of vitamin D. Specifically, it is now documented that healthy postmenopausal women with serum 25(OH)D levels averaging 86.5 nmol/l have calcium absorption efficiencies 65% greater than those with mean 25(OH)D levels of 50.1 nmol/l, even though both levels are within in the normal reference range.[70] Second, large randomized controlled trials have documented a significant reduction in fracture incidence among elderly given 800 IU D3 and calcium daily.

Chapuy and colleagues studied 3270 ambulatory elderly French women (mean age 84 years) with no serious medical conditions living in nursing homes or elderly apartments. Subjects were administered 1.2 g elemental calcium as tricalcium phosphate and 800 IU D3 daily. After the initial 18-month study period, there was a 43% reduction in hip fractures and a 32% reduction in all non-vertebral factures in the calcium and D group as compared to placebo. These benefits were sustained as an extension study ended with a 30% reduction in hip fractures and a 24% reduction in all nonverteral fractures at 36 months.[42] In a second placebo-controlled, randomized intervention study Dawson-Hughes and colleagues studied 389 healthy U.S. community dwelling women and men aged 65 years and older. Subjects were given 700 IU vitamin D3 and 500 mg elemental calcium as calcium citrate-malate in a 3-year study. The endpoints of the study were nonvertebral fractures and BMD changes. At 3 years the nonvertebral factures were reduced by 60%.[71]

Vitamin C

Vitamin C is required for the hydroxylation of lysine and proline necessary for collagen formation. Ascorbate also appears to stimulate osteoblast functioning, enhance calcium absorption, and enhance vitamin D's effect on bone metabolism and adrenal functioning. Epidemiological studies report a positive association between vitamin C intake and bone density[72] and those with the lowest vitamin C levels have been seen to lose bone at a greater rate than those with higher levels.[73] Additionally, a small U.S. cross-sectional study of elderly women ($N = 150$) found those with osteoporosis had markedly decreased antioxidant defenses as measured by vitamins C, A, and plasma glutathione peroxidase.[74]

As a premier antioxidant, vitamin C appears to protect bone against oxidant-mediated bone loss, particularly in current smokers. A large Swedish study found a three-fold increase in risk of hip fracture in current smokers with low intake of vitamins C and E.[75] Also vitamins C and E antioxidants were shown capable of nearly eliminating the structural damage to bone caused by heparin administration.[76]

While the RDA for vitamin C is minimal at 75 to 90 mg, there is a great deal of variation in individual biochemical need for this nutrient. Bleeding gums and bruising without cause are likely signs of inadequate vitamin C nutrition. Doses of 1000 to 3000 mg oral vitamin C generally correct these symptoms.

VITAMIN A

Deficiency of vitamin A limits calcium absorption, and results in a reduced number of osteoclasts. One might therefore conclude that vitamin A always promotes bone strength. This is not the case as presented by a landmark study in 1998. A Swedish population study with postmenopausal women reported an association between higher vitamin A intake and hip fracture risk.[77] Three of four cohort studies on vitamin A exposure and fracture suggested excess vitamin A exposure to be a risk factor for fracture.[78] New and colleagues suggest the proposed detrimental effect of vitamin A on bone could reflect a negative impact of oxidized fatty acids.[79] Overall, because the intake of vitamin A varies between countries and between studies, it is not yet possible to define an intake threshold associated with harm, although a recent Swedish fracture study among men suggests that serum retinal levels greater than 86 μg/dl may increase the risk of fracture. Barker and Blumsohn[80] offer a comprehensive review of the vitamin A skeletal health studies.

VITAMIN K

The only known role of vitamin K within the body is that of the required coenzyme for the conversion glutamic acid into gamma-carboxlyglutamic acid (Gla). Until the mid-1970s this coenzyme function was considered important only for blood coagulation. Now it is known that the vitamin K dependent γ-carboxylation process is important for the formation and proper functioning of the bone protein osteocalcin. If osteocalcin is properly carboxylated more mineral compounds are bound on to bone. If osteocalcin is undercarboxylated, bone is weakened and more susceptible to low trauma facture. Osteocalcin is the most studied Gla protein and the major noncollagenous bone protein.

Vitamin K deficiency prevents carboxylation of the Gla proteins, including osteocalcin. Vitamin K supplementation reduces under-carboxylated osteocalcin (ucOC), reduces urinary calcium excretion and decreases fracture risk. Several population studies correlate low vitamin K intakes and high ucOC with higher fracture rates. The large European EPIDOS Study found under-carboxylated osteocalcin (the measure of vitamin K adequacy) to be a major independent risk factor for hip fracture among healthy elderly women. Further, those women with both low BMD and high ucOC had a 5.5 risk of hip fracture, as compared to those with only low BMD or high ucOC levels.[81] Data from the Framingham Heart

Study revealed that those women and men in the highest quintile of vitamin K intake (250 µg/d) had one third the risk of hip fracture as those in the lowest quintile (75 µg/d). The Nurses Health Study ($N = 72,732$) also reported that the women in the lowest quintile of vitamin K intake had an increased risk of hip fracture. Equally, a study of elderly French institutionalized women found ucOC, but not conventional calcium metabolism parameters, predicts the subsequent risk of hip fracture.[82] In support of this vitamin K fracture link, clinical research in England found substantially depressed circulating levels of vitamin K1 in individuals who had suffered osteoporotic fractures as compared to age-matched controls.[83]

To date there appears to be only one reported long-term clinical trial investigating phylloquinone supplementation and bone mineral density. In this 3-year study a dietary supplement containing 1 mg phylloquinone, calcium, and vitamin D significantly reduced bone loss at the femoral neck in postmenopausal women aged 50 to 60 years, compared to a placebo or a supplement containing just calcium and vitamin D. No beneficial effect, however, was seen on lumbar BMD.[84] It is possible, and has been previously suggested, that vitamin K reduces fracture risk without substantially increasing BMD, as reviewed by Booth et al.[85]

Vitamin K is not a single nutrient, but the name given to a group of vitamins of similar composition. The two main groups of vitamin K that occur naturally are K1 (phylloquinone) and K2 (menaquinone). Vitamin K1 is found in vegetables (mostly green ones) and K2 is produced by bacteria in both fermented foods and the intestinal tract. Approximately 50% of the daily requirement of vitamin K is supplied by the gut flora, if in healthy balance. Hydrogenation of plant oils, as discussed by Dr. Enig in her chapter on fats, appears to decrease the absorption and biological effect of vitamin K in bone. Vitamin K (menadione) in a synthetic form is not recommended for supplemental use.

While the American consumption of vitamin K ranges between 56 and 250 µg/d, a recent study suggests that 1000 µg of phylloquinone daily is associated with optimal carboxylation of osteocalcin.[86,87]

B Vitamins

Vitamin B12 is essential for proper functioning of osteoblast cells, and anemia has been associated with osteoporosis. Most recently, vitamins B6, B12, and folic acid have been added to the list of important bone-protecting nutrients because of their role in the detoxification of homocysteine. The association between homocysteine and bone strength is discussed by Dr. Lamb in the chapter on osteoporosis.

Essential Fatty Acids

As it appears, essential fatty acids (EFAs), particularly eicosapentanoic acid (EPA), increase calcium absorption from the gut, in part by enhancing the effects of vitamin D. In fact, vitamin D and the EFAs synergistically improve calcium absorption and balance. In EFA deficiency, the effect of vitamin D in stimulation of calcium absorption and active calcium transport is greatly reduced, indicating that EFAs are absolutely required for normal vitamin D effects. EFAs are also known to influence the hydroxylation of vitamin D in the kidneys.[88]

EFAs also regulate and reduce urinary calcium excretion, possibly by reducing production of the inflammatory prostaglandins. EFAs have also been found to increase calcium deposition in bone, not an unlikely finding given that bone calcification has an absolute requirement for the presence of lipids in the form of phospholipids. Finally, essential fatty acids also appear to improve bone strength, possibly by fomenting collagen synthesis. EFA deficiency has been associated with loss of normal synthesis of bone connective tissue matrix, loss of normal cartilage and bone demineralization. The ratio of omega n-3 and n-6 fatty acids is important for inflammation reduction, heart and bone health, and that our contemporary diet contains an abundance of n-6 fats and a scarcity of n-3 fats. A recent study suggests that between 0.5 and 1 g/d of EPA plus DHA is an effective dose for reducing cardiovascular disease.[89] For bone, small human studies have seen benefits on 2 to 4 g of fish oils, containing approximately 666 to 1333 mg omega-3 fats. Increasing consumption of fish, fresh ground flax seed, and high-quality cod liver oil and other fish oils are a practical, safe way of increasing omega n-3 intake.

BASE-FORMING FOODS

Bone, and the hydration layer around bone, provides the only substantial reservoir of base available to titrate excess metabolic acids. For example, bone stores 99% of the body's calcium, 80% of its carbonate and citrate, 53 to 80% of the magnesium, and 35% of the sodium in various compounds. These buffering compounds are available for rapid exchange with the general extracellular fluid (ECF). The ECF of bone, for example, contains a potassium concentration 25 times that of general ECF, and thus is a major source from which the body can draw potassium. It is now documented that these base compounds found in bone provide a large reservoir of alkali readily available for the preservation of critical pH homeostasis.[63] Most explicitly, Bushinsky and colleagues have documented the mechanisms by which calcium, sodium, and carbonate are lost from bone in response to even a minor shift to a less alkaline pH. Also it is now clear that diet can influence systemic pH. The typical Western diet carries with it an excess of dietary acid precursors and a deficiency of base-precursors sufficient to cause a condition of chronic, low-grade metabolic acidosis.[29,90–92]

Foods are acid-forming because in the process of their being metabolized free hydrogen ions are generated. In general, meats, grains, sugar, flour, legumes, and dairy are acid-forming. Base-precursor foods are those whose final metabolic end products include a source of bicarbonate.[93] In general, vegetables, fruits, spices, nuts, and seeds are alkalinizing. This concept of biochemistry concerning the metabolic effect of foods is confusing and not always as it might appear. For

TABLE 25.3
Potential renal acid load (PRAL) of selected foods

Food or food group	PRAL (mEq/100 g edible portion)	Food or food group	PRAL (mEq/100 g edible portion)
Fruit and fruit juices		Dairy products and eggs	
Apples	−2.2	Milk (whole, pasteurized)	0.7
Bananas	−5.5	Yogurt (whole milk, plain)	1.5
Grape juice	−1.0	Cheddar cheese (reduced fat)	26.4
Lemon juice	−2.5	Cottage cheese	8.7
Orange	−2.7	Eggs (whole)	8.2
Vegetables		Whey	−1.6
Broccoli	−1.2	Meat and fish	
Carrots	−4.9	Beef (lean only)	7.8
Potatoes	−4.0	Chicken (meat only)	8.7
Onions	−1.5	Pork (lean only)	7.9
Zucchini	−4.6	Cod	7.1
Grain products:		Salmon	9.4
Bread (white wheat)	3.7	Beverages	
Cornflakes	6.0	Beer (draft)	−0.2
Rice (white)	4.6	Mineral water (Apollinaris)	−1.8
Spaghetti (white)	6.5	Red wine	−2.4
Wheat flour	8.2	White wine (dry)	−1.2

Notes:

1. Food with a negative value (mEq/100 g) exerts a base effect.
2. Food with a positive value (mEq/100 g) exerts an acid effect.
3. Calculations by Remer and Manz.[93] Copyright Institute for Prevention and Nutrition, D-85737 Ismaning.

example, some base-forming foods are acidic by the pH litmus-paper testing used in inorganic chemistry. Lemon is an example. Place litmus paper in lemon juice and the pH reading is acidic, however, send it through the human biochemical pathways and it emerges as bicarbonate-producing, metabolically base-forming food. A sample listing of base- and acid-forming foods is provided in Table 25.3.

Adults who consume a Western diet generate approximately 1 milliequivalent of acid/kg/d.[92,94] The acid load reduces carbonate buffers, as a result pH drops and low-grade metabolic acidosis ensues. Additional buffering is recruited from the hydration shell around bone and then from bone crystal itself.[95]

A variety of population-based studies now document the association between high intake of base-forming foods with bone mass, rates of bone loss, and fracture incidence. A beneficial effect on bone mass of fruit and vegetable intake, and the potassium and magnesium provided by these foods, has been shown in premenopausal, perimenopausal, postmenopausal, elderly women, and girls. Studies also indicated a similar beneficial effect for men.[96,97] Further, a large cross-cultural survey by Frassetto and colleagues found that the worldwide incidence of hip fracture varied directly with total protein and animal protein intake and inversely with vegetable protein intake. Those countries in the lowest third of hip fracture incidence had the lowest animal protein consumption and invariably the vegetable protein consumption exceeded the country's corresponding intake of animal protein.[23]

Double blind, placebo-controlled research shows that the increased urinary calcium loss and bone resorption caused by high sodium intake is reversible with potassium bicarbonate supplementation (90 mmol/d), the amount equivalent to seven or eight servings of potassium-rich fruits and vegetables. Net endogenous acid load was also neutralized on this amount of potassium citrate.[98] The DASH Intervention Trial found that simply increasing fruits and vegetables from 3.6 to 9.5 servings a day decreased urinary calcium excretion from 157 to 110 mg/d.[99] In a small intervention study Sebastian and colleagues[29] found that potassium promotes renal calcium retention. The administration of enough potassium bicarbonate to neutralize net endogenous acid loads resulted in improved calcium and phosphorus balance, increased serum osteocalcin (a marker of bone formation), and decreased urinary hydroxyproline (a marker of bone resorption).

Even though controlled clinical trials on the bone-enhancing effects of a diet high in fruits and vegetables are yet to be conducted, a large body of research documents the multifaceted health benefits of these food groups. Clinically, at a minimum, it is prudent to encourage a consumption of fruits and vegetables equal to that used in the DASH Intervention Trial, that is, 9.5 servings daily. This would provide for a total potassium intake near the current AI of 4700 mg potassium per day. It is additionally recommended to consume enough alkaline-forming foodstuffs to neutralize the individual's net endogenous acid production.

Net acid load can be approximated by measuring the pH of an "equilibrated urine," that is the first morning urine after at least 6 h sleep. This method was developed by Dr. Russell Jaffe[63] and verified by Whiting et al.[100] By this system a first morning urine pH reading of 6.5 to 7.5 suggests a favorable slightly alkaline pH tissue balance. Readings lower than 6.5 indicate low-grade metabolic acidosis. Consistent readings of 7.5 or above again suggest metabolic acidosis, but now from a catabolic state with associated tissue breakdown accompanied by the use of ammonia as a strong buffer. For an extended discussion you are referred to Brown and Jaffe.[63] An informative home urine pH test kit is available as per below.*

PHYTOESTROGENS

Phytoestrogen compounds are found in more than 300 plants and mimic estrogens in selected ways. The main phytoestrogens include isoflavones (as

---

*A pH test kit is available for the nonprofit Osteoporosis Education Project at www.betterbones.com under "OEP store," or 888-206-7119.

genistein, diadzein, and quercetin), coumestans, and lignans. The category of foods containing plant compounds known as phytoestrogens, and the isolated phytoestrogens themselves, are often suggested to promote bone health.

Because of their estrogen-like phenolic ring structure phytoestrogens may act as estrogen agonists or antagonists. Given this estrogen-like structure, and the lower fracture incidence among Asian populations consuming diets high in soy isoflavones, the soy isoflavones (genistein and diadzein) have been widely studied. Their mechanisms of action have been explored, dietary intake levels correlated with BMD and intervention studies conducted with conflicting results.

Some studies report isoflavones exert a minimal effect of slowing bone loss, but few have reported any gains in BMD. In one early study, pharmacological doses of 90 mg soy isoflavones (levels well exceeding Asian dietary intake) slightly increased spinal bone density, but not hip or total density, in post-menopausal women.[101] The largest, most controlled, and most recent inter-vention study found no benefits to the bone density of the spine or hip of postmenopausal women from supplementation with soy protein containing 99 mg isoflavones.[102]

As a word of caution it should be noted that super-dietary levels of isoflavone supplementation may carry important risks. Selected cell, animal and human studies document that isoflavone (as genistein) metabolites can act as an estrogen and play a role in tumor initiation and cell proliferation within estrogen-sensitive organs, particularly the breast. Moderate use of soy foods, particularly fermented soy foods as used in the Orient, seems prudent, while the safety of high-dose isoflavone supplements is unclear.

Ipriflavone is a synthetic isoflavone developed in Hungary from a research project looking for essential growth factors in animals. Between 1989 and 2000 there were reported 31 human clinical studies on ipriflavone and bone, conducted mainly in Italy and Japan.[103,104] The largest controlled intervention trial did not find ipriflavone (200 mg, thrice a day) to improve bone density or reduce fracture risk.[105] Since 12% of the 234 women using ipriflavone developed lymphopenia, compared to one woman among 240 in the control group, women using ipri-flavone should be monitored for WBC changes and those with lymphopenia should not use this compound.

WATER

Water is a nutrient upon which the body is totally dependent. By weight water comprises 60 to 70% of the body, and 25% of bone. In his chapter on water, Dr. Batmanghelidj offers additional perspective. Water insufficiency, he suggests, leads to histamine activated stimulation of PGE with increased PGE2 activity and increased bone resorption. As calcium is removed from the bone, collagen is exposed and made vulnerable for breakdown. Water reduces acidity and may also generate a form of hydroelectric energy across the cell membrane.

ANTINUTRIENTS

SALT (NaCl)

The movement of calcium and sodium through the renal tubules are intimately linked and a direct relationship exists between urinary sodium and calcium excretion. A high NaCl intake is considered deleterious to bone health by most, but not all authorities,[106] although some individuals show more pronounced effects than others.

It is estimated that on average, for every 500 mg increment in sodium intake, there is a 10 mg increase in urinary calcium loss. Given an average 25% calcium absorption rate, calcium intake must be raised 40 mg to compensate for a 500 mg increment in salt intake to compensate for calcium lost in the urine. High salt intake has been associated with reduced peak bone mass in children and a higher rate of bone mineral loss in postmenopausal women. Further, a study of postmenopausal women found an increasingly negative change in hip bone density with higher levels of urinary sodium (which can be equated with sodium intake). No bone loss occurred at the total hip site on a calcium intake of 1768 mg/d (44 nmol/d) or a urine sodium excretion of 2110 mg/d (92 nmol/d).[107] Reducing excessively high sodium intake appears to be an effective means of decreasing calcium loss, and thus calcium need, in both children and adults.

In the United States, salt intake averages 4000 to 4500 mg/d, but a more moderate intake of 2400 mg (one teaspoon or less) is generally recommended, particularly if the diet provides less than the AI for potassium as does the standard American diet.

CAFFEINE

Caffeine is a diuretic and stimulant that causes a short-term increase in urine calcium excretion and is linked by some studies, but not all, to increased bone mineral loss and susceptibility to fracture. The urinary loss of calcium from moderate caffeine consumption is generally held to be minor and easily compensated for by an increase in calcium intake. The negative impact of caffeine on calcium balance is more significant for those with low calcium intakes and high caffeine consumption. A study of postmenopausal women reported that consumption of two or more cups of coffee per day was associated with a lower bone mass in those who did not drink milk on a daily basis.[108] Further, a recent prospective study of elderly U.S. women reported that those who consumed 300 mg caffeine per day (equivalent to three 6-ounce cups of coffee) had a significantly higher rate of bone loss in the spine than those in the low-caffeine group.[109] Coffee consumption greater than two cups a day has also been associated with greater risk of hip fracture in elderly women.[110] Danish researchers report that coffee in excess of four cups a day could induce an extra urinary loss of 64 mg calcium per day.[111] Since only 25% of calcium is absorbed, an additional 256 mg/d of calcium would be needed to compensate for the caffeine-induced losses. Caffeine's potential to cause loss of other nutrients, or its contribution to chronic low-grade metabolic acidosis, has not been addressed.

ALCOHOL

High alcohol intake and alcoholism have long been identified as toxic to bone and associated with greatly increased fracture risk.[69] Moderate alcohol intake, however, does not appear to carry such risks and may benefit bone density.

SOFT DRINKS AND SODAS

Soft drinks consumption among U.S. children has increased from 5 to 12 fluid ounces per day between 1978 and 1998. Sodas increasingly replace water and nutrient dense beverages such as milk and juice. Caffeine, phosphoric acid, and sugar (and potentially artificial sweeteners) often contained in these beverages are adverse to bone health. With such a broad-sweeping public health topic focused on the nation's youth, one might expect that extensive research has been conducted. Yet, research is scant! A study of 14-year-old boys and girls reported a strong association between cola beverage consumption and bone fractures in girls (OR 3.59), but not in boys. In the same study, high dietary calcium consumption was protective of fractures.[112] In girls who consume soft drinks, a low calcium diet increases parathyroid hormone secretion, decreases bone mass, and increases fracture risk.[112–114] A study of Mexican children found a significant inverse correlation between soft drink consumption and serum calcium level.[115] Underlying causes for soft drinks' adverse effects include increased urine calcium loss from the associated caffeine and sugar; the additional acid load from the phosphoric acid components of colas and selected other soft drinks; and the displacement of water and more nutritious beverages from the diet.

MINERAL TOXINS

Heavy metals including mercury, cadmium, aluminum, and tin are human toxins commonly found as contaminants in the food and water of industrialized countries. Each has the potential to damage bone. See the chapter on xenobiotics by Dr. Jaffe.

Lead inhibits activation of vitamin D, limits calcium uptake, disrupts calcium-dependent signaling, and is directly toxic to osteoblasts and osteoclasts.[116] Bone is a repository for 90 to 95% of the lead in the body, where it displaces calcium. Thus, accelerated bone loss is accompanied by a release of lead into the blood. Several studies on American women have shown a significant increase in blood lead levels among all women during menopause as a result of bone breakdown freeing stored lead.[78,116,117] Animal studies suggest that high lead levels may distort BMD measurements. If this were shown to be true for humans it would be necessary to consider bone lead content when assessing bone density.[116]

Cadmium has a damaging effect on the kidneys and alters calcium metabolism. This toxic mineral can be found in pesticides, in the soil and air around cities and industrialized areas, in landfills, and in cigarette smoke.

Aluminum interferes with the mineralization process and modifies collagen production and bone formation in addition to lessening calcium resorption. Even small quantities of aluminum such as from aluminum-containing antacids can lead to negative calcium balance.[118] Major sources of aluminum exposure include aluminum-containing antacids, aluminum cookware and foil, tin cans, baking powder, food additives, soft water, and aluminum-containing antiperspirants, etc.

Tobacco

Tobacco use, whether ingested orally or smoked, is detrimental to bones in many ways and its use is associated with the development of osteoporosis, bone fracture, and tooth loss.[119–122]

SUMMARY CLINICAL GUIDELINES

- Encourage wholesome eating patterns, but keep in mind that nutritional supplementation is most often needed to assure adequate levels of all key bone nutrients.
- High-dose supplementation with a single nutrient such as calcium can be detrimental to the absorption of other minerals.
- Encourage daily consumption of 9 to 12 servings of fruits and vegetables to protect against bone erosion from chronic low-grade metabolic acidosis.
- Insure adequate protein consumption at the RDA level or somewhat above.
- If inadequate sunlight exposure is likely, start patients with 1000 IU of natural vitamin D3 and test the 25(OH)D level after 1 month of vitamin D3 use. Increase vitamin D supplementation in accordance with the test results, until nearing the high end of the normal range. This is reviewed by Dr. Holick.
- Consider the use of nutrient testing when nutrient status is questionable or the bone-building program ineffective. Useful tests include the D-penicillamine provocation test, RBC panels, and functional tests.
- The frail elderly are those at highest risk for fracture and those with lowest nutrient intakes. Increasing calories, protein, vitamin D, vitamins, and minerals reduces fracture risk and enhances fracture recovery among this population.

- Avoid bone antinutrients such as soft drinks, tobacco, excessive alcohol, excessive vitamin A, and exposure to toxic metals.
- A bone nutrition program is best implemented in conjunction with exercise and fall prevention program as discussed in the chapters on fractures and osteoporosis.

REFERENCES

1. Heaney, R.P., Bone biology in health and disease: a tutorial, in *Modern Nutrition in Health and Disease*, Shils, M.E., Olson, J.A., Shike, M., and Ross, C.A., Eds., Lippincott Williams & Wilkins, Baltimore, MD, 1999, pp. 1327–1338.
2. Frassetto, L., Morris, R.C., Jr., Sellmeyer, D.E., Todd, K., and Sebastian A., Diet, evolution and aging — the pathophysiologic effects of the post-agricultural inversion of the potassium-to-sodium and base-to-chloride ratios in the human diet, *Eur. J. Nutr.*, 200–213, 2001.
3. U.S. Department of Health and Human Services, *Bone Health and Osteoporosis: A Report of the Surgeon General*, U.S. Department of Health and Human Services, Office of the Surgeon General, Rockville, MD, 2004.
4. Morgan, K., Magnesium and calcium, *J. Am. Coll. Nutr.*, 4, 195–206, 1985.
5. Brown, J.E., *Nutrition Now*, 4th ed., Thomson Wadsworth, Belmont, CA, 2005.
6. Lakshmanan, F., Magnesium intakes, balances and blood levels of adults consuming self-selected diets, *Am. J. Clin. Nutr.*, 40, 1380–1389, 1984.
7. Pennington, J., Young, B., Wilson, D., Johnson, R., and Vanderveen, J., Mineral content of food and total diets: the selected minerals in foods survey, 1982 to 1984, *J. Am. Diet. Assoc.*, 86, 876–891, 1986.
8. Freeland-Graves, J., Manganese: an essential nutrient for humans, *Nutr. Today*, Nov./Dec., 13–19, 1988.
9. Klevay, L., Evidence of dietary copper and zinc deficiencies, *J. Am. Med. Assoc.*, 241, 1917–1918, 1979.
10. Nielsen, F., Hunt, C., and Mullen, L., Effect of dietary boron on mineral, estrogen, and testosterone metabolism in postmenopausal women, *FASEB J.*, 1, 394–397, 1987.
11. Hajjar, I.M., Grim, C.E., George, V., and Kotchen, T.A., Impact of diet on blood pressure and age-related changes in blood pressure in the US population: analysis of NHANES III, *Arch. Intern. Med.*, 161, 589–593, 2001.
12. http://www.pdrhealth.com/drug_info/nmdrugprofiles/nutsupdrugs/vit_0264.shtml.
13. Pao, E. and Mickle, S., Problem nutrients in the United States, *Food Technol.*, 58–64, 1981.
14. Feskanich, D., Singh, V., Willett, W.C., and Colditz, G.A., Vitamin A intake and hip fractures among postmenopausal women, *J. Am. Med. Assoc.*, 287, 47–54, 2002.
15. Serfontein, W.J., De Villiers, L.S., Ubbink, J., and Pitout, M.J., Vitamin B6 revisited. Evidence of subclinical deficiencies in various segments of the population and possible consequences thereof, *S. Afr. Med. J.*, 66, 437–441, 1984.
16. Booth, S.L. and Suttie, J.W., Dietary intake and adequacy of vitamin K, *J. Nutr.*, 128, 785–788, 1998.
17. Kakar, S. and Einhorn, T.A., Importance of nutrition in fracture healing, in *Nutrition and Bone Health*, Holick, M.F. and Dawson-Hughes, B., Eds., Humana Press, Totowa, NJ, 2004, pp. 85–103.

18. Rizzoli, R., Ammann, P., Bourrin, S., Chevalley, T., and Bonjour, J.P., Protein intake and bone homeostasis, in *Nutritional Aspects of Osteoporosis*, Burckhardt, P., Dawson-Hughes, B., and Heaney, R.P., Eds., Academic Press, San Diego, CA, 2001, 219–235.

19. Hannan, M.T., Tucker, K.L., Dawson-Hughes, B., Cupples, L.A., Felson, D.T., and Kiel, D.P., Effect of dietary protein on bone loss in elderly men and women: the Framingham Osteoporosis Study, *J. Bone Miner. Res.*, 15, 2504–2512, 2000.

20. Munger, R.G., Cerhan, J.R., and Chiu, B.C., Prospective study of dietary protein intake and risk of hip fracture in postmenopausal women, *Am. J. Clin. Nutr.*, 69, 147–152, 1999.

21. Hannan, M.T., Dietary protein and effects upon bone health in elderly men and women, in *Nutritional Aspects of Osteoporosis*, Burckhardt, P., Dawson-Hughes, B., and Heaney, R.P., Eds., Academic Press, San Diego, CA, 237–249, 2001.

22. Abelow, B.J., Holford, T.R., and Insogna, K.L., Cross-cultural association between dietary animal protein and hip fracture: a hypothesis, *Calcif. Tissue Int.*, 50, 14–18, 1992.

23. Frassetto, L.A., Todd, K.M., Morris. R.C., Jr., and Sebastian, A., Worldwide incidence of hip fracture in elderly women: relation to consumption of animal and vegetable foods, *J. Gerontol. A Biol. Sci. Med. Sci.*, 55, M585–M592, 2000.

24. Sellmeyer, D.E., Stone, K.L., Sebastian, A., and Cummings, S.R., A high ratio of dietary animal to vegetable protein increases the rate of bone loss and the risk of fracture in postmenopausal women. Study of Osteoporotic Fractures Research Group, *Am. J. Clin. Nutr.*, 73, 118–122, 2001.

25. Wengreen, H.J., Munger, R.G., West, N.A., et al., Dietary protein intake and risk of osteoporotic hip fracture in elderly residents of Utah, *J. Bone Miner. Res.*, 19, 537–545, 2004.

26. Eaton, S.B. and Nelson, D.A., Calcium in evolutionary perspective, *Am. J. Clin. Nutr.*, 54(1 Suppl.), 281S–287S, 1991.

27. Eaton, S.B. and Konner, M., Paleolithic nutrition. A consideration of its nature and current implications, *N. Engl. J. Med.*, 312, 283–289, 1985.

28. Sebastian, A., Frassetto, L.A., Sellmeyer, D.E., Merriam, R.L., and Morris, R.C., Jr., Estimation of the net acid load of the diet of ancestral preagricultural *Homo sapiens* and their hominid ancestors, *Am. J. Clin. Nutr.*, 76, 1308–1316, 2002.

29. Sebastian, A., Harris, S.T., Ottaway, J.H., Todd, K.M., and Morris, R.C., Jr., Improved mineral balance and skeletal metabolism in postmenopausal women treated with potassium bicarbonate, *N. Engl. J. Med.*, 330, 1776–1781, 1994.

30. Heaney, R.P. and Weaver, C.M., Calcium and vitamin D, *Endocrinol. Metab. Clin. North Am.*, 32, 181–194, vii–viii, 2003.

31. Prentice, A., What are the dietary requirements for calcium and vitamin D? *Calcif. Tissue Int.*, 70, 83–88, 2002.

32. Brown, S., *Better Bones, Better Body, A Comprehensive Self-Help Program for Preventing, Halting, and Overcoming Osteoporosis*, 2nd ed., Keats Publishing, Los Angeles, CA, 2000.

33. Melton, L. and Riggs, B., Epidemiology of age-related fractures, in *The Osteoporotic Syndrome: Detection, Prevention and Treatment*, Avioli, L., Ed., Grune and Stratton, New York, 1983, pp. 45–72.

34. Garn, S., Nutrition and bone loss: introductory remarks, *Fed. Proc.*, Nov./Dec., 1716, 1967.

35. Heaney, R.P., Calcium, dairy products and osteoporosis, *J. Am. Coll. Nutr.*, 19(2 Suppl), 83S–99S, 2000.

36. Cumming, R.G., Cummings, S.R., Nevitt, M.C., et al., Calcium intake and fracture risk: results from the study of osteoporotic fractures, *Am. J. Epidemiol.*, 145, 926–934, 1997.

37. Feskanich, D., Willett, W.C., Stampfer, M.J., and Colditz, G.A., Milk, dietary calcium, and bone fractures in women: a 12-year prospective study, *Am. J. Public Health*, 87, 992–997, 1997.

38. Michaelsson, K., Holmberg, L., Mallmin, H., et al., Diet and hip fracture risk: a case–control study. Study Group of the Multiple Risk Survey on Swedish Women for Eating Assessment, *Int. J. Epidemiol.*, 24, 771–782, 1995.

39. Strause, L., Saltman, P., Smith, K.T., Bracker, M., and Andon, M.B., Spinal bone loss in postmenopausal women supplemented with calcium and trace minerals, *J. Nutr.*, 124, 1060–1064, 1994.

40. Prentice, A., Diet, nutrition and the prevention of osteoporosis, *Public Health Nutr.*, 7, 227–243, 2004.

41. Heaney, R.P. and Nordin, B.E., Calcium effects on phosphorus absorption: implications for the prevention and co-therapy of osteoporosis, *J. Am. Coll. Nutr.*, 21, 239–244, 2002.

42. Chapuy, M.C., Arlot, M.E., Duboeuf, F., et al., Vitamin D3 and calcium to prevent hip fractures in the elderly women, *N. Engl. J. Med.*, 327, 1637–1642, 1992.

43. Rude, R.K., Magnesium deficiency: a possible risk factor for osteoporosis, in *Nutritional Aspects of Osteoporosis*, Burckhardt, P., Dawson-Hughes, B., and Heaney, R.P., Eds., Academic Press, San Diego, 2001, pp. 263–271.

44. Seelig, M.S., Altura, B.M., and Altura, B.T., Benefits and risks of sex hormone replacement in postmenopausal women, *J. Am. Coll. Nutr.*, 23, 482S–496S, 2004.

45. Stendig-Lindberg, G., Tepper, R., and Leichter, I., Trabecular bone density in a two year controlled trial of peroral magnesium in osteoporosis, *Magnes. Res.*, 6, 155–163, 1993.

46. Abraham, G.E., The importance of magnesium in the management of primary post-menopausal osteoporosis, *J. Nutr. Med.*, 2, 165–178, 1991.

47. Strause, L.G. and Saltman, P., Role of manganese in bone metabolism, in *Nutritional Bioavailability of Manganese*, Kies, C., Ed., American Chemical Society, Washington, DC, 1987, p. 46.

48. Strause, L.G., Hegenauer, J., Saltman, P., Cone, R., and Resnick, D., Effects of long-term dietary manganese and copper deficiency on rat skeleton, *J. Nutr.*, 116, 135–141, 1986.

49. Slemenda, C.W., Hui, S.L., Longcope, C., Wellman, H., and Johnston, C.C., Jr., Predictors of bone mass in perimenopausal women. A prospective study of clinical data using photon absorptiometry, *Ann. Intern. Med.*, 112, 96–101, 1990.

50. Reginster, J.Y., Strause, L.G., Saltman, P., and Franchimont, P., Trace elements and postmenopausal osteoporosis: a preliminary study of decreased serum manganese, *Med. Sci. Res.*, 116, 337–338, 1988.

51. [Vitrum osteomag in prevention of osteoporosis in postmenopausal women: results of the comparative open multicenter trial], *Ter. Arkh.*, 76, 88–93, 2004.

52. Atik, O.S., Zinc and senile osteoporosis, *J. Am. Geriatr. Soc.*, 31, 790–791, 1983.

53. Hyun, T.H., Barrett-Connor, E., and Milne, D.B., Zinc intakes and plasma concentrations in men with osteoporosis: the Rancho Bernardo Study, *Am. J. Clin. Nutr.*, 80, 715–721, 2004.

54. Elmstahl, S., Gullberg, B., Janzon, L., Johnell, O., and Elmstahl, B., Increased incidence of fractures in middle-aged and elderly men with low intakes of phosphorus and zinc, *Osteoporos. Int.*, 8, 333–340, 1998.

55. King, J.C. and Keen, C.L., Zinc, in *Modern Nutrition in Health and Disease*, Shils, M.E., Olson, J.A., Shike, M., and Ross, C.A., Eds., Lippincott Williams & Wilkins, Baltimore, MD, 1999, pp. 223–239.

56. Dawson-Hughes, B., Seligson, F.H., and Hughes, V.A., Effects of calcium carbonate and hydroxyapatite on zinc and iron retention in postmenopausal women, *Am. J. Clin. Nutr.*, 44, 83–88, 1986.

57. Wood, R.J. and Zheng, J.J., High dietary calcium intakes reduce zinc absorption and balance in humans, *Am. J. Clin. Nutr.*, 65, 1803–1809, 1997.

58. Lowe, N.M., Fraser, W.D., and Jackson, M.J., Is there a potential therapeutic value of copper and zinc for osteoporosis? *Proc. Nutr. Soc.*, 61, 181–185, 2002.

59. Eaton-Evans, J., McIlrath, E.M., Jackson, W.E., McCartney, H., and Strain, J.J., Copper supplementation and the maintenance of bone mineral density in middle-aged women, *J. Trace Elem. Exp. Med.*, 9, 87–94, 1996.

60. Strause, L., Saltman, P., Smith, K., and Andon, M., The role of trace elements in bone metabolism, in *Nutritional Aspects of Osteoporosis*, Burckhardt, P. and Heaney, R., Eds., Raven Press, New York, 1991, 223–233.

61. Turnlund, J.R., Copper, in *Modern Nutrition in Health and Disease*, Shils, M.E., Olson, J.A., Shike, M., and Ross, C.A., Eds., Lippincott Williams & Wilkins, Baltimore, MD, 1999, 241–252.

62. Bushinsky, D., Acid–base and the skeleton, in, *Acid–Base Metabolism: Nutrition — Health — Disease*, Oct. 6–7, 2000, Welhenstephan, Germany.

63. Brown, S. and Jaffe, R., Acid-alkaline balance and its effect on bone health, *Int. J. Integr. Med.*, 2, 7–15, 2000.

64. Frassetto, L., Morris, R.C., Jr., and Sebastian, A., Long-term persistence of the urine calcium-lowering effect of potassium bicarbonate in postmenopausal women, *J. Clin. Endocrinol. Metab.*, 90, 831–834, 2005.

65. Tucker, K.L., Hannan, M.T., Chen, H., Cupples, L.A., Wilson, P.W., and Kiel, D.P., Potassium, magnesium, and fruit and vegetable intakes are associated with greater bone mineral density in elderly men and women, *Am. J. Clin. Nutr.*, 69, 727–736, 1999.

66. New, S.A., Robins, S.P., Campbell, M.K., et al., Dietary influences on bone mass and bone metabolism: further evidence of a positive link between fruit and vegetable consumption and bone health? *Am. J. Clin. Nutr.*, 71, 142–151, 2000.

67. New, S.A. and Millward, D.J., Calcium, protein, and fruit and vegetables as dietary determinants of bone health, *Am. J. Clin. Nutr.*, 77, 1340–1341, 2003, author reply 1.

68. Jones, G., Riley, M.D., and Whiting, S., Association between urinary potassium, urinary sodium, current diet, and bone density in prepubertal children, *Am. J. Clin. Nutr.*, 73, 839–844, 2001.

69. New, S.A., Food groups and bone health, in *Nutrition and Bone Health*, Holick, M.F. and Dawson-Hughes. B., Eds., Humana Press, Totowa, NJ, 2004, pp. 235–248.

70. Heaney, R.P., Dowell, M.S., Hale, C.A., and Bendich, A., Calcium absorption varies within the reference range for serum 25-hydroxyvitamin D, *J. Am. Coll. Nutr.*, 22, 142–146, 2003.

71. Dawson-Hughes, B., Harris, S.S., Krall, E.A., and Dallal, G.E., Effect of calcium and vitamin D supplementation on bone density in men and women 65 years of age or older, *N. Engl. J. Med.*, 337, 670–676, 1997.

72. Weber, P., The role of vitamins in the prevention of osteoporosis — a brief status report, *Int. J. Vitam. Nutr. Res.*, 69, 194–197, 1999.

73. Kaptoge, S., Welch, A., McTaggart, A., et al., Effects of dietary nutrients and food groups on bone loss from the proximal femur in men and women in the 7th and 8th decades of age, *Osteoporos. Int.*, 14, 418–428, 2003.

74. Maggio, D., Barabani, M., Pierandrei, M., et al., Marked decrease in plasma antioxidants in aged osteoporotic women: results of a cross-sectional study, *J. Clin. Endocrinol. Metab.*, 88, 1523–1527, 2003.

75. Melhus, H., Michaelsson, K., Holmberg, L., Wolk, A., and Ljunghall, S., Smoking, antioxidant vitamins, and the risk of hip fracture, *J. Bone Miner. Res.*, 14, 129–135, 1999.

76. Turan, B., Can, B., and Delilbasi, E., Selenium combined with vitamin E and vitamin C restores structural alterations of bones in heparin-induced osteoporosis, *Clin. Rheumatol.*, 22, 432–436, 2003.

77. Melhus, H., Michaelsson, K., Kindmark, A., et al., Excessive dietary intake of vitamin A is associated with reduced bone mineral density and increased risk for hip fracture, *Ann. Intern. Med.*, 129, 770–778, 1998.

78. Symanski, E. and Hertz-Picciotto, I. Blood lead levels in relation to menopause, smoking, and pregnancy history, *Am. J. Epidemiol.*, 141, 1047–1058, 1995.

79. Macdonald, H.M., New, S.A., Golden, M.H., Campbell, M.K., and Reid, D.M., Nutritional associations with bone loss during the menopausal transition: evidence of a beneficial effect of calcium, alcohol, and fruit and vegetable nutrients and of a detrimental effect of fatty acids, *Am. J. Clin. Nutr.*, 79, 155–165, 2004.

80. Barker, M.E. and Blumsohn, A., Is vitamin A consumption a risk factor for osteoporotic fracture? *Proc. Nutr. Soc.*, 62, 845–850, 2003.

81. Vergnaud, P., Garnero, P., Meunier, P.J., Breart, G., Kamihagi, K., and Delmas, P.D., Undercarboxylated osteocalcin measured with a specific immunoassay predicts hip fracture in elderly women: the EPIDOS Study, *J. Clin. Endocrinol. Metab.*, 82, 719–724, 1997.

82. Szulc, P., Chapuy, M.C., Meunier, P.J., and Delmas, P.D., Serum undercarboxylated osteocalcin is a marker of the risk of hip fracture in elderly women, *J. Clin. Invest.*, 91, 1769–1774, 1993.

83. Hart, J.P., Shearer, M.J., and Klenerman, L., et al., Electrochemical detection of depressed circulating levels of vitamin K1 in osteoporosis, *J. Clin. Endocrinol. Metab.*, 60, 1268–1269, 1985.

84. Braam, L.A., Knapen, M.H., Geusens, P., et al., Vitamin K1 supplementation retards bone loss in postmenopausal women between 50 and 60 years of age, *Calcif. Tissue Int.*, 73, 21–26, 2003.

85. Booth, S.L. and Charette, A.M., Vitamin K, oral anticoagulants, and bone health, in *Nutrition and Bone Health*, Holick, M.F. and Dawson-Hughes, B., Eds., Humana Press, Totowa, NJ, 2004, pp. 457–478.

86. Binkley, N.C., Krueger, D.C., Kawahara, T.N., Engelke, J.A., Chappell, R.J., and Suttie, J.W., A high phylloquinone intake is required to achieve maximal osteocalcin gamma-carboxylation, *Am. J. Clin. Nutr.*, 76, 1055–1060, 2002.

87. Knapen, M.H., Hamulyak, K., and Vermeer, C., The effect of vitamin K supplementation on circulating osteocalcin (bone Gla protein) and urinary calcium excretion, *Ann. Intern. Med.*, 111, 1001–1005, 1989.

88. Kruger, M.C. and Horrobin, D.F., Calcium metabolism, osteoporosis and essential fatty acids: a review, *Prog. Lipid Res.*, 36, 131–151, 1997.

89. Harris, W.S. and Von Schacky, C., The Omega-3 Index: a new risk factor for death from coronary heart disease? *Prev. Med.*, 39, 212–220, 2004.

90. Remer, T. and Manz, F., Estimation of the renal net acid excretion by adults consuming diets containing variable amounts of protein, *Am. J. Clin. Nutr.*, 59, 1356–1361, 1994.

91. Morris, R.C., Jr., Frassetto, L.A., Schmidlin, O., Forman, A., and Sebastian, A., Expression of osteoporosis as determined by diet-disordered electrolyte and acid–base metabolism, in *Nutritional Aspects of Osteoporosis*, Burckhardt, P., Dawson-Hughes, B., and Heaney, R.P., Eds., Academic Press, San Diego, CA, 2001, pp. 357–378.

92. Bushinsky, D.A., Acid–base balance and bone health, in *Nutrition and Bone Health*, Holick, M.F. and Dawson-Hughes, B., Eds., Humana Press, Totowa, NJ, 2004, pp. 279–304.

93. Remer, T. and Manz, F., Potential renal acid load of foods and its influence on urine pH, *J. Am. Diet. Assoc.*, 95, 791–797, 1995.

94. Kurtz, I., Maher, T., Hulter, H.N., Schambelan, M., and Sebastian, A., Effect of diet on plasma acid–base composition in normal humans, *Kidney Int.*, 24, 670–680, 1983.

95. Bushinsky, D.A., Acid–base imbalance and the skeleton, *Eur. J. Nutr.*, 40, 238–244, 2001.

96. New, S.A., Impact of food clusters on bone, in *Nutritional Aspects of Osteoporosis*, Burckhardt, P., Dawson-Hughes, B., and Heaney, R.P., Eds., Academic Press, San Diego, CA, 2001, pp. 379–398.

97. McGartland, C.P., Robson, P.J., and Murray, L.J., et al., Fruit and vegetable consumption and bone mineral density: the Northern Ireland Young Hearts Project, *Am. J. Clin. Nutr.*, 80, 1019–1023, 2004.

98. Sellmeyer, D.E., Schloetter, M., and Sebastian, A., Potassium citrate prevents increased urine calcium excretion and bone resorption induced by a high sodium chloride diet, *J. Clin. Endocrinol. Metab.*, 87, 2008–2012, 2002.

99. Appel, L.J., Moore, T.J., Obarzanek, E., et al., A clinical trial of the effects of dietary patterns on blood pressure. DASH Collaborative Research Group [see comments], *N. Engl. J. Med.*, 336, 1117–1124, 1997.

100. Whiting, S., Bell, J., and Brown, S.E., First morning urine measured with pH paper strips reflects acid excretion, *ASBMR Meetings Abstract*, San Antonio, 2002.

101. Potter, S.M., Baum, J.A., Teng, H., Stillman, R.J., Shay, N.F., and Erdman, J.W., Jr., Soy protein and isoflavones: their effects on blood lipids and bone density in postmenopausal women, *Am. J. Clin. Nutr.*, 68(6 Suppl), 1375S–1379S, 1998.

102. Kreijkamp-Kaspers, S., Kok, L., Grobbee, D.E., et al., Effect of soy protein containing isoflavones on cognitive function, bone mineral density, and plasma lipids in postmenopausal women: a randomized controlled trial, *J. Am. Med. Assoc.*, 292, 65–74, 2004.

103. Katase, K., Kato, T., Hirai, Y., Hasumi, K., and Chen, J.T., Effects of ipriflavone on bone loss following a bilateral ovariectomy and menopause: a randomized placebo-controlled study, *Calcif. Tissue Int.*, 69, 73–77, 2001.

104. Somekawa, Y., Chiguchi, M., Ishibashi, T., Wakana, K., and Aso, T., Efficacy of ipriflavone in preventing adverse effects of leuprolide, *J. Clin. Endocrinol. Metab.*, 86, 3202–3206, 2001.

105. Alexandersen, P., Toussaint, A., Christiansen, C., et al., Ipriflavone in the treatment of postmenopausal osteoporosis: a randomized controlled trial, *J. Am. Med. Assoc.*, 285, 1482–1488, 2001.

106. Cohen, A.J. and Roe, F.J., Review of risk factors for osteoporosis with particular reference to a possible aetiological role of dietary salt, *Food Chem. Toxicol.*, 38, 237–253, 2000.

107. Devine, A., Criddle, R.A., Dick, I.M., Kerr, D.A., and Prince, R.L., A longitudinal study of the effect of sodium and calcium intakes on regional bone density in post-menopausal women, *Am. J. Clin. Nutr.*, 62, 740–745, 1995.

108. Barrett-Connor, E.M.D., et al., Coffee-associated osteoporosis offset by daily milk consumption, *J. Am. Med. Assoc.*, 271, 280–283, 1994.

109. Rapuri, P.B., Gallagher, J.C., Kinyamu, H.K., and Ryschon, K.L., Caffeine intake increases the rate of bone loss in elderly women and interacts with vitamin D receptor genotypes, *Am. J. Clin. Nutr.*, 74, 694–700, 2001.

110. Kiel, D.P., Felson, D.T., Hannan, M.T., Anderson, J.J., and Wilson, P.W., Caffeine and the risk of hip fracture: the Framingham Study, *Am. J. Epidemiol.*, 132, 675–684, 1990.

111. Hasling, C., Sondergaard, K., Charles, P., and Mosekilde, L., Calcium metabolism in postmenopausal osteoporotic women is determined by dietary calcium and coffee intake, *J. Nutr.*, 122, 1119–1126, 1992.

112. Wyshak, G. and Frisch, R.E., Carbonated beverages, dietary calcium, the dietary calcium/phosphorus ratio, and bone fractures in girls and boys, *J. Adolesc. Health*, 15, 210–215, 1994.

113. Calvo, M.S., Kumar, R., and Heath, H., Persistently elevated parathyroid hormone secretion and action in young women after four weeks of ingesting high phosphorus, low calcium diets, *J. Clin. Endocrinol. Metab.*, 70, 1334–1340, 1990.

114. Wyshak, G., Teenaged girls, carbonated beverage consumption, and bone fractures [see comments], *Arch. Pediatr. Adolesc. Med.*, 154, 610–613, 2000.

115. Mazariegos-Ramos, E., Guerrero-Romero, F., Rodriguez-Moran, M., Lazcano-Burciaga, G., Paniagua, R., and Amato, D., Consumption of soft drinks with phosphoric acid as a risk factor for the development of hypocalcemia in children: a case–control study, *J. Pediatr.*, 126, 940–942, 1995.

116. Puzas, J.E., Campbell, J., O'Keefe, R.J., and Rosier, R.N., Lead toxicity in the skeleton and its role in osteoporosis, in *Nutrition and Bone Health*, Holick, M.F. and Dawson-Hughes, B., Eds., Humana Press, Totowa, NJ, 2004, pp. 363–376.

117. Silbergeld, E.K., Schwartz, J., and Mahaffey, K., Lead and osteoporosis: mobilization of lead from bone in postmenopausal women, *Environ. Res.*, 47, 79–94, 1988.

118. Gaby, A.R.P.D., *Preventing and Reversing Osteoporosis*, Prima Publishing, Rocklin, 1994.

119. Law, M.R. and Hackshaw, A.K., A meta-analysis of cigarette smoking, bone mineral density and risk of hip fracture: recognition of a major effect, *Br. Med. J.*, 315, 841–846, 1997.

120. Slemenda, C.W., Cigarettes and the skeleton, *N. Engl. J. Med.*, 330, 430–431, 1994.

121. Nguyen, T.V., Kelly, P.J., Sambrook, P.N., Gilbert, C., Pocock, N.A., and Eisman, J.A., Lifestyle factors and bone density in the elderly: implications for osteoporosis prevention, *J. Bone Miner. Res.*, 9, 1339–1346, 1994.

122. Molloy, J., Wolff, L.F., Lopez-Guzman, A., and Hodges, J.S., The association of periodontal disease parameters with systemic medical conditions and tobacco use, *J. Clin. Periodontol.*, 31, 625–632, 2004.

26 Osteoporosis

Joseph J. Lamb, M.D.

CONTENTS

Editor's Note

Osteoporosis often lies undetected until severe bone loss is revealed by a fracture. Many medications and medical conditions predictably compromise bone density and strength. Clinicians familiar with the pathophysiology of osteoporosis, the lifestyle-related risk factors, and the consequences of medical therapeutics can offer patients prevention and early treatment of a formerly silent disease.

OSTEOPOROSIS — A SILENT DISEASE

Osteoporosis, literally "porous bone," is a reduction in the mass and quality of bone or is the presence of a fragility fracture. Osteoporosis is:

- the most common of all bone diseases in adults affecting 50% of women and 33% of men during their lifetimes.
- A disease that results in high morbidity and even mortality. One year mortality after hip fracture can be as high as 12 to 20% and up to half of survivors require long-term nursing care.
- Preventable. Appropriate lifestyle choices and risk factor modification can prevent the development of osteoporosis in identified at-risk patients.
- Diagnosable. The early stages of bone loss known as osteopenia can be diagnosed and the progression to frank osteoporosis can be prevented.

These hard facts beg the question of why osteoporosis remains a silent disease. Osteoporosis is currently a profound individual health challenge for many women and men and will be a profound societal health challenge for the next generation. Our patients' lifestyle choices regarding diet, exercise, and nutritional supplementation certainly play a role in their predisposition to osteoporosis. Additionally, health insurers' failure to reimburse for DEXA screening certainly compromises screening efforts. Yet, we must also be aware of our role in educating patients regarding lifestyle, identifying early primary osteoporosis, and strongly pursing the causes of secondary osteoporosis if we are to intervene in this modifiable health risk.

Some have considered the first fracture "a lucky break" as it creates an opportunity to treat osteoporosis. Unfortunately, once lost, bone mineral density (BMD) is very difficult to replace. Primary osteoporosis causes a slow bone loss of approximately 2% per year.[1] Secondary osteoporosis, on the other hand, has a much faster rate of loss; up to 8% in the spine and 5% in the hip per year. This rate of loss is very similar to that of early menopause.[2]

NEW DEFINITIONS FOR NEW UNDERSTANDINGS OF THE DISEASE PROCESS

Mild bone loss or osteopenia has been defined as a reduction in bone density to levels between 1.0 and 2.5 standard deviations below the mean average of a healthy young population. More severe bone loss or osteoporosis has been defined as a bone density less than 2.5 standard deviations below the mean. This definition acknowledges only the quality of mineralization in evaluating bone health. The now current National Institute of Health consensus on osteoporosis

TABLE 26.1
Causes of secondary osteoporosis (bone loss with etiologies other than aging)

Etiologic categories	Secondary causes
Endocrine	Hyperparathyroidism; thyrotoxicosis; insulin-dependent diabetes mellitus; acromegaly; hyperprolactinemia; Cushing's syndrome; perimenopause/menopause and other estrogen deficiency states including prolonged hypothalamic amenorrhea and anorexia nervosa; pregnancy and lactation
Nutritional and gastrointestinal	Leanness, low calcium intake secondary to malnutrition; parenteral nutrition; gastric or small bowel resection; maladsorption syndromes; end-stage liver disease including biliary cirrhosis
Rheumatological	Rheumatoid arthritis and ankylosing spondylitis
Hematologic and oncologic	Pernicious anemia; multiple myeloma; lymphomas and leukemias; malignancy associated parathyroid hormone production; mastocytosis; hemophilia; thalassemia
Genetic predispositions	Caucasian or Asian race; positive family history; inherited hypogondal states (Turner's and Klinefelter's syndromes); other inherited states (osteogenesis imperfecta, Marfan's syndrome, hemochromatosis, hypophosphatasia, glycogen storage disease, homocystinuria, Ehlers–Danos syndrome, and porphyria)
Drug induced	Excessive thyroxine, glucocorticoids, anticonvulsants, heparin, lithium, cyclosporine, aluminum, cytotoxic drugs, proton pump inhibitors, and gonadotrophin releasing hormone agonists
Miscellaneous	Short stature and short bones; immobilization; chronic obstructive pulmonary disease; scoliosis; multiple sclerosis; sarcoidosis; amyloidosis; endogenous stress response

defines osteoporosis as a decrease in bone strength creating a predisposition to a fragility fracture. Both bone density and bone quality are key determinants of bone strength.[3] While a patient's bone density can be assessed with diagnostic imaging, bone quality assessment remains problematic.

Primary osteoporosis has generally been viewed as the general decline in bone mass in women associated with aging and has been considered a natural consequence of aging. Secondary osteoporosis has been conventionally defined in the allopathic field of medicine as the development of osteoporosis because of a primary illness or as a side effect of a medication used to treat an illness. The causes of secondary osteoporosis are myriad. Even the broad categories are many. In broad allopathic terms, etiologies we need to consider include endocrine, nutritional and gastrointestinal, rheumatologic, hematologic and oncologic, genetic predispositions, drug induced, and a miscellaneous category (see Table 26.1).

It is now recognized that primary osteoporosis actually affects both men and women and may not be a natural consequence of aging. Instead, many of the traditionally labeled modifiable risk factors including cigarette smoking, failure to exercise, poor nutrition, alcohol abuse, and loss of muscle mass with aging are consequences of lifestyle choices interacting with predisposing antecedents and as such are causes of secondary osteoporosis. Individuals who have made these choices or have a genetic predisposition may also suffer with secondary conditions that are associated with decreased bone mineralization or increased bone loss resulting in a mixed picture of primary and secondary osteoporosis.

PHYSIOLOGY

An important part of understanding the development of osteoporosis is to understand the factors involved in the formation of healthy bone. Bone is a vibrant, metabolically active tissue providing the structural framework necessary for strength and mobility while also acting as a mineral reservoir for basic biochemistry. The average life expectancy of an osteoclast is just 12 days before death by apoptosis. Osteoblasts have a broader range of life expectancy lasting from just a few days up to 100. A significant minority of osteoblasts transforms into osteocytes and bone lining cells while the majority die by apoptosis.

The outer compartment is the dense cortical or compact bone that provides much of bone's inherent strength. The interior compartment is trabecular or cancellous bone, which is highly cellular and is interlaced with bone marrow.[4]

Bone quality is a measure of the functional status of the nonmineral component of bone. This component, also called the organic matrix, is composed primarily of collagen fibers with a 5 to 10% mix of proteoglycans (chondroitin sulfate and hyaluronic acid) and a variety of proteins.[5] This matrix is the substrate for the deposition of calcium and phosphorus. Once mineralized, it is the framework of strong healthy bones. Disruption of the organic matrix marked by changes in the type I collagen matrix and alterations in cross-linking between collagen fibers is one of the causes of osteoporosis.[6]

Bone density is a function of the adequacy of mineralization and is regulated primarily by the activity of three cell types — osteoblasts, osteoclasts, and osteocytes. Osteoblasts differentiate from stromal cell precursors in bone marrow. The primary function of osteoblasts is to secrete the organic matrix. Many growth factors influence osteoblast formation including insulin-like growth factors (IGFs), fibroblast growth factors, and transforming growth factors. Core binding Factor A1 (CBfA1) is a transcription factor expressed in osteoblast progenitors and stromal support cells that has been shown to be important in the control of osteoblast development. It regulates the expression of several osteoblast-specific genes including type 1 collagen, receptor-activator of NFKappaB (RANK) ligand also called osteoclast differentiation factor, osteocalcin, osteopontin, and bone sialoprotein. Osteoblasts, through secretion of RANK ligand (RANKL), actually promote differentiation and maturation of osteoclasts.

Interestingly, osteoblasts secrete osteoprotegerin, also called osteoclastogenesis inhibitory factor, which binds RANKL and acts as a receptor decoy to inhibit differentiation of osteoclasts.[7]

The osteoclasts are multinucleated cells derived from hematopoietic stem cells in the bone marrow, and are the primary agents of bone resorption. Stromal support cells secrete macrophage colony stimulating factor and RANKL to promote osteoclast differentiation and maturation. Locally produced growth factors and cytokines including gamma interferon, interleukins 1, 6, and 11 (IL-1, IL-6, IL-11), and tumor necrosis factor (TNF) play an important role in this maturation process by stimulating secretion of RANKL.

Mature osteocytes direct bone remodeling by sensing the mechanical forces exerted on bone by physical activity. Osteocytes also monitor the health of bone and can identify dysfunctional bone that is in need of repair. Exactly how osteocytes, osteoblasts, and osteoclasts communicate is not entirely defined, but as the multiplicity of locally active messenger molecules suggests bone formation is most responsive to local influences and to a lesser degree systemic influences. Systemic control is exerted by the influence of both parathyroid hormone (PTH) and 1,25-dehydroxy-vitamin D_3 directly on osteoclastic activity to maintain appropriate serum calcium and phosphorus levels.

Estrogen is another systemic influence on bone metabolism. Estrogen deficiency increases bone remodeling intensity, which exacerbates propensity to bone resorption in functionally challenged bone and certainly contributes to the development of primary osteoporosis in perimenopausal women. Though some experimental evidence reveals direct effects of serum levels of DHEA on cortical BMD and free testosterone on trabecular BMD,[8] other studies have demonstrated intracellular activity of aromatases converting DHEA to estrone[9] and postulated the primary role of estrogen rather than androgens in bone regulation.[10]

This interaction of cells communicating by growth factors and cytokines is the healthy norm of bone metabolism. Osteoporosis is the pathophysiologic disturbance of this process. Indeed, calcium insufficiency alone results in a different pathological process called osteomalacia. Thus, osteoporosis is characterized by derangements of mineral metabolism, of the healthy cellular matrix, and of cell-to-cell messaging of osteoblasts, osteocytes, and osteoclasts.

PATHOPHYSIOLOGY

As we explore the pathophysiology of osteoporosis, we find that underlying mechanisms rather than broad organ system classifications may cast more light on the underlying causes of osteoporosis. These broad mechanistic categories include diminished achievement of peak bone mass, decreased mineral availability, decreased osteoblast activity, increased osteoclast activity, abnormal protein metabolism, and systemic inflammation.

The discussion of pathophysiology of osteoporosis is dependent on knowing the particulars of an individual's health status as certain conditions may be considered either primary and secondary or both. In a postmenopausal woman, estrogen deficiency is the consequence of ovarian failure and may certainly be considered primary, but in an adolescent girl receiving a GnRH agonist as contraception or a premenopausal woman receiving chemotherapy for breast cancer, one would certainly consider their estrogen deficiency to be a secondary cause of osteoporosis. Complicating the task of separating etiologies into pathological categories is that many disease entities have broad effects and influence multiple pathophysiologic pathways. Cushing's syndrome, though thought to primarily inhibit osteoblast activity, has diverse effects also including impairment of matrix development, impairment of bone mineralization, growth factor disturbances, and increased osteocyte apoptosis.[2]

DECREASED PEAK BONE MASS

Before adulthood, bone forms by two separate mechanisms. Endochondral bone formation, typically involving the epiphysial growth plates, is the restructuring and replacing of previously calcified cartilage. Intermembranous bone formation, as occurs in skull bones, is *de novo* development without a calcified matrix.[6] Modeling is the creation of new bone during growth and development through adolescence, which culminates in the achievement of peak bone mass and the characteristic and optimal shape and structure. After adolescence, endochondral formation ceases. Peak bone mass must be achieved during adolescence or future BMD will be compromised as even relatively small incremental losses will have a proportionately greater affect on a lower peak bone mass.

Despite radioisotope studies that have demonstrated that 18% of calcium in bone turnovers per year — a good marker for the persistent metabolic activity in bone postadolescence — bone remodeling is a much slower process in adulthood. Remodeling is the maintenance of homeostasis as metabolic activity repairs microdamage within the skeleton, maintains skeletal strength, and supplies calcium to maintain serum levels. Specific associations include:

- Adolescent eating disorders, including both anorexia and bulimia, are conditions associated with failure to achieve peak bone mass. In addition to decreased mineral and protein availability because of insufficient intake, contributing factors to osteoporosis include secondary estrogen deficiency, secondary hyperparathyroidism, increased endogenous steroid production, and low levels of growth factors including IGF. Special attention to these metabolic consequences is required as studies do not demonstrate a full return to normal BMD after resolution of anorexia even during adolescence.[11]
- Use of Depo-Provera as contraception produces estrogen deficiency. In adolescents who are anorexic or on Depo-Provera, the primary

bone effect is failure to achieve expected peak bone mass.[11] With calcium supplementation in adolescents, some of potential loss, but apparently not all, can be ameliorated.

- Lead intoxication. A study in children with high lead exposure revealed significantly increased bone mineral density compared to normal controls. Despite the potential for heavy metals creating a false negative result in DEXA scanning because of x-ray absorption by lead and not calcium, the investigators postulated that lead exposure may actually accelerate boney maturation by inhibition of PTH. However, they went on to conclude that the accelerated rate of bone maturation results in a shorter period to accomplish mineralization and growth with a resultant decreased peak bone mass.[12]

Decreased Mineral Availability

Conditions that decrease mineral uptake from the gastrointestinal tract include:

- Malabsorption syndromes. Primary biliary cirrhosis with its resultant underlying fat malabsorption has been shown to contribute to insufficiencies of fat-soluble vitamins, specifically vitamin D and vitamin K.[13] Celiac disease, once thought to be quite rare, is diagnosed with increasing frequency. An ongoing inflammatory process secondary to an allergy to gluten containing grains, including wheat, rye, oats, kamut, spelt, and barley, results in marked mineral and calorie malabsorption. Indeed, one study revealed that 12% of menopausal women actually have antigliaden antibodies suggestive of asymptomatic celiac disease. Food intolerances mediated by IgG food allergies create a similar clinical presentation.
- Bariatric surgery. Surgical treatment for obesity has been associated with the development of osteoporosis in the postoperative period. Several factors are likely involved. Primarily, malabsorption plays a critical role with malabsorption of calcium, magnesium, protein, fat-soluble vitamins including vitamin D, B_{12}, folic acid all being reported. Additionally, secretion of stomach acid may be decreased, which contributes to the malabsorption of calcium. Given that obesity is actually protective against osteoporosis, correction may unmask an indolent predilection toward osteoporosis. Studies have demonstrated a greater decrease in BMD in surgically treated obesity compared to medically treated obesity though the overall weight loss in the surgical patients has been greater.[14]
- Generalized malnutrition.
- Gastric hypoacidity because of atrophy, proton pump inhibitors, and H_2 blockers. Calcium must be ionized to be optimally absorbed and ionization of calcium requires an acidic environment. Reduced gastric

acidity contributes to the failure to ionize calcium in the small intestine and decreases the bioavailability of calcium. Calcium carbonate is much more vulnerable to being malabsorbed as opposed to other forms of calcium including citrate, lactate, and gluconate as it is not already ionized. Acid deficiency has been shown to contribute to decreased protein and vitamin B_{12} absorption as well. Forty percent of postmenopausal women have been shown to be acid deficient.[1] Advancing age combined with the growing use of H_2 blockers and proton pump inhibitors now available over the counter for dyspepsia contribute to the magnitude of the problem.

Other conditions increase excretion of minerals, including high sodium diets, caffeine, high protein diets (although they also contain high amounts of calcium), and carbonated soft drink consumption (see Chapter 25).

DECREASED OSTEOBLAST ACTIVITY

Conditions that decrease osteoblast activity resulting in less bone formation include:

- Diabetes mellitus. Type I diabetes mellitus (DM) has been implicated as a cause of osteoporosis, but the relationship is controversial. One proposed mechanism is decreased levels of insulin and IGF-1, which are important trophic factors for osteoblasts. Another possible mechanism is increased renal losses secondary to osmotic diuresis. Reports on osteoporosis in type II DM are inconsistent. Given the rapidly increasing prevalence of DM in our population, surveillance for osteoporosis in diabetics may be of great importance.[11]
- Tobacco abuse. Cigarette smoking has been associated with osteoporosis. Tobacco has direct toxic effects on osteoblasts and also acts indirectly by modifying estrogen metabolism. Cigarette smokers on average reach menopause approximately 1 to 2 years earlier than nonsmokers. Tobacco abuse also increase overall illness and general frailty by decreasing exercise capacity and increasing the possible need for corticosteroid treatment of chronic obstructive pulmonary disease.[15]
- Alcohol abuse. Excessive alcohol has been shown to decrease osteoblast activity. And yet several studies have shown that moderate consumption has positive impact on bone health.[16] Higher consumption, especially in men, however, increased the rate of fracture, perhaps related to increased falls or nutritional compromise related to alcohol abuse. One drink per day for women and two drinks per day for men is a safe upper limit for consumption.
- Corticosteroid excess, whether exogenous or endogenous. Cushing's syndrome and corticosteroid excess have many deleterious effects on

healthy bone including principally an effect of decreasing osteoblast activity.[17] The profound effect of steroid excess is demonstrated by noting that it is the most common cause of secondary osteoporosis and is second only to menopause as a cause of overall osteoporosis. Fifty percent of patients on chronic corticosteroid administration for 6 months or longer develop osteoporosis. In fact, a daily dose of 2.5 to 5.0 mg of prednisone may be sufficient to cause osteoporosis.[2] Cushing's disease (endogenous corticosteroid excess) has been associated with rapidly progressive coxarthropathy associated with avascular necrosis and osteoporosis of the femoral head.[18] The onset of duration from diagnosis of Cushing's disease to diagnosis of osteonecrosis has varied from 8 months to 11 years in one small study.[19] However, the diagnosis of osteoporosis has also been presenting symptoms of Cushing's disease. Persistent physical and psychological stress can induce endogenous corticosteroid excess and increase BMD losses.

INCREASED OSTEOCLAST ACTIVITY

The following contribute to an increase in osteoclastic activity:

- Hyperparathyroidism predominately favors osteoclastic activity as a result of PTH's predominate effect of increasing mobilization of calcium. The primary effect of PTH is to maintain calcium and phosphorus in a narrow physiologic range. It does so by increasing activation of 25-hydroxy vitamin D_3 to 1.25-dehydroxy vitamin D_3 to increase serum calcium levels through increased absorption of calcium and by increasing bone resorption via increased osteoclast function. Secondary hyperparathyroidism is the response to any tendency to a lowered serum calcium level by an immediate increase in PTH levels and increased bone resorption. Lowered mineral availability because of calcium maladsorption, increased renal losses, or poor nutrition will induce a state of secondary osteoporosis. Chronic exposure to elevated levels results in increased osteoclast activity and osteoporosis. Interestingly, intermittent exposure to PTH actually leads to increases in BMD by favoring formation over resorption.[20]
- Calcineurin inhibitors, a class of immune suppressants used in transplant patients, directly increase osteoclast activity resulting in resorption.
- Postmenopausal estrogen deficiency and other hypogondal states, both primary and secondary. Estrogen deficiency increases the population of pre-B cells, a subset of bone marrow stromal cells, which in turn increase production of IL-1 and TNF. These cytokines induce cyclo-oxygenase 2 activity increasing prostaglandin E_2 production by osteoblasts and subsequent increase in RANKL expression and resultant osteoclastogenesis.[21] Androgen effects on bone appear to be

mediated by their aromatization to estrone. Many cancer therapies for breast, ovarian, and prostate cancer patients produce hypogonadal states. Treatment modalities for women include cytotoxic chemotherapy, oopherectomy, and radiation therapy to the ovaries. Tamoxifen has been shown to produce osteoporosis in premenopausal women. And obviously both aromatase inhibitors and GnRH agonists produce estrogen deficiency. In men, treatments include cytotoxic chemotherapies, orchiectomy, as well as antiandrogens and GNRH agonists. Estrogen levels approach the immeasurable in men after these procedures. Estrogen deficiency may also be associated with the genetic hypogonadal states such as Turner's syndrome and Klinefelter's syndrome.

- Heparin, a potent anticoagulant, stimulates both osteoclastic bone resorption as well as suppressing osteoblastic activity. Heparin doses of 15,000 units or greater daily for 6 months have been shown to induce osteoporosis.[11] Evidence regarding the osteoporotic effect of low molecular weight heparin is mixed with animal studies demonstrating greater safety than standard heparin yet one case has been reported of vertebral osteoporosis after 3 months of use.

- Inactivity, immobilization, and sarcopenia. Mature osteocytes by sensing the mechanical forces exerted on bone by physical activity directly influence bone remodeling. Recent evidence suggests that the osteocytes are uniquely positioned to detect areas of damaged or weakened bone that are in need of remodeling. Any condition that decreases these forces will have a negative impact on bone strength. Physical immobilization after trauma including fractures, cerebrovascular accident, or because of polio or multiple sclerosis has been associated with osteoporosis. A reduction in compressive mechanical forces because of immobilization reduces the canalicular fluid flow in bone with resultant osteocyte hypoxemia and death leading to increased osteoclast activity.[2] In spinal cord injury patients, the majority of losses occurs during the first year, but losses can continue for up to 15 years. The amount of loss related to immobilization can be quite impressive as studies of microgravity during space flight have demonstrated a 2% loss per month.

- Hyperthyroidism is associated with both increased osteoblastic and osteoclastic activities. Resorption is favored overall, however, as increased formation cannot keep pace with increased resorption. Treatment of thyrotoxicosis has been shown to increase bone density, but has not restored BMD to healthy norms. The effect of exogenous subclinical hyperthyroidism on BMD in women is unclear with mixed reports of normal and decreased BMD.[11] However, a small uncontrolled case series following women treated for thyroid hormone resistance with the development of exogenous subclinical hyperthyroidism manifested by modest suppression of TSH has revealed increased BMD with supplementation.[22]

- Cadmium intoxication. Low levels of chronic cadmium intoxication have been associated with the development of osteoporosis,[23] characterized by increased osteoclast activity.

IMPAIRED PROTEIN METABOLISM

The following conditions affecting protein metabolism have a very important role in the pathogenesis of osteoporosis as well:

- Cushing's syndrome whether primary or secondary to exogenous long-term administration of glucocorticoids can cause decreased deposition of protein throughout the body in addition to increasing protein catabolism. Though corticosteroid administration has profound effects on protein catabolism and likely alters protein substrate in the matrix and ground substance, this is not the primary effect of corticosteroids on osteoporosis.
- Increasing age is marked by decreasing levels of growth hormones and decreased protein anabolic activity.
- Deficiency of vitamin C, which is necessary for secretion of intercellular protein, interferes with formation of the matrix by osteoblasts.[24]
- Homocysteine has been shown to be elevated in the elderly and has a postulated role in the development of osteoporosis by interfering with the cross-linking of collagen in the organic matrix of bone. Indeed, folic acids levels have been found to be lower in women with osteoporosis compared to women with normal bone density. Folic acid, vitamin B_{12}, and vitamin B_6 are crucial nutrients in folic acid cycle metabolism and the formation of S-adenosyl methionine. Supplementation has been shown to reduce homocysteine levels, but has not yet been shown to increase bone density.
- Lead intoxication. Osteocalcins in the matrix bind lead preferentially to calcium with a resultant decrease in calcium binding opportunities and subsequent failure to bind hydroxyapatite. This decreases bone formation with the direct effect of lowering BMD.[25] Lead levels also increase by 25 to 30% in postmenopausal women with osteoporosis,[26] contributing to lead toxicity and resultant illnesses late in life.
- Warfarin. Vitamin K is a necessary cofactor for the conversion of inactivated osteocalcin to its active integral form in binding calcium to the organic matrix.[1] Warfarin, an oral anticoagulant, reduces vitamin K levels systemically. Though warfarin has inhibited bone formation *in vitro*, no clinical reports have been made.[11]

INFLAMMATION

Given the role of inflammatory messengers and cytokines in the cell-to-cell communication vital to the balanced remodeling process, it is clear that systemic inflammatory diseases with resultant increases in proinflammatory messengers have direct effects on bone ultimately resulting in the development of osteoporosis. These include:

- Inflammatory bowel disease is a good example of an inflammatory disease causing osteoporosis. Circulating proinflammatory cytokines increase osteoclast activity. Indeed, TNF alpha decreases differentiation of osteoblasts, increases differentiation of osteoclasts, and increases osteoclast survival by decreasing apoptosis. In fact, it has been proposed that osteoblast and osteoclast communication mediated by TNF is the final common pathway through which bone metabolism is altered.[27] High levels of IL-6 have been found in osteoporotic patients suffering from Crohn's disease compared to nonosteoporotic patients.[28] Intestinal and colonic dysbiosis impair production of vitamin K, which has been shown to be an important nutrient for bone metabolism. Additionally, acute intestinal inflammatory events produce central hypogonadism.[28]
- Calcineurin inhibitors (CIs), specifically cyclosporine A and tacrolimus, are potent immunomodulators used in transplant patients. Approximately 20,000 transplants are performed annually with more than 250,000 performed to date. These transplant patients are frequently in poor health and have osteoporosis prior to their surgery. Calcineurin inhibitors have multiple effects on bone including decreased bone formation, but the more important mechanism appears to be their effect on T-lymphocytes, which then produce osteoclast stimulatory cytokines. The overall loss in BMD in these patients is exacerbated by the frequent concurrent use with corticosteroids.
- Several chronic diseases of aging have been noted to be comorbid conditions with osteoporosis. These conditions, including atherosclerosis, osteoarthritis, and periodontal disease, share inflammation[29] as an underlying pathophysiological derangement. Osteoporosis of the spine, periodontal disease, and tooth loss has been associated in a cohort of postmenopausal women.[30]

UNCLEAR ETIOLOGIES

- Antiepileptic drugs (AEDs) have been associated with bone disease. Early reports on institutionalized patients were primarily of rickets and osteomalacia. But more recent reports, particularly in outpatients, have demonstrated evidence of osteoporosis. Mechanisms proposed include increased catabolism of vitamin D by the cytochrome P450 enzyme system, impairment of calcium absorption, impaired bone resorption and formation, and poor vitamin K status.[31] AEDs that induce the cytochrome P450 system enzyme system (phenobarbital, phenytoin, carbamazepine, and valproate) are most consistently implicated in the development of osteoporosis suggesting the importance of vitamin D metabolism. Newer AEDs (gabapentin, lamotrigine, topiramate, and vigabatrin) have been shown in one study to be safe. However, a few pediatric studies have noted short stature and low bone mass in children on lamotrigine. Certainly, the balance of studies suggests that polytherapy with AEDs increases the risk of osteoporosis compared to monotherapy.

- An interesting hypothesis has been proposed linking Gulf War Syndrome with osteoporosis. It has been noted that there might be a loss of immune tolerance to naturally occurring calcitonin gene related protein (CGRP), a vasoactive neuropeptide, following a variety of antigenic events including vaccination and exposure to sand fly vasodilating substance. Receptors for CGRP have been detected on osteoblasts.

BREAKING THE SILENCE

Osteoporosis has been called a silent disease because decreased bone strength is generally not discovered until a fragility fracture has occurred, a condition capable of causing osteoporosis is identified, or a diagnostic test has revealed evidence of osteoporosis. A review of the primary risk factors, our patients' lifestyle choices, and their overall health, including many of the conditions outlined earlier, allows one to assess a patient's individual risk for osteoporosis. Consideration of the pathophysiologic processes involved in the development highlights the interconnectedness of organ systems frequently considered to be separate in the standard allopathic approach. These interesting connections and the evolving and changing scope of our knowledge should demonstrate that osteoporosis cannot be considered a silent threat and that many individuals have easily recognizable clues to their at-risk state. Given the increasing prevalence of osteoporosis in the population and acknowledgment that 55% of the population over the age of 50 is at risk, we must view osteoporosis as a common condition. It is crucially important that we not only diagnose this disease early to begin timely treatment, we must also assist our patients early on to make choices crucial for the prevention of osteoporosis.

TREATMENT

Given the interrelatedness of primary and secondary osteoporosis, a common approach to these conditions is warranted. General nutritional and exercise-related recommendations are the basis on which to build a patient-specific regiment. Lifestyle modification and nutritional recommendations are specific to the underlying causes. If a disease is contributing to osteoporosis, closer management of the disease can be treatment. If a medication is contributing to osteoporosis through the pathways described earlier, alternate medications or alternative disease management to lessen the dosage required can be considered. For recalcitrant osteoporosis, one must consider the addition of standard allopathic therapies including biphosphonates and calcitonin to our integrative approach.

CALCIUM

A rich literature debates the pros and cons of the various forms of calcium available for supplementation. In general, chelated minerals, which are bound to organic acids, may be better absorbed than inorganic forms. Calcium citrate is better absorbed particularly in an environment of lowered acidity, common in both elderly patients and those taking acid-reducing medications, than is calcium carbonate. The chelated forms are generally more expensive. Natural sources, including bone meal, dolomite, and oyster shell, are frequently contaminated with lead. Calcium hydroxyapatite is essentially a purified bone meal and absorption may be significantly less than calcium carbonate or citrate. Coral calcium is expensive and the extensive health claims made for this product have not been substantiated.[32] Dietary sources are still considered the best, though the standard diet of western commerce generally falls far short of supplying adequate calcium. Good food sources for calcium are low-fat dairy products; green vegetables including broccoli, kale, collards; and calcium-fortified products including orange juice and soy products. Indeed, three to four servings of these foods per day can provide adequate dietary calcium intake. For clinical guidelines on calcium refer to Table 25.2 of Chapter 25.

MAGNESIUM

Epidemiological studies have shown a positive association of magnesium with bone density. Studies have shown that women with osteoporosis have lower bone magnesium content than women without osteoporosis. A small trial demonstrated a modest improvement in the magnesium supplemented group compared to controls. Indeed, these studies suggest that the importance of magnesium supplementation may currently be underestimated.[1] Supplementation with 400 to 800 mg of magnesium per day is recommended. Additional information on magnesium supplementation is provided in Chapter 9.

BORON

Boron is a trace element that influences vitamin D metabolism and enhances estrogenic activity in bone.[33] Given the inadequate daily fruit and vegetable intake of the average American, supplementation with 3 to 5 mg of boron per day is necessary to ensure adequate boron levels.[1] For testing boron using d-penicillamine, refer to Chapter 29.

Vitamin D

Vitamin D has received recent widespread attention as a very important cell signaling molecule, expanding its integral role in intestinal adsorption of calcium as well as modifying the speed of bone turnover. Vitamin D is discussed in Chapters 10 and 25.

Vitamin K

Vitamin K supplementation has been shown to play an important role in healthy bone formation. Broccoli and leafy greens, such as kale, collards, parsley, and lettuce, are a good source of vitamin K. Caution must be taken for those patients taking warfarin, though moderate intake is safe given frequent monitoring of prothrombin times.

Isoflavones

Of the herbals, isoflavones, found in soy and red clover, have attracted the most research interest to date for the prevention and treatment of osteoporosis. Epidemiologic studies have demonstrated beneficial effects in premenopausal and perimenopausal women, but not in postmenopausal women. The research demonstrated a dose-dependent benefit curve. Despite these findings, soy isoflavones have been marketed in relatively high doses with resultant concerns regarding their safety noted. Specifically at higher than dietary levels, there are concerns that because of their estrogenic effects they may be procarcinogenic as well as goitrogenic. However, research has shown that across a broad range of hormonal parameters including thyroid function tests, follicle stimulating hormone and luteinizing hormone levels, and total estrogen levels, one serving of soy food per day had no demonstrable negative effects. A semisynthetic isoflavone has been manufactured from daidzein called ipriflavone. It has been shown to affect postmenopausal bone density levels, but has also been found to adversely affect white blood cell levels. Given the current data, soy supplementation as a food would be considered an advantageous strategy, but supplementation with isolated isoflavones should be avoided.[16]

Dehydroepiandrosterone

Dehydroepiandrosterone (DHEA) is a natural occurring adrenal hormone that is a precursor to testosterone and estrogen. Available at compounding pharmacies and over the counter in health food markets, small studies have shown beneficial effects on bone density with topical applications of DHEA.[16] DHEA may, however, have profound effects on diverse hormonal levels and can be procarcinogenic. DHEA should only be administered under a physician's care.

CONCLUSION

The practitioner can use the concepts of osteoporosis' underlying pathophysiology to identify those patients most at risk for osteoporosis. This breaks the "silence" of the disease and perhaps offers patients life-saving treatment opportunities earlier than might have been the case otherwise. Treatment for affected individuals must be aimed at slowing ongoing loss of bone density and stimulating new bone formation with resultant new mineralization. Lifestyle choices, an appropriate diet, and wise nutritional supplementation can greatly augment conventional medical therapeutics.

REFERENCES

1. Murray, M.T. and Pizzorno, J.E., Jr., Osteoporosis, in *Textbook of Natural Medicine*, 2nd edn, Murray, M.T., Pizzorno, J.E., Jr., Eds, Churchill Livingston, Edinburgh, 1999, pp. 1453–1461.
2. Epstein, S., Inzerillo, A.M., Caminis, J., and Zaidi, M., Disorders associated with acute rapid and severe bone loss, *Journal of Bone and Mineral Research*, 18, 2083–2094, 2003.
3. *Osteoporosis Prevention, Diagnosis and Treatment*, NIH Consensus Statement 2000, March 27–29, 17(1), pp. 1–45.
4. Shoback, D.M. and Strewler, G.J., Disorders of the parathyroids & calcium metabolism, in *Pathophysiology of Disease, An Introduction to Clinical Medicine*, 3rd edn, McPhee, S.J., Lingappa, V.R., Ganong, W.F., and Lange, J.D., Eds., Lange Medical Books/McGraw-Hill, New York, 2000, pp. 405–415, 425–429.
5. Holick, M.F. and Krane, S.M., Introduction to bone and mineral metabolism, in *Harrison's Principles of Internal Medicine*, 15th edn, Braunwald, E., Fauci, A.S., Kasper, D.L., Hauser, S.L., Longo, D.L., and Jameson, J.L., Eds., McGraw-Hill, New York, 2001, pp. 2192–2205.
6. Russell, G., Pathogenesis of osteoporosis, in *Rheumatology*, 3rd edn, Hochberg, M.C., Silman, A.J., Smolen, J.S., Weinblatt, M.E., and Weisman, M.H., Eds., Mosby, Edinburgh, 2003, pp. 2075–2080.
7. Jilka, R.L., Biology of the basic multicellular unit and the pathophysiology of osteoporosis, *Medical and Pediatric Oncology*, 41, 182–185, 2003.
8. Tok, E.C., Ertunc, D., Oz, U., Candeuiren, H., Ozden, G., and Ditek, S., Effects of circulating androgens on bone mineral density in postmenopausal women, *Maturitas*, 48, 235–242, 2004.
9. Yanai, T., Suzuki, S., Gotu, K., Nomura, M., Okabe, T., Takaycnagi, R. and Noralie, H., Aromatase in bone: roles of vitamin D_3 and androgens, *Journal Steroid Biochemistry and Molecular Biology*, 86, 393–397, 2003.
10. Frank, G.R., Role of estrogen and androgens in pubertal skeletal physiology, *Medical and Pediatric Oncology*, 4, 217–221, 2003.
11. Stein, E. and Shane, E., Secondary osteoporosis, *Endocrinology and Metabolism Clinics of North America*, 32, 115–134, 2003.
12. Campbell, J.R., Rosier, R.N., Novotry, L., and Puzas, J.E., The association between environmental lead exposure and bone density in children, *Environmental Health Perspectives*, 112, 1200–1203, 2004.

13. Levy, C. and Lindor, K.D., Management of primary biliary cirrhosis, *Current Treatment and Opinions in Gastroenterology*, 6, 497–498, 2003.

14. *Surgical Treatment for Obesity*, Arbor Clinical Nutrition Update, 200, pp. 1–3, February 2005.

15. Lindsay, R. and Cosman, F., Osteoporosis, in *Harrison's Principles of Internal Medicine*, 15th edn, Braunwald, E., Fauci, A.S., Kasper, D.L., Hauser, S.L., Longo, D.L. and Jameson, J.L., Eds., McGraw-Hill, New York, 2001, pp. 2226–2237.

16. Shepherd, A.J., A review of osteoporosis, *Alternative Therapies in Health and Medicine*, 10, 26–33, 2004.

17. Saag, K.G., Glucocorticoid-induced osteoporosis, *Endocrinology and Metabolism Clinics of North America*, 32, 115–134, 2003.

18. Takada, J., Nagoya, S., Kuwabara, H., Kaya, M., and Yamashita, T., Rapidly destructive coxarthropathy with osteonecrosis and osteoporosis caused by Cushing's syndrome, *Orthopedics*, 27, 1111–1113, 2004.

19. Phillips, K.A., Nance, E.P., Jr., Rodriguez, R.M., and Kaye, J.J., Avascular necrosis of bone: a manifestation of Cushing's disease, *Southern Medical Journal,* 79, 825–829, 1986.

20. Potts, J.T., Jr., Diseases of the parathyroid gland and other hyper- and hypocalcemic disorders, in *Harrison's Principles of Internal Medicine*, 15th edn, Braunwald, E., Fauci, A.S., Kasper, D.L., Hauser, S.L., Longo, D.L., and Jameson, J.L., Eds., McGraw-Hill, New York, 2001, pp. 2205–2226.

21. Theriault, R.L., Pathophysiology and implications of cancer treatment — induced bone loss, *Oncology*, 18, 11–15, 2004.

22. Hurlock, D.G., Personal communication.

23. Altuer, T., Elinder, C.G., Carlsson, M.D., Grubb, A., Hellstrom, L., Persson, B., Pattersson, C., Spang, G., Schultz, A., Jarup, L., Low level chronic cadmium exposure and osteoporosis, *Journal of Bone and Mineral Research*, 5, 1579–1586, 2000.

24. Guyton, A.C. and Hall, J.E., Parathyroid hormone, calcitonin, calcium and phosphate metabolism, vitamin D, bone, and teeth, in *Textbook of Medical Physiology*, 10th edn, W.B. Saunders Company, Philadelphia, 2000, pp. 899–914.

25. Dowd, T.L., Rosen, J.F., Mirts, L., and Gundberg, C.M., The effect of Pb(2+) on the structure and hydroxyapatite binding properties of osteocalcin, *Biochimica Biophysica Acta*, 1535, 153–163, 2001.

26. Nash, D., Magder, L.S., Sherwin, R., Rubin, R.T., and Silbergeld, E.K., Bone density related predictors of blood lead levels among peri- and post-menopausal women in the United States, 3rd National Health Nutritional Examination Survey 1988–1994, *American Journal of Epidemiology*, 160, 901–911, 2004.

27. Harpavat, M., Keljo, D.J. and Regueiro, M.D., Metabolic bone disease in inflammatory bowel disease, *Journal of Clinical Gastroenterology*, 38, 218–224, 2004.

28. Siffledeen, J.S., Fedorak, R.N., Siminoski, K., Jen, H., Vaudan, E., Abraham, N., Seinhart, H., and Greenberg, G., Bones and Crohn's: risk factors associated with low bone mineral density in patient's with Crohn's disease, *Inflammatory Bowel Disease,* 10, 220–228, 2004.

29. Serhan, C.N., Clues for new therapeutics in osteoporosis and periodontal disease: a new role for lipoxygenase, *Expert Opinion and Therapeutic Targets,* 8, 643–654, 2004.

30. Mohammad, A.R., Bauer, R.l. and Yeh, C.K., Spinal bone density and tooth loss in a cohort of postmenopausal women, *International Journal of Prosthodontics*, 10, 381–385, 1997.

31. Pack, A.M., Gidal, B. and Vasquez, B., Bone disease associated with antiepileptic drugs, *Cleveland Clinic Journal of Medicine*, 71, s42–s48, 2004.
32. Weil, A., *Dr. Andrew Weil's Self Healing*, January 2003.
33. Minerals, in *Clinical Nutrition: A Functional Approach*, Bland, J.S., Costarella, L., Levin, B., Liska, D., Lukasczer, D., Schiltz, B. and Schmidt, M.A., Eds., The Institute for Functional Medicine, Gig Harbor, Washington, 1999.

27 Fractures

Craig Nadelson, D.O. and
Kevin Gebke, M.D.

CONTENTS

FUNCTIONS OF BONE

Bones provide mechanical function, which is rigidity and stiffness. This is necessary to move about on dry land, while resisting the natural forces of gravity. There is a fine balance between a skeleton that must resist these gravitational forces and one that would be too heavy to carry around. This homeostasis that needs to exist is directed by a negative-feedback loop. Mechanical sensors detect the exact amount of bending that occurs in bones during the forces and loads that the body sustains. When the level of bending is higher than the set point, a signal is sent to adjust the balance of resorption and formation, and initiate the bone remodeling process. Routinely, bones bend 0.1 to 0.15% in all dimensions.[1] If the amount of bend is a larger percentage than this range, the remodeling apparatus is signaled to increase the proportion of bone formation, so as to provide the increased rigidity necessary to resist gravity, as well as reduce the likelihood of fracture under normal forces. Conversely, if the percentage of bend is lower than this, the negative-feedback loop signals for a higher proportion of bone resorption, or breakdown, so that the skeleton is not too bulky and heavy for the normal functions that it is expected to perform.

The strength of bone is approximately proportional to the square of the bone density. This relationship helps to explain why bone strength is so sensitive to relatively small changes in density, and why fracture risk doubles at bone density values only 10 to 15% lower than normal.[1]

The second role of bone is to provide a homeostatic buffer. In particular, bones help to maintain a constant level of calcium in circulating fluids, as well as provide a reserve supply of phosphorus and other minerals. Electrolyte and pH balance are essential for minute-to-minute survival and are therefore maintained sometimes at the expense of bone health. This is covered in greater detail in the chapters on osteoporosis.

BONE STRUCTURE

Trabecular and cortical bone consist of the same cellular and noncellular components, but contain them in different ratios. Only 10 to 15% of the trabecular bone volume is calcified, while approximately 90% of the cortical bone volume is calcified.[2] A lattice structure allows a larger surface area of the trabecular bone to be in contact with the marrow space, and thus is available for metabolic activity and remodeling. By comparison, cortical bone is much more compact and makes up approximately 80% of the total skeletal mass, and thus plays a more critical mechanical role. However, because it makes up such a large percentage of skeletal mass, cortical bone also makes a substantial contribution to the metabolic activity of the skeleton.

Only 2 to 5% of bone comprises cellular tissue. It is the nonliving portion that contributes the mechanical properties of hardness, stiffness, and resiliency. This nonliving material is best described as a mineral-encrusted protein matrix, of which one-half, by volume, is protein matrix and the other half is bone mineral. The protein matrix determines the shape and three-dimensional structure of the bone, and it is also known as osteoid. It is 10% noncollagenous proteins, which are Gla-proteins, meaning glutamic acid residues that are carboxylated in a specific position. Among these Gla-proteins are osteocalcin, osteonectin, fibronectin, matrix Gla-protein, sialoprotein, and osteopontin.[1] The protein matrix consists of 90% type I collagen, which is a long fibrous protein, coiled as a triple helix. These fibers are cross-linked by the formation of tight covalent bonds formed between the various amino acid side chains projecting from collagen molecules. Collagen is also the predominant basis for dermis, tendons, and ligaments. The bone mineral is a carbonate-rich, imperfect hydroxyapatite. Its content is somewhat variable, with calcium comprising 37 to 40%, phosphate 50 to 58%, and carbonate 2 to 8%. The carbonate content is particularly sensitive to acid–base status in the body. In addition, bone mineral contains small amounts of sodium, potassium, magnesium, citrate, and other ions present in the extracellular fluid at the time the mineral is deposited.

Osteoblasts, osteoclasts, osteocytes, and lining cells are the four principal bone cells. In combination, these cells help contribute to the mechanical properties of bone, as well as mediate the calcium homeostasis between bone and the body.

Osteoblasts lay down bone and produce osteoid, the protein matrix. Osteoblasts synthesize and then secrete substances, such as collagen, which make up the osteoid. Then, they deposit and orient the fibrous proteins of the matrix. The matrix is laid down between and beneath the osteoblasts on the preexisting bony surface. Thus, the osteoblasts are pushing themselves backward as they add new bone.

Several days after initially depositing the matrix, mineralization is then directed by osteoblasts. Proteins are secreted into the osteoid matrix, and these proteins direct cross-linking of the collagen fibrils. The exact mechanism by which this occurs is still poorly understood. It is theorized, however, that the proteins help to create a three-dimensional structure that attracts calcium and phosphate ions and conjoins them into the apatite crystals. As mineral is deposited, the water within the original matrix is displaced. Organic phosphate compounds in the vicinity have the capability of inhibiting the mineralization process, but osteoblasts secrete an enzyme called alkaline phosphatase, which serves to hydrolyze these compounds. The process of mineralization itself takes several days.

Multiple things can occur to osteoblasts during the course of bone formation. A large proportion are encased into the newly mineralized bone and become osteocytes. Another portion will undergo programmed cell death, or apoptosis. Finally, a portion of the cells will remain as functioning osteoblasts.

The main cells directing bone resorption are osteoclasts. They do this by attaching to a microscopic bony surface at specific integrin receptor sites and walling off a small region of that surface. Acid and proteolytic enzymes are then secreted into this confined space and act to dissolve the mineral and digest the matrix. The breakdown products at the resorption site are released by the osteoclasts into the extracellular fluid and are eventually carried away by the circulating blood. The protein fragments are then metabolized by other areas of the body or excreted, while the calcium and phosphorus are either transported to other bone-forming sites in the skeleton or excreted. Unlike osteoblasts, all osteoclasts suffer the fate of apoptosis. This occurs after only a few short days of work.

Osteocytes, as mentioned above, are merely osteoblasts that become encased within the bone during the mineralization process. Other functioning osteoblasts continue to add new layers of osteoid matrix around and behind them. Osteocytes differ from their former osteoblast counterparts in that they no longer have the ability to synthesize protein matrix. They do, however, serve to monitor the amount of strain occurring in their local area when bone is mechanically loaded. The osteocytes communicate this information to the lining cells.

Lining cells are located on anatomic bone surfaces. These cells are in proximity to osteocytes for the purpose of receiving information on the amount of bend in their immediate location when mechanical forces are applied. The lining cells use this information to decide whether or not to initiate local bone remodeling projects.

BONE REMODELING AND COUPLING

The balance of bone formation and resorption within the body is known as bone remodeling. The temporal and spatial coordination of resorption and formation, the two phases of the remodeling cycle, is called coupling.[2] During normal physiologic conditions, resorptive activity is essentially equally balanced with formation activity through this coupling mechanism. At any given time, 2 to 4% of the human skeleton is undergoing remodeling.[2] To maintain the structural integrity of bone, old bone needs to be removed and replaced with new, healthy bone.

Resorption always precedes formation during the remodeling process. Howship's lacuna, also known as resorption pits, takes 7 to 10 days to reach full depth. This marks the end of the phase, and is a signal for the beginning of the formation phase. Osteoblasts lay down matrix, which eventually starts to mineralize after 10 days. The entire process of bone formation takes 3 to 4 months.[2]

FRACTURE CLASSIFICATION

By the simplest and broadest definition, a fracture is a break in the continuity of bone. There are several distinct ways by which fractures can be classified. For the purposes of this discussion, fractures will be classified by mechanism, or cause, which includes traumatic, pathologic, and stress fractures. Traumatic fractures are the more common type, and include fractures caused during motor vehicle accidents, falls, fights, sports, etc. These tend to be the types of fractures that the average person commonly thinks of when the term fracture is mentioned. Pathologic fractures occur because of an underlying pathology, or condition, such as metastatic bone cancer, osteoporosis, rickets, Paget's disease, etc. These fractures occur at levels of mechanical stress that would not normally fracture healthy bone. Because of the pathologic condition, bone formation and remodeling do not occur as they should. The result is bone that lacks the proper structural integrity to perform its normal bodily functions. Stress fractures are a distinct entity to be discussed in detail.

There are two competing theories that may explain how stress fractures develop. One theory suggests that during the initial increase in exercise or activity, the osteoblastic activity lags behind the osteoclastic activity by a few weeks, resulting in a period during which bones are more susceptible to injury. Microfractures can result from the torsional and bending stress forces applied to bone, and further repetitive use can eventually lead to a consolidation of these microfractures into a small macrofracture. A second theory suggests that strong, repetitive stress on bone at the insertion point of muscles results in focal bending, which generates stress greater than bone can tolerate. These two theories share a core central concept. Stress fractures occur as a result of a repetitive use injury that exceeds the intrinsic ability of bone to repair itself. Because of the unique pathophysiology by which stress fractures occur, they are not radiologically diagnosed in the same manner as other fractures. Stress fractures can be identified sooner and more accurately, using magnetic resonance imaging or three-phase bone scintigraphy instead of plain x-ray.

Two entities of stress fractures have also been described. Fatigue fractures occur when normal, healthy bone is exposed to repetitive, abnormal stresses. When normal forces are applied to abnormal, unhealthy bone, the fracture that might occur is an insufficiency fracture. Fatigue-type stress fractures tend to correlate with very specific anatomic areas, depending on the particular activity or sport, and what mechanical forces are applied to specific areas in the body. For example, running and jumping tend to cause tibial, navicular, and metatarsal stress fractures, whereas rowing could lead to the development of rib stress fractures.

There is evidence that stress fractures are a multifactorial disorder, with genetic and environmental factors affecting the final phenotype. Studies of stress fracture occurrence in monozygotic twins,[3,4] in children younger than 10 years of age,[3,5] and the association with a family history of osteoporosis,[3,6] all support a genetic predisposition to stress fractures.

A long list of risk factors for stress fractures exists. At the top of the list are poor prior to physical condition and rapid increase in physical activity or training program. "Too much, too soon" is the explanation for high rates of stress fractures in new military recruits during basic training.[7] Occurrence of a prior stress fracture is also a risk factor. According to Sanderlin et al., approximately 60% of those with stress fractures have had a previous stress fracture. Other risk factors include participation in sports that involve running and jumping, endurance sports, female gender (especially when accompanied by hormonal or menstrual disturbances),[8] low bone turnover rate, decreased cortical thickness of bone, decreased bone density, nutritional insufficiencies, extremes of body size and composition, inadequate muscle strength, inappropriate footwear, running on angled or irregular surfaces, and type "A" behavior.

Most often, stress fractures are best treated with conservative treatment. This includes rest, modification in exercise routine, ice, and depending on the location, possibly immobilization. If the cycle that led to the formation of the stress fracture is broken, the body's intrinsic ability to repair and form bone will be re-enabled, and the fracture will heal. If the cycle is not interrupted, stress fractures can develop into full-thickness fractures, which may require surgery. A more controversial aspect of treatment surrounds the use of nonsteroidal anti-inflammatory drugs (NSAIDs). An article in the *British Journal of Medicine,* February 2005,[9] that reviews this issue states that "there is evidence from animal studies that NSAIDs can adversely affect fracture healing, and that there is no conclusive evidence to document any effect of NSAIDs on stress fracture healing in humans." The article goes on to suggest that "until such evidence is produced, it is prudent to limit the use of NSAIDs in patients with proven stress fractures."

GENDER DIFFERENCES

Bone strength is influenced by numerous factors including bone mass, bone size, geometry, and microarchitecture. Many structural differences arise during pubertal development. The onset of puberty in males generally lags behind females by 2 years. It is during these two extra years of prepubertal growth that males have additional growth that contributes to increased long bone length.[10] By the end of puberty, males have achieved an overall greater bone size than females. Periosteum expands with little change in endocortical diameter in men, and as a result, there is increased cortical thickness and diameter. During female pubertal growth, periosteal expansion ceases, while endocortical bone formation continues. This leads to a thickened cortex, but at the expense of a decreased cortical diameter. Between the larger cortical diameter and the greater limb length it can be seen why males have achieved a larger peak bone mass and greater bone mineral density (BMD) at the end of puberty. Larger peak bone mass and BMD provide men with stronger bones than women, and thus, a smaller risk of fracture at equal applied forces. Women generally have smaller bones, smaller articular surfaces, and shorter leg length as a proportion of height.[11]

Fracture incidence among men and women shows a bimodal distribution with peaks occurring in youth and old age. The initial peak occurs in both boys and girls during the prepubescent growth spurt. While the prepubescent growth spurt is a time when girls and boys are physically active and sustain more trauma, it is also a time when the skeletal structure is more vulnerable, especially when nutrition is suboptimal. The second peak is due to fragility fractures.

The ratio of fractures in men and women changes with time. Prior to age 35, men suffer a higher rate of fracture, usually because of higher rates of trauma. Fracture incidence in women surpasses that of men by age 35. This is largely due to the rapid rise of fragility fractures by osteoporosis, to which women are more vulnerable. Therefore, the disparity in fracture incidence becomes even more pronounced in the postmenopausal period.

Editor's Note

Bone density, a clinical way to approximate bone strength, only needs to decrease by 10 to 15% to double the risk of a fracture. Fracture rates are increasing among children, adolescents, and the elderly, due to interrelated factors including more trauma, less physical activity, less vitamin D, smoking, longevity, and Western diets. Dietary trends are evident in the bones.

FRACTURES DURING INFANCY

During the first year of life fracture risk is low. The presence of recurrent fractures or a fracture with an unclear trauma should prompt the clinician to consider child abuse.[12] Spiral fractures, in particular, are commonly associated with abuse.

Since infancy is the time of rapid growth, suboptimal nutrition can be more readily detected in the bones. Infants whose mothers smoked during pregnancy and infants who are not breast-fed have lower bone mass.[13]

FRACTURE DURING CHILDHOOD

Roughly 55% of children break at least one bone before 18 years of age.[13] Injuries are the most common reason for hospitalization before the age of 14, and falls are the leading cause of morbidity. Victims of these injuries tend to be men (61%).[14] Although this age group may suffer from pathologic fractures, just as any other age group, most fractures occur via trauma. In youth, long bone fractures predominate because of this fact, and boys are more likely to suffer traumatic fractures than girls. Tall and heavy children are also at a higher fracture risk.[13] Stress fractures almost never occur in this age group because of the fact that bone turnover occurs so rapidly and aggressively in childhood. It should be noted that during this period, proper nutrition is essential to lay down strong, healthy bone for the future, and to help prevent some types of pathologic fractures, such as those associated with osteoporosis.

A landmark paper through the Mayo Clinic (Khosla et al.) showed a significant increase in the rate of distal forearm fractures during childhood over a 32 year period (1969 to 2001).[15,16] It is speculated that the reason for this increase is multifactorial. Among the likely causes are decreased activity in the population, decreased bone acquisition due to poor calcium intake, decreased vitamin D, Western diets, and increased trauma rates. Further studies are currently being pursued to help identify the exact causes for the increased childhood fracture rates. With the progression of modern technology, and the invention of larger and better televisions, computers, and video games, the children of today tend to be far more sedentary than the children of the 1970s. These children, who spend more time indoors, get less sunlight, and therefore less vitamin D. Also, the modern Western diet tends to be high in total fat and low in nutrients. A fast-paced society demands quick meals and relies too heavily on "fast food restaurants." For all of these reasons, we as clinicians need to address increasing physical activity and proper nutrition, especially in youth.

FRACTURES DURING ADOLESCENCE

Adolescence is a difficult period to define because it occurs at different times in different people. For simplicity, consider onset of adolescence to occur at age 10 in girls and 12 in boys, and age 17 as an end-point for both sexes. Usually, the growth spurt begins in boys at about age 12 to 13, peaks at 14 years, and is completed by 19 years of age. For girls, it usually begins at 10 to 11, peaks at 12, and is completed by age 15. Adolescence is a period of transition, both of body and of mind. Because competitors in sports are becoming bigger, stronger, faster, and are playing at a higher level of competition, this age group generally experiences more traumatic fractures and more severe fractures than they did as children playing sports. Adolescents begin driving privileges and for many reasons, adolescents have a high rate of motor vehicle accidents. Teenagers who smoke cigarettes on a regular basis have been shown to exhibit higher rates of fractures.[13]

Another significant issue that comes to the forefront during adolescence is body image. This confusing time of transition leads to constant evaluation of perceived attractiveness. Teenagers are keenly aware of the images of what is considered beauty in the society that surrounds them. It is this set of circumstances, along with the struggle for a personal sense of control in this group that makes the possibility of eating disorders a scary reality. Up until adolescence, a child is not faced with such circumstances. From the onset of adolescence, however, the possibility of disordered eating must be considered.

Eating Disorders and Fracture Risk, a Special Consideration during Adolescence

Disordered eating presents in several forms. Anorexia nervosa is essentially starvation and caloric deprivation. Excessive exercise, diuretic use, and laxative use may also accompany caloric deprivation. Binging and purging is known as bulimia. The two disorders can occur together as anorexic bulimia. Reduced BMD and eventually osteopenia are among the deleterious effects of anorexia and bulimia.[17] This is more prevalent in those with anorexia than those with bulimia or anorexic bulimia, as confirmed by Carmichael and Carmichael.[18] Because individuals with eating disorders vary so widely in their behavior, it is difficult to make a generalized statement. No direct correlation was found between BMD and body mass index, estrogen deficiency, tubular resorption of phosphorus, serum vitamin D, parathyroid hormone, or alkaline phosphatase levels during this study. However, they did establish that hypercortisolism was the best laboratory marker to assess the risk of osteopenia in these patients. Refer to the chapter on drug and disease induced osteoporosis for the mechanism by which cortisol decreases bone integrity.

In a large study[18,19] of 207 girls between the ages 9 and 18 years (an average of 2 to 4 years after menarche), researchers demonstrated that almost 99% of the maximal adult bone density is established by the age of 15. In another study[18,20] of 225 adult women, it was reported by authors that BMD significantly increases until the age of 35, at which time BMD decreases 1% per year until menopause. Both studies suggest that in the case of failure to establish critical peak bone mass by 15 to 35 years, as is likely with anorexia or bulimia, fracture risk is increased lifelong. It can also be inferred that if anorexia or bulimia precedes the adolescent growth spurt, bone development would be impaired and would lead to decrease in bone density, possible delays in normal bone maturation, and even interference in reaching full height potential. Even if the disordered eating is resolved, these effects are only partially reversible with time. Therefore, those with anorexia or bulimia are at a higher risk of all types of fractures, but especially of stress fractures.

Cobb et al.[21] studied the female triad, a syndrome composed of three interrelated conditions that influence each other. The triad is disordered eating, menstrual irregularity, and osteoporosis. The studies led researchers to three conclusions. First, disordered eating in runners is correlated with oligo/amenorrhea (defined as 0 to 9 menses per year). The second conclusion is that the association between oligo/amenorrhea and low BMD is independent of body weight and body composition. Third, disordered eating is associated with low BMD in eumenorrheic runners. The girls studied took the eating disorder index, which is a tested measurement of disordered eating. Those with elevated eating disorder index scores had a four-fold increase in risk for oligo/amenorrhea, even after authors controlled for other factors.

Because one of the main features of anorexia nervosa, and to a lesser degree anorexic bulimia and bulimia, is macro- and micronutrient deficiency, it would be expected that fracture healing would be more difficult and prolonged. As protein wasting becomes more severe with disordered eating over time, the necessary available proteins and amino acids used by the body in the process of bone formation are lacking. This can lead to slow and poor fracture repair, which can in turn lead to future fractures. A vicious cycle can ensue in this manner.

It is important to realize that boys and young men can suffer eating disorders like girls and young women, even though the prevalence is much lower. Boys who participate in endurance sports and sports that require a participant to be within a specific weight class are especially at risk. One example is the high school wrestler trying to lose weight for that day's match. He will do whatever it takes to meet the specific weight goal, including induced vomiting, starvation, purposeful dehydration, laxatives, and diuretics. Boys are also at risk of anabolic steroid use following puberty. Among the many detrimental effects of steroid use is bone pathology.[22,23] Users and abusers are at a much higher risk of pathologic fractures and several forms of bone cancer.

Obesity is multifactorial and is frequently associated with disordered eating. Initially, it was thought that the additional mass of exogenous fat promotes stronger bones, that obesity in adolescence may be protective of osteoporosis and fractures. Clinically, that theory is not substantiated. The diet of those obese may be high in macronutrients, but is often low in the bone-building nutrients described in the chapter on osteoporosis. The obese tend to exercise less, leading to less bone strength.

FRACTURES DURING YOUNG ADULTHOOD

Young adulthood is typically defined as age 18 to 35. During this period, the gender difference in fracture rates narrows down as men have fewer traumatic fractures by the close of this period and women develop osteoporosis. BMD no longer increases by the close of this period[21] apart from medical and nutritional interventions.

Fractures in Middle Adulthood

During this period, which will be described as age 36 to 64, the trend of higher overall fracture rates is skewed toward women. Following menopause, this holds true to an even larger degree because of the decline in circulating levels of estrogen, specifically, 17[β] estradiol.[11] Pathologic and insufficiency fractures continue to rise in both men and women and stress fractures still may occur, especially in relation to pathologic areas of bone.

Fractures in Older Adults

The final age group to be discussed is the most rapidly expanding segment of the population, and includes ages 65 and above. Those individuals over age 85 are a subset that is growing at an even faster rate. Older adults experience the highest percentage of pathologic and insufficiency fractures. This is a direct result of multiple factors, which include higher rates of disease states that interfere with bone formation, decreasing ability to absorb nutrients over time, progressively declining ability for the body to form bone as age increases, and in general, consumption of diets with fewer calories and worse nutrient content secondary to health problems, and less access to fresh foods.

Traumatic fractures are common, but for different reasons than earlier in life. Decreasing vision, decreasing sensation, decreasing proprioception, diminishing reflexes, widening base of gait, increasing joint stiffness, and muscle atrophy all contribute to traumatic fracture risk, along with decreased bone density. The increased rate of bones affected by pathology also causes an increased likelihood that fracture will occur as the result of a given injury. For these reasons, lifestyle modification must take place for this age group. Modifications should include exercise, use of a cane or walker when necessary, vitamin and calorie supplementation, or close dietary monitoring. Rehabilitation programs should be designed to increase strength, balance, proprioception, and range of motion, as well as incorporate protective devices, such as hip pads. Of note, elderly individuals who report being physically active are found to have a 20 to 40% lower incidence of hip fractures than those who report a sedentary lifestyle.[24–26]

EXERCISE FOR BONE HEALTH

Weight-bearing exercise contributes to bone strength and bone density throughout life. Animal studies demonstrate the osteogenic response to dynamic loading forces.[24,27]

Immobilization results in bone loss.[24,27] Ordinary bed rest also results in negative calcium, phosphorus, and potassium balance. Pitts found an 8% drop in fat-free weight, an increase in percent body fat, and a decrease in total body calcium in rats that spent 18 days in space. This further supports the need for weight-bearing exercise that requires gravity.[28]

Physical activity habits during childhood may have long-lasting benefits on bone health. Multiple small randomized, controlled trials have led to an exercise prescription that will augment bone mineral accrual in children and adolescents. Impact activities for 10 to 20 min done at high intensity in terms of bone-loading forces for at least 3 days a week is suggested.[24,26] Impact activities include plyometrics, gymnastics, jumping, resistance training, and combined running and jumping activities like basketball and soccer.

An exercise prescription for maintaining bone health during adulthood is 30 to 60 min/day of a combination of weight-bearing, endurance, and jumping activities three to five times per week.[24,26] Resistance exercises that target all major muscle groups two to three times per week, at a moderate to high intensity in terms of bone-loading forces, should also be included.[24,26]

Obese people who are active have lower mortality and morbidity than people whose weight is normal but are sedentary.[29] While the overall risk benefit ratio greatly favors a lifestyle with exercise, exercise does carry risks. Exercise is associated with increased risk of cardiac arrest, dehydration, osteoarthritis, and injuries including fractures.[30] Osteoarthritis is associated with the same forms of exercise that most benefit the bone. A study of 117 men former top-level athletes aged 45 to 65 (28 had been long distance runners, 31 soccer players, 29 weight lifters, and 29 shooters) looked at occurrence of knee osteoarthritis in activities with distinctly different loading conditions.[31] The prevalence in knee osteoarthritis was 31% in weight lifters, 29% in soccer players, 14% in runners, and only 3% in shooters. Prevalence directly correlated with the amount of loading force that occurs at the knee joint. The increased risk of premature osteoarthritis could only be partially explained by knee injuries in soccer players, and high body mass in weight lifters. Kujara concluded that all types of competitive athletes are at a slightly increased risk of requiring hospital care because of osteoarthritis of the knee, hip, or ankle when compared with the average population.[32] Power sports led to increased admissions for premature osteoarthritis, but in endurance athletes the admissions were at an older age. Obese persons, athletes, and others at high risk of osteoarthritis can use nutrition to strategically protect against osteoarthritis (Chapter 21).

NUTRITION FOR BONE HEALTH

Nutrients to improve bone health, resist fractures, and recover from fractures, and orthopedic surgery are very similar. The principles of dietary interventions and the nutrients most critical to bone health are described in Chapter 25 and can be applied across the life span.

SUMMARY

Fractures are the result of forces on bone that exceed the bone's ability to resist the forces. In trauma, bone is exposed to extremely great forces. In osteoporosis the bone has diminished ability to resist the forces. Most fractures throughout the life span are a combination of inadequate bone strength and increased forces. Clinicians can diagnose and treat the underlying causes of diminished bone strength. Exercise prescriptions and bone nutrition are recommended.

REFERENCES

1. Dawson-Hughes, B., Bone biology in health and disease: a tutorial, in *Modern Nutrition in Health and Disease*, Shils, M.E., Olson, J., Shike, M., Catharine, A., Eds., Lippincott Williams and Wilkins, Philadelphia, 1999.
2. Shoback, D. and Gross, C., Metabolic bone disease, in *Kelley's Textbook of Internal Medicine*, Humes, H.D., DuPont, H.L., Herbert, L., Gardner, L.B., Griffin, J.W., Harris, E.D., Hazzard, W.R., King, T.E., Loriaux, D.L., Nabel, E.G., Todd, R.F., and Traber, P.G., Eds., Lippincott Williams and Wilkins, Philadelphia, 2000.
3. Givon, U., Friedman, E., Reiner, A., Vered, I., Finestone, A., and Shemer, J., Stress fractures in the Israeli defense forces from 1995–1996, *Clin. Orthopaed. Relat. Res.*, 1, 227–232, 2000.
4. Singer, A., Ben-Yehuda, O., Ben-Ezra, Z., and Zaltzman, S., Multiple identical stress fractures in monozygotic twins, *J. Bone Joint Surg.*, 72B, 444–445, 1990.
5. Friedl, K.E., Nuovo, J.A., Patience, T.H., and Dettori, J.R., Factors associated with stress fracture in young army women: indications for further research, *Medicine*, 157, 334–338, 1992.
6. Meany, J.E.M. and Carty, H., Femoral stress fractures in children, *Skelet. Radiol.*, 21, 173–176, 1992.
7. Shabat, S., Mann, G., Constantini, N., Foldes, Y., and Nyska, M., Stress fractures among female athlete recruits undergoing basic training: reduced incidence following various interventions, *J. Bone Joint Surg. (Br.)*, 84-B (Suppl. III), 313, 2002.
8. Pollard, C.D., McKeown, K.A., Ferber, R., Davis, M., and Hamill, J., Selected structural characteristics of female runners with and without lower extremity stress fractures, *Med. Sci. Sports Exerc.*, 34 (Suppl. 1), S177, 2002.
9. Wheeler, P., Do non-steroidal anti-inflammatory drugs adversely affect stress fracture healing? *Br. J. Sports Med.*, 39, 65–69, 2005.
10. Stock, H., Schneider, A., and Strauss, E., Osteoporosis: a disease in men, *Clin. Orthopaed. Relat. Res.*, 1, 143–151, 2004.
11. Holschen, J., The female athlete, *South. Med. J.*, 97, 852–858, 2004.
12. Oral, R., Blum, K., Johnson, C., Fractures in young children: are physicians in the emergency department and orthopedic clinics adequately screening for possible abuse? *Pediatr. Emerg. Care*, 193, 148–153, 2003.
13. Jones, I.E., Williams, S.M., and Goulding, A., Associations of birth weight and length, childhood size, and smoking with bone fractures during growth: evidence from a birth cohort study, *Am. J. Epidemiol.*, 159, 343–350, 2004.
14. Kypri, K., Chalmers, D.J., Langley, J.D., and Wright, C.S., Child injury morbidity in New Zealand, 1987–1996, *J. Paediatr. Child Health*, 37, 227–234, 2001.

15. Khosla, S., Melton, L.J., Detukoski, M.B., Achenbach, S.J., Oberg, A.L., and Riggs, B.L., Incidence of childhood distal forearm fractures over 30 years: a population-based study, *J. Am. Med. Assoc.*, 290, 1479–1485, 2003.

16. Khosla, S., Melton, L.J., and Dekutoski, M.B., Increasing rates of forearm fractures in children, *J. Am. Med. Assoc.*, 290, 3193, 2003.

17. Putukian, M., The female athlete triad, *Curr. Opin. Orthopaed.*, 12, 132–141, 2001.

18. Carmichael, K. and Carmichael, D., Bone metabolism and osteopenia in eating disorders, *Medicine*, 74, 254–267, 1995.

19. Rigotti, N,A., Neer, R.M., and Jameson, L., Osteopenia and bone fractures in a man with anorexia nervosa and hypogonadism, *J. Am. Med. Assoc.*, 256, 385–388, 1986.

20. Rodin, A., Murby, B., Smith, M.A., Caleffi, M., Fentiman, I., Chapman, M.G., and Fogelman, I., Premenopausal bone loss in the lumbar spine and neck of the femur: a study of 225 Caucasian women, *Bone*, 11, 1–5, 1990.

21. Cobb, K., Bachrach, L., Greendale, G., Marcus, R., Neer, R., Nieves, J., Brown, B., Gopalakrishnan, G., Luetters, K., Tanner, H., Ward, B., and Kelsey, J., Disordered eating, menstrual irregularity, and bone mineral density in female runners, *Med. Sci. Sports Exerc.*, 35, 711–719, 2003.

22. Sturmi, J.E., and Diorio, D.J., Anabolic agents, *Clin. Sports Med.*, 17, 261–297, 1998.

23. Whitehead, R., Chillag, S., and Elliott, D., Anabolic steroid use among adolescents in a rural state, *J. Fam. Pract.*, 35, 401–406, 1992.

24. Kohrt, W., Bloomfield, S., Little, K., Nelson, M., and Yingling, V., Physical activity and bone health, Med. Sci. Sports Exerc., 36, 1985–1996, 2004.

25. Gregg, E., Pereira, M., and Caspersen, C.J., Physical activity, falls, and fractures among older adults: a review of the epidemiologic evidence, *J. Gerentol.*, 50, B97–B104, 1995.

26. Marks, R., Allagrente, M.C., and Lane, J.M., Hip fractures among the elderly: effects on dynamic strength, exercise capacity, muscle, and bone, *J. Gerentol.*, 50, B97–B104, 1995.

27. Deitrick, J.E., Whedon, G.D., and Shorr, E., *Am. J. Med.*, 4, 3–36, 1948.

28. Pitts, G.C., Ushakov, A.S., Pace, N. et al., *Am. J. Physiol.*, 244, R332–R337, 1983.

29. Bahr, R., Sports medicine, *Br. Med. J.*, 323, 328–331, 2001.

30. Melzer, K., Kayser, B., and Pichard, B., Physical activity: the health benefits outweigh the risks, *Clin. Nutr. Metab. Care*, 7, 641–647, 2004.

31. Kujara, U., Kettunen, J., Paananen, H., Aalto, T., Battie, M., Impivaara, O., Videman, T., and Sarna, S., Knee osteoarthritis in former runners, soccer players, weightlifters, and shooters, *Arthritis Rheum.*, 38, 539–546, 1995.

32. Kujara, U., Kaprio, J., and Sarna, S., Osteoarthritis of weight bearing joints of lower limbs in former elite male athletes, *Br. Med. J.*, 308, 231–234, 1994.

Section VII

Physical Stress

28 Preparing for Orthopedic Surgery

*Vilma A. Joseph, M.D., M.P.H. and
Ingrid Kohlstadt, M.D., M.P.H.*

CONTENTS

OVERVIEW

Orthopedic surgery is often elective, which offers time for presurgical preparation. The physical stress of surgery places demands on muscle, cartilage, and bone, the very tissues orthopedic surgery aims to heal. This chapter explains which herbal products should be discontinued before surgery. It reviews preprocedural fasting guidelines and safe preoperative weight reduction.

HERB–SURGERY INTERACTIONS

Consumer popularity of herbal supplements increased markedly in the 1990s. Based on longitudinal studies from Harvard, the use of self-prescribed herbal supplements in the U.S. general population was 12.1% in 1997[1] compared to the 2.5% prevalence found in 1990.[2] In a study of 3106 presurgical patients, 22% used herbal remedies, while a similar study of 755 found a report rate of 36%.[3] Use of herbal medicine was predominant in women and patients aged 40 to 60 years.[3,4] Between 20 and 44.4% of presurgical patients did not disclose their use of alternative medicine to their physicians.[3,5]

The popularity of herbal medicine among consumers is based on the false notion that herbal supplements can only be healthful or have no effect. Herbal supplements can be harmful, especially during surgery. While nutrients and nutritional supplements are chemicals on which metabolic processes depend, herbal supplements are chemical structures for which the body has no known requisite. Herbal supplements are concentrated beyond what could be consumed by diet alone, and concentrations of metabolically active components vary greatly. An analysis of 25 available ginseng products found a 15- to 200-fold variation in two markers, ginsenosides and eleutherosides.[6] Contamination can also occur. High levels of heavy metal have been found in 25% of 260 Asian patent medicines. In the same study, 7% of these medicines contained undeclared pharmaceuticals, such as steroids, hypoglycemics, and diuretics, to produce the desired effect.[7] From a period of 1990 to 1997, the most common heavy metals found in herbal medicines were mercury (66.7%), lead (19%), and copper (2.4%).[8]

Even though a patient may be presenting for an orthopedic procedure, the patient may be taking herbal medications, which could potentially cause them significant morbidity in the perioperative setting. Health care providers should consider a medication history incomplete until the patient is asked about the use of herbal medicines. Current recommendations by the American Society of Anesthesiology require that all patients are asked to stop taking herbal medicines 2 weeks prior to surgery. The goal is to avoid the platelet inhibition caused by many herbal medicines as well as to prevent herb–drug interactions, such as those given below and in Table 28.1 and Table 28.2. Ideally, patients will have an

TABLE 28.1
Examples of herbs and their potential effects

Herbs associated with electrolyte disturbances
American ginseng (↓ glucose)
Bitter melon (↓ glucose)
Fenugreek (↓ glucose)
Prickly pear (↓ glucose)
Licorice (↓ potassium)
Goldenseal (↓ potassium)

Herbs associated with enhanced bleeding potential

Ginger	Feverfew
Garlic	Fish oil
Ginseng	Danshen
Ginkgo	DongQuai

Herbs associated with prolongation of anesthesia
Valarian
Kava-kava
St. John's wort

TABLE 28.2
Reported herb–drug interactions

Herb + Drug = Effect

Herb	+ Drug	= Effect
Danshen	+ warfarin	= increased INR
Ginseng	+ digoxin	= ↑ digoxin levels
Ginkgo	+ thiazide diuretic	= hypertension
Ephedra	+ phenylzine	= severe monoamine oxidase inhibitor toxicity
Grapefruit juice	+ benzodiazepines	= increased drug bioavailability (↓ intestinal CYP3A4)
Licorice	+ diuretics	= exacerbated potassium loss, myopathy
Tamarind	+ aspirin	= increased absorption
Yohimbe	+ tricyclic antidepressants	= enhanced autonomic and central sympathomimetic effect

opportunity to discuss the health concern they are self-treating with herbs. For example, kava taken as a sleep aid may be replaced with a medication per the protocol outlined by Dr. Teitelbaum in his chapter on fibromyalgia. A person using St. John's wort may benefit from a prescription antidepressant during the weeks surrounding the surgery.

ECHINACEA

Uses: Mild sedative, antispasmodic, and antiseptic.

Drug–herb interaction: Hepatoxicity may occur with prolonged use and should not be taken with other hepatoxic drugs (anabolic steroids, amiodarone, methotrexate, or ketoconazole). Thus far, there have been no reported cases.[9]

FEVERFEW

Uses: Migraine prophylaxis.

Drug–herb interactions: Feverfew inhibits platelet activity and should be avoided with the use of warfarin and other anticoagulants.[9–11]

GARLIC

Uses: Hypercholesterolemia treatment.

Drug–herb interactions: Garlic decreases platelet aggregation, which may be exacerbated with the use of anticoagulants.[7,12,13]

GINGER

Uses: Antiemetic and antispasmotic.

Drug–herb interactions: Ginger acts as a potent thromboxane synthetase inhibitor.[9,14] Therefore, bleeding may be exacerbated in the presence of anticoagulants.

GINKGO

Uses: Dementia treatment.

Drug–herb interactions: Ginkgo is a potent inhibitor of platelet-activating factor and may cause bleeding with the concomitant use of aspirin, nonsteroidal anti-inflammatory agent (NSAID), heparin, and other anticoagulants.[7] Patients who use anticonvulsants and antidepressants should avoid using ginkgo. Since a neurotoxin, ginkgo toxin, is present in the ginkgo leaf and seed, it is advised that it should be avoided in epileptic patients.[9,11]

GINSENG

Uses: Treatment of type 2 diabetes, enhances heath and combats stress/disease.

Drug–herb interaction: Ginseng comes in several varieties (*Panax ginseng, Panax quinquefolius*, and *Panax pseudoginseng*). Falsely elevated digoxin levels in the absence of digoxin toxicity have been found in *P. pseudoginseng*. It is postulated that the eleutherosides may interact with the digoxin assay. The addition of ginseng to warfarin caused the normalization of a patient's international normalized ratio (INR) in *P. ginseng*.[9] Headache, tremulousness, and manic episodes have occurred in patients taking ginseng and phenelzine.[6,15]

KAVA

Uses: Sleep enhancer.
Drug–herb interaction: Kava and alprazolam used in combination may cause prolonged sedation.[7,16] This could cause prolongation of the sedative effects of anesthesia.

ST. JOHN'S WORT

Uses: Treatment of depression, anxiety, and sleep disorders.
Drug–herb interactions: Concomitant use of St. John's wort with piroxicam or tetracycline hydrochloride should be avoided, since it may cause photosensitivity. The use of selective serotonin reuptake inhibitors, such as fluoxetine and paroxetine, and St. John's wort may cause serotonin syndrome (headache, sweating, dizziness, and agitation).[9,16] Owing to the fact that the mechanism of action of St. John's wort may be characterized as a monoamine oxidase inhibitor, it may be prudent to avoid tyramine-containing foods like Swiss cheese, sauerkraut, or wine.[9]

VALERIAN

Uses: Treats insomnia.
Drug–herb interactions: The use of valerian and barbiturates (thiopental and pentobarbital) may cause prolonged sedation.[9] The use of alcohol should also be avoided until further studies are completed.

CAFFEINE

There are no specific recommendations on the use of caffeine in the perioperative setting. Caffeine, which is a methyxanthine, is found in a variety of products like teas, sodas, chocolate, soft drinks, and coffees. Most Americans consume some form of caffeinated beverage daily. The United States imports 30% of the world's coffee. Caffeine has been shown to increase systolic and diastolic blood pressure in men (4.1 and 3.8 mmHg, respectively) and women (4.5 and 3.3 mmHg, respectively).[17] In a case–control study of 713 patients, high-dose caffeine consumers were more likely to have chronic daily headaches (odds ratio 1.5, $p = .05$).[18] However, the abrupt withdrawal of caffeine leads to a caffeine physical dependence syndrome. This syndrome is characterized by headaches, muscle aches, nausea, and vomiting.[19] Caffeine-withdrawal headaches have been reported to occur if an individual ingests the equivalent of one cup of coffee per day, which depending on its strength may have between 96 and 136 mg of caffeine. Palpitations have been reported with the use of caffeine, and generally, if patients have a history of palpitations or panic disorder, they are instructed to avoid caffeine.[20] Caffeine avoidance is advisable for patients with hypertension. In the perioperative period, caffeine is better tapered 2 weeks prior to surgery, rather than discontinued abruptly the day of surgery.

PREOPERATIVE FASTING GUIDELINES

Aspiration of food from the stomach into the airways occurs when the laryngeal muscles are relaxed as is the case during various stages of anesthesia: general anesthesia, regional anesthesia, and sedation–analgesia (monitored anesthesia care).[21] Aspiration of solid material may cause an anatomic blockage of the airway. Aspirating gastric juices with a neutral pH may cause damage to the lung leading to a clinical picture of near drowning. Acidic gastric juices that are aspirated could potentially lead to an aspiration syndrome (Mendelson syndrome), characterized by dyspnea, cyanosis, and low-grade fever associated with diffuse rales, hypoxemia, and alveolar infiltrates in dependent lobes.[22] Mendelson syndrome is postulated to occur if the pH is less than 2.5 and the gastric volume is over 1.5 ml/kg. In an observational study of 318,880 surgical patients, the prevalence of aspiration pneumonia was approximately 1%[23] and associated mortality ranges from 10 to 71%.[21]

The American Society of Anesthesiologists (ASA) created practice guidelines for preoperative fasting with the intension of decreasing the complications associated with pulmonary aspiration of gastric contents. This is also commonly referred to as the *nil per os* (NPO) guidelines. The revised guidelines were created based on a literature review of over 3000 articles, a survey of attending anesthesiologists, and a task force analysis of the data. This was intended to improve the quality of anesthesia care and stimulate the evaluation of individual practices. Internationally, there has been a move to also adopt similar NPO guidelines.[24] Previously, patients were instructed to be NPO after midnight, which resulted in significantly more postoperative drowsiness, dizziness, and thirst ($p < .05$).[25] In fact, patients who ingested 150 ml of clear fluid more than 2 hours prior to a procedure had no significant effect on residual gastric volume and pH compared to those who had fasted overnight.[23]

The ASA has specific patient instructions for preoperative fasting of clear liquids, breast milk, infant formulae, and solid-food ingestion (see Figure 28.1). These guidelines apply to healthy, nonpregnant patients who are undergoing elective procedures.[26] Clear liquids should not be ingested within 2 hours of a procedure requiring general anesthesia, regional anesthesia, or sedation–analgesia (monitored anesthesia care). An infant should fast from breast milk for four or more hours prior to a procedure requiring general anesthesia, regional anesthesia, or sedation–analgesia. Infant formulae should not be ingested within 6 hours of a procedure where general anesthesia, regional anesthesia, or sedation–analgesia is utilized. A 6 hours or longer fast is recommended for a meal consisting of light

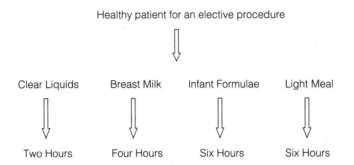

FIGURE 28.1 Pre-procedural fasting guidelines

solids or nonhuman milk prior to a general anesthetic, regional anesthetic, or sedation– analgesia. Patients should abstain from eating fatty, fried foods or meat 8 hours or more prior to a procedure requiring the administration of general anesthesia, regional anesthesia, or sedation–analgesia. Health care practitioners may need to modify NPO guidelines for persons at increased risk of pulmonary aspiration. Comorbidities include diabetes mellitus, obesity, emergency cases, bowel obstruction, hiatal hernia, or gastroesophageal reflux disease.[24]

Editor's Note

Surgery is a catabolic state where metabolism breaks down muscle and bone, the very tissues orthopedic surgery seeks to heal. Interventions that shorten catabolism and minimize oxidative damage could improve recovery and response to physical therapy. Effective nutritional interventions have been identified.

STRATEGIC NUTRITION

Nutritional status prior to surgery influences surgical outcomes. Furthermore, certain nutritional interventions have been shown to provide benefit in the perioperative setting in patients with suboptimal levels of these nutrients. One clinician's protocol for safely optimizing nutrition prior to orthopedic surgery is outlined in Table 28.3.

ANTIOXIDANTS

The body can store both water and fat-soluble antioxidants and draws on them during times of stress, such as orthopedic surgery. When antioxidants are in short

TABLE 28.3
A strategic nutrition protocol prior to orthopedic surgery

Step 1	Antioxidants
	Alkalinizing foods
	Amino acids
Step 2	Bone nutrients
	Biotics
Step 3	Correct deficiencies
	Comorbidities
	Carnitine
Step 4	Detoxify
	DHEA

supply, oxidative damage to lipids, proteins, and nucleic acids occurs resulting in tissue damage, muscle loss, and delayed wound healing. Refer to Dr. Harris' chapter on antioxidants. There has been research on the use of antioxidants (selenium, vitamin A, C, or E) to supplement feeding solutions, where antioxidants have been shown to decrease lipid peroxidase by 21% ($p < .05$).[27] Lipid peroxidase is a serum marker for high dietary lipids and oxidative stress. Deficiency in zinc has been linked to an increased susceptibility to wound infections.[28] Supplementation with zinc was evaluated to enhance wound healing. In a prospective study of 95 patients undergoing a hemiarthroplasty for a hip fracture, zinc levels of <95 µg/dl had an 11-fold increased risk of delayed wound healing.[28]

Vitamin C is of particular interest because it is a water-soluble antioxidant and also a vital nutrient for collagen synthesis, as described in Chapter 21. The physical stress of surgery can deplete marginal vitamin C stores, reducing the vitamin C levels needed for postsurgical healing. Individual vitamin C requirements can be determined by urine testing, as described in Chapter 25.

ALKALINIZING FOODS

Physical stress creates a metabolic acidosis, which is buffered by several organ systems including bone. Bone leaching from metabolic acidosis should be avoided, especially during orthopedic surgery, when metabolism would ideally support bone healing. Food selection influences metabolic processes. For example, fruits and vegetables, which are a rich source of antioxidants, also have the advantage of bone-sparing bicarbonate production. Refer to Chapter 25 for details on alkalinizing diets.

AMINO ACIDS

The role of dietary protein and some specialized amino acids is discussed at length in Chapters 6 and 18, and is presently applied to surgical patients. The National

Surgical Quality Improvement Project found that patients with an albumin level < 35 g/l were more likely to have a higher 30 day mortality rate than patients with an albumin over 35 g/l.[27,29] Loss of protein from protein–calorie malnutrition leads to decrease in wound tensile strength, T-cell function, phagocytic activity, and complement and antibody levels. These immune-related compromises of malnutrition correlate clinically with increased wound failure in lower-extremity amputations and bypass procedures.[28] A preoperative lymphocyte count of less than 1500 cells/unit was associated with a three times higher frequency of delayed wound healing.[30] Recommendations have been made for patients who are severely malnourished or have been NPO for over 3 days: enteral tube feeding or parenteral feeding for 7 to 15 days preoperatively is a means of nutritional supplementation if oral supplementation is not possible. Oral supplementation is less expensive and carries a smaller risk of infection and electrolyte abnormalities than parenteral feeding.[31] Supplementation with essential amino acids has been shown to be muscle sparing.[32] Most patients awaiting orthopedic surgery only need a reminder to eat breakfast and protein sources, such as lean meats, fish, nuts, organic eggs, and whey. Physical stress of surgery increases protein demand beyond the recommended dietary allowance of 0.8 g/kg body weight per day.

Certain amino acids are used individually to prepare a patient for surgery. Whey protein contains the three amino acids needed to synthesize the endogenous antioxidant, glutathione. L-Glutamine is used as a substrate for enterocytes and thereby appears to protect the mucuous membranes. L-Arginine is an amino acid that induces NO release and stimulates T-lymphocytes, which play an instrumental role in wound healing by promoting fibroplasias.[28] In addition to improving resistance to bacterial infections, arginine is cytoprotective during ischemia and reperfusion. It improves macrophage function after injury and inhibits the release of interleukin-2 (IL-2), IFNγ by Th1 lymphocytes.[33] One randomized control trial of 50 patients undergoing elective surgery found that those who received L-arginine along with ω-3-fatty acids and yeast ribonucleic acid for 5 days preoperatively showed an improvement in their delayed-type hypersensitivity response to recall antigens and serum IL-6 concentrations. Additionally, pneumonia was less prevalent in the treated group.[34] This clinician uses L-arginine 3 g twice daily in some patients with preexisting vascular disease. Most patients respond to choosing healthier protein sources.

BIOTICS

Antiobiotics commonly administered perioperatively alter the biotic environment of tissues. Friendly bacteria, such as *Acidophilus* and *Bifidobacteria*, protect the mucous membranes, making them more resistant to hospital-acquired microbes.[35] These same bacteria synthesize most of our B vitamins and vitamin K, and are themselves a fiber source.[36] Diverse probiotic strains may provide benefit beyond supplementation with a single strain; however, this clinician uses a single strain of *Bifidobacterium*, which can be cultured if a patient were to develop fever. Organic low-fat yogurt may provide additional probiotic benefit.

Bone Nutrients

Vitamin D, calcium, and anabolic steroids used in combination improved muscle mass, bone mineral density, and clinical function after hip fracture.[37] Vitamin D deficiency is prevalent and repletion has demonstrated benefits to both bone and muscle (see Chapters 10 and 25). Perioperatively, vitamin D can be supplemented at 1,000 IU daily. Calcium supplementation should be taken in a 2:1 ratio with magnesium, since the two minerals compete for absorption and preexisting low-magnesium stores are prevalent (see Chapters 9 and 25).

Correct Deficiencies

Suboptimal nutrient levels can be secondary to medications. Table 28.4 reviews common drug–nutrient interactions, pertinent to musculoskeletal health.

Comorbidities

Nutrition can be used as an adjunct to medical conditions, which need to be "tuned up" prior to surgery. Weight reduction plans for obesity may be considered

---

TABLE 28.4
Common medications known to alter nutrient status

Medication	Nutrient	Mechanism
Coumadin	Vitamin K	Blocks enzyme that synthesizes vitamin K
Iron	Chromium	Competitive absorption
Antibiotics	Vitamins K and B	Destroy intestinal flora, which synthesize these vitamins
Corticosteroids	Calcium, vitamin D, and chromium	Reduce active vitamin D, decrease calcium absorption, and increase chromium losses
Bile acid sequestrants	Fat-soluble vitamins	Decrease absorption
Diuretics	Magnesium, zinc	Increase urinary losses
Digoxin	Calcium and magnesium	Increase urinary losses
β-Blockers	Coenzyme Q10	Antagonize enzyme needed for synthesis
HMG-CoA reductase inhibitors	Coenzyme Q10	Block enzyme needed for synthesis
Sulfonylureas	Coenzyme Q10	Inhibit NADH-oxidase enzyme
Biguanides	Vitamin B_{12}	Competitive absorption
NSAIDs	Folate	Competes with enzymatic synthesis
H-2 blockers and proton pump inhibitors	Vitamin B_{12}, calcium, and protein	Decrease absorption by increasing gastric pH
Theophylline	Vitamin B_6	Inhibits enzyme
Anticonvulsants (most)	Vitamin D, folate, and L-carnitine	Interfere with metabolism, low serum levels

Source: Bralley, J.A. and Lord, R., *Laboratory Evaluations in Molecular Medicine*, The Institute for Advances in Molecular Medicine, 2001, p. 365; Hug, G. et al., *J. Pediatr.*, 119, 799–802, 1991; Physicians' Desk Reference, 2005.

---

an exception. Obesity is associated with many surgically managed orthopedic conditions. However, 2 weeks prior to surgery, treatment goals should shift to weight maintenance and muscle preservation.

Peripheral vascular disease is a comorbidity, which delays recovery from orthopedic surgery, especially of the affected extremity. Treatment of peripheral vascular disease can be augmented by nutrient supplementation. The amino acid L-arginine can improve endothelial vasodilation, primarily by increasing the release of nitric oxide. L-Arginine at a dose of 8 g twice daily can significantly reduce intermittent claudication.[38] Sustained release preparations are under development.[39] L-Carnitine at a dose of 2 g twice daily has also been shown to be effective in reducing symptoms of intermittent claudication.[40]

CARNITINE

L-Carnitine is an organic amine derived from both dietary sources and endogenous synthesis. L-Carnitine transports free fatty acid across the inner mitochondrial membrane, where the fatty acids are used for ATP synthesis. L-Carnitine availability can be a rate-limiting step for fat metabolism, especially during the elevated cortisol state of surgery. Supplementation with L-carnitine can prevent apoptosis of skeletal muscle cells and increase muscle mass.[41] This clinician recommends L-carnitine, 2 g, twice daily, 2 weeks pre- and postsurgery in persons with sarcopenia, insulin resistance, cardiovascular disease, congestive heart failure, or elevated triglycerides.[40] Vegetarians often benefit from supplementation because meat is the primary dietary source of L-carnitine.

DETOXIFICATION

Possibly more powerful and more difficult than adding nutrients may be subtracting antinutrients. Sugar and other highly refined carbohydrates spark unfavorable metabolic reactions, which actually cost the body nutrients. Although high-intensity sweeteners, such as aspartame, and sucralose have no calories per se, they are not metabolically inert; they interfere with nutrient absorption and metabolism. Stevia and sugar alcohols, such as xylitol, can be substituted.

Dietary *trans* fats should also be removed from the diet and the unrefined fats, described in Chapter 4, should be substituted. *Trans* fats alter cell-membrane chemistry and adversely modulate inflammation, just as healthful ω-3 fats can favorably modulate inflammation. Since ω-3 fats can interact with surgery and can be harmfully oxidized, initiating their use in supplemental doses prior to surgery is not advised. A diet that eliminates *trans* fats and is rich in organic, unrefined oils is strongly recommended.

DEHYDROEPIANDOSTRONE

Dehydroepiandostrone (DHEA) is an anabolic hormone available without medical prescription. Although it achieved consumer popularity among strength-building athletes, its primary benefit is among the frail. DHEA is released endogenously in a pulsatile fashion with cortisol. When stress increases, both cortisol and DHEA increase. However, on aging, endogenous DHEA production diminishes and is unable to increase with rising cortisol.[36,42,43] The presence of DHEA receptors on muscle tissue also suggests that DHEA has a muscle-sparing role in high-stress environments, apart from being a precursor for androgenic steroids. DHEA levels are correlated with serum L-carnitine levels, suggesting another potential mechanism of action.[44] DHEA supplementation at 100 mg for 6 months favorably increased body composition and muscle strength in men aged 50 to 65 years, but not in women.[45] DHEA supplementation of 50 mg for 6 months to 1 year increased bone density in women older than 70.[42,46] No adverse effects of DHEA were observed in these studies. Intramuscular anabolic steroids of higher potency were well tolerated among elderly women in a study that demonstrated muscle mass, bone mineral density, and clinical function after hip fracture.[37] Orthopedic surgery patients with osteoporosis and sarcopenia may receive muscle and bone-sparing benefit from a 6 month course of DHEA. Detailed discussions of anabolic steroid physiology can be found in Chapters 18 and 20.

CONCLUSION

A patient's nutritional status and the recent intake of dietary supplements and nutrients play an important role in the perioperative setting. Herbal medicines should be avoided 2 weeks prior to surgery. NPO guidelines must be explained to patients to avoid perioperative morbidity. Morbidity can occur from eating just prior to surgery and dehydration and protein catabolism can occur by not eating enough a few days before surgery. Strategic dietary and nutritional interventions enhance surgical outcomes and can be implemented using evidence-based protocols.

REFERENCES

1. Ernst, E., The risk-benefit profile of commonly used herbal therapies: ginkgo, St. John's wort, ginseng, echinacea, saw palmetto, and kava, *Ann. Intern. Med.*, 136, 42–53, 2002.
2. Eisenberg, D.M. et al., Trends in alternative medicine use in the United States, 1990–1997: results of a follow-up national survey, *J. Am. Med. Assoc.*, 280, 1569–1575, 1998.
3. Tsen, L.C. et al., Alternative medicine use in presurgical patients, *Anesthesiology*, 93, 148–151, 2000.
4. Skinner, C.M. and Rangasami, J., Preoperative use of herbal medicines: a patient survey, *Br. J. Anaesth.*, 89, 792–795, 2002.
5. Leung, J.M. et al., The prevalence and predictors of the use of alternative medicine in presurgical patients in five California hospitals, *Anesth. Analg.*, 93, 1062–1068, 2001.

6. Rotblatt, M. and Ziment, I., *Evidence-Based Herbal Medicine*, Hanley & Belfus, Philadelphia, 2002.

7. Bent, S. and Ko, R., Commonly used herbal medicines in the United States: a review, *Am. J. Med.*, 116, 478–485, 2004.

8. Kam, P.C. and Liew, S., Traditional Chinese herbal medicine and anaesthesia, *Anaesthesia*, 57, 1083–1089, 2002.

9. Miller, L.G., Herbal medicinals: selected clinical considerations focusing on known or potential drug–herb interactions, *Arch. Intern. Med.*, 158, 2200–2211, 1998.

10. Heptinstall, S. et al., Extracts of feverfew may inhibit platelet behaviour via neutralization of sulphydryl groups, *J. Pharm. Pharmacol.*, 39, 459–465, 1987.

11. Kaye, A.D., Kucera, I., and Sabar, R., Perioperative anesthesia clinical considerations of alternative medicines, *Anesthesiol. Clin. North America*, 22, 125–139, 2004.

12. Bordia, A., Effect of garlic on human platelet aggregation in vitro, *Atherosclerosis*, 30, 355–360, 1978.

13. Ackermann, R.T. et al., Garlic shows promise for improving some cardiovascular risk factors, *Arch. Intern. Med.*, 161, 813–824, 2001.

14. Backon, J., Ginger: inhibition of thromboxane synthetase and stimulation of prostacyclin: relevance for medicine and psychiatry, *Med. Hypotheses*, 20, 271–278, 1986.

15. Siegel, R.K., Ginseng abuse syndrome. Problems with the panacea, *J. Am. Med. Assoc.*, 241, 1614–1615, 1979.

16. Ang-Lee, M., Moss, J., Yuan, C., Herbal medicines and perioperative care, *J. Am. Med. Assoc.*, 286, 208–216, 2001.

17. Hartley, T.R., Lovallo, W.R., and Whitsett, T.L., Cardiovascular effects of caffeine in men and women, *Am. J. Cardiol.*, 93, 1022–1026, 2004.

18. Scher, A.I., Stewart, W.F., and Lipton, R.B., Caffeine as a risk factor for chronic daily headache: a population-based study, *Neurology*, 63, 2022–2027, 2004.

19. Kuczkowski, K.M., Anesthetic implications of drug abuse in pregnancy, *J. Clin. Anesth.*, 15, 382–394, 2003.

20. Abbott, A.V., Heart palpitations, *Am. Fam. Physician*, 71, 755–766, 2005.

21. Badellino, M.M. et al., Detection of pulmonary aspiration of gastric contents in an animal model by assay of peptic activity in bronchoalveolar fluid, *Crit. Care Med.*, 24, 1881–1885, 1996.

22. DePaso, W.J., Aspiration pneumonia, *Clin. Chest Med.*, 12, 269–284, 1991.

23. Hutchinson, A., Maltby, J.R., and Reid, C.R., Gastric fluid volume and pH in elective inpatients. Part I: coffee or orange juice versus overnight fast, *Can. J. Anaesth.*, 35, 12–15, 1988.

24. Scarlett, M., Crawford-Sykes, A., and Nelson, M., Preoperative starvation and pulmonary aspiration. New perspectives and guidelines, *West Indian Med. J.*, 51, 241–245, 2002.

25. Yogendran, S. et al., A prospective randomized double-blinded study of the effect of intravenous fluid therapy on adverse outcomes on outpatient surgery, *Anesth. Analg.*, 80, 682–686, 1995.

26. Pandit, S.K., Loberg, K.W., and Pandit, U.A., Toast and tea before elective surgery? A national survey on current practice, *Anesth. Analg.*, 90, 1348–1351, 2000.

27. Leite, J.F. et al., Value of nutritional parameters in the prediction of postoperative complications in elective gastrointestinal surgery, *Br. J. Surg.*, 74, 426–429, 1987.

28. Williams, J.Z. and Barbul, A., Nutrition and wound healing, *Surg. Clin. N. Am.*, 83, 571–596, 2003.

29. Moller, N. and Norrelund, H., The role of growth hormone in the regulation of protein metabolism with particular reference to conditions of fasting, *Horm. Res.*, 59 (Suppl. 1), 62–68, 2003.

30. Marin, L.A. et al., Preoperative nutritional evaluation as a prognostic tool for wound healing, *Acta. Orthop. Scand.*, 73, 2–5, 2002.

31. King, M.S., Preoperative evaluation, *Am. Fam. Physician*, 62, 387–396, 2000.

32. Volpi, E. et al., Essential amino acids are primarily responsible for the amino acid stimulation of muscle protein anabolism in healthy elderly adults, *Am. J. Clin. Nutr.*, 78, 250–258, 2003.

33. Alexander, J.W., Nutritional pharmacology in surgical patients, *Am. J. Surg.*, 183, 349–352, 2002.

34. Tepaske, R. et al., Effect of preoperative oral immune-enhancing nutritional supplement on patients at high risk of infection after cardiac surgery: a randomised placebo-controlled trial, *Lancet*, 358, 696–701, 2001.

35. Backhed, F. et al., Host-bacterial mutualism in the human intestine, *Science*, 307, 1915–1920, 2005.

36. Bralley, J.A. and Lord, R., *Laboratory Evaluations in Molecular Medicine*, The Institute for Advances in Molecular Medicine, Norcross, GA, 2001, p. 365.

37. Hedstrom, M. et al., Positive effects of anabolic steroids, vitamin D, and calcium on muscle mass, bone mineral density, and clinical function after a hip fracture. A randomised study of 63 women, *J. Bone Joint Surg. Br.*, 84, 497–503, 2002.

38. Boger, R.H. et al., Restoring vascular nitric oxide formation by L-arginine improves the symptoms of intermittent claudication in patients with peripheral arterial occlusive disease, *J. Am. Coll. Cardiol.*, 32, 1336–1344, 1998.

39. Boger, R.H. and Ron, E.S., L-Arginine improves vascular function by overcoming deleterious effects of ADMA, a novel cardiovascular risk factor, *Altern. Med. Rev.*, 10, 14–23, 2005.

40. Monograph L-carnitine, *Altern. Med. Rev.*, 10, 42–50, 2005.

41. Pistone, G. et al., Levocarnitine administration in elderly subjects with rapid muscle fatigue: effect on body composition, lipid profile, and fatigue. *Drugs Aging*, 20, 761–767, 2003.

42. Villareal, D.T., Holloszy, J.O., and Kohrt, W.M., Effects of DHEA replacement on bone mineral density and body composition in elderly women and men, *Clin. Endocrinol. (Oxf.)*, 53, 561–568, 2000.

43. Villareal, D.T., Effects of dehydroepiandrosterone on bone mineral density: what implications for therapy? *Treat. Endocrinol.*, 1, 349–357, 2002.

44. Chiu, K.M. et al., Correlation of serum L-carnitine and dehydro-epiandrosterone sulphate levels with age and sex in healthy adults, *Age Ageing*, 28, 211–216, 1999.

45. Morales, A.J. et al., The effect of six months treatment with a 100 mg daily dose of dehydroepiandrosterone (DHEA) on circulating sex steroids, body composition, and muscle strength in age-advanced men and women, *Clin. Endocrinol. (Oxf.)*, 49, 421–432, 1998.

46. Baulieu, E.E. et al., Dehydroepiandrosterone (DHEA), DHEA sulfate, and aging: contribution of the DHEAge study to a sociobiomedical issue. *Proc. Natl. Acad. Sci. USA*, 97, 4279–4284, 2000.

47. Hug, G. et al., Reduction of serum carnitine concentrations during anticonvulsant therapy with phenobarbital, valproic acid, phenytoin, and carbamazepine in children, *J. Pediatr.*, 119, 799–802, 1991.

48. Physicians' Desk Reference, 2005.

29 Xenobiotics: Managing Toxic Metals, Biocides, Hormone Mimics, Solvents, and Chemical Disruptors

Russell Jaffe, M.D., Ph.D.

CONTENTS

INTRODUCTION

Xenobiotics are biologically active chemicals in our environment, many of which compromise human health. The human cost of xenobiotics is a reduction of 8.8 years of life for the average person due to the effects of these toxicants.[1] This is 10% of most people's life span. The direct disease care costs induced by toxic metals, (TMs) for example, are calculated, in aggregate, to be in excess of $100 billion annually. A similar, yet less defined, burden is imposed by hormone disrupting persistent organic pollutants (POPs).[2] There has been a 1000-fold increase in TMs and persistent organic pollutants (POPs) in our environment due to anthropogenic effects. Indeed, over half of the TMs and POPs burden on the environment has been added within the last century. Bioaccumulation in mammals, including humans, is typically 100,000 to 200,000,000 times that of the environment. This is largely due to most mammals' ready uptake and impaired innate release (detoxification plus excretion) mechanisms when they lose homeostatic and innate antitoxic mechanisms. These innate mechanisms are designed to trap and facilitate the safer elimination of these toxins. Further, these mechanisms are inducible when we come in contact with small amounts of the toxicant and have the healthy resilience to induce elective, protective mechanisms. Today, too many people have lost those protective mechanisms and thus appear to be at greater (genetic) risk than their actual (phenotypic) situation. Still further, we know all too little about the interactions of toxins.

This chapter reviews the impact of better-studied, clinically known toxicant groups on musculoskeletal conditions. In addition, functional tests to determine body toxicant burden and immunotoxic reactivity are included because they improve diagnostic precision and clinical outcomes. Functional procedures such as penicillamine provocation for nutritional and TM status allow a noninvasive clinical window on cellular mineral and cellular buffering competencies. In addition, lymphocyte response assays (LRA) by ELISA/ACT method allow for patient-specific diagnostic testing and therapeutic monitoring. Taken together, these approaches to clinical management hasten more predictive, cost-effective, outcome-effective, integrative, and comprehensive clinical care.

Editor's Note

Many anthropogenic, human-sourced intoxicants bioaccumulate in the food chain. Since humans are a part of the food chain and toxins are stored primarily in fat, muscle, and bone, it follows logic that environmental toxins contribute to emerging and severe musculoskeletal conditions. Scientific evidence is also "bioaccumulating" for a clinical imperative to mitigate exposure where possible and to optimize host defenses, generally through strategic nutrition and functional adaptations.

PERSISTENT ORGANIC POLLUTANTS

POPs are a broad category of synthetic chemicals including polychlorinated biphenyls (PCBs), dioxin, chlordane, and DDT. POPs are pervasive chemicals, in that they persist in the environment due to limited ability of biota to metabolize or degrade them. POPs can be categorized as follows:

1. Hormone disruptor biocides (pesticides, fungicides, mitocides)
   - Cholinesterase inhibitor organophosphate pesticides
   - Halogenated pesticides.
2. Solvent residues
   - Chlorinated compounds (chloroform, methylene chloride, ethylene chloride)
   - Other halogenated compounds (brominated, fluorinated, iodinated) used most commonly as artificial food dye colorants, as radio-contrast agents, and art materials.

Even though some POPs have been banned or are restricted in use by some countries, POPs are, as their name suggests, persistent in the environment. They evaporate slowly into the atmosphere and aquifers and disperse around the globe. Living organisms then concentrate these fat-soluble chemicals in fatty tissues.

Adverse effects on human health can begin at thresholds below direct detection. In the case of dioxin, PCB, polybrominated biphenyl (PBB), and related compounds, human health risks emerge at the parts per trillion (ppt) level. This is in contrast to most laboratory tests that are only able to measure down to parts per million (ppm) levels of detection. In other words, we now routinely have biological health effects at amounts of materials in our bodies below our ability to detect them.

TOXIC METALS

While toxic metals with balanced electrons, such as metallic lead or mercury, are of low direct human toxicity,[3] their surprisingly ready conversion under physiological conditions to substantially more toxic biologically active forms (e.g., divalent methylmercury, dimethylmercury, mercuric sulfides, and other mercurous or mercuric compounds, ethyl-lead, etc.) continues to be a major public health risk.[4] Biologically active TMs are considered by Nriagu and Pacyna to be the most toxic of all the toxic anthropogenic exposures[5] in the biosphere even when compared with POPs and ionizing, xenobiotic radioisotopes.

The common TMs encountered in North America are lead (Pb^{2+}), mercury (Hg^{2+}), arsenic (As^{2+}), cadmium (Cd^{2+}), nickel (Ni^{2+}), and aluminum (Al^{3+}). Except for trivalent aluminum and exotic multivalent minerals, TMs are divalent. This predicts their transition state biochemistry.

Primary sources of TM exposure in humans include:

1. Medications and devices including amalgams and vaccines.
2. Metallic TMs in occupational or recreational settings.
3. Fungicides in interior environments or in agriculture.
4. Recreational exposures including from leaded glass decanters for beverages or ceramics used for food, ceramic glazes used by artists and commercial glazers, commercial uses of solders and fluxes.
5. Water and aerosol contamination.
6. Dietary sources including fish, fowl, such as commercially raised chicken, beef, and game. Generally, the higher up the food chain, the greater the contamination.

Living in an industrialized society exposes all inhabitants to metals and POPs in the environment. Substantial sources of highly toxic compounds can greatly enrich an environment in a toxicant without public awareness. These largely invisible depositions are bioidentical and just as toxic as the exposures of which we are aware. For example, while 200 to 600 tons of mercurial toxicants are annually added to the American ecosystem from all anthropogenic sources, an additional 100 tons of mercury is derived from trans-Atlantic tiny dust particles. Additional metric tons may be added by the trans-Pacific plumes of aerosol toxicants from the Pacific Rim. These are carried in the upper atmosphere and contain enough mercury and arsenic to qualify as mineable ore if only this dust could be trapped before it reaches the southern United States and Caribbean Basin.[6] This last environmental burden was unknown until as recently as 1990. This illustrates how substantial sources of "high toxic effects compounds" can greatly enrich an environment in a toxicant without general awareness of the influx of that toxicant. These largely invisible depositions are bioidentical and just as toxic as the exposures of which we are aware.

Toxic metals are potent metabolic, hormonal, immune, and gene toxins.[7] For example, continued exposures to TMs that bioaccumulate, above about 1 part per billion (ppb),[8,9] impose long-term human health risks, particularly for increased chronic autoimmune and cardiovascular illnesses.[10]

With regard to lead, the evidence base of pervasive subacute toxicities is particularly well documented and well reviewed elsewhere.[11]

Living in an industrialized society exposes all inhabitants to metals and POPs in the environment. Some minerals are essential for life. To some extent, beneficial minerals are antitoxic in that they block or compete with the TMs. In other words, people with adequate stores of buffering minerals block the uptake and facilitate the excretion of TMs from the body in all excretory pathways. These pathways of excretion include urine, stool, sweat, desquamated skin, hair, nails, and breath. The antitoxic minerals work best when the amounts, balance, and ratios provide ample reserve pools to draw upon. The particular minerals involved are potassium and sodium, calcium and magnesium, zinc and copper, chromium and vanadium, manganese and molybdenum, selenomethionine and iodides, etc.

Some minerals, like selenium, have proper, bioactive form (selenomethionine and selenocysteine) and can form stable, permanent, covalent links with biologically active mercury or arsenic (and probably other divalent TMs), thereby detoxifying them. These stable complexes are not easy to remove and may remain in the body for periods of years to decades. Their "balanced electron" relatively low toxicity reduces the priority placed on their removal from the host. In contrast, other forms of selenium commonly used in supplements do not have this beneficial property, yet are more toxic.

TMs and POPs are an acquired and reversible health risk for over 80 million Americans. The human cost is a reduction of 8.8 years of life for the average person due to the effects of these toxicants.[12] This is a biological tax of 10% of most people's life span. The direct disease care costs induced by TMs are calculated, in aggregate, to be in excess of $100 billion annually.[13]

This means that we could fund a transition from our current symptom-reactive, sick care focus to a proactive, intoxication prevention program out of savings from sick care costs not incurred. The public health risk from TMs is even greater due to observed but not extensively defined or replicated synergies of mineral toxicities.[14] Since TMs and POPs both bioaccumulate and bioconcentrate, the adventitious exposures are likely to increase greatly just at the time that internal reserve mineral and antioxidant protectors are at their highest. Chapter 25 addresses the importance of alkaline balance and of avoiding both metabolic acidosis and catabolic illness.

TMs and POPs are among "nature's mimics" in that they can bring to substantially greater intensity a wide variety of clinical conditions including fibromyalgia, rhabdomyolysis, chronic pain, osteoporosis, birth defects, and autoimmune syndromes. TMs and POPs potentiate these highly diverse conditions due to their common yet variable expressions of free radical pathology, made worse in the face of antioxidant deficits and metabolic acidosis.

Understanding this molecular pathophysiology allows us to enter a new era of clinical medicine where comprehensive, integrative care plays an important role. Identifying the role of clinical chronic subacute (low-level yet persisting) TM and POPs actions is integral to "identify and mitigate the causes rather than focus on relief from the symptomatic consequences" of philosophy of care that differentiates integrative and comprehensive care as a specialty from conventional internal medicine and family practice.

Among the effects of TMs and POPs are the following molecular consequences for cell functions:

1. *Metabolic uncoupler*: Inhibits cytochrome I to coenzyme Q_{10} transfer in the mitochondria, the cells energy producing detoxifying saprophytic organelle. This reduces ATP (high-energy compound) production, thus reducing the functionality of those parts of the cell consuming the most energy; generally, this means the most metabolically active and functionally important component of the cell becomes starved for energy.

2. *Hapten immunotoxins*: Small molecules that bind to and distort the structure of the body's own proteins, from globulins to insulin, from lipoproteins to macroglobulins, thus increasing the probability of autoimmune, chronic illness.

3. *Enzyme inhibitor*: For cell regulatory control kinases and other enzymes with cysteine or thiamine (B1) sulfhydryls at their active site. Phosphodiesterase, superoxide dismutase (SOD), and nucleotide binding protein (NBP) are examples of particularly vulnerable, functionally vital enzyme catalysts.

4. *Anti-antioxidants (pro-oxidants)*: TMs and POPs are pro-oxidants that induce excessive consumption and wasting of glutathione and ascorbate. These two antioxidants are at the center of the antioxidant recycling network that protects delicate cell components from free-radical oxidative damage when we are in physiologic homeostasis and immune tolerance. Once antioxidants are selectively depleted, free-radical damage can run rampant in oxidizing and making important cell systems dysfunctional. Chapter 7 by Harris and Baer addresses this in more detail.

5. *Bioconcentrate*: These toxicants bioaccumulate in critical and most unfortunate places within the body like the choroids plexus where spinal fluid is produced to the loop of Henle where the kidney concentrates toxins for excretion into the urine. This reduces the body's functionality and accelerates biological aging.

ABSENCE OF EVIDENCE IS NOT EVIDENCE OF ABSENCE

With regard to POPs and possible interactions among chemicals, of the 104,000 chemicals introduced into the environment through made-made novel synthesis, barely 4000 have been studied at all and barely a handful have been studied for their interactive toxicities. The absence of data is not a basis for assuming the data of absence exists.[15]

An example of absence of evidence is the immune system's response to toxins, even once removed. There are T-helper lymphocytes that are involved with delayed allergy reactions to haptenic[*] immunotoxins such as TMs. Clinically, this can be functionally measured by a classic memory enzyme linked immunosorbed assay (MELISA) modification of thymidine incorporation or by the LRA by ELISA/ACT tests that assay kinase activation prior to inducing thymidine incorporation and cell mitotic division. These technologies show us that even tiny amounts of internal or environmental exposure to a substance that induces an immunotoxic hypersensitivity reduces immune defense abilities and induces

---

[*]Haptenic substances (or haptens) are small molecules which, while not large enough to be recognized as foreign by the body, bind to the body's own proteins. This binding distorts the innate structure, rendering them "foreign" and immunoreactive in the body.

deferral of immune repair. When this becomes the usual condition, we become hospitable to "whatever is going around."

Another example of absence of evidence is the toxin's damage to energy production. Among the effects of TMs and POPs when they bioaccumulate in cells is apoptosis of mitochondria. After mitochondria commit this programmed cell suicide, the cell's overall death is not far off. In contrast, protection and rehabilitation of mitochondria is central to lifelong health maintenance, restoration, or enhancement.

The effects of TMs and POPs are more destructive when low cellular minerals (particularly potassium and magnesium) predispose the cell to metabolic acidosis. Intracellular depletion of potassium and magnesium can cause metabolic acidosis regardless of how well compensated the blood pH may be. The combination of metabolic acidosis and TMs and POPs accelerates mineral leaching from bone to buffer the excess acids the kidney needs to concentrate and excrete without damaging itself, to the extent possible. This means that osteopenia and osteoporosis are accelerated. Among the other effects are shifts within cells from elective production of structural proteins and Metallothionein to a survival mode for the cell such that only actions needed for the cell to avoid death are performed.

Elective and protective elements are no longer produced. Toxic effects of TMs are further potentiated in this situation. Unhealthy hormone metabolites may accumulate rather than be excreted owing to toxic damage or lack of cell energy required to "pump" toxicants out of the body and into urine, stool, and sweat while healthier hormone products, in contrast, may not be made. Further, we know too little about the interactions of low-level persistent TMs. What little we do know suggests there is synergy of toxic effects when two or more TMs are concurrently present.[16]

RISK OF BIOACCUMULATION OF TOXICANTS: A MATTER OF BALANCE AND HOMEOSTASIS

Bioaccumulation of TMs or POPs is a function of intake and output balance.

$$\text{Intake} - \text{Output} = \text{Residual (remainder in body)}$$

The integral of this simple input–output model determines individual body burden. For example, if

$$\text{Intake (high)} - \text{Output (low)} = \text{Increase in toxic burden}$$

1. Intake (high) − Output (high) = Steady state, high risk state
2. Intake (low) − Output (high) = Decrease in toxic burden
3. Intake (low) − Output (low) = Low exposure

$$\text{Goal: Intake (low)} - \text{Output (high)} = \text{Body burden reduction}$$

It is possible to reduce, but not avoid, intake as discussed earlier. It is also possible to increase output to reduce the residual, or total body burden. In other words, low intake and high capacity to excrete toxins is a feasible clinical evidence-based goal.

Note that high output is associated with elective synthesis of Metallothionein, polypeptides made largely of glycine and cysteine with zinc or magnesium as the counterion. When these biological detoxifiers are produced, substantial TM trapping capacity is observed in the gut, the plasma, and the cerebrospinal fluid.

INCREASING OUTPUT TO REDUCE BIOACCUMULATION

William Walsh of the Pfeiffer Treatment Center, Wheaton, IL, reports a link between the above basic science genetic and phenotypic data, suggesting a hereditary or xenobiotic pseudogenetic predisposition to mercury toxicity and T-lymphocyte hypersensitivity (DTH). The emerging data make thimerosal exposure at times of distress or impaired detoxification particularly troublesome. Thimerisal typically contains 5 to 7.5 μg of ethylmercury per vaccination dose.

High output of toxins from the human body is associated with elective synthesis of Metallothioneins. Under normal circumstances, there is a large concentration of the protein Metallothionein waiting in the intestines, as a sentinel, to interact with the mercury or other TM and detoxify it before it enters the body.

Each Metallothionein molecule has binding sites for seven atoms of zinc plus variable amounts of magnesium, selenomethionine, and glutathione. Structurally, it is a linear protein of 61 amino acids with 20 or more cysteine or cystine-active sulfhydryls. Its job is TM detoxification. It is present in high concentration in the GI tract and in the liver, but it is present in every cell in the body. When present, it protects the GI tract from all of the nasty things that TMs like mercury can do. However, its production is elective. Metallothionein production occurs only when the body is healthy, alkaline buffered, and in homeostatic equilibrium. In states of hormonal, neurochemical, or immune distress, Metallothionein production can be substantially downregulated.

> If you take somebody whose Metallothionein system is working well, however, the mercury forms covalent links to other, active sulfhydryl groups. The sulfhydryl groups in active site of certain enzymes in the gastrointestinal tract include the enzymes that break down casein from cow milk and gluten from wheat and other grains. A Metallothionein disorder, therefore, is often associated with major digestive and dysbiosis problems as well. Most typically, wheat and casein intolerances and other delayed T-cell mediated allergic hypersensitivities occur. These individuals are also prone to intestinal inflammation and enteropathy.
> Metallothionein is a family of four proteins (1,2,3, and 4). Metallothioneins 1 and 2 are ubiquitous and present in every cell in the body. Metallothioneins carry out innate antioxidant functions and deliver zinc wherever it is needed.[17]

Metallothioneins are also responsible for homeostasis between copper and zinc. These trace elements, in turn, are related to production of specific hormones, cytokines, and neurotransmitters. For example, for the zinc or copper requiring enzyme catalysts to convert the right amount of dopamine into norepinephrine, copper to zinc balance and sufficiency are required. This is discussed in more detail in Chapter 13.

Walsh and colleagues have used the plasma zinc–copper ratio as an indicator of properly functioning Metallothionein. They use it as an indicator of "toxic-coping ability." They report that, if you have a population of:

1. Obsessive–compulsive (OC) individuals, the ratio between plasma zinc and serum copper will be around 0.8.
2. The healthy range, based on nearly 100,000 individuals, is about 1.0.
3. Walsh et al. have examined 5700 individuals with attention-deficit disorder and the mean ratio is 1.17.
4. For children who exhibit violent behavior, the ratio is typically > 1.4.

Walsh suggests that impaired homeostasis for copper and zinc correlates with poor Metallothionein function. The detailed influence of supplementation on normalizing these ratios and their impact on function and performance are, as yet, unreported.[18]

Reducing Iatrogenic Input

If you study people with amalgams, many of them show few adverse effects. Similarly, most children who receive vaccinations containing thimerosal go through this experience without many notable adverse effects. Perhaps these are the individuals with adequate ascorbate and glutathione, magnesium and zinc, selenomethionine and sulfur from dietary sources (including breast milk from mothers whose antitoxic levels are high). These individuals are protected and are at relatively low risk. When zinc, selenomethionine, and magnesium are marginal or deficient, Metallothionein loses functionality.[19] Such individuals are sensitive and at high risk of the adverse consequences of TMs and POPs.

The Swedish experience is the most rigorous and extensive regarding toxicity from dental materials, particularly mercury amalgam. Lindh pioneered research using nuclear probe microscopy for minerals in biomedical analysis.[†] Neutrophil (granulocyte) mercury was compared between patients with mercury amalgams who were sick and controls (i.e., people with mercury amalgams who were not sick).

[†] Nuclear microscopy or PIXE is an advanced analytical tool that allows for the measurement of trace elements in small objects, such as the nucleus of the neutrophil granulocyte (with a detection limit of 0.5 μg/g dry substance). This is done by bombarding the cells and their organelles with protons (hydrogen atoms). Because each trace element has its own characteristic emission fingerprint, it is then possible to determine the amounts of a particular element in the various regions of the cell. This was based on the earlier work of Jaffe, Smith, and Costa.

The results showed that the patients who had amalgams and who were sick had detectable mercury in their cells and that the controls did not show bioaccumulation of mercury.

In addition, the concentrations of other elements such as magnesium, calcium, manganese, iron, and zinc were more than one standard deviation below in the patients and not in the asymptomatic controls. Examination of elements in the nucleus showed a maldistribution of zinc, which correlated with the presence of mercury in the nucleus of the neutrophils. There is a typical zinc distribution in the nucleus of the neutrophil granulocyte. In contrast to this normal situation, the patients who had mercury burdens showed an abnormal distribution and an invasion of mercury into delicate nuclear or nucleolar centers. Mercury in the nucleus correlated with the decreased zinc in those areas. Whether mercury caused the mineral aberrations or if preexisting mineral deficiencies predisposed to mercury remains to be determined. In summary, by using sensitive probes, Lindh clearly demonstrated the presence of mercury in the cells of patients who had amalgams and who were sick, and the absence of mercury above threshold levels in the cells of asymptomatic controls with amalgams.

The majority of metals that are used in dentistry belong to the transition group in the periodic table. A general characteristic of these elements is that they have an uncompleted electron shell, either in the natural or oxidative state. Since electrons always exist in pairs, transition metals form strong complexes with both organic and inorganic ligands. The memory cells are long-lived and can be detected in the blood of sensitive individuals, prior to the appearance of objectively documented clinical symptoms.

Stejskal and Lindh, elucidated the immune response that mercury may trigger. The research agrees that T-lymphocytes play a role in all types of allergic and autoimmune reactions.[20] This makes them evident candidates as markers for metal-induced sensitivity. After contact with an antigen, T- and B-lymphocytes that are antigen-specific for that substance correlate with inflammatory reactions that lead to cell damage when repair is delayed or blocked. Repeated exposure with the same or a chemically similar cross-reacting antigen will immediately induce a faster, secondary immunological reaction initiated by the memory cells. Cytokine release will activate other cell types and the result is either beneficial for the body when repair is facilitated or, in the case of repair deficient autoimmune diseases, a pathological consequence. Human lymphocytes can be stimulated *in vitro* with various foreign substances called mitogens. The lymphocyte stimulation test has been used for 30 years as routine analysis for evaluation of cellular immunity and clinical immunology, as well as for diagnoses of allergic reactions to medicines, metals, and other substances. Specific stimulation is based on the fact that every person's immune system remembers the antigen that it has previously been programmed to remember.[21] Such a reaction gives rise to memory T- and B-lymphocyte cells that circulate in the bloodstream and defend as needed the individual against foreign substances including:

1. Xenobiotics and other synthetic small molecules (mostly haptens).
2. Partially digested, immunoreactive food digestive remnants.
3. Pathogens including bacteria, parasites, viruses, or anything recognized by an individual as foreign to their immune system.

Other types of white blood cells are dendritic cells such as monocytes and macrophages, endothelial cells and fibroblasts, astrocytes and Kupfer cells. These cells perform various functions such as presentation of processed antigens to naive unprogrammed lymphocytes and removal of toxic substances; thus, they are termed "scavenger" or dendritic cells. They are short-lived with a typical life span of 8 to 12 hours in the body. Tests that employ changes in short-lived granulocytes are not using contemporary technology for functional immune system predictive response. At best they are looking "through a glass darkly" and over-interpreting aggregate particle changes as lymphocyte-specific changes, which they probably are not. The possibility to diagnose delayed allergy (hypersensitivity) with the help of lymphocyte stimulation tests rests on the fact that in the case of low molecular weight substances (haptens), antigen-specific memory cells are present in patients with allergy symptoms, but not in healthy exposed individuals. Further, since memory cells circulate through the body, the sensitization or allergy is always a systemic phenomenon. The term local allergy often used in the case of oral mucosal changes indicates ignorance of modern immunological principles. The majority of the lymphocytes that operate in cell-mediated reactions are T-lymphocytes. T-lymphocytes play a key role in the development of all types of allergic and autoimmune disorders. The identification of the antigenic structures (epitopes) involved in allergy and autoimmunity is a "hot field" in current research. One method of autoimmunity is that metals bind to the sulfhydryl groups on proteins and alter their three-dimensional structure. The immune system recognizes the altered proteins as foreign and an autoimmune process starts, often with condition-specific imbalances in Th1 and Th2 populations of lymphocytes. TMs and POPs can affect the immune system in several ways. In the oral cavity, high concentrations of metal ions may suppress the immune response and result in immunosuppression. This could explain why the oral mucosa contains only a low number of cells with the capability to present antigen to T-lymphocytes. This may also be why mucosal changes adjacent to metal fillings are rarely seen. Higher concentrations of metals can also upregulate immune reactions (called the polyclonal or nonspecific stimulation) and such responses are seen in individuals with intact immunity.

In contrast, in some hereditarily predisposed individuals, TMs may act as haptenic immune reactors. To be able to use the conventional lymphocyte stimulation test for diagnosis of metal-induced allergy, it was necessary to modify the test in such a way that only the antigen-specific reaction was measured. This was achieved by reducing the concentrations of the metals added to cultures. Since antigen-specific memory cells in the blood are relatively few, the number of lymphocytes in the metal cultures was increased, and the number of other cells that could affect the lymphocyte proliferation negatively was reduced. This version of the lymphocyte stimulation test is called MELISA. Another advanced lymphocyte response assay is the LRA by ELISA/ACT tests system.

In short, MELISA or LRA by ELISA/ACT enables individuals who are immunoreactive to mercury and other metals to be identified. Furthermore, after the removal of amalgam and replacement with nonmetal composites or the systematic reduction in immunoreactive exposures, the lymphocyte stimulation test often reverts to nonreactive. This "resetting" of immune responses typically takes 6 to 18 months. These changes parallel the decrease in concentrations of mercury inside the neutrophil granulocyte. The dental research in this regard in Sweden is well documented by Hudecek, a capable biological dentist. Following dental amalgam(s) removal, his data showed that 76% of patients reported long-term health improvement, 22% reported unchanged health, and 2% reported a worsening of symptoms.

Recently, Lindvall reported that at 1 to 2 years following amalgam removal, about a quarter of the patients had completely recovered from their chronic autoimmune or immune dysfunction syndromes, half were substantially improved, one fifth showed no change, and one twentieth (5%) were worse off than before. This latter group was mostly patients who had improper or premature amalgam removal.[22]

QUANTIFYING INDIVIDUAL EXPOSURE

Evaluation of a person suspected of chronic clinical metal toxicity and heavy metal sensitivity or POPs burden[23] can be based clinically on the following:

1. Determining the body exposure and burden of the TMs, POPs, and the relevant nutritional antitoxic metals on an appropriately provoked specimen is the current state of the art of testing and determining probably (?) clinical body burden at a sufficient level of precision to warrant clinical management based on the provoked urine quantitative information. In addition, unprovoked urine may be employed as a preprovocative testing screening assessment but is not routinely, clinically necessary.
2. Penicillamine (D-Pen™, Cupramine™) is an example of a mineral binding or chelating compounds that has been standardized for provocative testing and therapeutic monitoring. Penicillamine has been standardized as a challenge agent for cellular toxic and nutritional mineral content. Other chelators are in development, while a variety of selective chelators are currently available, varying with local regulatory practices.
3. Further, the timing of detoxification is best accomplished when host systems for sequestration and rapid elimination of toxin are facilitated. For example, removal of mercury containing amalgams (if needed) should follow a systematic program to enhance dietary intake of

detoxifying foods and to reduce the mobilizable burden of TMs or POPs. Examples of "detox" foods are garlic, onions and ginger, brassica sprouts, and eggs. Each of them can block uptake and bind (thereby detoxifying) TMs, most POPs, and other sources of biologically active sulfur compounds to accomplish the same effects. Individualized therapy by clinically experienced professionals is needed to guide supplementation, lifestyle changes, and attitudinal healing.

Confirmatory, follow-up testing is encouraged at 3 to 6 months following the initiation of therapy. In many cases, otherwise unexpected additional toxicants or essential nutritional mineral deficits will be revealed. It is cost-effective to engage these elements of comprehensive and integrative care. This reduction in human morbidity can be linked to the reduction of biologically active TMs/POPs and the enhancement of antioxidant, antitoxic stores in the person.

REMOVING TMs AND POPs

Now we will look at the practical aspects of identifying nutritional and TM body burden by provocation testing using penicillamine as an example of a validated oral protocol.

Penicillamine Protocol for Determining
Toxic and Nutritional Mineral Status in Cells by
Noninvasive Provocation into the Urine

Purpose: Determine the body's burden of mobilizable, potentially toxic metals and the divalent minerals altered when toxins are present.
Method: A 24 hours urine test during a short noninvasive provocation using oral d-penicillamine (Cupramine, D-Pen, dimethylcysteine, mercaptovaline) or acetyl-penicillamine, prescribed by a physician.
Protocol:

- The average-sized adult is prescribed 500 mg of penicillamine or *N*-acetyl-penicillamine with each meal and before bed for 3 days. Generally, two capsules of 250 mg each are taken four times a day. This is a total of 2 g each day. The dose is based on 30 mg/kg body weight. If weight is under 100 or over 300 lb, calculation of dose is recommended. For example, a 100 lb adult weighs 45.5 kg. A daily dose of 1590 mg (~1500 mg) is recommended. This would most easily be achieved by giving 2 × 250 mg capsules with breakfast, dinner, and at bedtime (2 capsules TID). By comparison, a 350 lb person weighs 160 kg. At 30 mg/kg, this calculates to a daily dose of 4800 mg (~4750 mg). This means taking 5 × 250 mg capsules with each of three meals plus 4 × 250 mg capsules at bedtime.

- This short course of penicillamine avoids the rare but important side effects of longer-term therapeutic doses of the drug as discussed in the *Physicians Desk Reference*. Inform patients to discontinue taking the medication until otherwise instructed if there is an adverse effect.
- Begin urine collection on the morning of the second day. This is 24 hours after initiating the penicillimine. Collect all urine in a heavy metal-free container, which is usually provided by the doctor or the laboratory. Urine must be collected for a full 24 hours cycle. If a urine sample is missed, the collection is incomplete and the protocol should be resumed 1 week later. Urine collected in an incomplete sample may be poured out and the same collection container reused.
- Take the completed urine collection to the laboratory promptly. The total volume is an important part of the information to be sent to the analytic laboratory. It is desirable, although not necessary, to keep the urine refrigerated during the collection period.
- Analyze the results. Typical penicillamine provocation reference ranges are included in Table 29.1.
- Please note that a third-day collection cannot be compared with the standardized second-day collection results. Because the specimen is provoked by d-penicillamine, it should not be used for mineral balance studies. The specimen may be used to check kidney function and to analyze for most hormones and neurotransmitter metabolites.
- If substantial total TM tissue burdens are documented, oral pulse therapy (2 days/week) with penicillamine is recommended. Use 7.5 mg/kg QID, on the two days each week for 3 months. After 3 months, retest the urine by the penicillamine provocation test to determine the residual TM being eliminated as well as for comparison of nutritional mineral status. For example, are they assimilating what is being given or do they have enteropathy with consequent reduction in mineral uptake? Do they have a particularly high need for particular minerals for their unique metabolic balance state, type, or condition based on functional tests?

The short course of penicillamine avoids the rare but important side effects of longer-term therapeutic doses of the drug as discussed in the *Physicians Desk Reference*. Patients should be advised to discontinue taking the medication if any adverse response is observed until otherwise instructed by a clinician.

Interpretation and Substantiation of Penicillamine Protocol

Each laboratory has an applicable reference range for each mineral assayed. Elevation above the range reported by that laboratory is indicative of increased tissue stores of that heavy metal. Tissue status of nutritional minerals may also be assessed in this way. Typical penicillamine provocation reference ranges are included in Table 29.1.

TABLE 29.1

Mineral value ranges for nutritional and toxic minerals in the second-day 24 h urine after d-penicillamine provocation, 7.5 mg/kg QID for 3 days (N = 200)

Mineral element	Reference range mg/g creatinine	Reference range mg/24 h sample
Nutritional		
Calcium	310–620	400–900
Magnesium	250–550	350–700
Zinc	0.8–1.3	1.1–1.5
Copper	0.04–0.06	0.06–0.08
Iron	0.20–0.30	0.24–0.36
Manganese	0.005–0.007	0.006–0.008
Molybdenum	0.11–0.14	0.13–0.19
Boron	4.1–5.6	5.8–6.7
Chromium	0.19–0.30	0.21–0.33
Cobalt	0.04–0.06	0.05–0.07
Selenium	0.25–0.31	0.24–0.35
Vanadium	0.02–0.03	0.03–0.04
Toxic	μg/gm creatinine	ug/24 h sample
Lead	<20	<25
Mercury	<7	<9
Arsenic	<120	<175
Nickel	<16	<25
Cadmium	<4	<6

Note: Values lower than the reference range in provoked specimens suggest deficiency of the above-needed essential minerals. Adequacy of supplemental intake to replenish deficits can be monitored by repeat d-penicillamine provocation every 3 months.

MANAGING MODEST AMOUNTS OF PROVOKED TMs

Patients are advised to follow the alkaline way diet. Eighty percent of this diet comprises alkaline-forming foods. Alkaline-forming foods add bicarbonate rather than hydrogen ions. One way patients can assess results of their diet is by monitoring urine pH. Refer to Chapter 25 for the alkaline way diet protocol.

This diet should be combined with sufficient amounts of antioxidants plus minerals (potassium, calcium, magnesium, and zinc as their fully ionized, fully soluble ascorbates, aspartates, citrates, malates, succinates, fumarates glycinates, or other fully soluble, nonallergenic mineral salts) to displace the TMs. Adequate herbal tea, mineral water, or spring water helps to "wash out" these toxins.

A repeat provocative urine minerals test after 3 to 6 months is recommended to confirm the reduction in available TMs.

MANAGING MORE THAN MODEST AMOUNTS OF PROVOKED TMs

Use penicillamine twice a week (e.g., Mondays and Thursdays) for 30 to 60 days at 7.5 mg/kg taken QID (500 mg/QID for most adults) with supplemental calcium, magnesium, and zinc particularly on the nonpenicillamine days to replace these minerals (which penicillamine will chelate along with the other divalent [double charged] minerals along with toxic or heavy metals).

Therapeutic doses of antioxidants are beneficial as described. They include:

1. Buffered ascorbate based on ascorbate calibration to determine physiological ascorbate need.[24] Flavonoid/flavanol combinations (e.g., a total of 1 to 30 g daily of quercetin dehydrate and soluble OPC) potentiate the benefits of buffered ascorbate. Their need increases in proportion to buffered ascorbate need as noted in the ascorbate calibration document.
2. Natural vitamin E (mixed tocopherols) 200 to 1600 IU/d with tocotrienols (polycosanols) and selenomethionine.
3. A balanced, high-potency, high-activity B complex including para-aminobenzoic acid (PABA) and selenomethionine.
4. A comprehensive micromineral supplement is recommended since micromineral deficits are pervasive. From magnesium and potassium to chromium and vanadium, from manganese and molybdenum to zinc and copper we can measure the relationships of these key nutritional minerals. Selenomethionine is the most active mineral form for combining with and inactivating TMs.
5. Sulfhydryl-rich foods such as garlic, ginger, and onions; eggs; and brassica vegetables (e.g., broccoli, cabbage, etc.). Make fresh ginger tea (with raw honey to taste) a staple beverage. A thumb-size piece of fresh ginger, finely chopped and steeped in hot water for 5 min contains over 5000 μg of TM-trapping sulfhydryl compounds. Ginger tea may be made up ahead of time and may be drunk cool or cold if preferred.
6. Probiotics (8 to 20 Bn/day) containing multiple human strains that have been cultured, harvested, and lyophilized (freeze dried) for maximum activity and potency.
7. Carotenoids (e.g., 25 to 100 mg daily of the carotenoid family including alphacarotene, betacarotene, lutein, cryptoxanthin, and pseudoxanthin) and vitamin D (600 to 2400 IU daily) for enhanced cell regulation and resilience.
8. Adequate beneficial, essential fats (e.g., 0.5 to 5 g daily of total omega-3 fatty acids intake) including conjugated linoleic acid, docosahexaenic acid, and eicosapentenoic acid (EPA) as discussed in detail in Chapter 4.

Enhancing antioxidant levels is demonstrated to improve flowing blood in metabolically and hormonally active cells, the blood–brain barrier and the choroid plexus, the enterocytes in the digestive tract, metabolically active nerve, endocrine, immune and hepatic cells, sexual function, and skin.

PENICILLAMINE IN CLINICAL PRACTICE

Penicillamine was found to bind copper in the body and safely mobilize it for excretion in the urine (and stool and sweat) of patients with Wilson's disease[25] for which it has remained the treatment of choice for almost half a century. Walsh has reported the safe and successful use of penicillamine in pregnant women, infants, the elderly, and the infirm.

In nonhuman species, lead in bone seems to be even more effectively mobilized by penicillamine than lead in soft tissues.[26,27] However, CaNa2 EDTA is reported to be a more effective lead chelator than penicillamine *in vitro* in tissue culture.[28] Questions have been raised about the safety of using any agent for low-level TM detoxification because some animal studies report that lead may redistribute into soft tissues such as the choroid plexus (where spinal fluid is produced) or the urine concentrating loop of Henle in the kidney after $CaNa_2$ EDTA therapy.[29] Concerns of this type have been raised about all oral chelators although less with regard to penicillamine than any other substance because of the tight bond between TMs and penicillamine.

LEAD, MERCURY, ARSENIC, CADMIUM, AND NICKEL MOBILIZATION BY PENICILLAMINE

Clinical benefits of penicillamine are described by Sachs *et al.*[30] and Vitale *et al.*,[31] but not by Marcus[32] (who administered penicillamine while the study subjects continued to live in lead exposed environs). This may well explain the less dramatic decline in blood lead levels in the Marcus study.

In Chisholm's study, children removed from further exposure and treated with penicillamine showed more rapid decline in blood lead levels and in the reversal of hematologic toxicity than the decline in toxicies resulting solely from eliminating the lead exposure sources.[33] In contrast, the study by Rogan et al.[34] did not confirm these findings. This study has been criticized as flawed in method because the environment of the children studies was not mitigated for continued TM exposure during the study period.[35] In other words, simple use of a chelator is insufficient if you leave the person in the intoxicated environment without mitigation.

In addition to lead, penicillamine also mobilizes and facilitates the safer excretion of TMs[36] including mercury,[37–44] arsenic,[45–50] cadmium,[51–53] and nickel.[54] Inconsistent reports of efficacy have been published. On balance, these may reflect lack of attention to sufficient reducing substance (ascorbate) to enhance TM mobilization and excretion while maintaining the more effective reduced form of penicillamine rather than its disulfide. An additional factor that reduces

TM mobilization is metabolic cellular acidosis. Correction of magnesium buffering deficit aids directly (by displacement) and indirectly (by correcting cellular acidosis) enhanced TM mobilization. Magnesium, as the second most prevalent mineral inside healthy mammalian cells, is a major contributor to cellular buffering and its absence induces cellular metabolic acidosis.[55]

The toxicity of penicillamine has been described based on its use for several indications in both adults and children. Toxicity of the racemic mixture used years ago to treat chronic arthritis in adults may account for the severity of some of these symptoms and should never be used. In children, nausea and vomiting appear more often at doses exceeding 60 mg/kg/d and may respond to a decrease in dosage.[56] This protocol uses 30 mg/kg doses for just 3 days for provocation.

When given daily and for prolonged periods (which we never recommend) adverse blood and skin effects seem to be idiosyncratic hypersensitivity reactions and are not dose related. Reversible leukopenia or mild thrombocytopenia is reported in less than 10% of children in one study,[57] but not with similar dosages in two other larger series.[58] This may have resulted from interaction between penicillamine and pyridoxine (B-6).[59] Supplemental B-6 is now routinely recommended as part of penicillamine therapy (not provocation). Eosinophilia (defined as $> 18\%$ eosinophils) has been noted in one fifth of high-risk children treated daily for an extended duration with the older, less pure preparations of d-penicillamine.[60]

Angioedema, urticaria, or maculopapular eruptions that require discontinuation of drug therapy are reported at a rate of 0.5 to 1%.[61] Still less commonly reported reactions are proteinuria, microscopic hematuria, and urinary incontinence.[62] All of these relate to increased tissue permeability due to inhibition of connective tissue cross-links when penicillamine is given on a continuing daily basis and not when it is given in the pulsed manner recommended here. All these problems are much less common today because of the higher purity of d-penicillamine and improved understanding of its mechanisms of action and how to separate them for clinical benefits.

Distribution in the body of penicillamine is widespread. Like amino acids such as cysteine of which penicillamine is the dimethyl analog, as also is mercaptovaline, it moves freely inside cells, subcellular organelles like the mitochondria and into deep tissue sites like the brain.[63–70]

Reactive foods or intestinal irritants such as ferrous sulfate[71] may reduce the peak level of penicillamine in blood by a third or more.[72] Antacids or functional hypochlorhydria[73] decreases penicillamine absorption by as much as two thirds.[74] As with all amino acids, peak blood levels are achieved when the amino acid is given on an empty stomach. For provocation and for therapy, mean blood levels are more important than peak blood levels. Thus, taking the penicillamine with food is acceptable. Compliance with this regimen, individually as suggested above, is high.

The recommended dose and duration of therapy with penicillamine have been empirically derived. Doses have ranged from 100 mg/kg/d (in earlier studies) to

20 to 40 mg/kg/d. Far fewer side effects are reported at the lower dosage range used in provocation and TM mobilization. The duration of the pulse therapy herein recommended is typically on Monday and Thursday for 3 to 6 months, depending on the pretreatment provoked urine TM concentration. When used in this pulsed fashion, penicillamine has become a first-line comprehensive care treatment of choice over the several decades of its increasingly widespread use.

Penicillamine has the additional benefit of serving as a source of nitric oxide, which facilitates cellular communication and improved vascular compliance.[75]

In addition, if substantial total TM tissue burdens are documented, oral pulse therapy (2 days/week) with penicillamine is recommended. Use 7.5 mg/kg qid, on the two days each week for 3 months. After 3 months, retest the urine by the penicillamine provocation test to determine residual TM being eliminated as well as comparison of nutritional mineral status. For example, are they assimilating what is being given or do they have enteropathy with consequent reduction in mineral uptake? Do they have a particularly high need for particular minerals for their unique metabolic balance state, type, or condition based on functional tests?

CONCLUSION: DIAGNOSING AND MANAGING MUSCULOSKELETAL CONDITIONS

This chapter focuses on TMs and POPs with emphasis on their clinical effects, their diagnostic assessment, and their safer detoxification. This is particularly true for the health of the body's frame (structure; bones, joints, and extracellular matrix), for metabolic balance (weight, obesity risk, insulin resistance), for managing such "mystery syndromes" as fibromyalgia or myofascial pain syndromes, as rhabdomyolosis or polymyalgica rheumatica, as chronic fatigue immune dysfunction syndrome (CFIDS) or adult failure to thrive syndrome; and for better ergonomic function (athletic ability and injury risk).

With regard to bone health, toxic metals intercalate in bone matrix, decreasing bone strength and falsely elevating apparent bone density. Further, many pollutants adjust pH downward, away from homeostasis and into cellular metabolic acidosis. As a consequence bone is dissolved to buffer and maintain serum acid–alkaline balance even at great metabolic cost to cells and body structures.

With regard to metabolic balance and weight management (obesity, leptin deficiency), TMs and POPs exacerbate the metabolic syndrome (syndrome X, insulin resistance). This is discussed in more detail in Chapter 14. Since most POPs are fat soluble (lipophilic), as one loses fat weight, toxins are released into the circulation. Increased toxin burden and inflammatory markers have been measured in clinically important amounts. The interaction (synergies) of these toxicants is largely unstudied.

With regard to fibromyalgia and myofascial pain syndromes, rhabdomyolosis (often induced by medications such as HMG-CoA reductase inhibitors or "statins") and polymyalgica rheumatica, CFIDS and adult failure to thrive syndrome — can be induced or exacerbated by TM excess, POPs. TMs and POPs are among nature's mimics in that they can bring to substantially greater intensity a wide variety of clinical conditions. This has been well demonstrated in "metal fume fever" in arc welders. Mitochondrial destruction leads to cell apoptosis.

With regard to ergonomics, ergogenics, and sports medicine, peak performance is decreased when muscle mitochondria are damaged or intoxicated (metabolically uncoupled). This makes the physical body more susceptible to repetitive motion injury or pain from a less than ideal office chair to sit in during the workday. This antiergonomic results links commonly with an antiergogenic effect. Some sports may even lead to increased toxicity when protective antioxidants and buffering minerals are insufficient to respond to the exercise challenge. An example is lead exposure and bioaccumulation in Motocross racers. In other cases, the artist or the draftsman, the computer programmer or the gardener get exposed to chemicals that inhibit muscle repair.

Our established presumption of safety deserves to give way to a prudent cautionary principle as is now being evolved in Europe and the Pacific Rim. This means that the burden of proving safety rests with the innovator. This is in contrast to our current presumption of safety and after-market surveillance to identify risks or toxicities. The potency, prevalence, and predictable interactions of modern synthetics/toxicant candidates, based on what we now know, has outstripped the ability of after-market surveillance to adequately protect public health and safety in a timely and cost-effective manner.

The informed clinician now remains the patient's advocate and safety net. Nutrition and detoxification are therfore fundamental to first-line comprehensive care.

REFERENCES

1. www.atsdr.cdc.gov/HEC/CSEM/lead/references_cited.html.
2. www.healthbenchmarks.org/mercury/.
3. www.nlm.nih.gov/medlineplus/mercury.html.
4. Toxic Mineral Monographs, ATSDR, CDC, USPHS, 1998–2002.
5. Nriagu, J.O. and Pacyna, J.M., Quantitative assessment of worldwide contamination of air, water, and soils by toxic metals, *Nature*, 333, 134–139, 1988.
6. Seba, D., personal communication, 2000–2001.
7. Arsenic Monograph, ATSDR, CDC, PHS, GOV, 2000.
8. EPA revised arsenic risk assessment, *Chem. Eng. News*, Jan. 8, 2001.
9. www.atsdr.cdc.gov/tfacts5.html.
10. Cohn, S.L. and Goldman, L., Preoperative risk evaluation and perioperative management of patients with coronary artery disease, *Med. Clin. North Am.*, 87, 111–136, 2003.
11. Needleman, H.L., Childhood lead poisoning: the promise and abandonment of primary prevention, *Am. J. Public Health*, 88, 1871–1877, 1998.

12. www.atsdr.cdc.gov/HEC/CSEM/lead/references_cited.html.
13. www.healthbenchmarks.org/mercury/.
14. Jaffe, R. and Morris, E., Medicine in Transition from Disease Treatment to Healthcare, HSC Report 100–14, 2000, Sterling, VA.
15. Sonawane, B., personal communication, May 2004.
16. Fowler, B. and Sonawane, B., ATSDR and EPA, personal communication, Oct. 16, 2001.
17. Presentation at the Princeton BioCenter, May 1990.
18. Walsh, W., personal communication, 1999.
19. Maret, W., Heffron, G., Hill, H.A., Djuicic, D., Jiang, L.J., and Vallee, B.L., The ATP/Metallothionein interaction: NMR and STM, *Biochemistry*, 41, 1689–1694, 2002.
20. Stejskal, V.D., Danersrund, A., Lindvall, A., Hudecek, R., Nordman, V., Yaqob, A., Mayer, W., Bieger, W., and Lindh, U., Metal-specific lymphocytes: biomarkers of sensitivity in man, *Neuroendocrinol. Lett.*, 20, 289–298, 1999.
21. Pelletier, L., Pasquier, R., Hirsch, F., Sapin, C., Druet, P., *In vivo* self-reactivity of mononuclear cells to T cells and macrophages exposed to HgCl2, *Eur. J. Immunol.*, 15, 460–465, 1985.
22. Lindh, U., Hudecek, R., Danesrund, A., Ericksson, S., and Lindvall, A., Removal of dental amalgam and other metal alloys supported by antioxidant therapy alleviates symptoms and improves quality of life in patients with amalgam-associated ill health, *Neuroendocrinol. Lett.*, 23, 459–482, 2002.
23. Second National Report on Human Exposure to environmental chemicals, CDCP, DHHS, Jan. 2003.
24. Jaffe, R., Determination of ascorbate physiologic need by calibration, *Health Studies Collegium Document 111*, Contact Client Services at 800-525-7372 for reprints.
25. Walshe, J.M., Penicillamine, a new oral therapy for Wilson's disease, *Am. J. Med.*, 21, 487–495, 1956.
26. Russell, J.C., Griffin, T.B., McChesney, E.W., and Coulston, F., Metabolism of airborne particulate lead in continuously exposed rats: effect of penicillamine on mobilization, *Ecotoxicol. Environ. Safety*, 2, 49–53, 1978.
27. Hammond, P.B., The effects of d-penicillamine on the tissue distribution and excretion of lead, *Toxicol. Appl. Pharmacol.*, 26, 241–246, 1973.
28. Rosen, J.F. and Markowitz, M.E., d-Penicillamine: its actions on lead transport in bone organ culture, *Pediatr. Res.*, 14, 330–335, 1980.
29. Klaassen, C.D., Heavy metals and heavy metal antagonists, in *The Pharmacological Basis of Therapeutics*, 7th ed., Gilman, A.G., Goodman, L.S, Rall, T.W., and Murad, F., Eds., MacMillan Publishing Co., New York, 1985, pp 1605–1627.
30. Sachs, H.K., Blanksma, L.A., Murray, E.F., and O'Connell, M.J., Ambulatory treatment of lead poisoning: report of 1155 cases, *Pediatrics*, 46, 389–396, 1970.
31. Vitale, L.F., Rosalinas-Bailon, A., Folland, D., Brennan, J.F., and McCormick, B., Oral penicillamine therapy for chronic lead poisoning in children, *J. Pediatr.*, 83, 1041–1045, 1973.
32. Marcus, S.M., Experience with d-penicillamine in treating lead poisoning, *Vet. Hum. Toxicol.*, 24, 18–20, 1982.
33. Chisolm, J.J., Jr., Chelation therapy in children with subclinical plumbism, *Pediatrics*, 53, 441–443, 1974.

34. Rogan, W.J., Dietrich, K.N., Ware, J.H., Dockery, D.W., Salganik, M., Radcliffe, J., Jones, R.L, Ragan, N.B., Chisolm, J.J., and Rhoads, G.G., The effect of chelation therapy with Succimer on neuropsychological development in children exposed to lead (the treatment of lead-exposed children trial group), *N. Engl. J. Med.*, 344, 1421–1426, 2001.

35. Shannon, M., Woolf, A., Binns, H., Mandelbaum, D.E., Rogan, W.J., Shaffer, T.R., and Dietrich, K.N., Chelation therapy in children exposed to lead the treatment of lead-exposed children trial investigators, *N. Engl. J. Med.*, 345, 1212–1213, 2001.

36. Chisolm, J.J., Jr., Poisoning due to heavy metals, *Pediatr. Clin. North Am.*, 17, 591–615, 1970.

37. Greenhouse, A.H., Heavy metals and the nervous system, *Clin. Neuropharmacol.*, 5, 45–92, 1982.

38. Satar, S., Toprak, N., Gokel, Y., and Sebe, A., Intoxication with 100 grams of mercury: a case report and importance of supportive therapy, *Eur. J. Emerg. Med.*, 8, 245–248, 2001.

39. Ozuah, P.O., Mercury poisoning, *Curr. Probl. Pediatr.*, 30, 91–99, 2000.

40. Rosenspire, A.J., Bodepudi, S., Mathews, M., and McCabe, M.J., Jr., Low levels of ionic mercury modulate protein tyrosine phosphorylation in lymphocytes, *Int. J. Immunopharmacol.*, 20, 697–707, 1998.

41. Finkelstein, Y., Vardi, J., Kesten, M.M., and Hod, I., The enigma of parkinsonism in chronic borderline mercury intoxication, resolved by challenge with penicillamine, *Neurotoxicology*, 17, 291–295, 1996.

42. Goyer, R.A., Cherian, M.G., Jones, M.M., and Reigart, J.R., Role of chelating agents for prevention, intervention, and treatment of exposures to toxic metals, *Environ. Health Perspect.*, 103, 1048–1052, 1995.

43. Schwartz, J.G., Snider, T.E., and Montiel, M.M., Toxicity of a family from vacuumed mercury, *Am. J. Emerg. Med.*, 10, 258–261, 1992.

44. Snodgrass, W., Sullivan, J.B., Jr., Rumack, B.H., and Hashimoto, C., Mercury poisoning from home gold ore processing. Use of penicillamine and dimercaprol, *J. Am. Med. Assoc.*, 246, 1929–1931, 1981.

45. Cullen, N.M., Wolf, L.R., and St. Clair, D., Pediatric arsenic ingestion, *Am. J. Emerg. Med.*, 13, 432–435, 1995.

46. Mahajan, S.K., Aggarwal, H.K., Wig, N., Maitra, S., and Chughm S.N., Arsenic induced neuropathy, *J. Assoc. Physicians India*, 40, 268–269, 1992.

47. Aaseth, J., Recent advance in the therapy of metal poisonings with chelating agents, *Hum. Toxicol.*, 2, 257–272, 1983.

48. Fesmire, F.M., Schauben, J.L., and Roberge, R.J., Survival following massive arsenic ingestion, *Am. J. Emerg. Med.*, 6, 602–606, 1988.

49. Watson, W.A., Veltri, J.C., and Metcalf, T.J., Acute arsenic exposure treated with oral D-penicillamine, *Vet. Hum. Toxicol.*, 23, 164–166, 1981.

50. Lyle, W.H., Penicillamine in metal poisoning, *J. Rheumatol.*, (Suppl. 7), 96–99, 1981.

51. Basinger, M.A., Jones, M.M., Holscher, M.A., and Vaughn, W.K., Antagonists for acute oral cadmium chloride intoxication, *J. Toxicol. Environ. Health.*, 23, 77–89, 1988.

52. Williams, D.R. and Halstead, B.W., Chelating agents in medicine, *J. Toxicol. Clin. Toxicol.*, 19, 1081–1115, 1982.

53. Freeman, H.C., Crystal structures of metal-peptide complexes, *Adv. Protein Chem.*, 22, 257–424, 1967.
54. Shi, X., Dalal, N.S., and Kasprzak, K.S., Generation of free radicals in reactions of Ni(II)-thiol complexes with molecular oxygen and model lipid hydroperoxides, *J. Inorg. Biochem.*, 50, 211–225, 1993.
55. Jaffe, R. and Brown, S., Acid-alkaline balance and its effect on bone health, *Int. J. Integrative Med.*, 4, 7–18, 2001.
56. Sachs, H.K., Blanksma, L.A., Murray, E.F., O'Connell, M.J., Ambulatory treatment of lead poisoning: report of 1155 cases, *Pediatrics*, 46, 389–396, 1970.
57. Shannon, M., Graef, J., Lovejoy, F.H., Jr., Efficacy and toxicity of d-penicillamine in low-level lead poisoning, *J. Pediatr.*, 112, 799–804, 1988.
58. Bartsocas, C.S., Grunt, J.A., Boylen, G.W., Jr., and Brandt, I.K., Oral d-penicillamine and intramuscular BAL + EDTA in the treatment of lead accumulation, *Acta Paediatr. Scand.* 60, 553–558, 1971; Chisholm, *ibid.*
59. Rothschild, B., Pyridoxine deficiency, *Arch. Intern. Med.*,142, 840, 1982.
60. Vitale, *op. cit.* and Marcus, *op. cit.*
61. Holt, G.A., *Food and Drug Interactions*, Precept Press, Chicago, 1998, p. 203.
62. Shannon, *op. cit.* and Chisholm, *op. cit.*
63. Willeit, J., Kiechl, S.G., Birbamer, G., Schmidauer, C., Felber, S., Aichner, F., Saltvari, L., Metzler, R., and Judmaier, G., Wilson's disease with primary CNS manifestation — current status in diagnosis and therapy, *Fortschr. Neurol. Psychiatr.*, 60, 237–245, 1992.
64. Meyer, B.U., Britton, T.C., and Benecke, R., Wilson's disease: normalisation of cortically evoked motor responses with (penicillamine) treatment, *J. Neurol.*, 238, 327–330, 1991.
65. Maurer, K., Ihl, R., and Dierks, T., The topography of P300 in neuropsychiatric pharmacotherapy. III. Cognitive P300 fields in an organic psychosyndrome (Wilson's disease) before and during treatment with d-penicillamine, *EEG EMG Z Elektroenzephalogr. Verwandte. Geb.* 19, 62–64, 1988.
66. Mizutani, N., Maehara, M., Negoro, T., and Watanabe, K., Serial changes of cranial computerized tomographic findings in Wilson disease during d-penicillamine therapy, *Brain Dev.* 5, 48–52, 1983.
67. Sack, G., Lossner, J., and Bachmann, H., Results of electroencephalographic and familial studies in Wilson's disease, *Psychiatr. Neurol. Med. Psychol. (Leipz)*, 27, 455–462, 1975.
68. Shimada, H., Fukudome, S., Kiyozumi, M., Funakoshi, T., Adachi, T., Yasutake, A., and Kojima, S., Further study of effects of chelating agents on excretion of inorganic mercury in rats, *Toxicology*, 77, 157–169, 1993.
69. Bluhm, R.E., Bobbitt, R.G., Welch, L.W., Wood, A.J., Bonfiglio, J.F., Sarzen, C., Heath, A.J., Branch, R.A., Elemental mercury vapour toxicity, treatment, and prognosis after acute, intensive exposure in chloralkali plant workers. Part I: history, neuropsychological findings and chelator effects, *Hum. Exp. Toxicol.*, 11, 201–210, 1992.
70. Kern, F., Roberts, N., Ostlere, L., Langtry, J., and Staughton, R.C., Ammoniated mercury ointment as a cause of peripheral neuropathy, *Dermatologica*, 183, 280–282, 1991.
71. Harkness, J.A.L. and Blake, D.R., Penicillamine nephropathy and iron, *Lancet*, ii, 368–369, 1982.

72. Osman, M.A., Patel, R.B., Schuna, A., Sundstrom, W.R., and Welling, P.G., Reduction in oral penicillamine absorption by food, antacid, and ferrous sulfate, *Clin. Pharmacol. Ther.*, 33, 465–470, 1983.
73. Threlkeld, D.S., Ed., Miscellaneous products, penicillamine, in *Facts and Comparisons Drug Information*, St. Louis, MO, 1996, pp. 714b–716b.
74. Ifan, A. and Welling, P.G., Pharmacokinetics of oral 500 mg penicillamine: effect of antacids on absorption, *Biopharm. Drug Dispos.*, 7, 401–405, 1986.
75. Stefano, G.B., Hartman, A., Bilfinger, T.V., Magazine, H.I., Liu, Y., Casares, F., and Goligorsky, M.S., *J. Biol. Chem.*, 270, 30290–30293, 1995.

30 Ergogenics: Maintaining Performance During Physical Stress

Luke R. Bucci, Ph.D.

CONTENTS

INTRODUCTION

This chapter will briefly describe which sports nutrition and dietary supplement products work and which do not work for enhancing physical performance. Physical activities require expenditure of metabolic energy over that required for existence. Desire to perform physical tasks better is a common human trait, especially in competitive sports.

Ergogenic aids are defined as agents capable of enhancing physical performance or work. Nutritional ergogenic aids use the broad field of nutrition as an agent to enhance physical performance. Nutritional ergogenic aids are ingested, and have five basic functions: (1) altering dietary intake; (2) adding macronutrients;

(3) adding specific micronutrients or metabolic intermediates; (4) adding specific micronutrients found in the diet but not the body, such as caffeine; and (5) combinations of functions. This chapter will rank nutritional ergogenic aids for (1) endurance exercise; (2) muscle mass, strength, or anaerobic exercise; and (3) sports skills and exercise-associated health concerns such as mental performance, muscle soreness, immune function, and musculoskeletal health. Effective daily doses or guidelines are given in the tables when applicable. Mechanisms of action will not be explored in this chapter.

The rather large amount of data are summarized in tables that have been divided into three categories depending on the degree of ergogenicity: (1) consistent ergogenic effects, which are sometimes conditional; (2) equivocal or limited ergogenic effects; and (3) consensus on lack of efficacy. Nutritional ergogenic aids are listed in alphabetical order within each class. Rating was assigned when a consensus of research was reached as estimated by this author. Consideration of ergogenicity was derived primarily from recent reviews, along with the weight of evidence based on experience in reviewing this field and individual articles when reviews were incomplete.

Supporting evidence is presented for nutritional ergogenic aids with consistent ergogenic effects. These nutritional ergogenic aids have either reached a consensus of efficacy from thorough reviews of multiple human studies or a majority of original studies have reproducibly shown ergogenicity. Nutritional ergogenic aids with equivocal or limited effects usually have some support for ergogenic actions in well-controlled human clinical trials. However, there may also be trials that did not find ergogenic actions, meaning a consensus is equivocal, and at this point in time, is not agreed upon by reviewers. It is possible that with further research, some nutrients may have reproducible and consistent ergogenic effects under certain conditions. Other nutrients in this category have fewer than three reports showing ergogenic effects. Some nutritional ergogenic aids are not considered ergogenic, nor is their status likely to change under any condition. A majority or consensus of human studies have not found improvements in performance from these ingredients as single agents. Ergogenic aids untested in human clinical trials are not listed.

As with any rating system, conclusions are only as valid as the input. Important research issues such as dose–response, statistical power, applicability of measurements, study design details, statistical analysis, investigator bias, and intrinsic variability of results affect the overall determination of efficacy. In the field of nutritional ergogenic aids, these issues are routinely suboptimal, leading to increased chance of type II errors (not finding a significant difference), and thus, any sweeping conclusion is probably pessimistic in nature. However, the available data, stressing controlled human clinical trials and reviews, have been expressed in these tables.

Evidence for or against ergogenicity of nutritional products ultimately lies in the hundreds of human clinical studies published in the peer-reviewed literature.

Most of these reports have been assessed for this chapter, but are not cited individually. However, when their number is not excessive, and there are few or no reviews on the topic, individual papers are cited. The primary source of evidence for this chapter is the large number of review articles, which in combination cite most original studies. Review articles may be "general," examining multiple nutrients, or "specific," focusing on one nutrient or nutrient category. Reviews represent expert opinions, and usually explore mechanisms of action not considered in this chapter. However, no single review is complete or comprehensive, and the level of thoroughness must be kept in mind when assessing conclusions. As an example, a recent meta-analysis on caffeine and exercise found 16 previous reviews on the subject, but each review only cited between 8 and 40 original articles each, whereas the meta-analysis examined 74 studies,[1] and this author has over 100 human studies accumulated. For some topics, there are more review articles than original reports. Nevertheless, review articles, book chapters, or books are important for the assessment of ergogenicity.

LONG-TERM ENDURANCE EXERCISE PERFORMANCE

Table 30.1 lists the nutritional ergogenic aids with evidence for improving long-term endurance exercise performance. For most conditions, sports drinks, carbohydrates, and caffeine are the most efficacious nutritional ergogenic aids for endurance performance. The primary goal of sports drinks is to prevent dehydration. Water can also accomplish prevention of dehydration in settings lasting less than 1 h or in the absence of excess sweating, and is the most important component of sports drinks. Antioxidants, mostly as tocopherols and combinations containing tocopherols, have conditional efficacy for maintaining endurance performance at high altitudes or hypoxic conditions.[2–10] Caffeine has improved aspects of endurance performance in a large number of studies.[1–7,11–30] Carbohydrates before, during, and after exercise remain the most studied and successful nutritional ergogenic aid for endurance performance.[2–7,11–14,16,18–20,31–42] Carnitine salts,[4,6,43–51] coenzyme Q_{10},[4,6,51–55] and ribose[56–60] improve exercise performance in persons with cardiovascular diseases, a topic largely ignored by most reviewers. Ephedrine and ephedrine–caffeine combinations are not assessed in this chapter because of the recently banned status of ephedrine by sports and government agencies. Persons with iron-deficiency anemia or low ferritin stores can return exercise performance to normal levels by iron supplementation; however, iron supplementation to nondeficient individuals has not met with success.[4,6,7,22,32,34,61–64] Sports drinks simultaneously administer water, electrolytes, and carbohydrates before and during exercise, and have become the mainstay of nutritional ergogenic aids for endurance performance.[3,4,6,7,11,15,18,19,32–34,36,38,65–71] When body water or electrolyte loss is high, fluids and sports drinks can prevent serious adverse consequences.

TABLE 30.1
Nutritional ergogenic aids for long-term endurance exercise performance

The majority of studies support maintenance of or improvements in endurance performance:

Nutrient	Effective daily doses	References
Antioxidants for high altitudes (tocopherols, specific combinations)	400 mg tocopherol	Comprehensive reviews: 2–7; specific reviews: 8–10
Caffeine	1.5–6 mg/kg 1 h before exercise	Comprehensive reviews: 2–7, 11–23; specific reviews: 1, 24–57
Carbohydrates (pre-, during, postexercise feedings)	300 g low-fiber, low-fat, complex carbohydrate meal 3–4 h before exercise; see sports drinks for during exercise; 50 g high-glycemic index carbohydrates within 1 h after exercise and every 2 h (500–700 g carbohydrates in 24 h)	Comprehensive reviews: 2–7, 11–14, 16, 18–20, 31–37; specific reviews: 38–42
L-Carnitine and salts (only for cardiopulmonary disease patients)	2.0–6.0 g	Comprehensive reviews: 4, 6; specific reviews: 43–51
Coenzyme Q_{10} (only for cardiovascular disease patients)	100–300 mg	Comprehensive reviews: 4, 6; specific reviews: 51–55
Ribose (only for cardiovascular ischemic disease patients)	10–60 g	Comprehensive reviews: 56, 57; specific reviews: 58–60
Iron (if anemia or low ferritin stores present)	18–100 mg	Comprehensive reviews: 4, 6, 7, 22, 32, 34; specific reviews: 61–64
Sports drinks (water, electrolytes, 6 to 8% carbohydrates)	200–400 ml before exercise, 100–150 ml every 15 min	Comprehensive reviews: 3, 4, 6, 7, 11, 15, 18, 19, 32–34, 36, 38; specific reviews: 61–64

Equivocal, conditional, or too few studies for adequate conclusions about endurance performance:

Antioxidants (N-acetyl-L-cysteine, ascorbate, beta carotene, carotenoids, coenzyme Q_{10}, glutathione, lipoic acid, selenium, soy isoflavones, tocopherols, and combinations), aspartate salts, branched chain amino acids (BCAAs), L-carnitine and salts, coenzyme Q_{10}, glycerol, herbals (singly or in blends — *Cordyceps sinensis, Eleutherococcus senticosus, P. ginseng, Rhodiola* spp.), beta-hydroxy-beta-methylbutyrate (HMB), hyperhydration, medium chain triglycerides (MCTs), minerals (iron, magnesium, zinc), nicotinamide adenine dinucleotide (NADH), omega-3 fatty acids, phosphates and other buffers (citrate)

The majority of evidence does not support improvements in endurance performance:

Bee pollen, calcium, choline, lecithin, phosphatidylcholine, creatine, dimethylglycine (DMG) and pangamic acid, fat loading, L-glutamine, multiple vitamin–minerals (200% daily value amounts or less), Niacin, octacosanol, ribose, royal jelly, selenium, single amino acids, spirulina (blue-green algae), succinate salts, vitamin B combinations, wheat germ oil

Editor's Note

Ergogenics studies athletic competition and maximizing sports performance, pushing the edge of human capacity a little further. Ergogenics differs from sports nutrition in that the outcome measure is not health, but enhanced performance. None-the-less, some ergogenic interventions improve overall nutritional status and confer health benefits, particularly for athletes with advanced age, restrictive diets, and preexisting health conditions.

MUSCLE MASS AND STRENGTH

Table 30.2 lists the nutritional ergogenic aids useful for increasing muscle mass, strength, and anaerobic exercise performance. Supramaximal cycling and tread-mill running are models for anaerobic exercise, rather than weightlifting, in the majority of the clinical studies cited. These studies demonstrate that large doses of sodium bicarbonate enhance short-term, intense anaerobic exercise perfor-mance.[2–4,6,7,13,14,17–19,36,56,72] Bicarbonate loading is not in common use, owing to high prevalence of gastrointestinal side effects. Calorie intake enhances body weight and muscle mass gain in resistance training programs.[3,6,11,14,18,19,37,56,73–81] The increased calorie intake in these studies was generally carbohydrate and protein combinations in the form of powders or drinks. Creatine has become the most studied, noncaloric nutritional ergogenic aid other than electrolytes and water. Creatine reproducibly increases body weight, lean mass, power, torque, strength, and repetitive, short-term anaerobic exercise performance.[2,3,6,7,11–14,16–19,21–23,27,36,37,56,73–95] Beta-hydroxy-beta-methylbutyrate, a leucine metabolite, has exhibited consistent effects on strength and anaerobic exercise performance.[3,6,16–18,22,34,36,56,75,76,78,96–99] Protein and amino acid mixtures are more effective than controls at maintaining nitrogen balance and muscle protein synthesis during intense training.[2–4,6,7,12–14,17–19,34,36,56,73–75,81,100–109] Deficiency of magnesium and zinc is not uncommon among exercising individu-als.[4,22,111–115] Magnesium and zinc salts have been shown to replete these nutrients and restore serum testosterone levels following overtraining.[6,22,56,110]

INDIRECT ERGOGENIC AIDS

The role of nutritional agents for promoting physical performance by indirect methods is not as well developed as for substances that affect physiological path-ways directly. Brief mention of nutritional manipulations of indirect effects is warranted because of the strong possibility of ergogenic properties, and the need for specific studies in physically stressed persons. Basic categories of mental effects, musculoskeletal integrity, immune function, and tissue repair play vital

TABLE 30.2
Nutritional ergogenic aids for strength, muscle mass, and anaerobic exercise

The majority of studies support maintenance of or improvements in muscle mass, strength, protein synthesis, or anaerobic exercise performance:

Nutrient	Effective daily doses	References
Bicarbonate	300–500 mg/kg body weight 1 h before the event	Comprehensive reviews: 2–4, 6, 7, 13, 14, 17–19, 36, 56; specific reviews: 72
Calories (usually carbohydrate–protein combinations, sometimes with other ingredients)	20–100 g of 1:4 protein–CHO combination 1 h before exercise 100–300 g of 1:4 to 1:1 protein–CHO combination 0.5 to 2 h after exercise	Comprehensive reviews: 3, 6, 11, 14, 18, 19, 37, 56, 73–81; specific reviews: none
Creatine	Loading dose 20 g/day for 5 days; maintenance dose 2–5 g/day; or 2–3 g/day long-term	Comprehensive reviews: 2, 3, 6, 7, 12–14, 16–19, 21–23, 27, 36, 37, 56, 73–81; specific reviews: 82–95
Beta-hydroxy-beta-methylbutyrate (HMB)	1.5–3.0 g	Comrpehensive reviews: 3, 6, 16–18, 22, 34, 36, 56, 75, 76, 78; specific reviews: 96–99
Protein and mixtures of amino acids	1.6–2.0 g/kg body weight	Comprehensive reviews: 2–4, 6, 7, 12–14, 17–19, 34, 36, 56, 73–75, 81; specific reviews: 100–109
Replenishing deficiencies of essential minerals (magnesium, zinc)	450 mg magnesium and 30 mg zinc	Comprehensive reviews: 6, 22, 56; specific reviews: 110

Equivocal, conditional, or too few studies for adequate conclusions about strength, muscle mass, or anaerobic exercise performance:

Antioxidants (N-acetyl-L-cysteine, ascorbate, carotenoids, coenzyme Q_{10}, glutathione, lipoic acid, soy isoflavones, selenium, tocopherols, and combinations), caffeine, L-carnitine, CLA, L-glutamine and L-ornithine-alpha-ketoglutarate (OKG), herbals (singly or in blends — e.g., *Eleutherococcus, P. ginseng, Rhodiola*), omega-3 fatty acids, vitamin C

Majority of evidence does not support improvements in muscle mass, strength, or anaerobic exercise performance:

Amino acid somatotropin secretagogues (arginine, arginine aspartate, arginine pyroglutamate, combinations, glutamine, glycine, 5-hydroxytryptophan, ornithine, tryptophan, tyrosine), antiestrogenic herbal compounds (chrysin, diindolylmethane, indole-3-carbinol), boron, calcium, carnosine, chromium, desiccated beef liver, glandulars (adrenal, liver, orchic, pituitary), herbals (*Coleus,* combinations, *Commiphora, Gymnema, Lagerstroemia, Tribulus*), inosine and other nucleotides (RNA, Brewer's yeast), MCTs, multiple vitamin–minerals (200% RDA amounts or less), myostatin inhibitors (*Cystoseira canariensis* algal extracts), nitric oxide inducers (arginine, arginine alpha-ketoglutarate, various herbals), octopamine (*Citrus aurantium* extracts, synthetic), phosphatidylserine, prohormones (DHEA, androstenedione, norandrostenediones, norandrostenediols, others), ribose, single antioxidants (selenium, vitamin C, vitamin E, herbal phenolics), sterols and interwoven roles in optimizing physical performance. At this time there are some suggestive areas of research that indicate nutritional ergogenic aids may enhance indirect effects, but practical guidelines for use are insufficiently developed for general recommendations. Thus, this chapter is intended to highlight or attract attention to some areas where evidence for changing indirect effects exists.

MENTAL EFFECTS

Mental effects comprise several large areas of study: (1) psychological factors such as mood, ambition, drive, aggressiveness, pain perception, or fatigue thresholds; (2) neurological factors such as reaction times and neuromuscular control; and (3) cognitive skills such as situational awareness, focus, and short-term memory.

Certain nutrients are known to improve mood and reduce depression and anxiety: B complex vitamins,[6,116–118] S-adenosyl-L-methionine,[119] and St. John's wort (*Hypericum perforatum*) extracts.[120–122] It is assumed that improvement of mood and reduction of anxiety indirectly improve performance and rehabilitation.[123–127] Stimulants such as caffeine improve many mental aspects important to physical functioning.[1,7] Some nutrients, such as DL-phenylalanine,[4,128] decrease perception of chronic pain in certain conditions. Ratings of fatigue perception during exercise have been lowered by fluid intake, carbohydrates, and caffeine during exercise. Administration of branched chain amino acids has also been studied with mixed results for effects on diminishing central fatigue.[2,35]

B vitamins (B complex, >500% daily value),[6,117,129–132] caffeine (100 to 500 mg),[1,7] *Panax ginseng* extracts (400 mg 4% ginsenosides),[133,134] and octacosanol (1 to 10 mg)[3,4,6,56,135,136] can improve neuromotor skills, primarily reaction times to auditory and visual stimuli.

B vitamins (B complex, >500% daily value),[117,129–132] caffeine (100 to 500 mg),[1,7] and *P. ginseng* extracts (400 mg 4% ginsenosides)[133,134] can improve cognitive skills under various conditions. Further research is needed to ascertain whether consistent and reliable effects can be obtained with these nutrients in physically stressed individuals.

Dyschronosis affects many traveling, competitive athletes. A Cochrane Review meta-analysis found reproducible and meaningful amelioration of jet lag, with accelerated acclimatization, after melatonin administration (0.5 to 5 mg before local bedtime).[137,138]

MUSCULOSKELETAL INTEGRITY

Another potential is prevention of or improved repair of musculoskeletal injuries.[139,140] Protease supplementation has a substantial literature for enhancing healing and reducing symptoms of acute, traumatic injuries, including sports injuries.[139,140] Glucosamine, chondroitin sulfates, and other nutrients discussed in Chapter 21 may enable persons suffering from arthritis to start, resume, or increase exercise training.[141–145] *S*-Adenosyl-ʟ-methionine and several herbal extracts have also shown reductions in symptoms in degenerative joint disease.[119,145,146]

Immune Function

Immune function is perhaps the most visible nonperformance means to enhance or maintain performance. However, even though several review books, many review chapters, and an entire journal (*Exercise Immunology Reviews*) are devoted to addressing this topic, there are relatively few studies testing whether specific nutrients reduce the incidence of upper respiratory tract illness and infections, especially in long-distance runners. Vitamin C (>1000 mg daily) is the nutrient with the most data on preventing infectious events in exercising individuals.[147–150] A primary reason antioxidant supplements are not studied in isolation is that they work synergistically with each other and with endogenously produced antioxidants (Chapter 7).

Tissue Repair and Recovery

Delayed onset muscle soreness has been reduced by chronic, high doses of vitamin C (400 to 3000 mg/day for at least 14 days).[151–157] Effects of nutritional agents with anti-inflammatory properties are poorly studied but do have sufficient rationale to suggest the studies are justified.

SUMMARY

One barometer of practical efficacy can be found in ingredients or products that stay in the marketplace. Factors such as convenience of use and cost influence what consumers continue to purchase, in spite of real or perceived efficacy. In other words, factors other than simple physical effects appear to be important to consumer usage, but seldom acknowledged. These factors should be kept in mind when assessing utility of nutritional ergogenic aids. Products that have stood the test of time are sports drinks, carbohydrate loading foods, caffeine sources, meal replacements, protein powders, carbohydrate–protein powders and bars. Creatine, antioxidant supplements, iron, and multiple vitamin–mineral supplements have conditional utility.

For endurance exercise, sports drinks and carbohydrates are effective, safe, and widely used (Chapters 8 and 5). The large majority of sales of nutritional ergogenic aids constitute these two product categories.[158] Caffeine in beverage and supplement form is also pervasive. For gaining strength and muscle mass, eating more calories, including protein, is commonly practiced and effective. Anaerobic muscular performance is augmented by creatine and HMB, which have been shown to be tolerable and safe with normal usage. However, a caveat for creatine must be added: long-term endurance exercise is not benefited, and in some cases may be compromised by the extra body mass caused by creatine.

Indirect effects of nutrients are less well studied than actual performance enhancers, but offer a promising area for future research. In spite of little attention, a few nutrients have accumulated enough data to suggest that they may aid sports performance in nonphysical ways.

Safety of ergogenic aids is of extreme importance, especially since some persons may be willing to optimize sports performance at cost to health. Excluding ephedrine–caffeine combinations and certain prohormones, there are few, if any, nutritional ergogenic aids that represent significant hazards. Those supplements that are foods (functional foods) or synthesized by the body are generally very safe. Supplementation may be used to restore healthy physiologic levels. Highly refined carbohydrates, processed *trans* fats, and high-intensity (artificial) sweeteners, which are not found in whole foods and are not endogenously produced, pose safety concerns discussed elsewhere in this text.

One aspect of safety seldom explored is the interaction and interplay of nutrient demands in the athlete. Short-term manipulations of nutrients may lead to additional nutrient demands that manifest as functional deficiencies. Future research should focus on children and adolescents, monitoring systems to observe for long-term effects, possible effects from combinations not seen from individual nutrients, and testing of products to forestall unintentional positive drug tests.

ACKNOWLEDGMENTS

The author wishes to thank Amy Turpin, Ann Grandjean, Brooke Bouwhuis, Bryan Haycock, Camilla Kragius, Charlotte Oler, Christina Beer, Douglas Kalman, E. Wayne Askew, Ira Wolinsky, Janet Sorensen, Jeff Feliciano, Jose Antonio, Judy Driskell, Stephanie Blum, and Trudy Day for their excellent technical assistance and insights.

REFERENCES

1. Doherty, M. and Smith, P.M., Effects of caffeine ingestion on exercise testing: a meta-analysis, *Int. J. Sport Nutr. Exerc. Metab.*, 14, 626–646, 2004.
2. Ahrendt, D.M., Ergogenic aids: counseling the athlete, *Am. Fam. Physician*, 63, 913–922, 2001.
3. Antonio, J. and Stout, J.R., *Sports Supplements*, Lippincott Williams and Wilkins, Philadelphia, 2001.
4. Bucci, L.R., *Nutrients as Ergogenic Aids for Sports and Exercise*, CRC Press, Boca Raton, 1993.
5. Juhn, M.S., Ergogenic aids in aerobic activity, *Curr. Sports Med. Rep.*, 1, 233–238, 2002.
6. Turpin, A.A., Talbott, S.M., Feliciano, J., and Bucci, L.R., Systematic and critical evaluation of benefits and possible risks of nutritional ergogenic aids, in *Nutritional Ergogenic Aids*, Wolinsky, I., Driskell, J.A., Eds., CRC Press, Boca Raton, 2004, pp. 469–504.
7. Williams, M.H., *The Ergogenics Edge: Pushing the Limits of Sports Performance*, Human Kinetics Publishers, Champaign, 1998.

8. Banerjee, A.K., Mandal, A., Chanda, D., and Chakraborti, S., Oxidant, antioxidant and physical exercise, *Mol. Cell Biochem.*, 253, 307–312, 2003.
9. Clarkson, P.M. and Thompson, H.S., Antioxidants: what role do they play in physical activity and health? *Am. J. Clin. Nutr.*, 72, 637S–646S, 2000.
10. Simon-Schnass, I., Vitamin E and high-altitude exercise, in *Vitamin E in Health and Disease*, Packer, L. and Fuchs, J., Eds., Marcel Dekker, New York, 1993, 455–463.
11. Antonio, J. and Stout, J.R., *Supplements for Endurance Athletes*, Human Kinetics, Champaign, 2002.
12. Applegate, E.A. and Grivetti, L.E., Search for the competitive edge: a history of dietary fads and supplements, *J. Nutr.*, 127, 869S–873S, 1997.
13. Applegate, E., Effective nutritional ergogenic aids, *Int. J. Sport Nutr.*, 9, 229–239, 1999.
14. Clarkson, P.M., Nutrition for improved sports performance. Current issues on ergogenic aids, *Sports Med.*, 21, 393–401, 1996.
15. Jeukendrup, A.E. and Martin, J., Improving cycling performance: how should we spend our time and money, *Sports Med.*, 31, 559–569, 2001.
16. Juhn, M., Popular sports supplements and ergogenic aids, *Sports Med.*, 33, 921–939, 2003.
17. Krcik, J.A., Performance-enhancing substances: what athletes are using, *Cleve. Clin. J. Med.*, 68, 283, 288–289, 295–297, 2001.
18. Maughan, R., The athlete's diet: nutritional goals and dietary strategies, *Proc. Nutr. Soc.*, 61, 87–96, 2002.
19. Maughan, R.J., King, D.S., and Lea, T., Dietary supplements, *J. Sports Sci.*, 22, 95–113, 2004.
20. Peters, E.M., Nutritional aspects in ultra-endurance exercise, *Curr. Opin. Clin. Nutr. Metab. Care*, 6, 427–434, 2003.
21. Rigassio Radler, D., Nutritional supplements, ergogenic aids, and herbals, *Dent. Clin. North Am.*, 47, 245–258, 2003.
22. Schwenk, T.L. and Costley, C.D., When food becomes a drug: nonanabolic nutritional supplement use in athletes, *Am. J. Sports Med.*, 30, 907–916, 2002.
23. Spriet, L.L. and Gibala, M.J., Nutritional strategies to influence adaptations to training, *J. Sports Sci.*, 22, 127–141, 2004.
24. Armstrong, L.E., Caffeine, body fluid-electrolyte balance, and exercise performance, *Int. J. Sport Nutr. Exerc. Metab.*, 12, 189–206, 2002.
25. Bohn, A.M., Khodaee, M., and Schwenk, T.L., Ephedrine and other stimulants as ergogenic aids, *Curr. Sports Med. Rep.*, 2, 220–225, 2003.
26. Graham, T.E. Caffeine, coffee and ephedrine: impact on exercise performance and metabolism, *Can. J. Appl. Physiol.*, 26, S103–S119, 2001.
27. Graham, T.E., Caffeine and exercise: metabolism, endurance and performance, *Sports Med.*, 31, 785–807, 2001.
28. Magkos, F. and Kavouras, S.A., Caffeine, in *Nutritional Ergogenic Aids*, Wolinsky, I., and Driskell, J.A., Eds., CRC Press, Boca Raton, 2004, pp. 275–324.
29. Paluska, S.A., Caffeine and exercise, *Curr. Sports Med. Rep.*, 2, 213–219, 2003.
30. Sinclair, C.J. and Geiger, J.D., Caffeine use in sports. A pharmacological review, *J. Sports Med. Phys. Fitness*, 40, 71–79, 2000.
31. Burke, L.M., Nutritional needs for exercise in the heat, *Comp. Biochem. Physiol.*, Part A 128, 735–748, 2001.
32. IOC Consensus Statement on Sports Nutrition, Lausanne, Switzerland, Jun. 13, 2003.

33. Manore, M.M., Barr, S.I., and Butterfield, G.E., Joint position statement: nutrition and athletic performance. American College of Sports Medicine, American Dietetic Association, and Dietitians of Canada, *Med. Sci. Sports Exerc.*, 32, 2130–2145, 2000.

34. Maughan, R., Sports nutrition: an overview, *Hosp. Med.*, 63, 136–139, 2002.

35. Petibois, C., Cazorla, G., Poortmans, J.R., and Deleris, G., Biochemical aspects of overtraining in endurance sports: a review, *Sports Med.*, 32, 867–878, 2002.

36. Talbott, S.M., Sports supplements and ergogenic aids, in *A Guide to Understanding Dietary Supplements*, Haworth Press, New York, 2003, 101–180.

37. Volek, J.S., Houseknecht, K., and Kraemer, W.J., Nutritional strategies to enhance performance of high-intensity exercise, *J. Strength Cond. Res.*, 11, 11–17, 1997.

38. Burke, L.M., Cox, G.R., Culmmings, N.K., and Desbrow, B., Guidelines for daily carbohydrate intake: do athletes achieve them? *Sports Med.*, 31, 267–299, 2001.

39. Doyle, J.A. and Papadopoulos, C., Simple and complex carbohydrates in exercise and sport, in *Energy-Yielding Macronutrients and Energy Metabolism in Sports Nutrition*, Driskell, J.A. and Wolinsky, I., Eds., CRC Press, Boca Raton, 2000, pp. 57–69.

40. Hargreaves, M., Pre-exercise nutritional strategies: effects on metabolism and performance, *Can. J. Appl. Physiol.*, 26 (Suppl.), S64–S70, 2001.

41. Ivy, J.L., Dietary strategies to promote glycogen synthesis after exercise, *Can. J. Appl. Physiol.*, 26 (Suppl.), S236–S245, 2001.

42. Jonnalagadda, A.A., Carbohydrate supplements in exercise and sport, in *Energy-Yielding Macronutrients and Energy Metabolism in Sports Nutrition*, Driskell, J.A. and Wolinsky, I., Eds., CRC Press, Boca Raton, 2001, pp 163–181.

43. Brass, E.P., Supplemental carnitine and exercise, *Am. J. Clin. Nutr.*, 72, 618S–623S, 2000.

44. Ferrari, R. and De Giuli, F., The propionyl-L-carnitine hypothesis: an alternative approach to treating heart failure, *J. Card. Fail.*, 3, 217–224, 1997.

45. Ferrari, R., Merli, E., Cicchitelli, G., Mele, D., Fucili, A., and Ceconi, C., Therapeutic effects of L-carnitine and propionyl-L-carnitine on cardiovascular diseases: a review, *Ann. N. Y. Acad. Sci.,* 1033, 79–91, 1994.

46. Gleim, G.G. and Glace, B., Carnitine as an ergogenic aid in health and disease, *J. Am. Coll. Nutr.*, 17, 203–204, 1998.

47. Goa, K.L. and Brogden, R.N., L-Carnitine. A preliminary review of its pharmacokinetics, and its therapeutic use in ischaemic heart disease and primary and secondary carnitine deficiencies in relationship to its role in fatty acid metabolism, *Drugs*, 34, 1–24, 1987.

48. Jackson, G., Combination therapy in angina: a review of combined haemodynamic treatment and the role for combined haemodynamic and cardiac metabolic agents, *Int. J. Clin. Pract.*, 55, 256–261, 2001.

49. Neumann, G., Effect of L-carnitine on athletic performance, in *Carnitine — Pathobiochemical Basics and Clinical Applications*, Seim, H.and Loster, H., Eds., Ponte Press Verlags-GmbH, Bochum, 1996, pp. 61–72.

50. Pauly, D.F. and Pepine, C.J., The role of carnitine in myocardial dysfunction, *Am. J. Kidney Dis.*, 41, S35–S43, 2003.

51. Witte, K.K., Clark, A.L., and Cleland, J.G., Chronic heart failure and micronutrients, *J. Am. Coll. Cardiol.*, 37, 1765–1774, 2001.

52. Langsjoen, P.H. and Langsjoen, A.M., Overview of the use of CoQ10 in cardiovascular disease, *Biofactors*, 9, 273–284, 1999.

53. Mortensen, S.A., Overview on coenzyme Q10 as adjunctive therapy in chronic heart failure. Rationale, design and end-points of "Q-symbio" — a multinational trial, *Biofactors*, 18, 79–89, 2003.

54. Rosenfeldt, F., Hilton, D., Pepe, S., and Krum, H., Systematic review of effect of coenzyme Q10 in physical exercise, hypertension and heart failure, *Biofactors*, 18, 91–100, 2003.

55. Tran, M.T., Mitchell, T.M., Kennedy, D.T., and Giles, J.T., Role of coenzyme Q10 in chronic heart failure, angina, and hypertension, *Pharmacotherapy*, 21, 797–806, 2001.

56. Antonio, J. and Stout, J.R., *Supplements for Strength-Power Athletes*, Human Kinetics, Champaign, 2002.

57. Talbott, S.M., Supplements for boosting energy levels, in *A Guide to Understanding Dietary Supplements*, Haworth Press, New York, 2003, pp. 181–216.

58. Pauly, D.F. and Pepine, C.J., D-Ribose as a supplement for cardiac energy metabolism, *J. Cardiovasc. Pharmacol. Ther.*, 5, 249–258, 2000.

59. Pauly, D.F., Johnson, C., and St Cyr J.A., The benefits of ribose in cardiovascular disease, *Med. Hypotheses*, 60, 149–151, 2003.

60. Pauly, D.F. and Pepine, C.J., Ischemic heart disease: metabolic approaches to management, *Clin. Cardiol.*, 27, 439–441, 2004.

61. Beard, J. and Tobin, B., Iron status and exercise, *Am. J. Clin. Nutr.*, 72, 594S–597S, 2000.

62. Beard, J.L., Iron biology in immune function, muscle metabolism and neuronal functioning, *J. Nutr.*, 131, 568S–579S, 2001.

63. Chatard, J.C., Mujika, I., Guy, C., and Lacour, J.R., Anaemia and iron deficiency in athletes. Practical recommendations for treatment, *Sports Med.*, 27, 229–240, 1999.

64. Haas, J.D. and Brownlie, T., Iron deficiency and reduced work capacity: a critical review of the research to determine a causal relationship, *J. Nutr.*, 131, 676S–688S, 2001.

65. American College of Sports Medicine, Position stand on exercise and fluid replacement, *Med. Sci. Sports Exer.*, 28, i–vii, 1996.

66. Holzheimer, L.A., Sports and energy drinks, *Diabetes Self Manag.*, 20, 96–101, 2003.

67. Kay, D. and Marino, F.E., Fluid ingestion and exercise hyperthermia: implications for performance, thermoregulation, metabolism and the development of fatigue, *J. Sports Sci.*, 18, 71–82, 2000.

68. Maughan, R.J., Food and fluid intake during exercise, *Can. J. Appl. Physiol.*, 26 (Suppl.), S71–S78, 2001.

69. Maughan, R.J., *Sports Drinks: Basic Science and Practical Aspects*, CRC Press, Boca Raton, 2001.

70. Rehrer, N.J., Fluid and electrolyte balance in ultra-endurance sport, *Sports Med.*, 31, 701–715, 2001.

71. Sawka, M.N. and Montain, S.J., Fluid and electrolyte supplementation for exercise heat stress, *Am. J. Clin. Nutr.*, 72, 564S–572S, 2000.

72. Haub, M.D., Buffers: bicarbonate, citrate and phosphate, in *Nutritional Ergogenic Aids*, Wolinsky, I., Driskell, J.A., Eds., CRC Press, Boca Raton, 2004, pp. 257–274.

73. Lambert, C.P., Frank, L.L., and Evans, W.J., Macronutrient considerations for the sport of bodybuilding, *Sports Med.*, 34, 317–327, 2004.

74. Aagaard, P., Making muscles "stronger": exercise, nutrition, drugs, *J. Musculoskelet. Neuronal Interact.*, 4, 165–174, 2004.

75. Clarkson, P.M. and Rawson, E.S., Nutritional supplements to increase muscle mass, *Crit. Rev. Food Sci. Nutr.*, 39, 317–328, 1999.

76. Fomous, C.M., Costello, R.B., and Coates, P.M., Symposium: conference on the science and policy of performance-enhancing products, *Med. Sci. Sports Exerc.*, 34, 1685–1690, 2002.

77. Lawrence, M.E. and Kirby, D.F., Nutrition and sports supplements: fact or fiction, *J. Clin. Gastroenterol.*, 35, 299–306, 2002.

78. Nissen, S.L. and Sharp, R.L., Effect of dietary supplements on lean mass and strength gains with resistance exercise: a meta-analysis, *J. Appl. Physiol.*, 94, 651–659, 2003.

79. Pecci, M.A. and Lombardo, J.A., Performance-enhancing supplements, *Phys. Med Rehab. Clin. North Am.*, 11, 949–960, 2000.

80. Rubinstein, M.L. and Federman, D.G., Sports supplements. Can dietary additives boost athletic performance and potential? *Postgrad. Med.*, 108, 103–106, 109–112, 2000.

81. Volek, J.S., Strength nutrition, *Curr. Sports Med. Rep.* 2, 189–193, 2003.

82. Benzi, G. and Ceci, A., Creatine as nutritional supplementation and medicinal product, *J. Sports Med. Phys. Fitness*, 41, 1–10, 2001.

83. Branch, J.D., Effect of creatine supplementation on body composition and performance: a meta-analysis, *Int. J. Sport Nutr. Exerc. Metab.*, 13, 198–226, 2003.

84. Casey, A. and Greenhaff, P.L., Does dietary creatine supplementation play a role in skeletal muscle metabolism and performance? *Am. J. Clin. Nutr.*, 72, 607S–617S, 2000.

85. Dempsey, R.L., Mazzone, M.F., and Meurer, L.N., Does oral creatine supplementation improve strength? A meta-analysis, *J. Fam. Pract.*, 51, 945–951, 2002.

86. Derave, W., Eijinde, B.O., and Hespel, P., Creatine supplementation in health and disease: what is the evidence for long-term efficacy? *Mol. Cell. Biochem.*, 244, 49–55, 2003.

87. Krämer, K., Weiss, M., and Liesen H., Creatine: physiology and exercise performance, in *Nutraceuticals in Health and Disease Prevention*, Krämer, K., Hoppe, P.-P., Packer, L., Eds., Marcel Dekker, New York, 2001, 165–186.

88. Kreider, R.B., Creatine supplementation in exercise and sport, in *Energy-Yielding Macronutrients and Energy Metabolism in Sports Nutrition*, Driskell, J.A. and Wolinsky, I., Eds., CRC Press, Boca Raton, 2000, pp. 213–242.

89. Kreider, R.B., Effects of creatine supplementation on performance and training adaptations, *Mol. Cell. Biochem.*, 244, 89–94, 2003.

90. Mesa, J.L., Ruiz, J.R., Gonzalez-Gross, M.M., Gutierrez Sainz, A., and Castillo Garzon, M.J., Oral creatine supplementation and skeletal muscle metabolism in physical exercise, *Sports Med.*, 32, 903–944, 2002.

91. Paoletti, R., Poli, A., and Jackson, A.S., *Creatine. From Basic Science to Clinical Application*, Kluwer Academic Publishers, Dordrecht, 2000.

92. Racette, S.B., Creatine supplementation and athletic performance, *J. Orthop. Sports Phys. Ther.*, 33, 615–621, 2003.

93. Terjung, R.L., Clarkson, P., Eichner, E.R., Greenhaff, P.L., Hespel, P.J., Israel, R.G., Kraemer, W.J., Meyer, R.A., Spriet, L.L., Tarnopolsky, M.A., Wagenmakers, A.J.M., and Williams, M.H., American College of Sports Medicine Roundtable. The physiological and health effects of oral creatine supplementation, *Med. Sci. Sports Exerc.*, 32, 706–717, 2000.

94. Wyss, M. and Kaddurah-Daouk, R., Creatine and creatinine metabolism, *Physiol. Rev.*, 80, 1107–1213, 2000.

95. Kreider, R.B., Leutholtz, B.C., and Greenwood, M., Creatine, in *Nutritional Ergogenic Aids*, Wolinsky, I. and Driskell, J.A., Eds., CRC Press, Boca Raton, 2004, pp. 81–104.

96. Alon, T., Bagchi, D., and Preuss, H.G., Supplementing with beta-hydroxy-beta-methylbutyrate (HMB) to build and maintain muscle mass: a review, *Res. Commun. Mol. Pathol. Pharmacol.*, 111, 139–151, 2002.

97. Gallagher, P.M., Carrithers, J.A., Godard, M.P., Schulze, K.E., and Trappe, S.W., Beta-hydroxy-beta-methylbutyrate ingestion, part I: effects on strength and fat free mass, *Med. Sci. Sports Exerc.*, 32, 2109–2115, 2000.

98. Nissen, S.L. and Abumrad, N.N., Nutritional role of the leucine metabolite beta-hydroxy beta-methylbutyrate (HMB), *Nutr. Biochem.*, 8, 300–311, 1997.

99. Slater, G.J. and Jenkins, D., Beta-hydroxy-beta-methylbutyrate (HMB) supplementation and the promotion of muscle growth and strength, *Sports Med.*, 30, 105–116, 2000.

100. Bucci, L.R. and Unlu, L.M., Proteins and amino acids supplements in exercise and sport, in *Energy-Yielding Macronutrients and Energy Metabolism in Sports Nutrition*, Driskell, J.A. and Wolinsky, I., Eds., CRC Press, Boca Raton, 2000, pp. 191–212.

101. Di Pasquale, M.G., Proteins and amino acids in exercise and sport, in *Energy-Yielding Macronutrients and Energy Metabolism in Sports Nutrition*, Driskell, J.A. and Wolinsky, I., Eds., CRC Press, Boca Raton, 2000, pp. 119–160.

102. Evans, W.J., Protein nutrition and resistance exercise, *Can. J. Appl. Physiol.* 26, S141–S152, 2001.

103. Fielding, R.A. and Parkington, J., What are the dietary protein requirements of physically active individuals? New evidence on the effects of exercise on protein utilization during post-exercise recovery, *Nutr. Clin. Care*, 5, 191–196, 2002.

104. Gibala, M.J., Nutritional supplementation and resistance exercise: what is the evidence for enhanced skeletal muscle hypertrophy? *Can. J. Appl. Physiol.*, 25, 524–535, 2000.

105. Lemon, P.W., Beyond the zone: protein needs of active individuals, *J. Am. Coll. Nutr.* 19, 513S–521S, 2000.

106. Millward, D.J., Protein and amino acid requirements of adults: current controversies, *Can. J. Appl. Physiol.* 26, S130–S140, 2001.

107. Tipton, K.D. and Wolfe, R.R., Exercise, protein metabolism, and muscle growth, *Int. J. Sport Nutr. Exerc. Metab.*, 11, 109–132, 2001.

108. Wolfe, R.R., Protein supplements and exercise, *Am. J. Clin. Nutr.*, 72, 551S–557S, 2000.

109. Wolfe, R.R., Regulation of muscle protein by amino acids, *J. Nutr.* 132, 3219S–3224S, 2002.

110. Brilla, L.R. and Conte V., Effects of a novel zinc-magnesium formulation on hormones and strength, *J. Exerc. Physiol. Online*, 3, 26–37, 2000.

111. Lukaski, H.C., Magnesium, zinc, and chromium nutriture and physical activity, *Am. J. Clin. Nutr.*, 72, 585S–593S, 2000.

112. Lukaski, H.C., Magnesium, zinc, and chromium nutrition and athletic performance, *Can. J. Appl. Physiol.*, 26, S13–S22, 2001.

113. Micheletti, A., Rossi, R., and Rufini, S. Zinc status in athletes: relation to diet and exercise, *Sports Med.*, 31, 577–582, 2001.

114. Newhouse, I.J., and Finstad, E.W., The effects of magnesium supplementation on exercise performance, *Clin. J. Sport Med.*, 10, 195–200, 2000.

115. Speich, M., Pineau, A., and Ballereau, F., Mineral, trace elements and related biological variables in athletes and during physical activity, *Clin. Chim. Acta*, 312, 1–11, 2001.

116. Benton, D., Haller, J., and Fordy, J., Vitamin supplementation for 1 year improves mood, *Neuropsychobiology*, 32, 98–105, 1995.

117. Benton, D., Griffiths, R., and Haller, J., Thiamine supplementation, mood and cognitive functioning, *Psychopharmacology*, 129, 66–71, 1997.

118. Carroll, D., Ring, C., Suter, M., and Willemsen, G., The effects of an oral multivitamin combination with calcium, magnesium, and zinc on psychological well-being in healthy young male volunteers: a double-blind placebo-controlled trial, *Psychopharmacology*, 150, 220–225, 2000.

119. Agency for Health Research Quality, *S*-Adenosyl-L-Methionine for Treatment of Depression, Osteoarthritis and Liver Disease, Evidence Report/Technology Assessment Number 64, U.S. Department of Health Human Services, Washington, DC, 2002.

120. Anon., Monograph. *Hypericum perforatum, Altern. Med. Rev.*, 9, 318–325, 2004.

121. Roder, C., Schaefer, M., and Leucht, S., Meta-analysis of effectiveness and tolerability of treatment of mild to moderate depression with St. John's Wort., *Fortschr. Neurol. Psychiatr.*, 72, 330–343, 2004.

122. Schulz, V., Clinical trials with hypericum extracts in patients with depression — results, comparisons, conclusions for therapy with antidepressant drugs, *Phytomedicine,* 9, 468–474, 2002.

123. Ahern, D.K. and Lohr, B.A., Psychosocial factors in sports injury rehabilitation, *Clin. Sports Med.*, 16, 755–768, 1997.

124. Astin, J.A., Shapiro, S.L., Eisenberg, D.M., and Forys, K.L., Mind-body medicine: state of the science, implications for practice, *J. Am. Board Fam. Pract.*, 16, 131–147, 2003.

125. Fava, G.A. and Sonino, N., Psychosomatic medicine: emerging trends and perspectives, *Psychother. Psychosom.*, 69, 184–197, 2000.

126. Harter, M., Weisser, B., Reuter, K., and Bengel, J., Prevalence and risk factors of psychological burden and mental disorders in patients with musculoskeletal diseases — a review of empirical studies, *Schmerz*, 17, 50–59, 2003.

127. Roux, C.H., Guillemin, F., Boini, S., Longuetaud, F., Arnault, N., and Hercberg, S., Briancon, S., The impact of musculoskeletal disorders on quality of life: an inception cohort study, *Ann. Rheum. Dis.*, 64: 604–611, 2004.

128. Russell, A.L. and McCarty, M.F., DL-Phenylalanine markedly potentiates opiate analgesia — an example of nutrient/pharmaceutical up-regulation of the endogenous analgesia system, *Med. Hypotheses*, 55, 283–288, 2000.

129. Benton, D., Fordy, H., and Haller, J., The impact of long-term vitamin supplementation on cognitive functioning, *Psychopharmacology*, 117, 298–305, 1995.

130. Bonke, D. and Nickel, B., Improvement of fine motorific movement control by elevated dosages of vitamin B1, B6, and B12 in target shooting, *Int. J. Vitam. Nutr. Res.* (Suppl. 30), 198–204, 1989.

131. Heseker, H., Kubler, W., Pudel, V., and Westenhofer, J., Interaction of vitamins with mental performance, *Bibl. Nutr. Dieta*, 52, 43–55, 1995.

132. Bucci, L.R. and Turpin, A.A., Introduction, in *Handbook of Sports Nutrition: Vitamins and Trace Minerals*, Driskell, J.A. and Wolinsky, I., Eds., CRC Press, Boca Raton, 1999, pp. 3–17.

133. Bucci, L.R., Selected herbals and exercise performance, *Am. J. Clin. Nutr.*, 72, 624S–636S, 2000.

134. Bucci, L.R., Turpin, A.A., Beer, C., and Feliciano, J., Ginseng, in *Nutritional Ergogenic Aids*, Driskell, J.A. and Wolinsky, I., Eds., CRC Press, Boca Raton, 2004, pp. 379–410.

135. Brozek, B., Soviet studies on nutrition and higher nervous activity, *Ann. N. Y. Acad. Sci.*, 93, 665–671, 1963.

136. Saint-John, M. and McNaughton, L., Octacosanol ingestion and its effects on metabolic responses to submaximal cycle ergometry, reaction time and chest and grip strength, *Int. Clin. Nutr. Rev.*, 6, 81–89, 1986.

137. Herxheimer, A. and Petrie, K.J. Melatonin for the prevention and treatment of jet lag. *Cochrane Database Syst. Rev.*, 2, CD001520, 2002.

138. Atkinson, G., Drust, B., Reilly, T., and Waterhouse, J., The relevance of melatonin to sports medicine and science, *Sports Med.*, 33, 809–831, 2003.

139. Bucci, L.R., *Nutrition Applied to Injury Rehabilitation and Sports Medicine*, CRC Press, Boca Raton, 1994.

140. MacKay, D. and Miller, A.L., Nutritional support for wound healing, *Altern. Med. Rev.*, 8, 359–377, 2003.

141. Jackson, D.W., The role of chondroitin sulfate in the management of osteoarthritis, *Orthop. Today Monogr.*, Jun., 1–18, 2003.

142. McAlindon, T.E., LaValley, M.P., Gulin, J.P., and Felson, D.T., Glucosamine and chondroitin for treatment of osteoarthritis. A systematic quality assessment and meta-analysis, *J. Am. Med. Assoc.*, 283, 1469–1475, 2000.

143. Richy, F., Bruyere, O., Ethgen, O., Cucherat, M., Henrotin, Y., and Reginster, J.Y., Structural and symptomatic efficacy of glucosamine and chondroitin in knee osteoarthritis: a comprehensive meta-analysis, *Arch. Intern. Med.*, 163, 1514–1522, 2003.

144. Towheed, T.E., Anastassiades, T.P., Shea, B., Houpt, J., Welch, V., and Hochberg, M.C., Glucosamine therapy for treating osteoarthritis, *Cochrane Database Syst. Rev.*, 1, CD002946, 2001.

145. Soeken, K.L., Selected CAM therapies for arthritis-related pain: the evidence from systematic reviews, *Clin. J. Pain*, 20, 13–18, 2004.

146. Soeken, K.L., Lee, W.L., Bausell, R.B., Agile, M., and Berman, B.M., Safety and efficacy of S-adenosyl methionine (SAMe) for osteoarthritis, *J. Fam. Pract.*, 51, 425–430, 2002.

147. Gleeson, M., Nieman, D.C., and Pedersen, B.K., Exercise and immune function, *J. Sports Sci*, 22, 115–125, 2004.

148. Nyman, D.C. and Pedersen, B.K., Exercise and immune function. Recent developments, *Sports Med.*, 27, 73–80, 1999.

149. Peters, M.E., Vitamin C, neutrophil function, and upper respiratory tract infection risk in distance runners: the missing link, *Exerc. Immune Rev.*, 3, 32–52, 1997.

150. Pedersen, B.O., Broussard, H., Jensen, M., Krzywkowski, K., and Ostrowski, K., Exercise and immune function: effect of ageing and nutrition, *Proc. Nutr. Soc.*, 58, 733–742, 1999.

151. Kaminski, M. and Boal, R., An effect of ascorbic acid on delayed-onset muscle soreness, *Pain*, 50, 317–321, 1992.

152. Jakeman, P. and Maxwell, S., Effect of antioxidant vitamin supplementation on muscle function after eccentric exercise, *Eur. J. Appl. Physiol.*, 67, 426–430, 1993.

153. Thompson, D., Nicholas, C.W., McGregor, S.J., McArdle, F., Jackson, M.J., and Williams, C., Muscle soreness and damage following two weeks vitamin C supplementation, *Med. Sci. Sports Exerc.*, 32, S171, 2000.

154. Thompson, D., Williams, C., Kingsley, M., Nicholas, C.W., Lakomy, H.K., McArdle, F., and Jackson, M.J., Muscle soreness and damage parameters after prolonged intermittent shuttle-running following acute vitamin C ingestion, *Int. J. Sports Med.*, 22, 68–75, 2001.

155. Thompson, D., Williams, C., McGregor, S.J., Nicholas, C.W., McArdle, F., Jackson, M.J., and Powell, J.R., Prolonged vitamin C supplementation and recovery from demanding exercise, *Int. J. Sport Nutr. Exerc. Metab.*, 11, 466–481, 2001.

156. Bryer, S.C. and Goldfarb, A.H., The effect of vitamin C supplementation on blood glutathione status, DOMS & creatine kinase, *Med. Sci. Sports Exerc.*, 33, S122, 2001.

157. Bailey, D.M., Williams, C., Hurst, T., and Powell, J., Recovery from downhill running following ascorbic acid supplementation, *Med. Sci. Sports Exerc.*, 33, S122, 2001.

158. Turpin, A.A., Feliciano, J., and Bucci, L.R., Nutritional ergogenic aids: introduction, definitions and regulatory issues, in *Nutritional Ergogenic Aids*, Wolinsky, I. and Driskell J.A., Eds., CRC Press, Boca Raton, 2004, pp. 3–17.

31 Terrestrial Extremes: Nutritional Considerations for High-Altitude and Cold and Hot Climates

Matthew A. Pikosky, Ph.D., R.D. and
Andrew J. Young, Ph.D.

CONTENTS

INTRODUCTION

Millions of people live, work, and play in regions of the world where weather is intemperate or at terrestrial elevations where ambient oxygen pressure is less than at sea level. Exposure to extremes of heat, cold, or hypobaric hypoxia can elicit a variety of physiological responses in humans, which assist the body to re-establish and/or maintain homeostasis under the influence of new environmental conditions. Those physiological responses can have nutritional implications.

The three environmental stressors of greatest physiological importance are hypoxia, cold, and heat. This chapter will, for each, review the environmental characteristics constituting the biologically significant stress, the physiological adjustments elicited, and the potential nutritional implications of those adjustments. It is worth noting that the environmental extremes that people usually experience do not elicit responses approaching physiological limits in people resting quietly, and probably have little impact on nutritional requirements of sedentary people. In contrast, physiological stress of physical activity often elicits responses approaching physiological limits, and that stress can be greatly compounded by exposure to extreme environmental conditions. Since responses to exercise can be a major factor influencing nutritional requirements, this chapter will examine environmental effects on nutritional requirements from the perspective of physically active persons engaging in strenuous activities.

NUTRITIONAL NEEDS DURING HIGH-ALTITUDE SOJOURNS

THE HYPOXIC ENVIRONMENT AND THE OXYGEN TRANSPORT "CASCADE"

The weight of the atmosphere causes air to be denser at sea level than at higher elevations, and barometric pressure (P_B, mmHg) decreases from sea level ($P_B = 760$ mmHg) to the summit of Mount Everest ($P_B = 253$ mmHg), as Figure 31.1 shows. Atmospheric gas concentrations are constant over the earth. When water vapor is absent, oxygen (O_2) comprises 20.93% of the air at all elevations, and the partial pressure of oxygen (PO_2, mmHg) in the atmosphere can be calculated as $P_B \times 0.2093$. Thus, ambient PO_2 falls with P_B as elevation

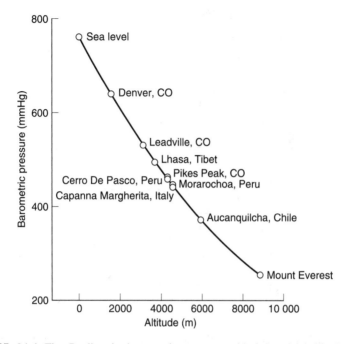

FIGURE 31.1 The Decline in barometric pressure with increasing altitude. (From Young, A.J. and Reeves, J.T., in *Medical Aspects of Harsh Environments*, Vol. 2., Pandolf, K.B. and Burr, R.E., Eds., Department of the Army, The Office of The Surgeon General, Washington, DC, 2002, pp. 647–683.)

increases. The atmospheric PO_2 (in dry air) is 159 mmHg at sea level (760×0.2093) and 53 mmHg on the summit of Mount Everest (253×0.2093). When the air is inspired, it is warmed to body temperature and saturated with water vapor. The partial pressure of water (PH_2O) of saturated inspired air at 37°C body temperature is 47 mmHg, which is also a component of the total pressure of the inspired air. Therefore, addition of water vapor reduces oxygen pressure of inspired air (P_IO_2) below ambient PO_2, and $P_IO_2 = (P_B - 47) \times 0.2093$. The P_IO_2 is 149 mmHg ($[760 - 47] \times 0.2093$) at sea level and 43 mmHg ($[253 - 47] \times 0.2093$) on the summit of Mount Everest.

To sustain metabolism, O_2 is continuously transported down a series of steps in which PO_2 falls sequentially from the atmosphere to the mitochondria: (1) ventilation, whereby respiratory bellows action transports O_2 from ambient air to the alveolus; (2) lung diffusion, whereby O_2 passively diffuses through the alveolar–capillary membrane into the blood; (3) circulation, in which O_2 moves convectively via cardiac action to capillaries; and (4) tissue diffusion whereby O_2 passively diffuses through tissues to mitochondria. Figure 31.2 illustrates the PO_2

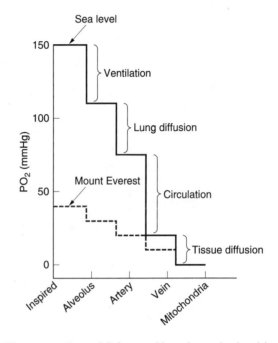

FIGURE 31.2 The oxygen "cascade" from ambient air to mitochondria at sea level and the summit of Mount Everest. (From Young, A.J. and Reeves, J.T., in *Medical Aspects of Harsh Environments*, Vol. 2., Pandolf, K.B. and Burr, R.E., Eds., Department of the Army, The Office of The Surgeon General, Washington, DC, 2002, pp. 647–683.)

fall for each step in the cascade during near maximal exercise.[1] The overall PO_2 pressure gradient driving O_2 down the transport chain during heavy exercise at sea level is approximately 150 mmHg from inspired air to the mitochondria. The overall PO_2 gradient driving O_2 transport at the summit of Mount Everest is about 43 mmHg from inspired air to the mitochondria, because of the low atmospheric PO_2. Nevertheless, men have ascended Mount Everest successfully without supplemental O_2. Clearly, humans have a great capacity for physiological compensation for hypoxia, and these compensations can influence nutrition.

PHYSIOLOGICAL ADJUSTMENTS TO EXERCISE AT HIGH ALTITUDE

Respiratory Exchange

One of the principal physiological responses to hypoxia is increased pulmonary ventilation. Ventilation increases within seconds of hypoxic exposure under control of carotid-body chemoreceptors sensing falling arterial O_2 pressure of (P_aO_2). The subsequent time-dependent changes in ventilation are complex and are considered in detail elsewhere.[1] Briefly, a period of several hours ensues in which hypocapnic responses and centrally mediated hypoxic ventilatory depression limit the increase in ventilation rate, and it is somewhat lower than the initial acute response. A period of ventilatory acclimatization follows, when ventilation progressively rises over the first few weeks of continuing altitude exposure. The ventilatory response to acute hypoxia is greater during exercise than rest, but acclimatization effects are less pronounced during exercise than rest.

The increased ventilation with hypoxia enables alveolar O_2 concentration to be maintained higher for any given P_IO_2 than would be possible without the increase. Although, P_IO_2 is independent of ventilation rate, increased ventilation increases CO_2 removal from the alveolus relative to the rate that it diffuses in from the blood. This hyperventilation lowers partial pressure of alveolar CO_2 (P_ACO_2), and there is a corresponding rise in alveolar partial pressure of O_2 (P_AO_2), enhancing the gradient driving O_2 diffusion across the lung into the blood.[1] However, this ventilatory response to hypoxia comes at the "cost" of an increased energy requirement that contributes to the increase in basal or resting metabolic rate and total daily energy expenditure observed in sojourners at high altitude.[2]

After reaching the alveolus, O_2 diffuses passively across lung membranes and into the red cells of the pulmonary capillary. Notwithstanding increased ventilation, the P_AO_2 in high-altitude sojourners remains less than at sea level (see Figure 31.2) during both rest and exercise. Therefore, the partial pressure of O_2 in arterial blood (P_aO_2) must also fall. Inside red cells, hemoglobin binds O_2 according to concentration-dependent kinetics such that the percent of hemoglobin bound or "saturated" by O_2 (S_aO_2) varies with P_aO_2. The amount of O_2 contained in a volume of blood (blood O_2 content, C_aO_2) is determined by: $C_aO_2 = S_aO_2 \times$ [Hb] $\times A$, where [Hb] is the blood hemoglobin concentration, and the constant A defines the maximal amount of O_2 that can bind to a unit of hemoglobin (~1.35 ml O_2 per gram).

Systemic O_2 Transport

The decline in S_aO_2 and CaO_2 that lowlanders experience with ascent to high altitude necessitate adjustments in systemic O_2 transport to maintain sufficient O_2 delivery to sustain metabolism. Metabolic rate determines systemic O_2 transport requirements, as defined by the Fick equation: $VO_2 = Q_c \times (C_aO_2 - C_vO_2)$, where VO_2 is the O_2 uptake, Q_c is the cardiac output, C_aO_2 is the arterial O_2 content, and C_vO_2 is the mixed venous O_2 content. Neglecting efficiency changes, a given physical activity requires the same metabolic energy at altitude as sea level. Thus, steady-state muscle and whole-body VO_2 during submaximal exercise is the same at altitude and sea level.[1,3–5] However, the reduction in C_aO_2 at high altitude necessitates an increased O_2 extraction by metabolically active tissues (i.e., achieving lower C_vO_2), and more importantly, increased O_2 delivery to active tissue by an increased Q_c.[1,3,5] This increased Q_c is achieved by an increased heart rate.[3] While

Q_c for a given submaximal level of activity is elevated, maximal Q_c remains unchanged from sea-level values and is achieved at lower exercise intensities at altitude.[3] Hence, maximal O_2 uptake (VO_2 max) declines with ascent, with little or no decline below 500 m, only a small decrement between 1000 and 2000 m, and about a 10% decrement for every 1000 m ascended, thereafter.[4] The increased Q_c and tachycardia elicited when lowlanders first ascend to altitude occur at the expense of added cardiac work, myocardial O_2 uptake and coronary blood flow.[1] These effects contribute to the decreased endurance and increased metabolic rates experienced on arrival at high altitude.

In lowlanders who remain at high altitude and acclimatize, the "acute" responses are progressively replaced by physiological adjustments that alleviate strain while still allowing systemic O_2 transport requirements to be sustained. An important effect of altitude acclimatization is a reduction in Q_c, which is apparent at rest and during exercise. This reduction begins developing as early as the second day after ascent and continues developing over the next week to 10 days.[5] The reduction in Q_c with altitude acclimatization primarily results from reduced stroke volume[5] mediated by hemodynamic adjustments associated with a hemo-concentration during the first 7 to 14 days of acclimatization.[6] Sometimes mistakenly attributed to an increase in circulating red blood cells, the hemocon-centration during the first weeks of altitude acclimatization results from a loss of plasma; erythrocyte volume remains unchanged, so blood volume decreases.[7] As a result, blood hemoglobin concentration increases and, thus, C_aO_2 also increases. In lowlanders acclimatizing for several months, hemoconcentration is replaced by expansion of erythrocyte volume which sustains the increased C_aO_2, and, in com-bination with a partial recovery of lost plasma volume, restores normovolemia or may even expand blood volume.[8] Also contributing to the increased C_aO_2, is a concomitant rise in S_aO_2 due to the ventilatory acclimatization discussed earlier.[1] Thus, a key factor enabling systemic O_2 transport requirements to be achieved with a lower cardiac output for a given VO_2 after altitude acclimatization, is an increased O_2 extraction, primarily due to an increased C_aO_2. This adjustment enables exercise and other activity to be performed with lower cardiac work and less cardiovascular strain.

Energy Metabolism — The Lactate Paradox

The energy demands of contracting skeletal muscle are supplied by the break-down of biochemical compounds containing high-energy phosphate bonds. Acute hypoxia and altitude acclimatization have pronounced effects on the metabolic processes involved in the breakdown and regeneration of these high-energy phos-phate compounds during exercise. The collective manifestation of these effects is a phenomenon known as the "lactate paradox." This phenomenon (illustrated in Figure 31.3), first reported by Dill et al.[9] and confirmed most recently by Pronk et al.,[10] is characterized by higher blood lactate concentrations during exercise at altitude than at sea level in unacclimatized persons, but lower blood lactate levels

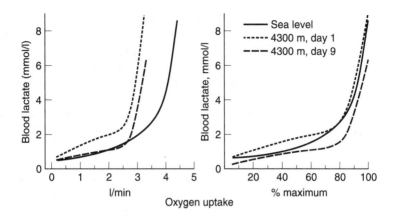

FIGURE 31.3 Effect of high altitude (4300 m) on blood lactate concentration during exercise at different absolute and relative intensities. (From Young, A.J. and Reeves, J.T., in *Medical Aspects of Harsh Environments*, Vol. 2., Pandolf, K.B. and Burr, R.E., Eds., Department of the Army, The Office of The Surgeon General, Washington, DC, 2002, pp. 647–683.)

in acclimatized persons, sometimes even lower than at sea level. The paradox arises because it is assumed that hypoxia accelerates lactate production at altitude via the Pasteur effect, but acclimatized persons exhibit decreased blood lactate accumulation despite continuing hypoxia. The increased blood lactate during acute hypoxic exercise reflects increased lactate release from active muscle not decreased lactate clearance, and probably results from accelerated muscle glycolytic rate fueled by enhanced uptake of blood glucose.[1,11] The decreased blood lactate during hypoxic exercise after acclimatization reflects decreased muscle lactate release since lactate clearance decreases following altitude acclimatization,[11] and may result from diminished muscle glycogenolysis.[12] The mechanism regulating accelerated muscle glycolysis and lactate accumulation during hypoxic exercise, and subsequent reversal of this effect remains unresolved, but is unlikely to be due to the Pasteur effect.[1] Current theory is that changes in muscle energy metabolism during high-altitude exposure are mediated by concomitant changes in epinephrine responses to exercise.[13,14]

Work Capacity and Physical Performance

As described earlier, VO_2 max is markedly reduced as elevation increases. However, most physical activities elicit VO_2 well below maximal, and thus performance of these activities is not limited by VO_2 max, at sea level or high altitude. Only after ascending to very extreme altitudes is the reduction in VO_2 max sufficient that the VO_2 required for activities such as walking approaches maximal. Nevertheless, endurance for many submaximal activities is impaired in unacclimatized lowlanders at high altitude, presumably reflecting the strain from increased cardiac output, accelerated glycolysis and greater lactate accumulation during exercise. With as little as 12 to 16 days of acclimatization, endurance during submaximal exercise increases 40 to 60%, even though maximal O_2 uptake remains decremented.[1,4,5] The improved endurance with acclimatization is probably attributable to the diminished cardiac work associated with the lower cardiac output compared to initially after arriving at high altitude.[15] The development of glycogen sparing adaptations and blunted lactate accumulation further contributes to the improvement in performance. Thus, in unacclimatized lowlanders ascending to high altitude, maximal performance appears limited by respiratory factors, whereas submaximal performance is limited by nonrespiratory factors. However, with acclimatization, both respiratory and non-respiratory factors appear to contribute importantly to performance improvements.

NUTRITION DURING SOJOURNS AT HIGH ALTITUDE

High-Altitude Weight Loss: Energy and Water Balance

Lowlanders who ascend to high altitude and remain for more than a few days typically lose weight. The magnitude of weight loss varies from 80 to nearly 500 g/day.[16–18] Hypohydration and negative energy balance are the principal factors accounting for this weight loss.

Most lowlanders experience a reduction in total body water when they ascend to high altitude.[18] However, this effect may not be experienced by sedentary persons.[19] The degree to which water balance (i.e., intake vs. losses) becomes disrupted at high altitude probably depends on the sojourner's overall level of activity and energy expenditure.[18,19] For example, hypoxia-stimulated ventilation leads to increased respiratory water loss, but this effect may be less pronounced in sedentary than active persons. Similarly, hypoxia can lead to greater sweat losses during exercise than at sea level,[1] but this effect would be minimal for sedentary persons. Unacclimatized lowlanders also usually experience hormonally mediated diuresis at altitude.[18,20,21] Both thirst and appetite are diminished in lowlanders ascending to altitude,[16,18] which could exacerbate the mismatch between water loss and intake when drinking is *ad libitum*. Specific drinking requirements to replace water losses in lowlanders sojourning at altitude will vary considerably among individuals depending on environmental conditions, activity level and a host of other factors. Eventually, however, with acclimatization, body fluid regulatory mechanisms re-establish homeostasis, and studies of lowlanders acclimatized at altitude for at least 10 weeks suggest that total body water is not reduced.[22]

Just as at sea level, negative energy balance can contribute to weight loss during high-altitude sojourn. However, avoiding negative energy balance may be more challenging during sojourns at altitude than at sea level. Energy intake may be constrained under hypoxic conditions. Gastrointestinal macronutrient absorption is unaffected, but anorexia develops in many lowlanders who ascend to altitude.[16] In reviewing the limited number of investigations accurately comparing *ad libitum* energy intake of subjects at sea level and again at high altitude, the consistent finding is that food intake typically declines 10 to 50% during acute altitude exposure.[16,23] This is particularly noticeable among those experiencing acute mountain sickness (AMS), a transient but debilitating syndrome (headache, nausea, vomiting, insomnia, lassitude, and malaise) experienced by 25% of lowlanders who ascend above 3000 m. However, anorexia can persist even after acclimatization when AMS abates,[16] suggesting that hypoxia may directly contribute to appetite suppression.[24]

A reduction in energy intake during high-altitude sojourns may be compounded by an increase in energy requirements. Most people's total daily energy expenditures increase during altitude sojourns compared to sea level. Lowlanders experience a 7 to 17% increase in basal metabolic rate (BMR),[16,25] mediated at least in part by changes in circulating thyroid hormones, but also reflecting energy costs of cardiorespiratory responses to hypoxia.[1] Some investigators suggest that the increase in BMR is transient, with BMR returning to sea level values within 3 to 7 days.[26] However, in those studies, volunteers were fed *ad libitum*, consumed less energy than expended, and lost weight. In contrast, when subjects were fed a diet with energy intake matched to energy expenditure, weight loss was prevented and the 17% increase in BMR measured initially after arriving at high altitude was maintained throughout 3 weeks of sojourn.[25] Therefore, the increase in BMR experienced by lowlanders ascending to high altitude is probably not transient, as long as an increase in energy intake balances the increased energy expenditure, and prevents the loss of metabolically active body tissue. Another likely contribution to increased total daily energy expenditure in high-altitude sojourners is an increase in the energy expenditure of activity. Even though the energy required to sustain a given activity is the same at high altitude as at sea level, most lowlanders ascending to high altitudes engage in more strenuous activities than they do while living at sea level, and that increases daily energy expenditure. For example, Westerterp et al.[27] calculated that daily energy expenditures increased by 880 to 1200 kcal/day over sea level values (1.5 to 2.4 times SL BMR) in subjects climbing to 6542 m. Further, energy requirements of soldiers in mountainous regions reportedly increase by approximately 800 to 2900 kcal/day (2.1 to 3.5 times SL BMR) above sea-level requirements.[28,29]

Thus, decreased fluid and energy intake, increased energy expenditure, or both contribute to the inability of lowlanders sojourning at high altitude to maintain proper hydration and energy balance when diet is *ad libitum*. The magnitude and composition (i.e., water, fat, lean tissue) of the weight lost will depend on the severity of water and energy imbalance. However, countermeasures can be instituted to ameliorate these effects, minimize dehydration and cachexia, and sustain body mass during altitude sojourns, at least at moderate elevations below 5000 m.[16,25]

Macronutrient Requirements at High Altitude

It is widely accepted that consuming a high-carbohydrate diet is advantageous while sojourning at high altitude. As described earlier, glycolytic and glycogenolytic energy metabolism appears to be accelerated during exercise at altitude as compared to at sea level. Furthermore, high carbohydrate diets are often recommended to reduce the symptoms associated with AMS. The exact mechanism by which carbohydrate exerts a beneficial effect is not completely understood, but is generally accepted to be attributable to the increased ventilation produced by the higher respiratory quotient (RQ) of carbohydrate metabolism. A number of studies have demonstrated that this increase in ventilation induced by a high carbohydrate diet subsequently results in a greater arterial PO_2 both during rest[30] and exercise.[31] However, the evidence for an associated alleviation in AMS is scant. Consolazio et al.,[32] reported that subjects consuming a high (70%) carbohydrate diet after arriving at 4300 m from sea level were less nauseated, more energetic, and less depressed than subjects consuming a diet containing a "normal" carbohydrate content diet (35%). However, recent studies have failed to confirm the notion that high carbohydrate diets ameliorate AMS symptoms.[30,31] Nevertheless, benefits of high carbohydrate diets for improving physical performance of lowlanders sojourning at altitude have been confirmed,[33,34] and on that basis, it seems that, at a minimum, lowlanders sojourning at high altitude should consume at least as much carbohydrate in their diet as recommended for physically active individuals living at sea level, that is, ~55% of total caloric intake, or in the range of 6 to 8 g of carbohydrate per kg body weight per day.[35]

There has also been speculation that dietary protein and amino acid requirements may increase during sojourns at high altitude. Body weight loss during high-altitude sojourns was more pronounced from lean than fat mass in some investigations.[24,36] At sea level, negative energy balance increases catabolism of body protein stores, primarily skeletal muscle, as a metabolic fuel, while at the same time reducing skeletal muscle protein synthesis. Negative energy balance at high altitude would have the same effects. Negative nitrogen balance is commonly observed in lowlanders at high altitude, at least transiently.[2,16] Synthesis of skeletal muscle protein appears impaired in hypoxic or high-altitude conditions,[37,38] and some,[37] but not all[38] studies suggest that muscle protein breakdown is increased. Those observations raise the possibility that dietary protein intake should be higher at altitude than sea level. However, investigations manipulating dietary protein content and providing amino acid supplements to lowlanders sojourning at high altitude have yielded mixed results, both in terms of effects on lean mass as well as physical performance.[39–41] On the other hand, investigators observed that when the energy intake of subjects living at 4300 m was sufficient to match daily energy expenditure, and body weight remained unchanged, nitrogen balance was also maintained,[2,25] implying the maintenance of protein mass and thus lean body mass. Collectively, the available research suggests that dietary protein supplementation is not necessary to preserve muscle protein content during high-altitude exposures, as long as dietary energy is consumed in balance with energy expenditure, and protein intake is consistent with recommendations for active persons at sea level, that is, 1.2 to 1.7 g/kg body weight per day.[35]

Micronutrient Requirements at High Altitude

There is little scientific basis to expect that micronutrient requirements of lowlanders would be much affected with ascent to high altitudes,[42] although admittedly, this aspect has not received nearly as much research attention as macronutrient nutrition. The two possible exceptions to this generalization may be with respect to antioxidant vitamins and iron. Oxidative stress may be increased at high altitude, particularly for physically active persons, raising the possibility that dietary supplementation with antioxidant vitamins could be warranted. One field study suggests that antioxidant supplementation mitigates symptoms of AMS, compared to placebo treatment,[43] but a rigorous placebo-controlled research study found no effect of antioxidant supplementation on biomarkers of oxidative stress in lowlanders sojourning 2 weeks at 4300 m.[44]

As described previously, the increase in hematocrit exhibited by lowlanders during the first 2 weeks or so following ascent to high altitude is attributable to hemoconcentration. However, for those who remain longer, increased erythropoetic activity stimulates increased red blood cell production and hemoglobin synthesis.[1] Most healthy, well-nourished lowlanders will not need to supplement iron intake to sustain this response, since several studies indicate that lowlanders consuming an *ad libitum* diet while at high altitude increase their iron intake without supplementation, and intestinal iron absorption may be increased by hypoxia.[45] Iron-deficient individuals, especially athletes, fail to demonstrate the erthrythropoetic response to altitude fully,[46] and, therefore, may need supplementation to achieve 15 (men) to 20 (women) milligrams per day intake.[45]

NUTRITIONAL NEEDS IN HOT AND COLD ENVIRONMENTS

REGULATION OF THERMAL BALANCE

Biophysics of Heat Exchange Between Humans and Environment

People experience thermal stress due to the combined effects of temperature, humidity, sun, wind, rain/water exposures, insulation worn, and body heat produced. The breakdown of biochemical energy to sustain muscular contraction and other physiological processes produces metabolic heat that is transferred from the active tissues to blood, and then distributed convectively throughout the body. The balance between internal heat production and its transfer to the environment determines body temperature. These relationships are described by the heat balance equation: $S = M - (\pm W) \pm (R + C) \pm K - E$, in which S = rate of body heat storage;

M = rate of metabolic energy (heat) production; W = mechanical work, either concentric (positive) or eccentric (negative) exercise; $R + C$ = rate of radiant and convective energy exchanges; K = rate of conduction (important only when in direct contact with an object, such as clothing, or a substance, such as water; and E = rate of evaporative loss.[47] The sum of these, heat storage, represents heat gain if positive, or heat loss if negative. Body temperature increases when S is positive, decreases when S is negative and remains constant when S is zero.

"Body" temperature is most commonly assessed by the measurement of body core temperature. There is no one "true" core temperature because temperature varies among different sites reflecting differences in local tissue metabolic rate, regional blood flow, and temperature gradients between contiguous regions. Core temperature is often measured at the esophagus, rectum, mouth, tympanum, and auditory meatus. Considerable temperature gradients exist between and within the different sites. Measurement methods employed for each of these sites and the relative advantages and disadvantages of each are discussed in detail by Sawka and Young.[48]

Human Thermoregulatory Control System

The human thermoregulatory system normally regulates core temperature within a narrow range (35 to 41°C) through behavioral and physiological responses to thermal stress. Body temperature alterations above and below these "normal" levels can be lethal, but even small fluctuations within that range may degrade performance. Behavioral temperature regulation operates through conscious actions to minimize or avoid thermal stress by modifying activity levels, changing clothes and seeking shade or shelter. When behavior cannot completely negate thermal stress, physiological responses are activated that, depending on whether the thermal stress is heat or cold, enhance dissipation or conservation of body heat stores through mechanisms to alter metabolic rate (shivering), blood flow between the core to the skin (vasoconstriction or vasodilation), and sweating. Thermal receptors in the body core and skin send information about their temperatures to a central integrator, and any deviation between the controlled variable (body temperature) and a reference variable ("set-point") constitute a "load error" generating a "thermal command signal" that participates in the control of sweating, vasodilation, vasoconstriction, and shivering.[49] These responses, which operate until heat balance and body temperatures return to normal, produce physiological strain that can influence nutritional requirements.

Exercise and fever both affect core temperature, even when environmental conditions are temperate or cold. Acute exercise does not involve a set-point increase, whereas fever does.[48] During exercise, core temperature (T_c) increases because metabolic heat production increases. The set-point temperature (T_{set}) is unchanged, so heat-dissipating responses are elicited as core temperature increases. When exercise stops, heat loss exceeds heat production, so core temperature declines towards the set-point. This diminishes the signal eliciting the heat dissipation responses, which leads, in turn, to a decline in the response back to baseline levels, as the pre-exercise thermal balance is re-established. This increase in body temperature during exercise is called hyperthermia. In fever, the set-point temperature increases, causing a negative load or error signal. Heat-dissipating responses are inhibited and heat production is stimulated (shivering) until core temperature increases enough to correct the error signal and establish a new thermal balance in which heat production and heat loss are near (or slightly above) their values before the fever. When fever abates and set-point returns to "normal," the heat-dissipating responses are increased and heat production reduced until pre-fever thermal balance is re-established.

COLD STRESS

Physiological Responses During Cold Exposure

The principal cold-stress determinants outdoors in cold weather are air temperature and wind speed. Most body heat loss during cold exposure occurs via conductive and convective mechanisms. When ambient temperature is colder than body temperature, the thermal gradient favors body heat loss, and wind exacerbates heat loss (i.e., wind-chill) by facilitating convection at the body.[48] Wind-chill effects are greatly reduced by wearing windproof clothing and engaging in strenuous exercise. Water has a much higher thermal capacity than air, and the heat transfer coefficient in water is 25 times greater than in air. Therefore, heat conduction away from the body, is greater during exposure to cold air when skin and clothing are wet (e.g., from rain) than dry. The enhancement of conductive heat loss is more pronounced during full or partial immersion, thus swimmers experience considerable body heat loss even in relatively mild water temperatures. Regardless of the severity of cold, body temperature changes will depend on the balance between heat loss and heat production.

When behavioral thermoregulation provides inadequate protection from the cold, physiological responses are elicited. The two principal physiological responses exhibited by humans exposed to cold are a peripheral vasoconstriction and thermogenesis.[48] Peripheral vasoconstriction decreases peripheral blood flow, which reduces convective heat transfer between the body's core and shell (skin, subcutaneous fat, and skeletal muscle) increasing insulation. Since heat is now being lost from the body surface faster than it is replaced, skin temperature declines. Thus, the vasoconstrictor response to cold retards body heat loss, but at the expense of declining peripheral tissue temperature. In humans, cold-induced thermogenesis is attributable to skeletal muscle contractile activity. Humans initiate thermogenesis voluntarily by increasing activity (exercise, increased "fidgeting," etc), or through involuntary shivering, which consists of repeated, rhythmic muscle contractions, the intensity of which varies according to the severity of cold. As more muscles are recruited and shivering intensity increases, whole-body VO_2 increases, typically reaching about 600 to 700 ml/min during resting exposure to cold air, but often exceeding 1000 ml/min during resting immersion in cold water. While certain animals exhibit a cold-induced, nonshivering thermogenesis by noncontracting tissues, humans lack this mechanism.

Factors Modifying Physiological Responses to Cold

Two factors commonly thought to influence thermoregulatory responses to cold are physical fitness and acclimatization state. In fact, however, physical training and fitness level have only minor influences on thermoregulatory responses to cold, aside from those actually attributable to anthropometric effects associated with fitness training.[48] Persons chronically or repeatedly exposed to cold exhibit adjustments in thermoregulation considered to represent cold acclimatization.[50] However, physiological adjustments to cold acclimatization are less pronounced, slower to develop and less practical in terms of relieving thermal strain, defending normal body temperature, and preventing thermal injury compared to the effects heat acclimatization that will be discussed later in this chapter. Therefore, cold acclimatization probably has little impact on nutritional requirements for optimal health in cold environments.

All external factors being equal (i.e., environment, clothing, and physical activity level), anthropometric differences account for most of the variability between individuals in their thermoregulatory responses and capability to maintain normal body temperature during cold exposure.[51] Convective heat transfer at the skin surface is the principal heat loss vector in cold-exposed humans,[47] therefore, persons with the largest surface area to mass ratios experience the greatest declines in body temperature in the cold. While all body tissues provide insulation to the body, adipose tissue's thermal resistivity is greater than other tissues, so persons with more adipose tissue experience smaller body temperature changes and shiver less during cold exposure than lean persons.[48] Gender-associated differences in thermoregulatory responses and the ability to maintain thermal balance during cold exposure are almost entirely attributable anthropometric differences, and no definitive scientific evidence substantiates the existence of significant gender-associated differences in thermoregulatory responses to cold.[51]

As mentioned earlier, voluntary physical activity or exercise will influence thermal balance during cold exposure. Exercise elicits both thermogenesis and an increased peripheral blood flow (skin and muscles).[48] The increase in peripheral blood flow facilitates body heat loss to the cold environment by enhancing convective heat transfer from the central core to peripheral shell. However, during exposure to cold air, exercise-induced thermogenesis is usually sufficiently pronounced that the increased metabolic heat production matches or exceeds any exercise-related facilitation of heat loss. In contrast, because of the greater convective heat transfer coefficient during water immersion than in air, the exercise-associated increase in heat loss during immersion can be so great that metabolic heat production during even intense exercise can be insufficient to maintain thermal balance.

Metabolic heat production can increase more during physical activity or exercise than shivering. Oxygen uptake of young men resting and shivering in cold air

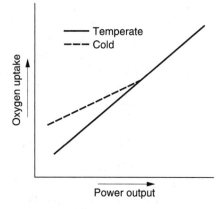

FIGURE 31.4 Effect of cold exposure and shivering on oxygen uptake during exercise. (From Young, A.J., Sawka, M.N., and Pandolf, K.B., in *Nutritional Needs in Cold and in High-Altitude Environments*, Marriott, B.M. and Carlson, S.J., Eds., National Academy Press, Washington, DC, 1996, pp. 127–147.)

averaged 600 to 700 ml/min (15% VO_2 max),[52] and 1 l/min, (25 to 30% VO_2 max),[53] but exercise can increase VO_2 and metabolic rate much higher. The thermogenic effect of exercise or other voluntary activity can partially or even completely obviate the shivering response to cold, depending on the exercise intensity, as schematically illustrated in Figure 31.4. At low exercise intensities in the cold, metabolic heat production is not high enough to prevent shivering, thus VO_2 is higher than for the same exercise in warm conditions, with the increase representing the added VO_2 requirement for shivering activity. As metabolic heat production rises with increasing exercise intensity, core and skin temperatures are maintained warmer and the afferent stimulus for shivering declines. Therefore, the shivering-associated component of total VO_2 during exercise also declines with increasing exercise intensity. At high intensities, metabolism is high enough to completely prevent shivering, and VO_2 during exercise is the same in cold and warm conditions. The exercise intensity at which metabolic heat production is sufficient to prevent shivering will depend on the severity of cold stress.

Fatigue due to exertion, sleep restriction, and underfeeding impair an individual's ability to maintain thermal balance in the cold.[54,55] This syndrome has been referred to as "hiker's hypothermia," and the simplest etiological explanation proposed is that prolonged exercise produces fatigue, thus the exercise intensity and rate of metabolic heat production that can be sustained declines, and if ambient conditions are sufficiently cold, negative thermal balance and declining core temperature ensue. When underfeeding is a factor, effects probably result from development of hypoglycemia, since acute hypoglycemia impairs shivering through a central nervous system mediated effect. Also, declining peripheral carbohydrate stores probably contribute to an inability to sustain exercise or activity, and the associated exercise-induced thermogenesis during cold exposure. Studies also indicate that shivering and peripheral vasoconstriction responses to cold may themselves be *directly* affected, that is, impaired, following strenuous exercise,[56] repeated or prolonged cold exposure,[57] or both in combination. Irrespective of mechanism, when strenuous exercise produces acute or chronic fatigue, ability to maintain thermal balance appears to be degraded, and that in turn can further limit performance.

Impact of Cold Exposure on Nutritional Requirements

Cold exposure is widely thought to influence body fluid balance. Behavioral responses to cold can constrain fluid intake, as thirst sensation may be blunted in cold persons, and cold environments often present practical constraints on voluntary drinking (frozen drinking supplies, desire to avoid urinating outdoors in cold climates). In contrast, physiological responses to cold exposure can exacerbate fluid losses. For example, a widely recognized effect of cold exposure is an increased urine flow rate, that is, cold-induced diuresis (CID), produced by blood-pressure mediated increase in filtration and decrease reabsorption of water and solute by the kidney.[58] However, CID is self-limiting, producing 1 to 2 l fluid loss at most. Furthermore, exercise prevents CID,[58] and people often maintain a vigorous activity level when they are cold. Breathing cold air has also been suggested to exacerbate respiratory water loss during exercise, since cold air has lower water content than warmer air, but studies actually show *less* water lost in exhaled air when breathing cold than warm air.[59] The most significant avenue of fluid loss during exercise in cold conditions is probably the same as in warm conditions, that is, sweating. Even in cold environments, metabolic heat production can exceed heat loss, with the resulting heat storage initiating thermoregulatory sweating which can substantially increase the fluid replacement requirements. If those increased fluid requirements go unmet, dehydration will ensue, with physiological and performance consequences. Otherwise, there is little evidence that cold exposure has any unique impact on body fluid regulation.[60]

While it is widely accepted that total energy requirements are greater in cold weather than temperate conditions, this may not always be the case.[48] Cold exposure can increase energy requirements due to the additional energy required to support thermoregulatory responses to cold, principally shivering thermogenesis. Therefore, if clothing and body insulation or exercise thermogenesis are sufficient to maintain body heat storage constant without initiating shivering, there will be no additional thermoregulatory contribution to total energy requirements due to shivering. The other factor potentially increasing energy requirements in cold compared to temperate environments relates to the energy cost of activity. Often, cold-exposed persons engage in more vigorous activity than they might normally undertake in a temperate climate. Also, energy costs for a given activity can be greater in cold than temperate weather, simply because locomotion can be more difficult through snow, ice, and mud common to cold climates compared to locomotion on dry terrain. Additionally, the hobbling effect of heavy, cold-weather protective clothing can further increase energy costs of a given activity. Whether cold conditions really affect total energy requirements, therefore, will depend on whether the environment, clothing, anthropometric, and exercise-intensity factors interact to elicit additional physiological strain. As has been noted (Ref.[61]), "man in a cold environment is not necessarily a cold man."

Cold exposure has also been thought to affect macronutrient requirements. A widely held view is that a high-fat, and high-protein diet is optimal for persons engaged in cold-weather activities. This concept probably originates from early observations of primitive circumpolar residents whose natural diet was comprised primarily of fat and protein.[42] However, those diets simply reflected regional food availability rather than any nutritional advantage for cold climates, and now circumpolar residents consume a diet similar to the U.S. population.[62] High-fat diets are also the usual choice for expeditioners traversing circumpolar regions,[63,64] but this choice is primarily to maximize dietary energy density while minimizing weight and cube of the food carried, rather than to achieve any thermoregulatory benefit. Lastly, a critical review of the available information indicates no affect of cold exposure on macronutrient preferences of persons who can freely select their food.[65]

On the other hand, metabolic energy requirements of active skeletal muscle may provide a basis for recommending a high carbohydrate diet for persons experiencing cold exposure. Lactate accumulation and muscle glycogen depletion can be more pronounced during low intensity (e.g., below 25% VO_2 max) exercise in the cold when VO_2 levels were elevated compared to similar exercise intensity and duration performed under temperate conditions.[11] However, glycogen depletion is the same when higher intensity exercises are compared.[11] Earlier interpretations of that observation were that added energy requirements of shivering during low intensity exercise increased glycogen breakdown, and that shivering activity preferentially metabolized muscle glycogen as an energy source. However, recent findings instead show that shivering, like low intensity exercise, relies on lipid as the predominant metabolic substrate, but blood glucose, muscle glycogen, and even protein are metabolized in significant amounts as well.[66] Therefore, the current hypothesis to explain accelerated glycogen depletion during shivering is that muscle motor unit recruitment during shivering activity favors fast, glycolytic fibers.[67] Regardless of whether cold-induced shivering increases glycogen depletion rate, the ability to sustain high-intensity activity during cold exposure will, as in temperate conditions, be limited by muscle glycogen and blood glucose availability. Thus, a high-carbohydrate diet (i.e., ~55% total energy intake) will probably be optimal for physically active people exposed to cold weather.

Other nutritional strategies have been proposed to improve overall comfort and perhaps even prevent or delay hypothermia during cold exposure. For example, diets high in protein produce greater thermogenic effects of food (TEF) than diets with equivalent caloric content, but less protein and higher fat content.[68,69] Whether manipulating TEF by altering macronutrient content can affect body temperature during cold exposure has not been tested. However, in subjects consuming an energy balanced diet of 49% carbohydrate, 15% protein, and 36% fat, TEF increases more when subjects were exposed to 16°C ($+13\%$ total energy expenditure) than when exposed to 22°C ($+8\%$ total energy expenditure).[70] This suggests that TEF might contribute more to total energy expenditure during cold than warm conditions, and might be more important than thought for heat balance.

Another dietary approach suggested for augmenting thermogenic responses to cold is to consume foods containing methylxanthines. By itself, the most common naturally occurring methylxanthine in food, caffeine, does not provide any thermoregulatory advantage during cold exposure, even when administered in dosages triple that of a typical serving of coffee.[71,72] However, when ephedrine was ingested in combination with a dose of caffeine approximately equivalent to that typical for a serving of coffee, thermogenic response to cold was enhanced and warmer skin and core temperatures were maintained during cold exposure compared to placebo treatment.[73] Although the health risks of consuming ephedrine would preclude its use as a food additive, the apparent mechanism for the thermogenic effect, an enhancement of carbohydrate oxidation rate, may suggest safer nutritional strategies for further research. So, for example, subjects in another investigation experienced much smaller declines in core temperature during cold exposure after consuming theophylline, the principal methylxanthine in tea, than placebo trials, which the investigators theorized resulted from a shift in metabolic substrate utilization.[74] Additional research on the intriguing possibility that nutritional strategies can enhance thermoregulation and thermal balance during cold exposure is needed.

With respect to micronutrient requirements, the Institute of Medicine's review of the scientific literature concluded that there is no need for any adjustments to the recommended daily intakes of any vitamin or mineral micronutrients for people exposed to cold.[42] However, the review also noted that research on the topic was limited, and additional study was warranted. Further, the Institute of Medicine's invited expert on micronutrient requirements noted in the report that increased high-intensity exercise/activity typically undertaken by people exposed to cold weather accelerates energy metabolism and exacerbates oxidative stress, thus optimal intakes of vitamin E, thiamin, folic acid, iron, and zinc could be higher during cold exposure than in temperate environments.[45] However, this remains to be demonstrated.

HEAT STRESS

Physiological Responses to Heat Stress

Climatic heat stress and exercise interact synergistically to increase requirements for sweating and circulatory responses to dissipate body heat. The wet bulb globe temperature (WBGT) is an empirical index of climatic heat stress widely used to assess the risk of heat injury. It is calculated as: outdoor WBGT = 0.7 natural wet bulb + 0.2 black globe = 0.1 dry bulb, or indoor WBGT = 0.7 natural wet bulb + 0.3 black globe. High WBGT values can be achieved either through high humidity, as reflected in high wet bulb temperature, or through high air (dry bulb) temperature and solar load, as reflected in black globe temperature. This index, originally developed for predicting resting comfort conditions, does not consider clothing or exercise intensity (metabolic rate). Therefore, WBGT cannot predict heat exchange between a person and the climate, or the physiological strain of thermoregulation.[48] WBGT underestimates heat-injury risk for humid conditions, and must be used more conservatively to guide allowable activity in high than low humidity climates. Climatic heat stress can be categorized as *compensated* or *uncompensated*. Compensated heat stress exists when thermoregulatory responses can achieve heat dissipation at a rate balancing heat production, so that a steady-state core temperature can be maintained. Uncompensated heat stress occurs when the individual's cooling requirements exceed the environment's cooling capacity (e.g., when high humidity or clothing limit evaporative and convective heat transfer to the environment, even with maximal thermoregulatory response), so steady-state core temperature cannot be maintained, and core temperature rises progressively as long as exercise continues.

As described previously, exercise-induced hyperthermia elicits an increased skin blood flow and sweating, which work in tandem to dissipate heat.[48] Raising skin blood flow facilitates convective heat transfer from the deep body tissues to the skin surface, where it can be transferred to the environment via convective, conductive, and evaporative transfer. In conditions in which sweating occurs, the tendency of skin blood flow to warm the skin is approximately balanced by the tendency of sweat evaporation to cool the skin. The increase in sweating closely parallels increasing body temperature. Sweat on the skin surface causes cooling when it evaporates from liquid to water vapor. When a gram of sweat is vaporized at 30°C, 2.43 kilojoules (kJ) of heat energy becomes kinetic energy (latent heat of evaporation). Therefore, after sweating has begun, skin blood flow serves primarily to deliver to the skin the heat that is being removed by sweat evaporation.

During exercise-heat stress, sustaining sufficient cardiac output to simultaneously support high skin blood flow for heat dissipation and high muscle blood flow for metabolism strains the cardiovascular system. During mild exercise-heat stress, cardiac output can be increased, relative to comparable exercise in temperate conditions, in order to satisfy both metabolic and thermoregulatory demands. However, the average adult's skin blood flow can approach 8 l/min during exercise in heat-stress conditions.[48] Maintaining such high skin blood flow can reduce cardiac filling, right atrial pressure and stroke volume, thereby necessitating a higher heart rate to maintain cardiac output.[48] A compensatory reduction in visceral blood flow allows cardiac output to be diverted to skin and exercising muscle, but during severe exercise-heat stress, cardiac output may decline below levels observed during comparable exercise in temperate conditions, and skin and muscle blood flow might be compromised.[75,76]

Heat stress modestly increases the metabolic rate elicited to perform a given level of submaximal exercise, possibly because the rate of ATP utilization to develop a given muscle tension is increased as muscle temperature increases.[11] Aerobic metabolism and muscle total adenine pool may decrease, while oxygen debt, blood and muscle lactate accumulation, skeletal muscle glycogen utilization, and inosine 5-monophosphate concentration may all increase during exercise with higher muscle temperatures.[11,77] The increased glycogen utilization is probably mediated by elevated epinephrine and muscle hyperthermia.[78] In addition, lactate uptake and oxidation by the liver (and probably nonexercising muscle) are impaired during exercise-heat stress.[11]

Factors Modifying Physiological Responses to Heat Stress

Anthropometric factors can influence heat balance during heat stress exposure. Body mass index (BMI) influences risk of heat injury,[79] but it is not easy to quantify the difference in risk for being overfat vs. being heavy muscled at the same BMI. Whole-body insulation (i.e., resistance to conductive heat transfer from core to skin surface) is affected by the thickness of the peripheral tissue layer (fat, muscle, skin). In addition, fat has a lower specific heat than muscle tissue, so this will tend to cause greater heat storage in fatter persons, compared to leaner persons of equal total body mass. However, those differences in heat transfer properties may not have practical effects during exercise-heat stress. Sweat rates of small and large people are the same if conditions produce similar heat storage and similar rise in core temperature, but that usually only happens in controlled experimental conditions. Thus, even if the fatter person does store more heat than a leaner person, a higher sweat rate will result and enable enhanced evaporative cooling, if the environmental conditions allow it. Compared to small people, big people produce more heat at a given absolute exercise intensity, but they also dissipate more heat by virtue of their larger surface area. Where these effects "crossover" is a factor of absolute metabolic rate, adiposity, and acclimation status, all of which will vary among individuals.[80] Further, when given the opportunity, big people adopt a slower self paced work rate than smaller people exposed to the same heat stress conditions, and that tends to equalize the thermoregulatory effects.

Aerobic fitness and heat acclimatization both have very significant effects that can reduce physiological strain and improve exercise capabilities in the heat. Exercise training increases the sensitivity of sweating responses such that a given change in core temperature produces a more pronounced increment in sweating rate than in the untrained state, and skin blood flow responses to heat stress change in a similar manner after exercise training. As a result, evaporative heat loss increases, and skin temperatures are lower during exercise-heat stress. However, thermoregulatory improvements produced by exercise training in temperate conditions are modest compared to those obtained by heat acclimatization. Heat acclimatization develops through about 7 to 10 days of repeated heat exposures that are sufficiently stressful to elevate core and skin temperatures, and provoke perfuse sweating. The three classical signs of heat acclimatization are lower heart rate and core temperature, and higher sweat rate during exercise-heat stress.[48] Exercise in the heat produces the most pronounced acclimatization, but even resting in the heat induces some acclimatization.

In contrast, dehydration counteracts the thermoregulatory benefits associated with high aerobic fitness and heat acclimatization, increasing physiological strain and degrading both physical and cognitive performance in hot weather.[48] Persons dehydrate (sustain a body water deficit) when fluid intake fails to adequately replace fluid lost through sweating, urination, and respiration. When dehydrated, sweating and skin blood flow responses to exercise are reduced, and impaired heat dissipation exacerbates the elevation of core temperature. The cardiovascular strain of exercise in the heat is exacerbated by dehydration which induces hypovolemia and a sympathetically mediated tachycardia, both of which compromise cardiac filling, making it more difficult to sustain cardiac output. During severe exercise-heat stress, dehydration mediates a reduction in cardiac output, and skeletal muscle blood flow can be, but is not always, decreased. Muscle glycogenolysis and lactate production during exercise are also accelerated by dehydration, either due to exacerbated hyperthermia (Q_{10} effect) or greater catecholamine responses to exercise. The effects of dehydration manifest even at small water deficits (equivalent to 2% body weight or less), and progressively worsen as the level of dehydration increases.[48]

Hyperhydration, or greater than normal body water, has been suggested to improve, above euhydration levels, thermoregulation and exercise-heat performance. It was theorized that an increase in body water might reduce cardiovascular and thermal strain of exercise by expanding blood volume and reducing blood tonicity, thereby improving exercise performance. A few studies purport to support that theory, including some in which glycerol was added to the drinking water to "enhance" fluid retention and the resulting hyperhydration. However, those studies all suffer from a variety of confounding factors. Carefully controlled studies show no thermoregulatory advantages with hyperhydration during exercise-heat stress, whether achieved by ingesting water alone or water with glycerol.[48]

Impact of Heat Stress on Nutritional Requirements

As described, fluid intake must balance fluid loss to prevent dehydration. During exercise in the heat, renal water losses will be minimal and respiratory water losses will usually be offset by metabolic water production. Therefore, for physically active persons exposed to hot weather, sweating is the primary determinate of water needs. Also, since sweat contains electrolytes (primarily sodium and chloride) prolonged periods of sweating can lead to electrolyte deficits, which must also be replaced.

Climatic conditions, clothing and exercise intensity are the primary factors determining an individual's sweating rate. Sweating rates of 0.3 to 1.0 l/h are observed in persons engaged in routine occupational activities in hot-weather

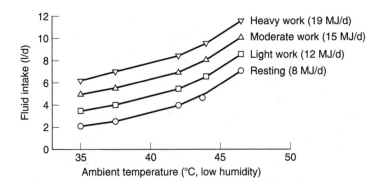

FIGURE 31.5 Effects of increase in work intensity on daily fluid requirements at different ambient temperatures. (From Sawka, M.N., Montain, S.J., and Latzka, W.A., *Comp. Biochem. Physiol. A Mol. Integr. Physiol.*, 128, 679–690, 2001.)

climates,[81] and 1.0 to perhaps as high as 2.5 l/h in athletes exercising intensely in the heat.[48] However, usually people only sustain high sweating rates for several hours per day, and the remainder of time, when more sedentary, they will have lower sweating rates. For competitive athletes training hot weather, daily fluid requirements might range from 4 to 12 l, whereas daily fluid requirements of less active or sedentary persons would fall nearer the bottom of that range.[48,82] Figure 31.5 illustrates the effect of increasing daily energy expenditure on daily fluid requirements over a range of hot weather conditions. Notwithstanding the potential for daily water requirements to be quite high in hot weather, people often ignore thirst.[83] *Ad libitum* drinking often does not fully replace body water losses, and body water deficits of ~2% body weight are often observed following athletic competition.[83,84] As a result, during exposure to hot weather, some dehydration is likely to occur throughout the course of a day, particularly during and after exercise. Most people, however, will usually fully rehydrate at meals, when taking fluids is stimulated by consuming food.

Sweating also results in electrolyte loss, primarily sodium chloride, but also lesser amounts of potassium, calcium, magnesium, and other trace minerals. Sweat sodium concentrations average 50 mEq/l, but vary widely over a range from 10 to 70 mEq/l.[83] However, a lot of factors influence sweat composition, including the specific sweating rate, diet, hydration, and heat acclimation status. Therefore, daily electrolyte requirements for hot climates are difficult to predict with precision. General guidance is that sodium requirements in hot climates may be somewhat higher than the 4 g/day recommended for cool environments, ranging from 6 g/day for people engaged in light or sedentary activities, to as high as 12 g/day for persons performing extremely strenuous activities in a very hot climates. Overall, during a typical 24 h recovery period when meals are consumed *ad libitum*, supplementation is not necessary because adjustments in an individual's salt appetite correct for changes in sodium stores.[85] Furthermore, when individuals increase their level of physical activity, *ad libitum* caloric intake usually increases, with a concomitant increment in sodium intake sufficient to compensate for any increased loss due to the additional exercise.[86] Sweat potassium, calcium, and magnesium concentrations are typically 3 to 15, 0.3 to 2, and 0.2 to 1.5 mmol/l, respectively. Thus, sweat losses are much lower than for sodium, and the impact of hot weather on daily requirements for those electrolytes is probably negligible.

Symptomatic hyponatremia (serum sodium concentration of 125 to 130 mEq/l) has been observed during prolonged ultramarathon competition, military training and recreational activities,[87] but is not common.[48] The primary causative event is drinking excessively large quantities of hypotonic fluids for many hours. However, excessive electrolytes losses (sweating and other), nausea (which increases vasopressin levels) and heat/exercise stress (which reduce renal blood flow and urine output) can exacerbate hyponatremia when excessively large volumes of fluids are consumed. In order to become hyponatremic, total body water will usually need to be markedly increased with hypotonic fluids and significant sodium loss will need to occur.[87]

As mentioned, metabolic rate elicited by submaximal exercise in hot conditions is higher than during equivalent exercise in temperate conditions.[11] This might suggest that total daily energy requirements might be greater during hot than temperate weather. However, in most situations, the impact of any elevation in metabolic rate during exercise in the heat is probably offset by a compensatory reduction in the amount and intensity of other self-selected activities. Thus, total daily energy expenditure and daily energy requirements are unlikely to be increased by hot weather, and may even be lower than in cooler conditions. On the other hand, the increased reliance on glycolytic muscle metabolism[11,77] indicates optimal dietary carbohydrate intakes for physically active persons are likely to be as high or higher (> 55% total daily energy requirement) during hot weather as in temperate conditions.

SUMMARY

When humans are exposed to environmental extremes, physiological and behavioral responses to changes in ambient oxygen tension and temperature may influence energy metabolism, body fluid regulation, and electrolyte balance. The nutritional significance of these effects are probably more significant for physically active than sedentary persons. At high altitude and in the cold, both physiological and behavioral effects can increase total daily energy requirements, which, if not met, can lead to loss of body mass and diminished performance. Energy requirements for most people are likely to be the same or somewhat less in hot than cool weather, unless conditions do not allow activity levels to be self-paced. Current recommendations for physically active persons in temperate environments are to consume between 55–65% of total caloric intake as carbohydrate, or in the range of 6 to 8 g of carbohydrate per kg body weight per day.[35]

For people exposed to extremes of heat, cold or high altitude, optimal dietary carbohydrate intake is probably at the upper end of that range, both because of the physiological responses to the environmental stress, and because, at least in cold and/or high altitude conditions, most people will also be engaged in activities that elevate total energy expenditure well above normal levels. Exposure to extremes of altitude and temperature probably has little or no effect on dietary protein requirements, although the possibility that high protein meals or snacks might enhance thermogenesis and comfort in cold weather deserves further study. Similarly, micronutrient requirements of well-nourished people are not likely to be affected by exposure to environmental extremes if they consume a balanced and unrestricted diet, although additional study is probably warranted. The possible exception to that generalization might be for those people sustaining extremely vigorous activity levels (e.g., athletes in training) for periods longer than several weeks at high altitude (iron supplementation), or during hot weather (sodium supplementation). Fluid intake requirements to maintain body water balance will probably increase during exposure to all environmental extremes, but the increment may be especially pronounced for active people during hot weather. Blunting of appetite and thirst at high altitude and in hot or cold weather will make it difficult for people to maintain energy and water balance when food and fluid intake is strictly *ad libitum*. However, preplanned diet and hydration strategies can provide effective countermeasures to prevent weight loss and dehydration in extreme conditions.

DISCLAIMER

The opinions or assertions contained herein are the private views of the authors and are not to be construed as official or as reflecting the views of the Army or Department of Defense. Citations of commercial organizations and trade names in this report do not constitute an official Department of the Army endorsement or approval of the products or services of these organizations.

Approved for public release; distribution unlimited.

REFERENCES

1. Young, A.J. and Reeves, J.T., Human adaptation to high terrestrial altitude, in *Medical Aspects of Harsh Environments*, Vol. 2., Pandolf, K.B. and Burr, R.E., Eds., Department of the Army, The Office of The Surgeon General, Washington, DC, 2002, pp. 647–683.
2. Mawson, J.T., Braun, B., Rock, P.B., Moore, L.G., Mazzeo, R., and Butterfield, G.E., Women at altitude: energy requirement at 4,300 m, *J. Appl. Physiol.*, 88, 272–281, 2000.
3. Stenberg, J., Ekblom, B., and Messin, R., Hemodynamic response to work at simulated altitude, 4000 m, *J. Appl. Physiol.*, 21, 1589–1594, 1966.
4. Fulco, C.S., Rock, P.B., and Cymerman, A., Maximal and submaximal exercise performance at altitude, *Aviat. Space Environ. Med.*, 69, 793–801, 1998.

5. Grover, R.F., Weil, J.V., and Reeves, J.T., Cardiovascular adaptation to exercise and high altitude, in *Exercise and Sport Sciences Reviews*, Pandolf, K.B., Ed., Macmillan, New York, 1986, pp. 269–302.

6. Calbet, J.A.L., Radegran, G., Boushel, R., Sondergaard, H., Saltin, B., and Wagner, P.D., Plasma volume expansion does not increase maximal cardiac output or VO2 max in lowlanders acclimatized to altitude, *Am. J. Physiol. Heart Circ. Physiol.*, 287, H1214–H1224, 2004.

7. Sawka, M.N., Young, A.J., Rock, P.B. et al., Altitude acclimatization and blood volume: effects of erythrocyte volume expansion, *J. Appl. Physiol.*, 81, 636–642, 1996.

8. Ward, M.P., Milledge, J.S., and West, J.B., *Haematological Changes and Plasma Volume*, Chapman & Hall, London, 1989.

9. Dill, D.B., Edwards, H.T., Folling, A., Oberg, S.A., Pappenheimer, A.M., and Talbot, J.H., Adaptations of the organism to changes in oxygen pressure, *J. Physiol.*, 71, 47–63, 1931.

10. Pronk, M., Tiemessen, I., Hupperets, M.D.W. et al., Persistence of the lactate paradox over 8 weeks at 3800 m, *High Alt. Med. Biol.*, 4, 431–443, 2003.

11. Young, A.J., Energy substrate utilization during exercise in extreme environments, in *Exercise and Sports Sciences Reviews*, Pandolf, K.B. and Holloszy, J.O., Eds., Williams and Wilkens, Baltimore, MD, 1990, pp. 65–117.

12. Young, A.J., Evans, W.J., Cymerman, A., Pandolf, K.B., Knapik, J.J., and Maher, J.T., Sparing effect of chronic high-altitude exposure on muscle glycogen utilization, *J. Appl. Physiol.*, 52, 857–862, 1982.

13. Young, A.J., Young, P.M., McCullough, R.E., Moore, L.G., Cymerman, A., and Reeves, J.T., Effect of beta-adrenergic blockade on plasma lactate concentration during exercise at high altitude, *Eur. J. Appl. Physiol.*, 63, 315–322, 1991.

14. Mazzeo, R. and Reeves, J.T., Adrenergic contribution during acclimatization to high altitude: perspectives from Pikes Peak, *Med. Sci. Sports Exerc.*, 31, 13–18, 2003.

15. Grover, R.F., Lufschanowski, R., and Alexander, J.K., Alterations in the coronary circulation of man following ascent to 3100 m altitude, *J. Appl. Physiol.*, 41, 832–838, 1976.

16. Butterfield, G.E., Maintenance of body weight at altitude: in search of 500 kcal/day, in Marriot, B.M. and Carlson, S.J., Eds., National Academy Press, Washington, DC, 1996, pp. 357–378.

17. Hoyt, R.W. and Honig, A., Environmental influences on body fluid balance during exercise: altitude, in Buskirk, E.R., Ed., CRC Press, New York, 1996, pp. 183–196.

18. Hoyt, R.W. and Honig, A., Body fluid and energy metabolism at high altitude, in *Handbook of Physiology: Section 4, Environmental Physiology*, Vol. II, Fregley, M.J. and Blatteis, C.M., Eds., Oxford University Press, New York, 1995, pp. 1277–1289.

19. Westerterp, K.R., Energy and water balance at high altitude, *News Physiol. Sci.*, 16, 134–137, 2001.

20. Westerterp, K.R., Robach, P., Wouters, L., and Richalet, J.P., Water balance and acute mountain sickness before and after arrival at high altitude of 4,350 m., *J. Appl. Physiol.*, 80, 1968–1972, 1996.

21. Raff, H., Janowski, B.M., Engel, W.C., and Oaks, M.K., Hypoxia in vivo inhibits aldosterone synthesis and aldosterone synthase mRNA in rats, *J. Appl. Physiol.*, 81, 604–610, 1996.

22. Anand, I.S., Chandrashekhar, Y., Rao, S.K. et al., Body fluid compartments, renal blood flow and hormones at 6,000 m in normal subjects, *J. Appl. Physiol.*, 74, 1234–1239, 1993.

23. Askew, E.W., Nutrition and performance in hot, cold, and high-altitude environments, in *Nutrition in Exercise and Sport*, Wolinsky I., Ed., CRC Press, Boca Raton, 1998, pp. 608–613.

24. Rose, M.S., Houston, C.S., Fulco, C.S., Coates, G., Sutton, J.R., and Cymerman, A., Operation Everest. II: nutrition and body composition, *J. Appl. Physiol.*, 65, 2545–2551, 1988.

25. Butterfield, G.E., Gates, J., Fleming, S., Brooks, G.A., Sutton, J.R., and Reeves, J.T., Increased energy intake minimizes weight loss in men at high altitude, *J. Appl. Physiol.*, 72, 1741–1748, 1992.

26 Hannon, J.P. and Sudman, D.M., Basal metabolic and cardiovascular function of women during altitude acclimatization, *J. Appl. Physiol.*, 34, 471–477, 1973.

27. Westerterp, K.R., Kayser, B., Wouters, L., Le Trong, J.L., and Richalet, J.P., Energy balance at high altitude of 6,542 m, *J. Appl. Physiol.*, 77, 862–866, 1994.

28. Hoyt, R.W., Jones, T.E., Baker-Fulco, C.J. et al., Doubly labeled water measurement of human energy expenditure during exercise at high altitude, *Am. J. Physiol.*, 266, R966–R971, 1994.

29. Worme, J.D., Lickteig, J.A., Reynolds, R.D., and Deuster, P.A., Consumption of a dehydrated ration for 31 days at moderate altitudes: energy intakes and physical performance, *J. Am. Diet. Assoc.*, 91, 1543–1549, 1991.

30. Lawless, N.P., Dillard, T.A., Torrington, K.G., Davis, H.Q., and Kamimori, G., Improvement in hypoxemia at 4600 meters of simulated altitude with carbohydrate ingestion, *Aviat. Space Environ. Med.*, 70, 874–878, 1999.

31. Swenson, E.R., MacDonald, A., Vatheuer, M. et al., Acute mountain sickness is not altered by a high carbohydrate diet nor associated with elevated circulating cytokines, *Aviat. Space Environ. Med.*, 68, 499–503, 1997.

32. Consolazio, C.F., Johnson, H.L., Krzywicki, H.J., and Daws, T.A., Metabolic aspects of acute altitude exposure (4,300 meters) in adequately nourished humans, *Am. J. Clin. Nutr.*, 25, 23–29, 1972.

33. Fulco, C.S., Kambis, K.W., Freidlander, A.L., Rock, P.B., Muza, S.R., and Cymerman, A., Carbohydrate supplementation improves time-trial cycle performance at 4300 m altitude, *J. Appl. Physiol.*, 99: 867–876, 2005.

34. Askew, E.W., Food for high-altitude expeditions: Pugh got it right in 1954 — a commentary on the report by L.G.C.E. Pugh: "Himalayan rations with special reference to the 1953 expedition to Mount Everest," *Wilderness Environ. Med.*, 15, 121–124, 2004.

35. American College of Sports Medicine ADAaDoC, Joint Position Statement: nutrition and athletic performance, *Med. Sci. Sports Exerc.*, 32, 2130–2145, 2000.

36. Kayser, B., Nutrition and energetics of exercise at altitude. Theory and possible practical implications, *Sports Med.*, 17, 309–323, 1994.

37. Rennie, M.J., Babij, P., Sutton, J.R. et al., Effects of acute hypoxia on forearm leucine metabolism, *Prog. Clin. Biol. Res.*, 136, 317–323, 1983.

38. Narici, M.V. and Kayser, B., Hypertrophic response of human skeletal muscle to strength training in hypoxia and normoxia, *Eur. J. Appl. Physiol. Occup. Physiol.*, 70, 213–219, 1995.

39. Bigard, A.X., Lavier, P., Ullmann, L., Legrand, H., Douce, P., and Guezennec, C.Y. Branched-chain amino acid supplementation during repeated prolonged skiing exercises at altitude, *Int. J. Sport Nutr.*, 6, 295–306, 1996.

40. Bigard, A.X., Satabin, P., Lavier. P., Canon, F., Taillandier, D., and Guezennec, C.Y., Effects of protein supplementation during prolonged exercise at moderate altitude on performance and plasma amino acid pattern, *Eur. J. Appl. Physiol. Occup. Physiol.*, 66, 5–10, 1993.

41. Schena, F., Guerrini, F., Tregnaghi, P., and Kayser, B., Branched-chain amino acid supplementation during trekking at high altitude. The effects on loss of body mass, body composition, and muscle power, *Eur. J. Appl. Physiol. Occup. Physiol.*, 65, 394–398, 1993.

42. Committee on Military Nutrition Research, A review of the physiology and nutrition in cold and in high altitude environments, in *Nutritional Needs in Cold and in High-Altitude Environments*, Marriot, B.M. and Carlson, S.J., Eds., National Academy Press, Washington, DC, 1996, pp. 3–57.

43. Bailey, D.M. and Davies, B., Acute mountain sickness; prophylactic benefits of antioxidant vitamin supplementation at high altitude, *High Alt. Med. Biol.*, 2, 21–29, 2001.

44. Subudhi, A.W., Jacobs, K.A., Hagobian, T.A. et al., Antioxidant supplementation does not attenuate oxidative stress at high altitude, *Aviat. Space Environ. Med.*, 75, 881–888, 2004.

45. Reynolds, R.D., Effects of cold and altitude on vitamin and mineral requirements, in *Nutritional Needs in Cold and in High-Altitude Environments*, Marriot, B.M. and Carlson, L.D., Eds., National Academy Press, Washington, DC, 1996, pp. 215–244.

46. Levine, B.D. and Stray-Gundersen, J., A practical approach to altitude training: where to live and train for optimal performance enhancement, *Int. J. Sports Med.*, 13 (Suppl. 1), S209–S212, 1992.

47. Gagge, A.P. and Gonzalez, R.R., Mechanisms of heat exchange: biophysics and physiology, in *Handbook of Physiology: Section 4, Environmental Physiology*, Fregly, M.J. and Blatteis, C.M., Eds., Oxford University Press, New York, 1996, pp. 45–84.

48. Sawka, M.N. and Young, A.J., Physiological systems and their responses with exposure to heat and cold, in *ACSM Advanced Exercise Physiology Textbook*, Tipton, C.M. and Tate, C.A., Eds., Lippincott, Williams & Wilkins, Baltimore, 2005, pp. 535–563.

49. Sawka, M.N., Wenger, C.B., and Pandolf, K.B., Thermoregulatory responses to acute exercise-heat stress and heat acclimation, in *Handbook of Physiology: Section 4, Environmental Physiology*, Fregly, M.J. and Blatteis, C.M., Eds., Oxford University Press, New York, 1996, pp. 157–185.

50. Young, A.J., Homeostatic responses to prolonged cold exposure: human cold acclimatization, in *Handbook of Physiology: Section 4, Environmental Physiology*, Fregley, M.J. and Blatteis, C.M., Eds., Oxford University Press, New York, 1996, pp. 419–438.

51. Young, A.J., Sawka, M.N., and Pandolf, K.B., Physiology of cold exposure, in *Nutritional Needs in Cold and in High-Altitude Environments*, Marriott, B.M. and Carlson, S.J., Eds., National Academy Press, Washington, DC, 1996, pp. 127–147.

52. Young, A.J., Muza, S.R., Sawka, M.N., Gonzalez, R.R., and Pandolf, K.B., Human thermoregulatory responses to cold air are altered by repeated cold water immersion, *J. Appl. Physiol.*, 60, 1542–1548, 1986.

53. Young, A.J., Sawka, M.N., Neufer, P.D., Muza, S.R., Askew, E.W., and Pandolf, K.B., Thermoregulation during cold water immersion is unimpaired by low muscle glycogen levels, *J. Appl. Physiol.*, 66, 1809–1816, 1989.

54. Young, A.J., Castellani, J.W., O'Brien, C. et al., Exertional fatigue, sleep loss, and negative energy balance increase susceptibility to hypothermia, *J. Appl. Physiol.*, 85, 1210–1217, 1998.

55. Pugh, L.G.C.E., Cold stress and muscular exercise, with special reference to accidental hypothermia, *Br. Med. J.*, 2, 333–337, 1967.

56. Castellani, J.W., Young, A.J., Kain, J.E., Rouse, A., and Sawka, M.N., Thermoregulation during cold exposure: effects of prior exercise, *J. Appl. Physiol.*, 87, 247–252, 1999.

57. Castellani, J.W., Young, A.J., Sawka, M.N., and Pandolf, K.B., Human thermoregulatory responses during serial cold-water immersions, *J. Appl. Physiol.*, 85, 204–209, 1998.

58. Freund, B. and Young, A.J., Environmental influences on body fluid balance during exercise: cold exposure, in *Body Fluid Balance*, Buskirk, E. and Puhl, S.M., Eds., CRC Press, New York, 1996, pp. 159–181.

59. McFadden, E.R., Jr., Nelson, J.A., Skowronski, M.E., and Lenner, K.A., Thermally induced asthma and airway drying, *Am. J. Respir. Crit. Care Med.*, 160, 221–226, 1999.

60. O'Brien, C., Young, A.J., and Sawka, M.N., Hypohydration and thermoregulation in cold air, *J. Appl. Physiol.*, 84, 185–189, 1998.

61. Bass, D.E., Metabolic and energy balances in men in a cold environment, in *Cold Injury*, Horvath, S.M., Ed., Josiah Macy, Jr. Foundation, New York, 1960, pp. 317–338.

62. Nobmann, E.D., Byers, T., Lanier, A.P., Hankin, J.H., and Jackson, M.Y., The diet of Alaska native adults: 1987–1988, *Am. J. Clin. Nutr.*, 55, 1024–1032, 1992.

63. Frykman, P.N., Harman, E.A., Opstad, P.K., Hoyt, R.W., DeLany, J.P., and Friedl, K.E., Effects of a 3-month endurance event on physical performance and body composition: the G2 trans-Greenland expedition, *Wilderness Environ. Med.*, 14, 240–248, 2003.

64. Stroud, M.A., Nutrition and energy balance on the 'Footsteps of Scott' expedition 1984–86, *Hum. Nutr. Appl. Nutr.*, 41, 426–433, 1987.

65. Jones, P.J.H. and Lee, I.K.K., Macronutrient requirements for work in cold environments, in *Nutritional Needs in Cold and in High-Altitude Environments*, Marriot, B.M. and Carlson, S.J, Eds., National Academy Press, Washington, DC, 1996, pp. 189–202.

66. Haman, F., Peronnet, F., Kenny, G.P. et al., Effect of cold exposure on fuel utilization in humans: plasma glucose, muscle glycogen, and lipids, *J. Appl. Physiol.*, 93, 77–84, 2002.

67. Haman, F., Legault, S.R., and Weber, J.M., Fuel selection during intense shivering in humans: EMG pattern reflects carbohydrate oxidation, *J. Physiol.*, 556, 305–313, 2004.

68. Westerterp-Plantenga, M.S., Rolland, V., Wilson, S.A., and Westerterp, K.R., Satiety related to 24 h diet-induced thermogenesis during high protein/carbohydrate vs high fat diets measured in a respiration chamber, *Eur. J. Clin. Nutr.*, 53, 495–502, 1999.

69. Westerterp-Plantenga, M.S., Wijckmans-Duijsens, N.E., Verboeket-van de Venne, W.P., De Graaf, K., Weststrate, J.A., and van het Hof, K.H., Diet-induced thermogenesis and satiety in humans after full-fat and reduced-fat meals, *Physiol. Behav.*, 61, 343–349, 1997.

70. van Marken Lichtenbelt, W.D., Schrauwen, P., van de Kerckhove, S., and Westerterp-Plantenga, M.S., Individual variation in body temperature and energy expenditure in response to mild cold, *Am. J. Physiol. Endocrinol. Metab.*, 282, E1077–E1083, 2002.

71. MacNaughton, K.W., Sathasivam, P., Vallerand, A.L., and Graham, T.E., Influence of caffeine on metabolic responses of men at rest in 28 and 5 degrees C, *J. Appl. Physiol.*, 68, 1889–1895, 1990.

72. Graham, T.E., Sathasivam, P., and MacNaughton, K.W., Influence of cold, exercise, and caffeine on catecholamines and metabolism in men, *J. Appl. Physiol.*, 70, 2052–2058, 1991.

73. Vallerand, A.L., Jacobs, I., and Kavanagh, M.F., Mechanism of enhanced cold tolerance by an ephedrine–caffeine mixture in humans, *J. Appl. Physiol.*, 67, 428–444, 1989.

74. Wang, L.C., Man, S.F., and Belcastro, A.N., Metabolic and hormonal responses in theophylline-increased cold resistance in males, *J. Appl. Physiol.*, 63, 589–596, 1987.

75. Gonzales-Alonso, J., Teller, C., Anderson, S.L., Jensen, F.B., Hyldig, T., and Nielsen, B., Influence of body temperature on the development of fatigue during prolonged exercise in the heat, *J. Appl. Physiol.*, 86, 1032–1039, 1999.

76. Gonzales-Alonso, J., Mora-Rodriguez, R., and Coyle, E.F., Stroke volume during exercise: interaction of environment and hydration, *Am. J. Physiol.*, 278, H321–H330, 2000.

77. Febbraio, M.A., Does muscle function and metabolism affect exercise performance in the heat? *Exerc. Sport Sci. Rev.*, 28, 171–176, 2000.

78. Febbraio, M.A., Alterations in energy metabolism during exercise and heat stress, *Sports Med.*, 31, 47–59, 2001.

79. Kark, J.A., Burr, P.Q., Wenger, C.B., Gastaldo, E., and Gardner, J.W., Exertional heat illness in Marine Corps recruit training, *Aviat., Space Environ. Med.*, 67, 354–360, 1996.

80. Havenith, G., Luttikholt, V.G., and Vrijkotte T.G., The relative influence of body characteristics on humid heat stress response, *Eur. J. Appl. Physiol. Occup. Physiol.*, 70, 270–279, 1995.

81. Adolph, E.F., *Associates. Physiology of Man in the Desert*, Intersciences, Inc., New York, 1947.

82. Sawka, M.N., Montain, S.J., and Latzka, W.A., Hydration effects on thermoregulation and performance in the heat, *Comp. Biochem. Physiol. A Mol. Integr. Physiol.*, 128, 679–690, 2001.

83. Sawka, M.N. and Montain, S.J., Fluid and electrolyte supplementation for exercise heat stress, *Am. J. Clin. Nutr.*, 72 (Suppl. 2), 564S–572S, 2000.

84. Greenleaf, C.J. and Wade, C.E., Mechanisms controlling fluid ingestion: thirst and drinking, in *Body Fluid Balance*, Buskirk, E. and Puhl, S.M., Eds., CRC Press, New York, 1996, pp. 3–18.

85. Convertino, V.A., Armstrong, L.E., Coyle, E.F. et al., American College of Sports Medicine position stand. Exercise and fluid replacement, *Med. Sci. Sports Exerc.*, 28, i–vii, 1996.

86. Sawka, M.N., Montain, S.J., and Latzka, W.A., Hydration effects on thermoregulation and performance in the heat, Comp. Biochem. Physiol. A Mol. Integr. Physiol., 128, 679–690, 2001.

87. Montain, S.J., Sawka, M.N., and Wenger, C.B., Hyponatremia associated with exercise: risk factors and pathogenesis, *Exerc. Sport Sci. Rev.*, 29, 113–117, 2001.

Index

A

Acarbose, 218

Acetyl-L-carnitine, 106, 420

N-Acetylcysteine (NAC), 106

Acidity
amino acids and, 96
base-forming foods, *See* Alkalinizing foods
bone and, 445, 454–455, 459–461, 479–480
gastric hypoacidity, 479–480
human ancestral diet, 448
presurgical nutrition issues, 514
xenobiotics and, 527, 538

Acidophilus, 515

Acidosis, *See* Metabolic acidosis

Acne, 371, 417

Actin, 96

Activities of daily living, age-related muscle dysfunction and, 308

Acupuncture, 346–349

Acute phase muscle strain, 340–341

Adenosine, 84

Adenosine triphosphate (ATP), 35, 84
magnesium and, 137, 143
phosphorous malnutrition and, 293
protein metabolism and, 96
xenobiotic effects, 525

Adenosyl methionine, *See* S-adenosyl methionine

Adipocytokines, 34, 220

Adiponectin, 220

Adipose tissue, 6
CT pixel intensity values, 16
starvation effects, 284
thermal resistivity, 576

Adiposity rebound, 255

Adolescence
anabolic steroid effects, 376
BMI standards, 9

body image and, 498
bone development, 496
bone fractures and, 497–498
critical period for obesity risk, 255–256
eating disorders and bone health, 498
fat cell number, 74
growth spurt, 496, 498

Adrenal insufficiency, fibromyalgia/chronic fatigue syndrome and, 414–415

Adrenocorticotrophic hormone (ACTH), 348

Advanced glycosylation end products (AGEs), 91

Advanced strengthening phase, 343

Advertising, 262–263

Aerobic exercise, *See also* Exercise
age and peak capacity, 308
mitochondrial function and, 310
resting metabolic rate and, 198
sarcopenia and, 310

African Americans
obesity and, 232–233
resting metabolic rate, 196
women's fat intake, 235

Age-related muscle loss, *See* Sarcopenia

Aging, *See also* Elderly and older persons
body composition and resting metabolic rate, 195–196
body composition changes, 19, 306
definition, 29
lifestyle and nutrition roles, 29
mitochondrial dysfunction, 308
muscle hypertrophy limitation, 359
muscle loss as marker, 305, *See also* Sarcopenia
nutrigenomics and, 36
osteoarthritis risk, 392
oxidative stress model, 122
primary osteoporosis, 475

O